Manual of Cardiovascular Disease in Women

Angela H.E.M. Maas • Eva Gerdts
Editors

Manual of Cardiovascular Disease in Women

Springer

Editors
Angela H.E.M. Maas
Department of Cardiology, route 616
Radboud University Medical Center
Nijmegen, The Netherlands

Eva Gerdts
Department of Clinical Science
University of Bergen
Bergen, Norway

ISBN 978-3-031-65954-6 ISBN 978-3-031-65952-2 (eBook)
https://doi.org/10.1007/978-3-031-65952-2

This Springer imprint is published by the registered company Springer Nature Switzerland AG
The registered company address is: Gewerbestrasse 11, 6330 Cham, Switzerland

If disposing of this product, please recycle the paper.

Preface

In the past decades, it has become clear that there are important sex and gender differences in cardiovascular disease of great relevance to clinical practice. Differences in underlying pathophysiology and risk factors affect disease presentation, diagnosis, treatment and outcomes throughout all areas of cardiovascular disease. Although women are still underrepresented in basic research and clinical trials, evolving insights are increasingly acknowledged. This needs to be communicated to all caregivers involved in women's (cardiovascular) health. We need to tailor our clinical decisions more to each individual patient with respect to gender and diversity. The life-course of women has many unique aspects that interfere with their future cardiovascular risk, such as prior hypertensive pregnancy disorders and an early menopause. Collaboration between various medical disciplines is therefore key. Progress and innovation are at the crossroads of different angles of evolving knowledge in many fields of healthcare.

This *Manual of Cardiovascular Disease in Women* is a unique collaborative project of experts in women's health, written with the latest insights from their various medical disciplines. This e-book provides many practice tools for cardiovascular specialists, trainees, and nurse practitioners. As prevention should start early in life, considering women's health along a horizontal life-approach can be helpful to distinguish between low- and high-risk women.

We hope that this book adds to the knowledge of all those who aim to improve cardiovascular care in women.

Nijmegen, The Netherlands — Angela H.E.M. Maas
Bergen, Norway — Eva Gerdts
January 2024

Contents

Global Perspective of Cardiovascular Disease in Women 1
Angela H.E.M. Maas and Eva Gerdts

Part I Traditional CVD Risk Factors in Women

Obesity and Cardiovascular Disease in Women 17
Gabriele Riccardi and Giovanni de Simone

Tobacco Use and Cardiovascular Risk in Women 31
Maja-Lisa Løchen and Sweta Tiwari

Nutrition, Exercise and Alcohol Use 41
Johanna M. Geleijnse

Dyslipidemia in Women 55
Jeanine E. Roeters van Lennep and Kirsten B. Holven

Diabetes in Women 65
Carola Deischinger, Jürgen Harreiter,
and Alexandra Kautzky-Willer

Hypertension Along Women's Life Course 77
Ester A. Kringeland and Eva Gerdts

Hypertensive Cardiovascular Organ Damage 91
Costantino Mancusi and Eva Gerdts

Part II Non-traditional CVD Risk Factors in Women

Cycle Abnormalities and Cardiometabolic Health 109
M. P. Nadine Daan, Angela H.E.M. Maas,
and Bart C. J. M. Fauser

Hypertensive Disorders of Pregnancy and Cardiovascular Disease Risk 119
Anne Cathrine Staff, Ralf Dechend, and Daniel Pitz Jacobsen

Menopause and Cardiovascular Changes: A Unique Opportunity for Risk Assessment 143
Renata Cifkova and Angela H.E.M. Maas

Hormone Replacement Therapy (And Other Options to Treat Menopausal Symptoms) 153
Irene Lambrinoudaki, Eleni Armeni, and Elina Silionga

Migraine and Cardiovascular Risk in Women 169
Linda Al-Hassany and Antoinette MaassenVanDenBrink

Rheumatic and Autoimmune Disorders and CVD Risk in Women 181
Helga Midtbø and Marie Wahren-Herlenius

Psychosocial Risk in Women with Heart Disease 191
Dinah van Schalkwijk, Paula M. C. Mommersteeg, and Nina Kupper

Domestic Violence, Psychosocial Stress, Socio-Economic Status and CVD Risk in Women 207
Nicole van Gelder and Sabine Oertelt-Prigione

Cardiovascular Health Issues in Transgender Persons 217
C. C. van Bunderen and H. L. Claahsen- van der Grinten

Part III Heart Disease in Women

Valvular Heart Disease in Women 231
Shauna L. Newton and Catherine M. Otto

Stable Ischaemic Heart Disease, Including Obstructive CAD, INOCA and Coronary Vasomotor Disorders 245
Michael Lawless, Graziella Pompei, Mila Kovacevic, and Vijay Kunadian

Acute Coronary Syndromes in Women Including MINOCA 267
Valeria Paradies, Giulia Botti, and Alaide Chieffo

SCAD in Acute and Chronic Phase and Work Up for FMD 281
Teresa Bastante, David del Val, and Fernando Alfonso

Atrial Fibrillation in Women 297
Amelie H. Ohlrogge and Renate B. Schnabel

Stroke in Women 315
Virginia Cancelloni, Ilaria Leone de Magistris, and Valeria Caso

Heart Failure in Women 331
Tiny Jaarsma, Joanna-Maria Papageorgiou, and Anna Strömberg

Takotsubo Syndrome 341
Anenta Ratneswaren and Juan Carlos Kaski

Peripartum Cardiomyopathy 353
Milos Kubanek and Tereza Schimerova

Cardiac Rehabilitation in Women 363
Lis Neubeck, Robyn Gallagher, and Tone M. Norekvål

Part IV Miscellaneous Topics in Cardiology for Women

Cardiotoxicity in Breast Cancer Treatment 377
Berlinde A. von Kemp

Cardiovascular Genetics in Women 393
Yilong Lin and Nabila Bouatia-Naji

Aortic Pathology and Peripheral Arterial Disease in Women 409
M. Teraa and C. E. V. B. Hazenberg

Cardiovascular Therapy in Women with Hypertension or Heart Failure 419
Juan Tamargo and Eva Delpón

Sex Differences in Pharmacokinetics, Pharmacodynamics, and Adverse Drug Reactions of Cardiovascular Drugs 445
A. Evelo, E. Leegwater, and L. E. Visser

Global Perspective of Cardiovascular Disease in Women

Angela H.E.M. Maas and Eva Gerdts

Abstract

Cardiovascular diseases (CVD) remain the most important causes of morbidity and mortality in women worldwide. Overall, one in three women die from CVD, and 45% of adult women have some form of CVD. Ischemic heart disease is the dominant cause of CVD mortality in women worldwide, followed by stroke. Over the past three decades, a decline in CVD mortality in women has been observed in many regions but remained unchanged in Oceania and Sub-Saharan Africa and increased in Central Asia. Aging, ongoing urbanization, and differences in access to care and in socio-economic factors contribute to these regional variations. Uncontrolled metabolic risk factors (high blood pressure, high low density lipoprotein cholesterol, and obesity) are now the main drivers of CVD in women. Early detection and management of these risk factors and better attention to female-specific CVD risk factors remain paramount to reduce CVD morbidity and mortality in women. Furthermore, better understanding of how under-recognised risk factors like psychological and socio-cultural factors, socio-economic status, and health literacy contribute to CVD in women worldwide is spoken for. Integration of these factors in standard CVD risk assessment is necessary to improve CVD prevention in women.

Keywords

Global · Cardiovascular disease · Women
Health literacy

Test your learning and check your understanding of this book's contents: use the "Springer Nature Flashcards" app to access questions.
To use the app, please follow the instructions below:

1. Go to https://flashcards.springernature.com/login
2. Create a user account by entering your e-mail address and assigning a password.
3. Use the following link to access your SN Flashcards set: ▶ https://sn.pub/51ny7m

If the link is missing or does not work, please send an e-mail with the subject "SN Flashcards" and the book title to customerservice@springernature.com

A. H.E.M. Maas
Department of Cardiology, route 616, Radboud University Medical Center, Nijmegen, The Netherlands
e-mail: angela.maas@radboudumc.nl

E. Gerdts (✉)
Department of Clinical Science, University of Bergen, Bergen, Norway
e-mail: eva.gerdts@uib.no

A. H.E.M. Maas, E. Gerdts (eds.), *Manual of Cardiovascular Disease in Women*,
https://doi.org/10.1007/978-3-031-65952-2_1

1 Introduction

Cardiovascular diseases (CVD) remain the leading causes of morbidity and mortality for women worldwide [1]. Overall, one in three women die from CVD, and 45% of adult women have some form of CVD. Globally, 75% of deaths from CVD in women before the age of 70 years occur in low- and middle-income countries (LMIC) [2]. Among women, the highest age-standardized rates of disability adjusted life years (DALYs) were found in Central Asia, Oceania, North Africa, the Middle East and in Eastern Europe, while the lowest rates were found in High-Income Asia Pacific, Australasia, and Western Europe [2]. These regional and national differences in CVD morbidity and mortality reflect differences in prevalence of CVD risk factors, access to health care and socio-economic factors [2, 3]. The continuous global increase in CVD result from population growth, aging, and ongoing urbanization particularly in Northern Africa, central Sub-Saharan Africa, Asia, Latin-America and the Caribbean [4]. While CVD mortality has declined in women in countries with high socio-demographic index (a composite measure of development defined from the rankings of the incomes per capita, average educational attainment, and fertility rates, as defined by the Global Burden of Disease), the highest rates of CVD mortality has shifted from men to women in countries with a low socio-demographic index [2, 3]. In 2019, ischemic heart disease (IHD) was the primary cause of CVD mortality in women worldwide, followed by stroke [3]. Recent research has pointed out the diversity in CVD risk factors and clinical presentation of IHD between women and men [5–8]. Still, CVD remain understudied, under-recognised, underdiagnosed, and undertreated in women [3], in part as a consequence of lack of implementation of modern knowledge about CVD in women in guidelines and health politics. Thus, a distinct sex and gender perspective is necessary for more effective prevention and management of CVD worldwide [9]. The present chapter gives an overview of CVD in women and barriers to diagnosis and treatment in a global perspective.

2 Theory

Traditional, women-specific and under-recognized risk factors as well as sociocultural factors contribute to the CVD burden in women (Fig. 1).

2.1 Traditional CVD Risk Factors in Women

Uncontrolled metabolic risk factors like high blood pressure (BP, hypertension), high low-density lipoprotein (LDL) cholesterol, obesity and type 2 diabetes are the main drivers of CVD morbidity and premature mortality in women today [3]. Hypertension, obesity, diabetes and smoking are all more damaging to the cardiovascular organs in women compared to men. Globally, hypertension is the most important contributor, followed by obesity in most regions, and high LDL cholesterol in Europe, East and South Asia, Australasia and high-income Asia-Pacific. Tobacco smoking still remains an important contributor in women in the Western Europe and high-income Asia-Pacific regions, and global smoking prevalence among women was 6.8% in 2019 [2]. Early detection and management of these traditional CVD risk factors remain paramount for improving women's health and reduce CVD morbidity and premature mortality in women.

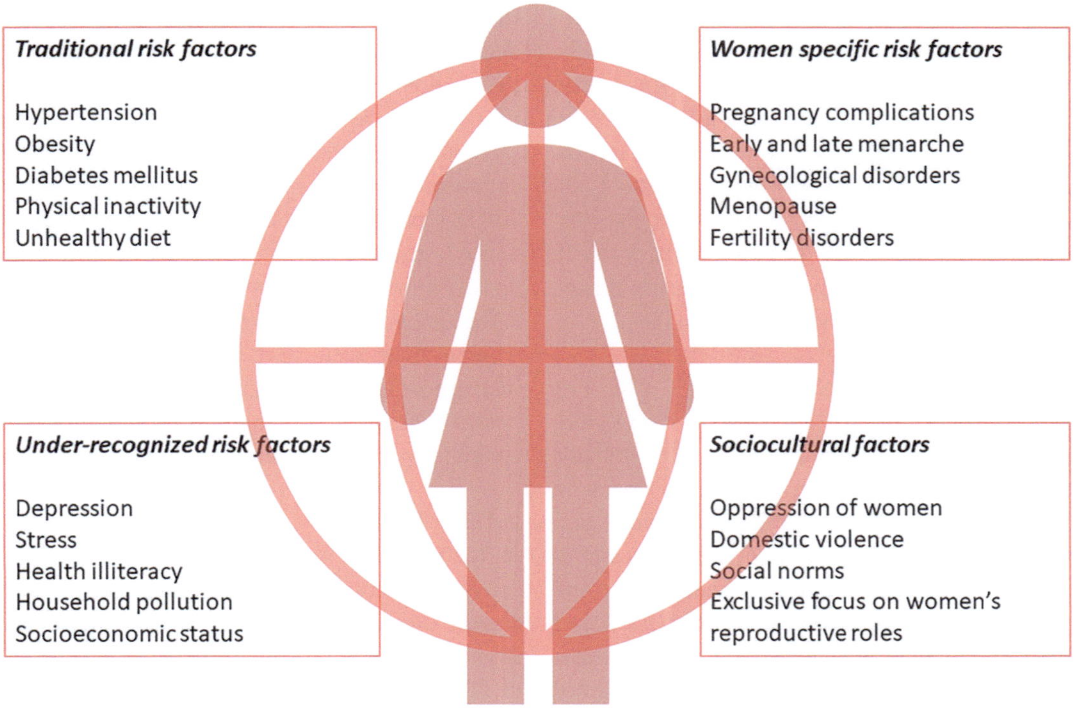

Fig. 1 Traditional, women-specific and under-recognized risk factors as well as sociocultural factors that contribute to the global CVD burden in women

2.1.1 Hypertension

Hypertension is the leading global risk factor for CVD in women, being the main cause of premature death in women and the main contributor to DALYs in women above 55 years [10]. The age-adjusted global prevalence of hypertension is 32%. Women in LMIC have higher prevalence of hypertension than women in HIC across all age groups [11]. The age-adjusted hypertension prevalence has been stable over the past three decades, reflecting that the decline in hypertension prevalence in high-income countries (HIC) is balanced by an increase of hypertension in LMIC [12]. However the number of women with hypertension has more than doubled during this period as a consequence of aging and population gain. Data from 201 studies in 184 countries covering 99% of the world's population with 104 million participants aged 30–79 years have documented that hypertension was undiagnosed in 41% of women compared to in 51% men, pointing to the need for better screening [12]. In that study, higher rates of treatment and BP control was found in women. Still, BP was controlled (<140/90 mmHg) in less than half of those treated [12]. In contrast, a recent Canadian national survey reported lower BP awareness, and a concerning rise in uncontrolled treated hypertension in older women over the past decade [13].

2.1.2 Obesity

The global obesity epidemic is increasing, and prevalence of obesity (body mass index ≥30 kg/m^2) has tripled since 1975. In 2018, the World Health Organization [14] reported that 15% of adult women were obese compared to 11% of men. In women, the prevalence of obesity peaks around age 60–64 years. The United States of America, the National Health and Nutrition Examination Survey (NHANES) from 2013–2014 found obesity in 40.5% of women, and the prevalence was highest in women of Hispanic ethnicity [15]. Data from the European Social Survey Round 7, performed in 20 European countries, found 15.9% of women to be obese, and the highest prevalences were found in the United Kingdom and the East-European countries [16]. Globally, obesity has higher impact on DALYs for women at older ages, and in the regions of Oceania, Central Asia, North and Sub-Saharan Africa, Middle East, Eastern Europe, Central Latin America and the Caribbean. However, the age-standardized death rate for obesity was lower in women than in men. The highest obesity-related death rate is found in the Middle East [17].

2.1.3 Diabetes Mellitus

The prevalence of type 2 diabetes is rising globally because of the obesity epidemic. Globally, the prevalence of diabetes is slightly lower in women than men. The overall prevalence of diabetes is 8.5%. Diabetes is associated with a twofold increase in risk of coronary heart disease and stroke, and is a major cause of blindness, lower limb amputations and end-stage renal disease. From 2000 to 2019 the global age-standardized mortality rate due to diabetes increased by 3%, and up to 13% in LMIC [10]. The impact of diabetes on DALYs increases with age and is higher in Oceania and Central Asia. The relative CVD protection in pre-menopausal women is significantly reduced by diabetes. Diabetes increases relative CVD risk more in women compared to in men, by 44% for coronary heart disease and by 27% for stroke [3, 18, 19]. The highest excess risk is observed in women <40 years with diabetes. In type 1 diabetes initiating before the age of 10 years, women had a 6 times higher risk of myocardial infarction compared to men in the Swedish Nation Diabetes Registry [20]. In Uganda, it is demonstrated that urbanization contributes to the obesity epidemic as well as to the increase in type 2 diabetes [21].

2.1.4 High LDL-Cholesterol

At the global level, burden of LDL-cholesterol related disease remains lower in women than men [2]. In post-menopausal women, LDL-cholesterol levels are comparable to that of men at similar age, and DALYs attributed to high LDL-cholesterol increase also in women from age 60 years forward. Age-standardized DALYs due to high LDL-cholesterol are highest in Eastern Europe, North Africa, the Middle East, Oceania and Central Asia and track with tobacco use [2]. Serum lipid types and development over the life course differ between women and men [22]. The INTERHEART study, which was performed in 52 countries across the world, found that the ratio of APOB (apolipoprotein B) to APOA1 (apolipoprotein A1) and the ratio of total cholesterol to high density lipoprotein cholesterol were both stronger associated with incident myocardial infarction in women than men [23]. However, 1 mmol/L increase in LDL-cholesterol has similar risk for coronary heart disease, myocardial infarction and stroke in women and men [14].

2.1.5 Smoking

In 2020, 7.8% of women globally were smokers, and 80% of these live in LMIC. Tobacco smoking and the use of electronic cigarettes are increasing in young women [3]. Data from the Global Burden of Disease study showed a global age-standardized prevalence of smoking of 5% among women, but higher prevalences were found in many European countries. Tobacco smoking kills 50% of it's users. The risk of CVD associated with smoking is 25% higher in women [3].

2.2 Female-Specific CVD Risk Factors

Recent research has documented the influence of X-chromosomes, female sex hormones, reproductive events, infertility and menopause for CVD risk in women [7]. While traditional CVD risk factors dominate in middle-aged and older women, female-specific risk factors and inflammatory disorders are particular important for CVD risk in young and middle-aged women [24].

2.2.1 Pregnancy Complications

Recurrent pregnancy loss, preterm delivery, small for gestational age newborns, gestational diabetes mellitus and hypertensive pregnancy complications are all associated with increased maternal CVD risk [24]. WHO report that hypertensive pregnancy complications occur in up to 10% of pregnancies, and the prevalence increases with maternal age and metabolic comorbidities and is higher in regions with low calcium intake. However, the global perspective has focused more on maternal mortality reduction during pregnancy and labour, and DALYs due to delivery-related urogenital complications. Between 2016–2020 the global maternal mortality remained stable. It decreased in South-East Asia, and increased in Europe, the Americas and in Western Pacific. The lifetime risk of maternal death is 1 in 49 in LMIC, compared to 1 in 5300 in HIC. The stillbirth rate is an important marker of quality of care in pregnancy and childbirth. The global stillbirth rate was 13.9 per 1000 births in 2021. The highest stillbirth rate was found in Sub-Saharan Africa and Southern Asia. The maternal deaths are mainly caused by severe bleeding or infection after birth, and by preeclampsia.

Maternal CVD complicates 1–4% of pregnancies, and accounts for 15% of maternal mortality worldwide. Data from the European Society of Cardiology Registry of pregnancy and cardiac disease identified congenital heart disease as the most prevalent type of CVD in pregnancy, followed by valvular heart disease. In HIC, access to surgery and medical treatment of women with congenital heart disease has led to an increase in pregnancies among women with congenital heart diseases. Furthermore, multidisciplinary pregnancy care has improved outcome in these women. The increasing maternal age of pregnancy in HIC leads to higher risk of stable or unstable IHD during pregnancy. A recent report from the European Society of Cardiology Registry of Pregnancy and Cardiac disease, using data from 5739 pregnancies in women with CVD during 2008–2028, congenital heart disease and rheumatic heart disease were the most prevalent types of CVD, while IHD was present in 4% [25].

2.2.2 Menopause

Most women experience menopause between the age of 45 and 55 years as a natural part of biological aging. Menopause is caused by the loss of ovarian follicular function. Natural menopause is deemed to have occurred after 12 consecutive months without menstruation for which there are no other medical reason. The proportion of postmenopausal women is growing globally and was 26% of all women and girls in 2021. Despite the lower risk of CVD in premenopausal women, the risk increases substantially after menopause following reduction in the female sex hormones oestrogen and progesterone. The increase in CVD risk after menopause is mostly explained by increases in BP, dyslipidaemia, and obesity because of reduced oestrogen inhibition of the sympathetic nervous system, renin-angiotensin system, reduced vascular nitric oxide bioavailability, reduced progesterone blockade of aldosterone effects, and oestrogen-loss related reduction in energy spenditure. The Study of Women Across the Nation followed 3302 American women across the perimenopausal period. The study demonstrated that 35% developed hypertension within one year after menopause. New onset hypertension was particularly associated with weight-gain, abdominal obesity, diabetes and more pronounced vasomotor symptoms [26]. In a study of 218 Finnish women, menopause also led to an average 11% increase in LDL-cholesterol, 7% increase in APOB and a 3% increase in triglycerides [27]. Menopause is also associated with a switch from subcutaneous to abdominal fat storage with more adverse inflammatory characteristics [24].

2.3 Under-Recognised CVD Risk Factors

Women are more likely than men to be subject to health disparities that arise from sociocultural and socioeconomic factors [3]. WHO state that unequal power relations between women and men, social norms that decrease education and paid employment opportunities, and the exclusive focus on women's reproductive roles are major sociocultural factors that prevent women to benefit from quality health service and attain the best possible level of cardiovascular health.

2.3.1 Psychosocial Risk Factors

Globally, an estimated 5% of adults suffer from depression. Disproportionally more women suffer from depression and anxiety. Depression is an independent risk factor for both non-obstructive and obstructive coronary artery disease in women and associated with worse outcome after myocardial infarction [3]. Younger and middle-aged women report higher level of perceived stress after myocardial infarction [28]. Stress induces a stronger activation of heart-brain crosstalk in women, which initiates and promotes systemic inflammation and atherosclerosis [29].

2.3.2 Health Literacy

Health literacy refers to an individual's motivation and ability to gain access to, understand, and use information to promote good health. Inadequate health literacy is more common in women and associated with increased risk of CVD [3]. Globally, illiteracy, lack of education and oppression of women are main contributors to lower health literacy in women, as reflected in the United Nation Sustainable Development Goals. Owning a mobile phone has been shown to be an important tool to empower women and enable them to access information and services, pointing to the importance of digital competence. In a national assessment of adult literacy in the United States of America in 2006, 12% of women had less than basic health literacy [3].

2.3.3 Social Determinants of Health

Risk factors that are related to social and economic development, including living conditions, education, income, employment status, food insecurity, discrimination, and access to affordable quality health services, may account for 30-35% of health outcomes globally. The WHO acknowledges that unequal power relationships between women and men, social norms that decrease education and paid employment opportunities for girls and women, and an exclusive focus on women's health as reproductive roles, all contribute to reduced cardiovascular health in women. The Global Burden of Disease study found that women have twofold higher age-adjusted mortality than men in countries with low socio-demographic index [2]. However, this has also been reported for women with minority ethnicity living in poverty in HIC. Low income, low levels of education and living in disadvantaged areas were associated with low cardiovascular health to a greater magnitude in women than in men in the Jackson Heart Study [30]. The lower cost of unhealthy food promotes obesity, hypertension, type 2 diabetes and dyslipidaemia in these women. Women with low socioeconomic status also more often suffer from depression, chronic stress, intimate partner violence and domestic abuse, all recognized as CVD risk factors in women [3].

2.3.4 Environmental Factors

Air pollution is the leading environmental risk factor for global health, and the fourth largest risk factor for global mortality [2]. The risk of CVD is strongly associated with exposure to environmental stressors like air pollution, noise, artificial light at night and climate change [4]. Of note, CVD accounted for 51.5% of the total DALYs attributable to particulate matter with an aerodynamic diameter smaller than 2.5 μm ($PM_{2.5}$), and 31.5% of the total DALYs attributable to household air pollution from the use of solid fuels for cooking, respectively. Worldwide in 2019, the DALYs attributable to $PM_{2.5}$ was higher in men, while the exposure to household air pollution was more similar for women and men. The highest rates of DALYs attributable to household air pollution is seen in Sub-Saharan Africa, South Asia and Oceania [2].

2.4 CVD in Women in a Global Perspective

CVD are the leading causes of death globally, representing 32% of deaths, of which ¾ takes place in LMIC. 85% of CVD deaths are due to IHD and strokes [2]. One in three women die from CVD, and 45% of adult women in the world have some form of CVD [2].

2.4.1 Ischemic Heart Disease

Ischemic heart disease is the leading cause of death in women worldwide. Myocardial infarction is less prevalent in women than in men throughout the lifespan [31]. The pathophysiology, clinical presentation, risk factors, quality of care and outcomes differ substantially between women and men with IHD in publications from HIC [2, 32]. Interestingly, a recent publication from the Kerala region in India among 21,374 patients (24% women) hospitalized with acute coronary syndrome found the same sex disparities [33]. Women were older with higher prevalences of diabetes and hypertension, and lower prevalence of smoking. Furthermore, women were admitted later, received less treatment with aspirin and less percutaneous coronary intervention for ST-elevation myocardial infarction, developed more heart failure and had a higher in-hospital and 30-days mortality also when adjusted for the co-morbidities [33].

Women more often have myocardial ischemia with no obstructive coronary artery disease (INOCA). Among women with INOCA, about 1/3 have non-obstructive coronary artery disease [34, 35]. Other underlying factors include microvascular dysfunction or hypertensive heart disease causing arterial-muscular mismatch and relative myocardial ischemia [36, 37]. Also 10–20% of women with acute myocardial infarction have no obstructive coronary artery disease (MINOCA). In young women, MINOCA is caused by a spontaneous coronary artery dissection (SCAD) in up to 35%, and in up to 43% of myocardial infarctions occurring during or just after pregnancy [38]. In contrast SCAD is a rare cause of myocardial infarction in men, found in 1–4%. The pathophysiology of SCAD may include fibromuscular dysplasia, connective tissue disorders, systemic inflammatory disease, pregnancy, emotional stress and use of illicit drug [38].

2.4.2 Rheumatic Heart Disease

Rheumatic heart disease is the most commonly acquired heart disease in people under 25 years of age globally and mostly affects children and adolescents in LMICs [39]. Girls above age 15 years, and young women are disproportionally affected [2]. According to WHO, rheumatic heart disease claimed 288,348 lives worldwide in 2019, due to lack of adequate health care in endemic countries. However, it only accounts for about 2% of global CVD deaths. Although the disease has been eradicated by effective treatment in many parts of the world, it remains prevalent in sub-Saharan Africa, Central and South Asia, the Middle East and the South Pacific. The prospective Global Rheumatic Heart Disease registry which included 3343 patients (66% women) from 25 hospitals in 12 African countries, India and Yemen, found that in young girls, mitral regurgitation dominated, but from the second decade, mixed mitral and aortic valve disease was the dominant valve pathology [40]. A high prevalence of complications were found, including atrial fibrillation, pulmonary hypertension, left ventricular dysfunction and stroke [40].

2.4.3 Hypertensive Heart Disease

Hypertensive heart disease is defined as heart failure symptoms due to longstanding hypertension which has caused left ventricular hypertrophy, left atrial enlargement, or left ventricular systolic or diastolic dysfunction [5]. The global prevalence of hypertensive heart disease has risen over the past three decades and is a major cause of DALYs and death, and is particularly common in women above 70 years of age [2]. The highest age-standardized rates of DALYs due to hypertensive heart disease are noted in Africa, and is particularly high in women living in Central and Eastern Sub-Saharan Africa.

2.4.4 Heart Failure

The overall incidence of heart failure is similar in women and men [41]. The lifetime risk for heart failure by age 40 years in the Framingham Heart Study was about 20% in both women and men, while the risk of heart failure without an antecedent myocardial infarction was higher in women (15% vs. 11% in men) [42]. The overall prevalence of heart failure in Europe is 1–2% of adults, but the prevalence increases with age, and is >10% in those above 70 years of age [43]. Current guidelines group heart failure into three classes based on left ventricular ejection fraction (EF): heart failure with preserved ejection fraction (HFpEF) (EF >50%), heart failure with mildly reduced EF (EF 40–59%) and heart failure with reduced EF (EF <40%, HFrEF) [43]. HFpEF is twice as common in women, found in around 60% of women compared to 30% of men [44]. The types of heart failure reflect the differences in underlying pathophysiology, hypertension being the most common cause of HFpEF, while IHD is the most common cause of HRrEF. Data from the Swedish heart Failure Registry reported that women were more symptomatic but had lower mortality across heart failure subtypes [45]. In contrast, in the PURSUIT-HFpEF study (Prospective Multicenter Observational Study of patients with HFpEF) performed in East Asia, women had higher risk of combined death and hospitalization for heart failure than men when adjusted for co-morbidities [44]. Obesity is a strong risk factor for HFpEF in women.

Cardiomyopathies are important causes of heart failure. In women, peripartum cardiomyopathy is a feared complication of pregnancy with subsequent heart failure and maternal death. An analysis of the National Inpatient Sample database in the USA reported a prevalence of peripartum cardiomyopathy of 33.5 per 100,000 livebirths in women aged 15–35 years, and a twofold higher prevalence was found in older women [46]. Globally, the incidence of peripartum cardiomyopathy varies between countries, with the highest rates in Nigeria (1 in 102 births) and lowest in Japan (1 in 15,533 births) [47]. Maternal and neonatal outcomes are dependent on socioeconomic factors and access to quality health care [48].

Cardiomyopathies and heart failure may also be caused by infectious agents (Chagas disease and endomyocardial fibrosis), hemoglobinopathies (Thalassemia and Sickle Cell disease) and nutritional deficiencies (BeriBeri, selenium deficiency or hypocalcemia) which traditionally have been more prevalent in tropical regions [49]. These types of heart failure now re-appear in HIC as a consequence of migration and refugees from these regions. Chagas disease may transmit from mother to fetus during pregnancy.

2.4.5 Stroke

Stroke is the second most common cause of CVD death in women. According to WHO 15 million people suffered a stroke in 2021, of whom 30% died and another 30% were left permanently disabled. Around 62% of these strokes were ischemic strokes, 28% intracerebral haemorrhages and 10% subarachnoid haemorrhages. The increase in global stroke burden is mainly due to population increase and aging [2]. The highest age-standardized rates of stroke death and DALYs are found in Oceania, Central Asia, Southeast and East Asia, Eastern Europe and Sub-Saharan Africa. Stroke incidence increases with aging and is higher in women than men among the elderly, above the age of 80 years. Pregnancy, postpartum and menopause are life periods with an increased stroke risk for women [50]. In a systematic review of 19 studies assessing stroke among 18–45 years old individuals, stroke was 44% more common among women in the group <35 years of age, suggesting that female-specific risk factors like migraine, oral contraception, pregnancy and postpartum period may have contributed beyond traditional risk factors [51].

3 Clinical Practice

3.1 Global Perspectives in Prevention of CVD in Women

Although overall awareness about CVD disease in women has increased over the past decade, most health care providers and patients still tend to underestimate CVD risk in women [6]. Hypertension, obesity, diabetes and smoking all have a more deleterious effect on the cardiovascular organs in women than in men.

3.1.1 Hypertension

Although treatment and control rates have improved in most regions over the past three decades, little improvement has been found in Sub-Saharan Africa and Oceania [12]. Women are more at risk for hypertension complications

[52, 53], and the risk of CVD initiates at a lower BP level in women [54, 55]. An analysis from the UK Biobank cohort found women to have higher risk of stroke with increasing severity of hypertension than men. Several publications have documented that the CVD risk initiates at a lower BP level in women both for myocardial infarction and for stroke [54, 55]. Taken together, the proportion of CVD that can be prevented by BP control is likely higher among women.

Women and men differ in their BP development over the life course [56]. A more exaggerated BP increase is observed in women already from the third decade. Thus, regularly BP measurement in adult women is recommended, and in women at the time of CVD risk incidences like hypertensive pregnancy complications and menopause. Annual BP measurement is recommended in women after a hypertensive pregnancy complication [24]. Women in LMIC may have little access to risk-assessment both before and after a hypertensive pregnancy complication. However, opportunistic BP measurement in women bringing their children for vaccination, or elderly house-hold members to health care facilities may help detect hypertension early. Postmenopausal women and black people are more salt sensitive, and low sodium intake is recommended to avoid BP increase and incident hypertension. In the DASH (Dietary Approaches to Stop Hypertension) trial, women had better BP lowering effect of low sodium intake compared to men [57]. However, the majority of women with hypertension will need drug therapy for management and control of BP [58]. Antihypertensive drug treatment recommendations are the same in women and men.

3.1.2 Obesity

Compared to men, a similar increase in body mass index in women is associated with a larger increase in BP and CVD. Obesity is also associated with adverse outcome in pregnancy and with infertility. Weight control is therefore an essential part of prevention of hypertension and CVD in women, and in management of hypertension [58]. WHO recommend limiting energy intake from total fats and sugars, and increase consumption of fruit, vegetables, legumes, whole grains and nuts to control body weight. Furthermore, 60 min daily physical activity is recommended for girls and 20–30 min a day for adult women. However, low income and poverty may limit compliance with these recommendations. In LMIC obesity may be taken as a sign of wealth, an attitude that should be combated.

3.1.3 Tobacco Use

There is no safe level of smoking or exposure to second-hand smoke. E-cigarettes should not be recommended as a smoking cessation strategy in women.

3.2 Global Perspectives in Improving Management of CVD in Women

3.2.1 Refocus of Health Administration

Health administrators in LMIC have traditionally focused on communicable diseases, and now must increase their focus on non-communicable diseases. WHO have identified CVD, diabetes, chronic obstructive lung diseases and cancer as the main non-communicable diseases. Communication about female-specific CVD risk factors is important to educate health professionals and empower women to retain good cardiovascular health. The WHO has developed a series of fact sheets freely available for this purpose. However, many of these fact sheets could be improved by including sex and gender informed health information. Sex-specific strategies are urgently needed to provide optimal health care for women worldwide. Electronic health information to women could also be provided through mobile phones. However, although mobile phones are increasingly common in LMIC, and may empower women and improve health literacy, many users do not have access to internet through their phone due to costs. Also in HIC, electronic health information may be less effective in elderly women, due to low digital competence.

Worldwide, the focus on women's health remains limited to reproduction and organs that fit in the bikini. In reality, modern research has demonstrated that women's health relates to the whole body, and CVD play a major role for women's health. Because of the high prevalence, better prevention and management of CVD in women is a prerequisite for social and cultural progress and sustainable development of all societies. Despite the large body of knowledge on sex differences in risk factors, symptoms and clinical presentation of CVD [3], sex and gender informed health information is often not presented on official webpages. In 2023, a Norwegian official report from the Women's Health Commission was submitted to the government, listing 75 action points to improve women's health (https://www.regjeringen.no/en/aktuelt/womens-health-commission-submits-report/id2965065/). Key points included updated public health websites to include sex specific information, mandatory presentation of sex and gender informed information from national health registries, inclusion of sex and gender aspects in all levels of health care and increasing public funding of research on under-recognized risk factors for CVD in women (Fig. 1). Also, by increasing the number of women in leading positions within health care and supporting their unique values, all themes connected with women's cardiovascular health will be put higher on the agenda [59].

3.2.2 Implementation of Sex and Gender Aspects in Health Profession Education

Knowledge changes practice. CVD remain understudied, underdiagnosed and undertreated in women [3]. Inclusion of sex and gender aspects in CVD in the national curricula of health profession educations is paramount for future health workers to include these aspects into clinical practice both in primary and specialised health care, in nursing and in information given by the pharmacists. Implementation of modern knowledge on prevention and management of CVD in women must parallel an increased and adequately powered research focus on closing knowledge gaps on CVD in women. Previous awareness campaigns targeting lay women, have paid little attention to the role of physicians and other health care providers in assessing and managing CVD risk [6]. Exposing students in health profession educations to the important knowledge of biological and cultural sex for CVD risk and optimal management as well as to current knowledge gaps, will provide future health workers with better tools for diagnosis, prevention and treatment of CVD in women, and for delivering a better standard of care for women. In parallel, organization of cardiovascular health care at all levels must incorporate sex and gender aspects to optimize information to women with CVD and ensure better diagnosis and management.

4 Conclusions

Globally, CVD causes one out of three deaths in women, and 45% of women live with CVD. IHD and strokes causes 85% of CVD death in women. Female-specific risk factors, risk factors that predominate in women and the larger impact of hypertension, obesity, diabetes and smoking are not accounted for in international risk scores recommended for CVD prevention. Sex-specific strategies are urgently needed to take these factors as well as under-recognized factors and sociocultural factors into account to provide optimal care for women (Fig. 1). An increased awareness and focus on CVD in women is called for not only in medical practice and research, but in health care administration and organization, education of health professionals, and in health communication across the world.

Key Issues

- One out of three women die from CVD globally
- 85% of CVD death in women is caused by IHD and stroke
- CVD mortality has declined in HIC and increased in LMIC
- Metabolic risk factors drive CVD in women
- Hypertension is the number one cause of premature death in women globally

- Hypertensive pregnancy complications are more prevalent in women with metabolic comorbidities and in regions with low calcium intake
- Depression, stress, health literacy and socio-economic factors are under-recognised CVD risk factors in women
- Unequal power relations between women and men, social norms that decrease education and paid employment opportunities for women, and the exclusive focus on women's reproductive roles are major sociocultural factors that reduce cardiovascular health in women

Questions and Answers

1. What is the percentage of death in women <70 years of age that are caused by CVD
   (A) 25%
   (B) 45%
   (C) 32%
   (D) 63%
   Comment: The correct answer is C. In 2019, The Global Burden of Disease Study reported that 32% of deaths in women <70 years of age were caused by CVD. Death before the age of 70 years is referred to as premature death.
2. What is the global number one risk factor for CVD in women?
   (A) Menopause
   (B) Diabetes
   (C) Hypertensive pregnancy complications
   (D) Hypertension
   Comment: The correct answer is D. Hypertension is the global number one risk factor for CVD in women. About 50% of women that develop hypertension do so during menopausal transition. Hypertensive pregnancy complications occur in up to 10% of pregnancies and predispose for development of hypertension later in life.
3. What is the most common cause of CVD death in women globally?
   (A) Stroke
   (B) Heart failure
   (C) Cardiomyopathies
   (D) IHD
   Comment: The correct answer is D. IHD contributes to ~50% of CVD mortality in women globally according to the Global Burden of Disease Study in 2019. 85% of global CVD mortality is attributed to stroke and IHD combined.
4. Which of these factors may obstruct diagnosis of CVD in women?
   (A) Unequal power relationships between women and men
   (B) Social norms that decrease education and employment
   (C) Exclusive focus on women's health related to reproduction
   (D) All of the above
   Comment: The best answer is D. Unequal power relationships between women and men, social norms the oppress women and decrease education and paid employment opportunities, and the exclusive focus on women's health as related to reproductive roles are all identified by the WHO as socio-cultural factors that prevent women and girls to benefit from quality health care and attain the best possible level of cardiovascular health.
5. Do hypertension, obesity, diabetes and smoking all have a more deleterious effect on the cardiovascular organs in women than in men?
   (A) Yes
   (B) No
   Comment: A is correct. The relative impact of these CVD risk factors is larger in women than in men.

6. CVD remain understudied, under-recognized, underdiagnosed, and undertreated in women. What is the reason for this is:
   (A) Women with CVD are more often asymptomatic
   (B) The male pattern of CVD is the norm in medicine
   (C) Elderly women have fewer co-morbidities than men
   (D) Women live longer in better health
   Comment: B is correct. Medicine is still considered from the male perspective.
7. A lower socio-economic status (SES) leads to more health problems and reduces life expectancy. Which of these social determinants are the main contributors to CVD in women?
   (A) Unhealthy food and mental stress
   (B) Poorer housing conditions
   (C) Lower income and access to health care
   (D) All above factors contribute
   Comment: D is correct. A low SES affects many determinants of heath, including nutrition, lifestyle factors, education, access to care, as well as issues related to power and control.

References

1. Cho L, Davis M, Elgendy I, Epps K, Lindley KJ, Mehta PK, et al. Summary of updated recommendations for primary prevention of cardiovascular disease in women: JACC state-of-the-art review. J Am Coll Cardiol. 2020;75(20):2602–18.
2. Roth GA, Mensah GA, Johnson CO, Addolorato G, Ammirati E, Baddour LM, et al. Global burden of cardiovascular diseases and risk factors, 1990-2019: update from the GBD 2019 study. J Am Coll Cardiol. 2020;76(25):2982–3021.
3. Vogel B, Acevedo M, Appelman Y, Bairey Merz CN, Chieffo A, Figtree GA, et al. The Lancet women and cardiovascular disease Commission: reducing the global burden by 2030. Lancet. 2021;397(10292):2385–438.
4. Munzel T, Hahad O, Sorensen M, Lelieveld J, Duerr GD, Nieuwenhuijsen M, et al. Environmental risk factors and cardiovascular diseases: a comprehensive expert review. Cardiovasc Res. 2022;118(14):2880–902.
5. Gerdts E, Sudano I, Brouwers S, Borghi C, Bruno RM, Ceconi C, et al. Sex differences in arterial hypertension. Eur Heart J. 2022;43(46):4777–88.
6. Bairey Merz CN, Andersen H, Sprague E, Burns A, Keida M, Walsh MN, et al. Knowledge, attitudes, and beliefs regarding cardiovascular disease in women: the women's heart alliance. J Am Coll Cardiol. 2017;70(2):123–32.
7. Bartz D, Chitnis T, Kaiser UB, Rich-Edwards JW, Rexrode KM, Pennell PB, et al. Clinical advances in sex- and gender-informed medicine to improve the health of all: a review. JAMA Intern Med. 2020;180(4):574–83.
8. Perrino C, Ferdinandy P, Botker HE, Brundel B, Collins P, Davidson SM, et al. Improving translational research in sex-specific effects of comorbidities and risk factors in ischaemic heart disease and cardioprotection: position paper and recommendations of the ESC Working Group on Cellular Biology of the Heart. Cardiovasc Res. 2021;117(2):367–85.
9. Hay K, McDougal L, Percival V, Henry S, Klugman J, Wurie H, et al. Disrupting gender norms in health systems: making the case for change. Lancet. 2019;393(10190):2535–49.
10. Collaborators GBDRF. Global burden of 87 risk factors in 204 countries and territories, 1990-2019: a systematic analysis for the Global Burden of Disease Study 2019. Lancet. 2020;396(10258):1223–49.
11. Ahmad A, Oparil S. Hypertension in women: recent advances and lingering questions. Hypertension. 2017;70(1):19–26.
12. Collaboration NCDRF. Worldwide trends in hypertension prevalence and progress in treatment and control from 1990 to 2019: a pooled analysis of 1201 population-representative studies with 104 million participants. Lancet. 2021;398(10304):957–80.
13. Leung AA, Williams JV, McAlister FA, Campbell NR, Padwal RS, et al. Worsening hypertension awareness, treatment, and control rates in Canadian women between 2007 and 2017. Can J Cardiol. 2020;36(5):732–9.
14. Group WCRCW. World Health Organization cardiovascular disease risk charts: revised models to estimate risk in 21 global regions. Lancet Glob Health. 2019;7(10):1332–45.
15. Flegal KM, Kruszon-Moran D, Carroll MD, Fryar CD, Ogden CL. Trends in obesity among adults in the United States, 2005 to 2014. JAMA. 2016;315(21):2284–91.
16. Marques A, Peralta M, Naia A, Loureiro N, de Matos MG. Prevalence of adult overweight and obesity in 20 European countries, 2014. Eur J Pub Health. 2018;28(2):295–300.
17. Chong B, Jayabaskaran J, Kong G, Chan YH, Chin YH, Goh R, et al. Trends and predictions of malnutrition and obesity in 204 countries and territories: an analysis of the Global Burden of Disease Study 2019. EClinicalMedicine. 2023;57:101850.
18. Peters SA, Huxley RR, Woodward M. Diabetes as risk factor for incident coronary heart disease in women compared with men: a systematic review and meta-analysis of 64 cohorts including 858,507 indi-

viduals and 28,203 coronary events. Diabetologia. 2014;57(8):1542–51.
19. Al-Salameh A, Chanson P, Bucher S, Ringa V, Becquemont L. Cardiovascular disease in type 2 diabetes: a review of sex-related differences in predisposition and prevention. Mayo Clin Proc. 2019;94(2):287–308.
20. Rawshani A, Sattar N, Franzen S, Rawshani A, Hattersley AT, Svensson AM, et al. Excess mortality and cardiovascular disease in young adults with type 1 diabetes in relation to age at onset: a nationwide, register-based cohort study. Lancet. 2018;392(10146):477–86.
21. Mayega RW, Guwatudde D, Makumbi F, Nakwagala FN, Peterson S, Tomson G, et al. Diabetes and pre-diabetes among persons aged 35 to 60 years in eastern Uganda: prevalence and associated factors. PLoS One. 2013;8(8):e72554.
22. Roeters van Lennep JE, Tokgozoglu LS, Badimon L, Dumanski SM, Gulati M, Hess CN, et al. Women, lipids, and atherosclerotic cardiovascular disease: a call to action from the European Atherosclerosis Society. Eur Heart J. 2023;44(39):4157–73.
23. McQueen MJ, Hawken S, Wang X, Ounpuu S, Sniderman A, Probstfield J, et al. Lipids, lipoproteins, and apolipoproteins as risk markers of myocardial infarction in 52 countries (the INTERHEART study): a case-control study. Lancet. 2008;372(9634):224–33.
24. Maas A, Rosano G, Cifkova R, Chieffo A, van Dijken D, Hamoda H, et al. Cardiovascular health after menopause transition, pregnancy disorders, and other gynaecologic conditions: a consensus document from European cardiologists, gynaecologists, and endocrinologists. Eur Heart J. 2021;42(10):967–84.
25. Roos-Hesselink J, Baris L, Johnson M, De Backer J, Otto C, Marelli A, et al. Pregnancy outcomes in women with cardiovascular disease: evolving trends over 10 years in the ESC Registry of Pregnancy and Cardiac Disease (ROPAC). Eur Heart J. 2019;40(47):3848–55.
26. Samargandy S, Matthews KA, Brooks MM, Barinas-Mitchell E, Magnani JW, Thurston RC, et al. Trajectories of blood pressure in midlife women: does menopause matter? Circ Res. 2022;130(3):312–22.
27. Karppinen JE, Tormakangas T, Kujala UM, Sipila S, Laukkanen J, Aukee P, et al. Menopause modulates the circulating metabolome: evidence from a prospective cohort study. Eur J Prev Cardiol. 2022;29(10):1448–59.
28. Xu X, Bao H, Strait KM, Edmondson DE, Davidson KW, Beltrame JF, et al. Perceived stress after acute myocardial infarction: a comparison between young and middle-aged women versus men. Psychosom Med. 2017;79(1):50–8.
29. Rossi A, Mikail N, Bengs S, Haider A, Treyer V, Buechel RR, et al. Heart-brain interactions in cardiac and brain diseases: why sex matters. Eur Heart J. 2022;43(39):3971–80.
30. Joseph JJ, Williams A, Azap RA, Zhao S, Brock G, Kline D, et al. Role of sex in the association of socioeconomic status with cardiovascular health in Black Americans: the Jackson heart study. J Am Heart Assoc. 2023;12(23):e030695.
31. Albrektsen G, Heuch I, Lochen ML, Thelle DS, Wilsgaard T, Njolstad I, et al. Risk of incident myocardial infarction by gender: interactions with serum lipids, blood pressure and smoking. The Tromso study 1979-2012. Atherosclerosis. 2017;261:52–9.
32. Regitz-Zagrosek V, Oertelt-Prigione S, Prescott E, Franconi F, Gerdts E, et al. Gender in cardiovascular diseases: impact on clinical manifestations, management, and outcomes. Eur Heart J. 2016;37(1):24–34.
33. Khraishah H, Alahmad B, Alfaddagh A, Jeong SY, Mathenge N, Kassab MB, et al. Sex disparities in the presentation, management and outcomes of patients with acute coronary syndrome: insights from the ACS QUIK trial. Open Heart. 2021;8(1):1470.
34. Reynolds HR, Shaw LJ, Min JK, Spertus JA, Chaitman BR, Berman DS, et al. Association of sex with severity of coronary artery disease, ischemia, and symptom burden in patients with moderate or severe ischemia: secondary analysis of the ISCHEMIA randomized clinical trial. JAMA Cardiol. 2020;5(7):773–86.
35. Shaw LJ, Merz CN, Pepine CJ, Reis SE, Bittner V, Kip KE, et al. The economic burden of angina in women with suspected ischemic heart disease: results from the National Institutes of Health–National Heart, Lung, and Blood Institute–sponsored Women's Ischemia Syndrome Evaluation. Circulation. 2006;114(9):894–904.
36. Eskerud I, Gerdts E, Larsen TH, Lonnebakken MT. Left ventricular hypertrophy contributes to myocardial ischemia in non-obstructive coronary artery disease (the MicroCAD study). Int J Cardiol. 2019;286:1–6.
37. Mehta PK, Huang J, Levit RD, Malas W, Waheed N, Bairey Merz CN. Ischemia and no obstructive coronary arteries (INOCA): a narrative review. Atherosclerosis. 2022;363:8–21.
38. Stanojevic D, Apostolovic S, Kostic T, Mitov V, Kutlesic-Kurtovic D, Kovacevic M, et al. A review of the risk and precipitating factors for spontaneous coronary artery dissection. Front Cardiovasc Med. 2023;10:1273301.
39. Remenyi B, Carapetis J, Wyber R, Taubert K, Mayosi BM, World Heart F. Position statement of the World Heart Federation on the prevention and control of rheumatic heart disease. Nat Rev Cardiol. 2013;10(5):284–92.
40. Zuhlke L, Engel ME, Karthikeyan G, Rangarajan S, Mackie P, Cupido B, et al. Characteristics, complications, and gaps in evidence-based interventions in rheumatic heart disease: the Global Rheumatic Heart Disease Registry (the REMEDY study). Eur Heart J. 2015;36(18):1115–22.
41. Lala A, Tayal U, Hamo CE, Youmans Q, Al-Khatib SM, Bozkurt B, et al. Sex differences in heart failure. J Card Fail. 2022;28(3):477–98.
42. Lloyd-Jones DM, Larson MG, Leip EP, Beiser A, D'Agostino RB, Kannel WB, et al. Lifetime risk for

developing congestive heart failure: the Framingham Heart Study. Circulation. 2002;106(24):3068–72.
43. McDonagh TA, Metra M, Adamo M, Gardner RS, Baumbach A, Bohm M, et al. 2021 ESC Guidelines for the diagnosis and treatment of acute and chronic heart failure. Eur Heart J. 2021;42(36):3599–726.
44. Sotomi Y, Hikoso S, Nakatani D, Mizuno H, Okada K, Dohi T, et al. Sex differences in heart failure with preserved ejection fraction. J Am Heart Assoc. 2021;10(5):e018574.
45. Stolfo D, Uijl A, Vedin O, Stromberg A, Faxen UL, Rosano GMC, et al. Sex-based differences in heart failure across the ejection fraction spectrum: phenotyping, and prognostic and therapeutic implications. JACC Heart Fail. 2019;7(6):505–15.
46. Ijaz SH, Jamal S, Minhas AMK, Sheikh AB, Nazir S, Khan MS, et al. Trends in characteristics and outcomes of peripartum cardiomyopathy hospitalizations in the United States Between 2004 and 2018. Am J Cardiol. 2022;168:142–50.
47. Isogai T, Kamiya CA. Worldwide incidence of peripartum cardiomyopathy and overall maternal mortality. Int Heart J. 2019;60(3):503–11.
48. Sliwa K, van der Meer P, Viljoen C, Jackson AM, Petrie MC, Mebazaa A, et al. Socio-economic factors determine maternal and neonatal outcomes in women with peripartum cardiomyopathy: a study of the ESC EORP PPCM registry. Int J Cardiol. 2023;398:131596.
49. Sliwa K, Viljoen CA, Hasan B, Ntusi NAB. Nutritional heart disease and cardiomyopathies: JACC Focus Seminar 4/4. J Am Coll Cardiol 2022. https://doi.org/10.1016/j.jacc.2022.08.812.
50. Kremer C, Gdovinova Z, Bejot Y, Heldner MR, Zuurbier S, Walter S, et al. European Stroke Organisation guidelines on stroke in women: management of menopause, pregnancy and postpartum. Eur Stroke J. 2022;7(2):I–XIX.
51. Leppert MH, Burke JF, Lisabeth LD, Madsen TE, Kleindorfer DO, Sillau S, et al. Systematic review of sex differences in ischemic strokes among young adults: are young women disproportionately at risk? Stroke. 2022;53(2):319–27.
52. Yusuf S, Hawken S, Ounpuu S, Dans T, Avezum A, Lanas F, et al. Effect of potentially modifiable risk factors associated with myocardial infarction in 52 countries (the INTERHEART study): case-control study. Lancet. 2004;364(9438):937–52.
53. Gerdts E, Izzo R, Mancusi C, Losi MA, Manzi MV, Canciello G, et al. Left ventricular hypertrophy offsets the sex difference in cardiovascular risk (the Campania Salute Network). Int J Cardiol. 2018;258:257–61.
54. Ji H, Niiranen TJ, Rader F, Henglin M, Kim A, Ebinger JE, et al. Sex differences in blood pressure associations with cardiovascular outcomes. Circulation. 2021;143(7):761–3.
55. Kringeland E, Tell GS, Midtbo H, Igland J, Haugsgjerd TR, Gerdts E. Stage 1 hypertension, sex, and acute coronary syndromes during midlife: the Hordaland Health Study. Eur J Prev Cardiol. 2022;29(1):147–54.
56. Ji H, Kim A, Ebinger JE, Niiranen TJ, Claggett BL, Bairey Merz CN, et al. Sex differences in blood pressure trajectories over the life course. JAMA Cardiol. 2020;5(3):19–26.
57. Sacks FM, Svetkey LP, Vollmer WM, Appel LJ, Bray GA, Harsha D, et al. Effects on blood pressure of reduced dietary sodium and the dietary approaches to stop hypertension (DASH) diet. DASH-Sodium Collaborative Research Group. N Engl J Med. 2001;344(1):3–10.
58. Williams B, Mancia G, Spiering W, Agabiti Rosei E, Azizi M, Burnier M, et al. 2018 ESC/ESH guidelines for the management of arterial hypertension. Eur Heart J. 2018;39(33):3021–104.
59. Maas A. Empower women in healthcare to move Women's Health forward. Maturitas. 2020;136:22–4.

Part I

Traditional CVD Risk Factors in Women

Obesity and Cardiovascular Disease in Women

Gabriele Riccardi and Giovanni de Simone

Abstract

Obesity is a serious chronic condition of epidemic proportions, increasing incidence of cardiovascular (CV) disease (CVD) and other morbid conditions. Women are particularly affected by the obesity epidemic. The greater prevalence of obesity in women becomes only manifested in adulthood, with peak prevalence occurring between 60 and 64 years of age. The sex-related difference in obesity prevalence have been attributed to nutrition, lifestyle, behavior, and environment. The association of CVD and obesity is particularly relevant in women, being their leading cause of death. Nondiabetic premenopausal women are protected against CVD when compared with age-matched men. However, once obese and insulin resistant, women exhibit worsened CVD outcomes. The increased CV risk in obese women is largely due to coexistence with diabetes, hyperlipidemia, and hypertension. Since overweight and obesity are associated with increased prevalence of CV risk factors and incidence of CVD events, weight loss in obese women is expected both to benefit long-term survival and to have many beneficial effects on CV risk factors. Therapy for obesity is based on lifestyle changes, drugs, and bariatric surgery. Lifestyle modifications include low calorie diets and moderate-intensity physical activity. The most effective weight reducing drugs are GLP-1 (glucagon-like peptide-1) receptor agonists, which can induce a weight loss greater than 10% in most individuals, more pronounced in females. Metabolic surgery can induce an average weight loss of up to 20% for as much as 20 years. Matched-pair cohort analysis demonstrated that bariatric surgery results in comparable short- and mid-term efficacy in men and women.

Keywords

Obese women · Cardiovascular risk · Weight loss · Treatment

G. Riccardi (✉)
Diabetes, Nutrition and Metabolism Unit, Federico II University, Naples, Italy
e-mail: riccardi@unina.it

G. de Simone
Department of Advanced Biomedical Sciences, Federico II University, Naples, Italy
e-mail: simogi@unina.it

A. H.E.M. Maas, E. Gerdts (eds.), *Manual of Cardiovascular Disease in Women*,
https://doi.org/10.1007/978-3-031-65952-2_2

Test your learning and check your understanding of this book's contents: use the "Springer Nature Flashcards" app to access questions using ▶ https://sn.pub/51ny7m
To use the app, please follow the instructions in chapter 1.

1 Introduction

Overweight and obesity are pathophysiologic conditions responsible for chronic diseases and risk factors, especially impacting cardiovascular (CV) system and causing about 60% of deaths worldwide. The GBD (Global Burden of Disease) Obesity Collaborators estimated that 39% of the world's population (2.8–3.5 billion people) is overweight or obese, with obesity prevalence doubling between 1980 and 2015 in 73 countries and continuously increasing in most of the other countries. Over recent decades, body mass index (BMI, i.e., weight, in kg, divided by squared height, in m^2) has increased substantially worldwide not only in adults but also in children and adolescents. In addition, the GBD investigators found increasing burden of high BMI, accounting for 4.0 million deaths in 2015, more than two-thirds of which were caused by CV disease (CVD), even after accounting for smoking and other diseases [1].

2 Theory

2.1 Epidemiology of Overweight and Obesity

Women are particularly affected by the obesity epidemic. Between 1980 and 2015, the global prevalence of overweight (a body mass index (BMI) $\geq$ 25 kg/m^2) rose from 27.8 to 39.4% in women, and from 25.4 to 38.5% in men [2]. In Europe, in 2020, 29.3% of adult women were obese, compared to 24.1% of adult men. This trend seems consistent across all regions of Europe [3].

The greater prevalence of obesity in women becomes only manifested in adulthood, with peak prevalence occurring between 60 and 64 years of age. These sex-related differences have been attributed to nutrition, lifestyle, behavior, and environment [2].

Results from the analysis of pooled data from 19 prospective studies, including 1.46 million white adults, 19–84 years old, followed up for 10 years, demonstrate a J-shaped relationship between obesity and all-cause mortality, with the highest risk in the lowest and the highest categories of BMI. A possible reason of the relation between underweight and mortality could be coexisting undetected diseases and/or smoking, as smoking is associated with a lower BMI and increased risk of CV, respiratory, and neoplastic death. The HR was 1.51 (1.46–1.56) for men versus 1.30 (1.26–1.33) for women (heterogeneity $p < 0.0001$). Hence, a given increase in BMI is associated with a far greater absolute mortality increase in men than in women. Moreover, males with a higher waist-to-hip ratio (WHR), a measure of central obesity, have a disproportionately higher risk of mortality than females. Thus, assessing and targeting WHR may have greater relevance in males. Since female adiposity distribution is drastically different than that in males, the relatively higher abdominal obesity in males may explain the sex-specific difference in mortality [4].

Obesity, and in particular central obesity, affects lifespan in both men and women [5] (Fig. 1), mostly because it is associated with an increased risk of metabolic, CVD and oncologic events. Mendelian randomization analyses suggest a linear relation between BMI and mortality in never-smokers and a J-shaped relation in ever-smokers [5].

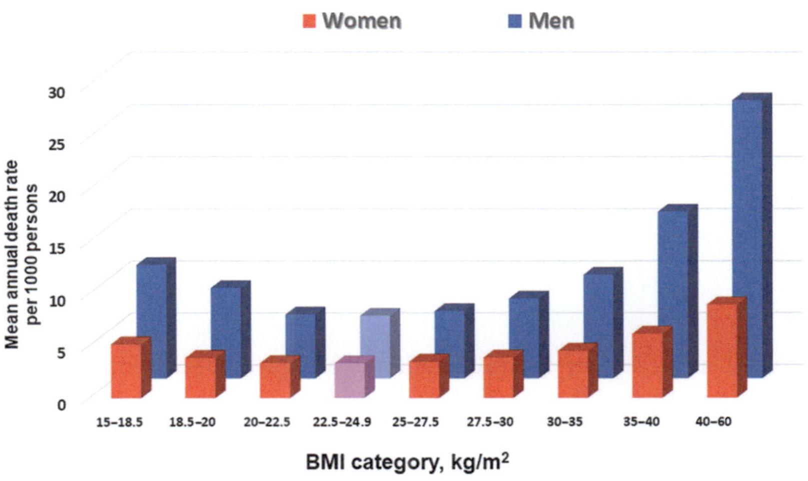

Fig. 1 Mean annual deathrate per 1000 person in BMI categories for women and men

However, there is a large body of evidence indicating that moderate excess of body weight is associated with a lower risk for adverse events in patients with CVD, including heart failure. This phenomenon has been identified as the "obesity paradox". In particular, observational studies consistently show that overweight or obese patients with heart failure or a myocardial infarction have a significantly lower mortality risk compared with those with normal weight.

Some studies have shown that in comparison with normal weight subjects, obese men with established CVD have an increased risk of CVD events and death, while the risk is reduced in obese women. These findings may potentially explain some of the variation in the outcomes in previous studies reporting on the obesity paradox [6].

The underlying cause of the obesity paradox is still unclear. The paradox may be explained by the observation that patients with overweight or obesity develop CVD earlier in their lifetime or are tested earlier for CVD than patients with normal weight, resulting in earlier diagnoses and treatment and confounding differences in outcomes. Also, the so-called cardiac cachexia can largely explain the paradox in heart failure because wasting has been demonstrated as a potent, independent predictor of outcome in non-edematous patients [7].

In addition, differences in cardiorespiratory fitness may explain more favorable CVD outcomes regardless of BMI. Different potential explanations behind the paradoxical findings have been postulated and highlight the inherent limitations of assessing adiposity by BMI alone. In fact, in studies categorizing patients based on BMI, the possibility exists that groups exhibiting benefit may have a relative healthier fat distribution and higher muscle mass. This hypothesis is supported by the observation that the obesity paradox is not observed if the presence of adiposity is evaluated by measuring WHR [6].

2.2 Markers of Pre-clinical CVD in Women with Overweight, Obesity, and Central Obesity

Both cross-sectional studies and prospective studies have shown a strong relationship between excessive body fat and premature CV morbidity and mortality. In the 1980s, the Framingham Heart Study showed that the degree of overweight was an important predictor of CVD. The association of CVD with obesity is particularly relevant in women.

Table 1 Relative risk of CVD events in obese men and women and contribution of the CV Risk factors to the excess risk

	CVD events	CV risk factors		
		Type 2 diabetes	Hypertension	Dyslipidemia
Men	⇧	⇧	⇧	⇧
Women	⇧⇧	⇧⇧	⇧⇧	⇧⇧

CVD is the leading cause of death for women in developed countries and in most of the developing ones (Table 1). Data from the Framingham Heart Study shows that obesity increases the risk of coronary artery disease by 64% in women compared with 46% in men [8]. Nondiabetic premenopausal women are protected against CVD when compared with age-matched men. However, women with obesity and insulin resistance exhibit worsened CV outcomes [2]. One aspect that needs attention is the CV profile of women at higher risk of major adverse CVD events.

In the FATCOR study, most overweight and obese participants presented potent markers of what is called preclinical CVD [9], which contributes to the impaired prognosis observed in obese women. In this study women had a higher prevalence of left atrial dilatation than men (74% vs. 56%, $p < 0.001$), while men had a higher prevalence of abnormal left ventricular geometry (30% vs. 21%, $p = 0.011$). In multivariate logistic regression analysis, female sex was associated with a twofold higher risk of subclinical cardiac disease, in particular left atrial dilatation (confidence interval [CI] 1.67–3.49, $p < 0.001$) after adjusting for confounders [10]. Obesity is also a critical condition for development of LV hypertrophy, even in the context of arterial hypertension. In the Campania Salute Network, an Italian registry for arterial hypertension, probability of LV hypertrophy increased more than fivefold in the presence of obesity, by >50% in women, and greater than twofold with diabetes [11]. In the Strong Heart Study, obesity influences LV geometry substantially more in women than in men, possibly due to biological factors specifically associated with female adiposity, namely adipose absolute mass and body fat distribution [12].

Although BMI is routinely used in both clinical and research settings to stratify at-risk individuals, it does not accurately reflect the actual location of excess adiposity. Strong evidence indicates that distribution of adiposity influences CV morbidity [2, 13] especially in women, explaining why waist-hip ratio (WHR) works better than BMI, as the expression of abdominal (visceral) fat, normalized by hip (subcutaneous) fat for prediction of cardio-metabolic diseases. Therefore, the prevalence of at-risk women in relation to their adiposity is likely more elevated than what is currently recognized by measuring BMI alone [2].

In addition to considerations on body fat distribution, also general adiposity is very different in men and women (Fig. 2). At a given BMI, the amount of fat-free mass is substantially higher in men than in women, implying that the fat component is much higher in women.

Thus, compared to men, as BMI increases women tend to become relatively sarcopenic [14]. In a recent study using a conservative and relatively method-independent definition of sarcopenia, an obesity phenotype, characterized by relative fat-free mass deficiency (RFFMD), could be identified [15], which was typical in the feminine obesity (90%). Despite this relative deficiency, those women exhibited increased LV chamber dimension and mass (even normalized for fat-free mass) and signs of hemodynamic volume overload. In this context, the condition of RFFMD was a potent determinant of the variance of LV mass index, independent of aging, blood pressure, history of hypertension, anthropometric measures of adiposity, diabetes, and renal function. We can speculate that part of the estimated echocardiographic LV mass is just fat infiltrated into the myocardium, as well documented also in advanced imaging studies [16].

2.3 Causative CV Risk Factors in Women with Overweight, Obesity, and Central Obesity

Because the excessive increase in fat-mass, obesity causes alterations in the profile of hormones secreted by adipose tissue (adipokines).

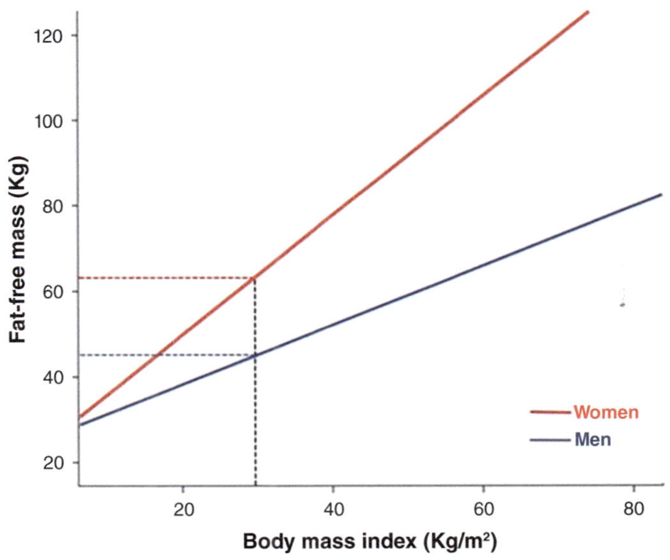

Fig. 2 Relationship between body mass index and fat free mass by bioimpedance analysis in men and women from the Strong Heart Study cohort. At the current cutoff for obesity (30 kg/m^2), there are bear 20 kg fat-free mass difference between men and women, indicating substantial difference in body composition that increases with increasing BMI

Moreover, obesity is associated with an increase in adipocyte secretion of other chemokines, which promote macrophage infiltration and activation, and negatively impact insulin sensitivity (the so-called *Inflammation Hypothesis*) [17]. Women are known to have higher levels of inflammatory markers, which is well fitting with their specific body composition: data from the Dallas Heart Study show that women have significantly higher levels of CRP compared with men (3.3 vs. 1.8 mg/l), and that the elevation in CRP associated with obesity is greater for women than for men [18]. However, the role of CRP as a causative agent of the CV complications of obesity in women is unclear [2], despite some evidence that CRP and fibrinogen increase risk of incident heart failure (HF), especially when associated with metabolic syndrome in a population with high prevalence of obesity [19].

People with higher BMI have a greater risk of HF occurrence in a lifetime also due to association with hypertension, insulin resistance and dyslipidemia. When obesity is combined with female sex, HF with preserved ejection fraction (HFpEF) is more often present. Women demonstrate a stronger correlation than men of obesity associated cardiometabolic abnormalities, such as insulin resistance, with incident HFpEF [20]. Clinical manifestations of HF in obese women also differ from obese men, since they present a worse quality of life due to greater fatigue, dyspnea, and decreased exercise capacity compared with their male counterparts. Women have been underrepresented in earlier clinical trials concerning HF. These observations warrant the need to establish female-specific outlines in the approach, diagnosis, and treatment of HF [2].

The classical protection against CVD in premenopausal lean women has been attributed to the effects of oestrogen on the vasculature. However, this protection declines when conditions such as obesity, insulin resistance, and type 2 diabetes are concurrently present and, in particular, the classical beneficial effects of oestrogens are lost in conditions of overnutrition. Specifically, the abrogation of the protective vascular effects of oestrogen in the setting of obesity and insulin resistance appears to be mediated by activation of sodium channels in endothelial cells [21].

Increased adiposity is also characterized by elevated aldosterone levels and enhanced activation of mineral-corticoids. Both preclinical and clinical investigations support a greater role for these hormones in the etiology of vascular disease in insulin resistant overweight women [22].

Excessive fat, especially if visceral, is associated with many important CV risk factors, such as insulin resistance and prediabetes, hypertriglyceridemia, small LDL particles, low HDL levels, in addition to hypertension and low-grade inflammation. Association of a more atherogenic profile with arterial hypertension explains the excess of major adverse CVD events (MACE) in individuals with visceral obesity, regardless of their weight [23]. Thus, obesity should be regarded not as a risk factor in the traditional sense, but rather as a CV risk booster, by the effect, both direct and indirect, on CVD risk. A substantial part of CVD risk is in fact mediated by the three major CV risk factors, often coexisting in obese individuals: diabetes, hypertension, and hyperlipidemia (Table 1).

Coexistence of central obesity with hyperglycemia, insulin resistance, hypertension, dyslipidemia represents a complex clinical presentation, called metabolic syndrome [8], which is associated with incident CVD in the presence or absence of type 2 diabetes [24].

Taken altogether, these findings bring the conclusion that metabolic syndrome might be more harmful in women than in men, a suggestion that seems recently supported by an Iranian study [25]. The importance of CV risk factors in modulating the increased CVD risk observed in women is also supported by findings in a population-based cohort study, from UK Biobank: the excess CVD risk attenuated and become more similar between men and women after adjusting for clinical and lifestyle factors particularly obesity and antihypertensive or statin use [26]. Most probably the sex-differences suggested on epidemiological scale are mainly the consequence of differently prevalent components of the syndrome, while differences disappear when analyses are performed separately in men and women [27].

Interestingly, sex-related differences in the prescription of medications and adherence to treatment also have been postulated to contribute to this sex-related divergent effect [28].

2.3.1 Overweight, Obesity, and Diabetes

Obesity is strictly related with type 2 diabetes mellitus. Longitudinal studies have demonstrated that higher BMI is a strong predictor of development of type 2 diabetes, with a linear increase in diabetes risk across the whole spectrum of BMI, but highest in subjects with BMI >30 kg/m^2. Compared with adult onset, men who experienced adolescent obesity are more likely to develop diabetes during young adulthood (Fig. 3) [29].

Type 2 diabetes is strongly associated with increased adiposity and sex-related differences have been identified in the relationships among elevated BMI, type 2 diabetes, and CVD. Compared with men, women with type 2 diabetes are more often obese, have higher cen-

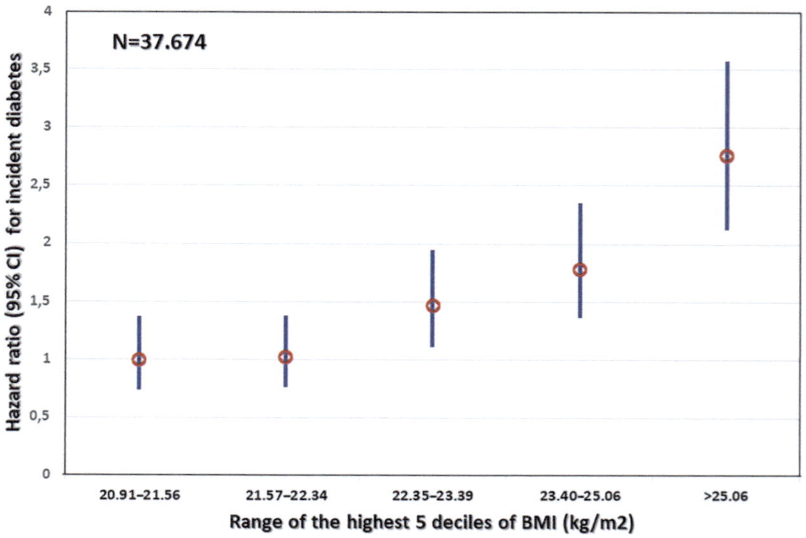

Fig. 3 Incident diabetes in relation to deciles of BMI in 37,674 apparently healthy young men. Hazard of diabetes in the highest 5 deciles of BMI, adjusted for age, family history of diabetes, blood pressure, physical activity, fasting glucose and triglycerides levels

tral adiposity indices, and more severe CV risk profile, compared to males, also including higher prevalence of hypertension [30]. For a given BMI, abdominal fat distribution increases the risk of metabolic abnormalities, and, in particular of type 2 diabetes. Prospective studies have shown that measures of central adiposity, namely waist circumference, are better predictors of risk of developing diabetes than most of the other measures of adiposity [2].

A possible mechanism underlying the increased burden of CVD among diabetic women is represented by the clustering of adiposity, elevated triglycerides, and the influence of sex hormones. Women accumulate greater fat mass before developing type 2 diabetes in comparison to men and this can potentially result in more frequent cardiometabolic alterations, endothelial dysfunction, and hypercoagulability.

2.3.2 Overweight, Obesity and Hypertension

Obesity is recognized as one of the most important risk factors for the development of hypertension. The relation between adiposity and blood pressure seems to be linear. Obese individuals show higher levels of office as well as ambulatory blood pressure. Higher blood pressure values in obese than in non-obese individuals are observed in the normotensive range also in children and adolescents [31]. In the Framingham Heart Study, the prevalence of hypertension in obese individuals was twice compared to normal weight subjects. This relationship was observed in both sexes, in all age groups, and in different ethnic groups. Obesity is a modifiable risk condition that is clearly associated with hypertension similarly in both men and women. An analysis of the Framingham cohort showed that the attributable risk for hypertension related to overweight (BMI $\geq$25 kg/m^2) was 26% in men and 28% in women [8], a finding that was further confirmed in other population studies.

However, women are relatively protected from hypertension until menopause, a phenomenon mainly related to the vasodilatory and anti-inflammatory effects of oestrogens, which also improve insulin sensitivity. Also, progesterone might concur to this protective effect, through its natriuretic effect and vascular protection [32]. However, exogenous oestrogen therapy in post menopause does not result in improved blood pressure (BP) control and exogenous progesterone has been associated with hypertension (possibly due to androgenic activity). Obesity partially offsets oestrogen benefits, since BMI and age of onset of hypertension are negatively related [2].

It should also be considered that BP-attributable risk for acute coronary syndromes and HF increases at a lower level of BP in women than in men, suggesting that the definition of arterial hypertension should be reconsidered especially in the setting of high CV risk. Even high normal BP (130–139/80–89 mmHg) is associated with an up to twofold higher risk of CVD events during midlife in women, but not in men [33]. In addition, using guidelines cutoffs for arterial hypertension in either sex, women have more LV hypertrophy than men and, in a large Italian registry of hypertensive patients, the presence of LV hypertrophy offsets the sex-difference in the risk of incident MACE [34].

2.3.3 Overweight, Obesity and Dyslipidemia

The primary dyslipidemia related to obesity is characterized by increased triglycerides, decreased HDL levels, and abnormal LDL composition. The pathogenesis of the dyslipidemia of obesity seems to be closely related to insulin resistance. The dyslipidemia associated with obesity certainty plays a major role in the development of atherosclerosis and CVD in women. All components of dyslipidemia, including higher triglycerides, decreased HDL levels, and increased small, dense LDL particles, have been shown to be atherogenic. Obesity in women is also associated with decreased high-density lipoprotein (HDL) cholesterol. An average difference in 10 mg/dl in HDL has been found between normal weight and obese women [35].

The effects of obesity on low-density lipoprotein (LDL) concentrations are less consistent, whereas several studies have demonstrated that obesity is associated with a change in LDL composition: LDL particles are smaller and more dense, and therefore more atherogenic. This is particularly relevant in obese women with increased waist circumference [35].

3 Clinical Practice

3.1 Clinical Evaluation of Women with Obesity

We have already underlined that an appropriate clinical evaluation of obese women cannot be limited to measure BMI, but also the WHR and waist circumference should be recorded. Body composition with reliable methods like the dual-energy X-ray absorptiometry (DXA), if available, or bioelectrical impedance analysis (BIA) may be useful. Other evaluations include accurate dietary assessment and physical activity record, as well as measurements of cardiometabolic risk factors [36]. However, to have a more precise evaluation of the context and the severity of the obese condition, multiple biological, clinical, psychological and sociological parameters should be acquired. This is important not only to establish the disease-associated risk, but also to choose the most appropriate treatment strategy. To this aim, some staging criteria have been developed which allow a comprehensive assessment of the severity of the disease condition, over and above the degree of weight excess (Table 2).

In this context, the Kings Obesity Staging Criteria (Table 2) was designed to allow a practical and simplified assessment of obesity-related complications and risk of mortality to minimize inter-operator variability. It grades 12 aspects of obesity-related morbidity. For each domain, a person's health is assigned a score of 0 (normal health), 1 (at risk), 2 (established disease) or 3 (advanced disease). This staging system uses quantifiable measures wherever possible, to reduce the bias of subjective measures. A benefit of the King's Criteria is that separate scores can

Table 2 Clinical evaluation of overweight women in relation to the global health risk

Criteria	Stage 0	Stage 1	Stage 2	Stage 3
Airway sleep	Normal	Snoring	Apnea require continuous positive airway pressure (CPAP)	Cor pulmonale
BMI (kg/m^2)	<30	30–35	35–50	>50
Cardiovascular	<25% risk	>25% risk	Heart disease	Heart failure
Diabetes	Normal	Impaired glucose regulation	Type 2 diabetes	Uncontrolled type 2 diabetes
Economic	Normal	Suffered discrimination	Unemployed due to obesity	Requires financial support
Functional	Can manage 3 flights of stairs	Manage 1 or 2 flights of stairs	Manage <1 flight of stairs or requires walking aids	Housebound
Gonadal	Normal	Irregular periods	Polycystic ovary syndrome (PCOS)	Infertility
Health status	Normal	Low mood or quality of life	Moderate depression or poor quality of life	Severe depression
Image	Normal	Does not like looking in mirror	Avoid mirrors/body image dysphoria	Severe eating disorder
Gastroesophageal junction	Normal	Heartburn	Esophagitis	Barrett esophagus
Kidney	Normal	Proteinuria	GFR <60 mL/min	GFR <30 mL/min
Liver	Normal	Raised liver function tests/non-alcoholic fatty liver disease (NAFLD)	Non-alcoholic steatohepatitis (NASH)	Liver failure

be tracked for each domain, which allows for a more holistic and specific assessment of treatment [37].

The Edmonton Obesity Staging System (EOSS) classifies the impact of obesity on an individual into five stages of severity. Stage 0 represents the obese phenotype with no co-morbidities. With increasing severity of the obesity condition, the staging score rises up to 4, which characterizes a condition for which surgical interventions are contraindicated. This staging system, in contrast with the Kings classification, is particularly focused to the choice of an appropriate treatment strategy rather than on a prognostic evaluation [38].

3.2 Benefits of Weight Reduction on CVD Events in Overweight Women

Since overweight and obesity are associated with decreased lifespan, increased prevalence of CV risk factors and CVD events, weight loss might be expected to benefit both long-term survival and to have many intermediate effects on CV risk factors. The relationship between weight loss and mortality is debated, with observational studies suggesting no change, or reduced mortality subsequent to weight loss. This discrepancy concerning the effects of weight loss on mortality has been related particularly to inability of observational studies to distinguish intentional from unintentional weight loss. Thus, when unintentional, weight loss might be the consequence of conditions that lead to death rather than the cause of increased mortality.

The association between weight loss and increased mortality is more pronounced among men; in a recent study all-cause mortality was 8.4% among men keeping a consistent weight over a mean of 4.4 ± 1.7 years vs 30.1% among those decreasing weight by more than 10%; for women, the equivalent mortality rates were 5.5% and 12.6%, respectively [39]. The observation that weight loss was associated with a lower mortality among women than among men may be the result of the different body composition. For men, a higher proportion of body mass is represented by muscle and bone mass, whereas for women, a higher proportion of body mass is fat. If weight loss in men is predominantly loss of muscle mass and bone mass, it could explain their higher mortality when loosing weight. Thus, when unintentional, weight loss might be the consequence of conditions that lead to death rather than the cause of increased mortality. Typical example is cardiac cachexia occurring in the end-stage HF [7]

The therapeutic approaches used for the treatment of obesity are lifestyle changes (diet and physical activity), drug treatment and bariatric surgery (Table 3).

Table 3 Efficacy of different treatment strategies on weight reduction in overweight men and women

	Lifestyle	GLP1 RA	Metabolic surgery
Men	++	++	+++++
Women	+	+++	+++++

GLP1 RA glucagon like peptide receptor agonist

3.2.1 Lifestyle

Weight loss obtained with lifestyle interventions has been shown to be effective in reducing the incidence of diabetes and other CV risk factors. A modest decrease (5–10%) in body weight can increase insulin sensitivity and, therefore, improve the metabolic derangements and CV risk factors clustering insulin resistance. Comparing the difference in absolute weight loss in men and women for diet-only, exercise-only or combined diet and exercise interventions, absolute weight loss is significantly greater in men on diet-only or diet plus exercise interventions than in women. However, this sex-specific effect might be at least partially due to some regression toward the mean rather than specific lifestyle interventions (men exhibit greater baseline weight than women). In most studies, women had clinically significant weight loss; this indicates that lifestyle interventions including dietary and exercise prescription are effective for both men and women (Table 3) [40]. Unfortunately, there are no data on possible differences between males and females on the effects of weight reducing diets on CVD risk.

There are indications that men lose more weight, fat mass, and lean mass on low carbohydrate diets, compared to low fat diets, whereas women achieved similar weight loss on both types of diet. In addition, within the low carbohydrate group, men lost significantly more weight than women, which was not true for the low-fat diet [41].

At this time, there is little evidence that men and women should adopt different weight loss strategies and the differences in weight loss seen in the short term may have little significance in the long run. To facilitate weight loss in overweight and obese men and women, health professionals need to focus on the inclusion of both diet and exercise in weight loss attempts and need to provide support for individuals to assist with implementation of programs which has the potential to increase long-term success.

3.2.2 Drug Treatment

The addition of pharmacotherapy produces greater weight loss and weight-loss maintenance compared with lifestyle therapy alone. The use of semaglutide, liraglutide, phentermine-topiramate ER, and naltrexone-bupropion ER (based on moderate certainty evidence), and phentermine and diethylpropion (based on low certainty evidence), are usually recommended for long-term management of overweight and obesity in patients with weight related complications not achieving an adequate weight loss with lifestyle alone [42].

The most effective weight reducing drugs are glucagon like peptide-1 receptor agonist (GLP-1 RA) which can induce weight loss greater than 10% in most individuals; cumulative evidence suggests that weight reduction due to GLP-1 RAs is more pronounced in females (Table 3) This disproportionate response of women was evident in a cohort study in which after a 12-month period of exenatide treatment, 33% of women achieved weight loss targets compared to 17% of men. Studies that used different molecules of the class, such as dulaglutide and liraglutide, obtained similar findings [43]. Although several studies have indicated that sex may represent a predictor of HbA_{1c} reduction after the initiation of treatment, other studies have not confirmed this finding, and therefore a definitive conclusion has not yet been drawn on this matter.

In studies on the efficacy of GLP-1 RA on CV outcomes, a remarkable reduction in MACE has been observed in both sexes. This was further supported by a meta-analysis demonstrating that the effect of GLP-1 RA on MACE was similar between men and women ($p = 0.375$) [44]. While it is evident that the male and female responses to GLP-1 RAs differ at some level with respect to the achievement of weight loss such a difference could be partly attributed to sex specific pharmacodynamics of GLP-1 RA: women have lower body mass and therefore are exposed to relatively higher drug levels than men. Specific hormonal profiles can play a role in this dissimilarity. Eventually the greater adiposity of women may favor the efficacy of this class of drugs. Unfortunately, at this time, clinical trials do not always provide sufficient sex-specific data, which is of paramount importance to shed more light on the sex-specificity of the GLP-1 RA action. Sex-disaggregated data should always be provided in clinical trials on this topic, to allow the achievement of more accurate evidence-based conclusions and optimize the management of obesity, particularly in type 2 diabetic patients [43].

For the choice of the most appropriate weight reducing drug, risk of adverse effects should always be considered. A recent study in 16 million patients reported that the use of GLP-1 RA for weight loss was associated with an increased risk of pancreatitis, gastroparesis, and bowel obstruction in comparison with the use of bupropion-naltrexone [45]. However, the observational nature of this study does not allow to draw definite conclusions.

3.2.3 Bariatric Surgery

Bariatric surgery has a beneficial impact on several medical comorbidities and is considered the only medical intervention offering a clinically relevant weight loss and health benefits for morbid obesity in the long-term. Bariatric surgery is associated with remission of type 2 diabetes, remission of arterial hypertension, reduced cancer incidence, and improved all-cause mortality. Emerging data also suggest a role in the reduction of CVD risk.

Several retrospective studies have consistently reported improved long-term survival in bariatric surgery populations when compared to severely obese control groups. The reduced mortality seems to be due mainly to CVD and diabetes. In the Swedish Obese Subjects (SOS) Study, focused primarily on long-term mortality following bariatric surgery, involving 4047 obese participants, 2010 who had bariatric surgery (vertical banded gastroplasty, gastric banding, and gastric bypass) and 2037 matched controls who received conventional weight loss therapy. After 10 years from randomization, the surgical group had greater remission of diabetes, hypertriglyceridemia, low levels of HDL cholesterol, and hypertension when compared to the control group. Over a 15-year follow-up, bariatric surgery was associated with a reduction in the number of CV deaths and first time CVD events (fatal and nonfatal) after controlling for the cardiometabolic risk profile at baseline. Compared with controls the adjusted hazard ratio of bariatric surgery for total CVD events was 0.67 (95% CI 0.54–0.83, $p < 0.001$); for fatal CVD events, the adjusted hazard ratio was 0.47 (95% CI 0.29–0.76, $p < 0.02$) [46]. A rapid improvement of markers of preclinical CVD has also been reported, as a proxy of improved CVD risk burden [47].

Matched-pair cohort analysis demonstrated that bariatric surgery results in comparable short- and mid-term efficacy in men and women and is associated with similar rates and severity of postoperative complications between sexes, similar total weight loss, BMI and percentage of excess BMI reduction at 12, 24, and 36 months postoperatively in either sex, with no difference in remission of diabetes mellitus, hypertension and dyslipidemia at 12 months (Table 3) [48].

4 Conclusions

Obesity is associated with decreased lifespan in both men and women and causes biological changes that reduce or even eliminate the relative protection in CVD risk that women exhibit at every age. Weight loss is, therefore, expected to restore their relative CV protection, to improve their long-term survival and to have beneficial effects on their CVD risk. Lifestyle modifications include modest weight loss and moderate-intensity physical activity. A low-fat (low saturated fat), low-sugar diet rich in fruit and vegetables, as well as legumes and whole grains, should be advised for its beneficial impact on weight and CVD risk. The use of weight reducing drugs should be considered within a global strategy to treat obesity and its associated diseases; it seems very effective but long-term clinical data are so far scanty. Bariatric surgery represents an effective treatment in cases of severe (morbid) obesity. Prevention of overweight and obesity at the population level will probably play a major role in fighting against the present obesity epidemic. Combining different intervention strategies is probably the best choice for maximizing the effects and minimizing the costs.

Key Issues

- Women are more affected by the obesity epidemic. The greater prevalence of obesity in women becomes evident in adulthood and peaks at 60–64 years of age
- Obesity and insulin resistance in women is associated with worsened cardiovascular prognosis
- Weight reducing regimens promote beneficial effects on CV risk factors and improved survival in obese women
- Obesity therapy includes lifestyle changes, drug treatment and bariatric surgery
- GLP-1 receptor agonists are more effective weight reducing drugs in women, and a >10% weight loss is achieved in most individuals
- Bariatric surgery has comparable short- and midterm efficacy in women and men

Questions and Answers

1. What is the global prevalence of a BMI ≥25 kg/m^2 in women?
   (A) Less than 20%
   (B) Between 20 and 30%
   (C) Between 30 and 40%
   (D) More than 40%
   The correct answer is C

2. What is the correct statement about the risk of CVD in obese women?
   (A) Generally lower than in men
   (B) Lower than in men only after the menopause
   (C) Generally higher than in men
   (D) Higher than in men only after the menopause
   The correct answer is D
3. At a similar level of BMI, the amount of fat free mass in women is
   (A) Lower than in men
   (B) Higher than in men
   (C) Roughly the same as in men
   (D) Roughly the same as in men only if BMI >30 kg/m^2
   The correct answer is A
4. The impact of treatment with a GLP-1 receptor agonist on weight reduction in overweight women is
   (A) Higher than in men but only with semaglutide
   (B) Higher than in men with all GLP-1 receptor agonists
   (C) Lower than in men
   (D) Roughly the same as in men
   The correct answer is B
5. The efficacy of bariatric surgery on weight reduction in obese women is
   (A) Higher than in men
   (B) Lower than in men
   (C) Roughly the same as in men
   (D) Roughly the same as in men but only with gastric by-pass
   The correct answer is C

References

1. GBD 2015 Obesity Collaborators. Health effects of overweight and obesity in 195 countries over 25 years. N Engl J Med. 2017;377:13–27. https://doi.org/10.1056/NEJMoa1614362.
2. Manrique-Acevedo C, Chinnakotla B, Padilla J, Martinez-Lemus LA, Gozal D. Obesity and cardiovascular disease in women. Int J Obes. 2020;44:1210–26. https://doi.org/10.1038/s41366-020-0548-0.
3. World Health Organization. Regional Office for Europe. WHO European Regional Obesity: Report 2022. n.d.
4. Khan I, Chong M, Le A, Mohammadi-Shemirani P, Morton R, Brinza C, et al. Surrogate adiposity markers and mortality. JAMA Netw Open. 2023;6:e2334836. https://doi.org/10.1001/jamanetworkopen.2023.34836.
5. Di Angelantonio E, Bhupathiraju SN, Wormser D, Gao P, Kaptoge S, de Gonzalez AB, et al. Body-mass index and all-cause mortality: individual-participant-data meta-analysis of 239 prospective studies in four continents. Lancet. 2016;388:776–86. https://doi.org/10.1016/S0140-6736(16)30175-1.
6. Powell-Wiley TM, Poirier P, Burke LE, Després JP, Gordon-Larsen P, Lavie CJ, et al. Obesity and cardiovascular disease a scientific statement from the American Heart Association. Circulation. 2021;143:e984–e1010. https://doi.org/10.1161/CIR.0000000000000973.
7. Anker SD, Ponikowski P, Varney S, Chua TP, Clark AL, Webb-Peploe KM, et al. Wasting as independent risk factor for mortality in chronic heart failure. n.d.
8. Turpie AGG, Bauer KA, Eriksson BI, Lassen MR. Overweight and obesity as determinants of cardiovascular risk: the Framingham experience. Arch Intern Med. 2002;162:1867. https://doi.org/10.1001/archinte.162.16.1867.
9. Devereux RB, Alderman MH. Role of preclinical cardiovascular disease in the evolution from risk factor exposure to development of morbid events. n.d.
10. Halland H, Lønnebakken MT, Pristaj N, Saeed S, Midtbø H, Einarsen E, et al. Sex differences in subclinical cardiac disease in overweight and obesity (the FATCOR study). Nutr Metab Cardiovasc Dis. 2018;28:1054–60. https://doi.org/10.1016/j.numecd.2018.06.014.
11. Mancusi C, Gerdts E, Losi MA, D'Amato A, Manzi MV, Canciello G, et al. Differential effect of obesity on prevalence of cardiac and carotid target organ damage in hypertension (the Campania Salute Network). Int J Cardiol. 2017;244:260–4. https://doi.org/10.1016/j.ijcard.2017.06.045.
12. de Simone G, Devereux RB, Chinali M, Roman MJ, Barac A, Panza JA, et al. Sex differences in obesity-related changes in left ventricular morphology: The Strong Heart Study. J Hypertens. 2011;29:1431–8. https://doi.org/10.1097/HJH.0b013e328347a093.
13. Ross R, Neeland IJ, Yamashita S, Shai I, Seidell J, Magni P, et al. Waist circumference as a vital sign in clinical practice: a Consensus Statement from the IAS and ICCR Working Group on Visceral Obesity. Nat Rev Endocrinol. 2020;16:177–89. https://doi.org/10.1038/s41574-019-0310-7.
14. Roubenoff R. Sarcopenic obesity: the confluence of two epidemics. Obes Res. 2004;12:887–8. https://doi.org/10.1038/oby.2004.107.
15. de Simone G, Pasanisi F, Ferrara AL, Roman MJ, Lee ET, Contaldo F, et al. Relative fat-free mass deficiency and left ventricular adaptation to obesity: The Strong Heart Study. Int J Cardiol. 2013;168:729–33. https://doi.org/10.1016/j.ijcard.2012.09.055.
16. Kimura F, Matsuo Y, Nakajima T, Nishikawa T, Kawamura S, Sannohe S, et al. Myocardial fat at car-

diac imaging: how can we differentiate pathologic from physiologic fatty infiltration? Radiographics. 2010;30:1587–602. https://doi.org/10.1148/rg.306105519.
17. Wu H, Ballantyne CM. Metabolic inflammation and insulin resistance in obesity. Circ Res. 2020;126:1549–64. https://doi.org/10.1161/CIRCRESAHA.119.315896.
18. Gupta NK, De Lemos JA, Ayers CR, Abdullah SM, McGuire DK, Khera A. The relationship between C-reactive protein and atherosclerosis differs on the basis of body mass index: the Dallas heart study. J Am Coll Cardiol. 2012;60:1148–55. https://doi.org/10.1016/j.jacc.2012.04.050.
19. Barac A, Wang H, Shara NM, de Simone G, Carter EA, Umans JG, et al. Markers of inflammation, metabolic risk factors, and incident heart failure in American Indians: The strong heart study. J Clin Hypertens. 2012;14:13–9. https://doi.org/10.1111/j.1751-7176.2011.00560.x.
20. Savji N, Meijers WC, Bartz TM, Bhambhani V, Cushman M, Nayor M, et al. The association of obesity and cardiometabolic traits with incident HFpEF and HFrEF. JACC Heart Fail. 2018;6:701–9. https://doi.org/10.1016/j.jchf.2018.05.018.
21. Padilla J, Woodford ML, Lastra-Gonzalez G, Martinez-Diaz V, Fujie S, Yang Y, et al. Sexual dimorphism in obesity-associated endothelial ENaC activity and stiffening in mice. Endocrinology. 2019;160:2918–28. https://doi.org/10.1210/en.2019-00483.
22. Shukri MZ, Tan JW, Manosroi W, Pojoga LH, Rivera A, Williams JS, et al. Biological sex modulates the adrenal and blood pressure responses to angiotensin II. Hypertension. 2018;71:11087. https://doi.org/10.1161/HYPERTENSIONAHA.117.11087.
23. Abraham TM, Pedley A, Massaro JM, Hoffmann U, Fox CS. Association between visceral and subcutaneous adipose depots and incident cardiovascular disease risk factors. Circulation. 2015;132:1639–47. https://doi.org/10.1161/CIRCULATIONAHA.114.015000.
24. de Simone G, Devereux RB, Chinali M, Best LG, Lee ET, Galloway JM, et al. Prognostic impact of metabolic syndrome by different definitions in a population with high prevalence of obesity and diabetes: the strong heart study. Diabetes Care. 2007;30:1851–6. https://doi.org/10.2337/dc06-2152.
25. Ramezankhani A, Azizi F, Hadaegh F. Gender differences in changes in metabolic syndrome status and its components and risk of cardiovascular disease: a longitudinal cohort study. Cardiovasc Diabetol. 2022;21:227. https://doi.org/10.1186/s12933-022-01665-8.
26. Rentsch CT, Garfield V, Mathur R, Eastwood S V, Smeeth L, Chaturvedi N, et al. Sex-specific risks for cardiovascular disease across the glycaemic spectrum: a population-based cohort study using the UK Biobank. 2023.
27. Pradhan AD. Sex differences in the metabolic syndrome: implications for cardiovascular health in women. Clin Chem. 2014;60:202549. https://doi.org/10.1373/clinchem.2013.202549.
28. Lyon A, Jackson EA, Kalyani RR, Vaidya D, Kim C. Sex-specific differential in risk of diabetes-related macrovascular outcomes. Curr Diab Rep. 2015;15:85. https://doi.org/10.1007/s11892-015-0662-x.
29. Tirosh A, Shai I, Afek A, Dubnov-Raz G, Ayalon N, Gordon B, et al. Adolescent BMI trajectory and risk of diabetes versus coronary disease. N Engl J Med. 2011;364:1315–25. https://doi.org/10.1056/nejmoa1006992.
30. Du T, Fernandez C, Barshop R, Guo Y, Krousel-Wood M, Chen W, et al. Sex differences in cardiovascular risk profile from childhood to midlife between individuals who did and did not develop diabetes at follow-up: The Bogalusa Heart Study. Diabetes Care. 2019;42:66–74. https://doi.org/10.2337/dc18-2029.
31. Chinali M, de Simone G, Roman MJ, Lee ET, Best LG, Howard BV, et al. Impact of obesity on cardiac geometry and function in a population of adolescents. The strong heart study. J Am Coll Cardiol. 2006;47:2267–73. https://doi.org/10.1016/j.jacc.2006.03.004.
32. Regitz-Zagrosek V, Gebhard C. Gender medicine: effects of sex and gender on cardiovascular disease manifestation and outcomes. Nat Rev Cardiol. 2023;20(4):236–47. https://doi.org/10.1038/s41569-022-00797-4.
33. Gerdts E, de Simone G. Hypertension in women: should there be a sex-specific threshold? Eur Cardiol Rev. 2021;16:e38. https://doi.org/10.15420/ECR.2021.17.
34. Gerdts E, Izzo R, Mancusi C, Losi MA, Manzi MV, Canciello G, et al. Left ventricular hypertrophy offsets the sex difference in cardiovascular risk (the Campania Salute Network). Int J Cardiol. 2018;258:257–61. https://doi.org/10.1016/j.ijcard.2017.12.086.
35. Gerdts E, Regitz-Zagrosek V. Sex differences in cardiometabolic disorders. Nat Med. 2019;25:1657–66. https://doi.org/10.1038/s41591-019-0643-8.
36. Garvey WT, Mechanick JI, Brett EM, Garber AJ, Hurley DL, Jastreboff AM, et al. American association of clinical endocrinologists and American college of endocrinology comprehensive clinical practice guidelines for medical care of patients with obesity. Endocr Pract. 2016;22:1–203. https://doi.org/10.4158/EP161365.GL.
37. Whyte MB, Velusamy S, Aylwin SJB. Disease severity and staging of obesity: a rational approach to patient selection. Curr Atheroscler Rep. 2014;16:456. https://doi.org/10.1007/s11883-014-0456-7.
38. Kuk JL, Ardern CI, Church TS, Sharma AM, Padwal R, Sui X, et al. Edmonton obesity staging system: association with weight history and mortality risk. Appl Physiol Nutr Metab. 2011;36:570–6. https://doi.org/10.1139/h11-058.
39. Hussain SM, Newman AB, Beilin LJ, Tonkin AM, Woods RL, Neumann JT, et al. Associations of

change in body size with all-cause and cause-specific mortality among healthy older adults. JAMA Netw Open. 2023;6:e237482. https://doi.org/10.1001/jamanetworkopen.2023.7482.
40. Williams RL, Wood LG, Collins CE, Callister R. Effectiveness of weight loss interventions - is there a difference between men and women: a systematic review. Obes Rev. 2015;16:88–98. https://doi.org/10.1111/obr.12241.
41. Aronica L, Rigdon J, Offringa LC, Stefanick ML, Gardner CD. Examining differences between overweight women and men in 12-month weight loss study comparing healthy low-carbohydrate vs. low-fat diets. Int J Obes. 2021;45:225–34. https://doi.org/10.1038/s41366-020-00708-y.
42. Grunvald E, Shah R, Hernaez R, Chandar AK, Pickett-Blakely O, Teigen LM, et al. AGA Clinical practice guideline on pharmacological interventions for adults with obesity. Gastroenterology. 2022;163(5):1198–225. https://doi.org/10.1053/j.gastro.2022.08.045.
43. Rentzeperi E, Pegiou S, Koufakis T, Grammatiki M, Kotsa K. Sex differences in response to treatment with glucagon-like peptide 1 receptor agonists: opportunities for a tailored approach to diabetes and obesity care. J Pers Med. 2022;12:30454. https://doi.org/10.3390/jpm12030454.
44. Raparelli V, Elharram M, Moura CS, Abrahamowicz M, Bernatsky S, Behlouli H, et al. Sex differences in cardiovascular effectiveness of newer glucose-lowering drugs added to metformin in type 2 diabetes mellitus. J Am Heart Assoc. 2020;9:e012940. https://doi.org/10.1161/JAHA.119.012940.
45. Sodhi M, Rezaeianzadeh R, Kezouh A, Etminan M. Risk of gastrointestinal adverse events associated with glucagon-like peptide-1 receptor agonists for weight loss. JAMA. 2023;330(18):1795–7. https://doi.org/10.1001/jama.2023.19574.
46. Sjöström L. Review of the key results from the Swedish Obese Subjects (SOS) trial - a prospective controlled intervention study of bariatric surgery. J Intern Med. 2013;273:219–34. https://doi.org/10.1111/joim.12012.
47. Damiano S, De Marco M, Del Genio F, Contaldo F, Gerdts E, De Simone G, et al. Effect of bariatric surgery on left ventricular geometry and function in severe obesity. Obes Res Clin Pract. 2012;6:175–262. https://doi.org/10.1016/j.orcp.2012.02.008.
48. Mousapour P, Tasdighi E, Khalaj A, Mahdavi M, Valizadeh M, Taheri H, et al. Sex disparity in laparoscopic bariatric surgery outcomes: a matched-pair cohort analysis. Sci Rep. 2021;11:12809. https://doi.org/10.1038/s41598-021-92254-4.

Tobacco Use and Cardiovascular Risk in Women

Maja-Lisa Løchen and Sweta Tiwari

Abstract

Smoking is a significant contributor to the incidence, mortality, and risk factors for cardiovascular disease (CVD) in women. Smoking is the most important preventable cause of CVD in women younger than 55 years, with sevenfold increased risk. Women are shown to be more at risk from long-term smoking than men. It is unclear if biological factors or differences in smoking behavior account for the sex differences. According to some authors, absorption, or pathophysiological effects of toxins from cigarette smoke might be greater in women. However, more research is needed into the mechanisms that contribute to this elevated risk and to the possible sex differences. A non-linear dose–response relationship exists between smoking and the risk of CVD and mortality. There is no safe lower limit for smoking and all forms, including occasional smoking, passive smoking, snuffing, and electronic cigarettes, are harmful. Quitting smoking is the most effective strategy for CVD prevention. Equal access to therapies based on recommendations and resources to aid in quitting smoking should be provided to both men and women and they should receive the same access to guideline-based treatments. In smokers, offering follow-up support, nicotine replacement therapy, varenicline, and bupropion individually or in combination should be considered. Smoking cessation may contribute to an increase in obesity in the population, but it is still advised to stop smoking regardless of weight gain because the advantages of quitting for CVD are not diminished by weight gain.

Keywords

Daily smoking · Occasional smoking
Passive smoking · Snuffing · Electronic cigarettes

M.-L. Løchen (✉) · S. Tiwari
Department of Clinical Medicine, UiT The Arctic University of Norway, Tromsø, Norway
e-mail: maja-lisa.lochen@uit.no; sweta.tiwari@uit.no

A. H.E.M. Maas, E. Gerdts (eds.), *Manual of Cardiovascular Disease in Women*,
https://doi.org/10.1007/978-3-031-65952-2_3

Test your learning and check your understanding of this book's contents: use the "Springer Nature Flashcards" app to access questions using ▶ https://sn.pub/51ny7m To use the app, please follow the instructions in chapter 1.

1 Introduction

Smoking is the second leading cause of disability adjusted life-years after high systolic blood pressure. Cigarette smoking is responsible for 50% of all preventable deaths in smokers, with cardiovascular disease (CVD) accounting for 50% of these deaths. A lifetime smoker has a 50% probability of dying from smoking, and on average loses 10 years of life. The CVD risk in smokers under 50 years is five-fold higher than in non-smokers. Long-term smoking is found to be more hazardous for women than men [1]. There is a significant socioeconomic gradient in smoking. About 26% of women with basic education are daily smokers compared to about 2% daily smokers among women with higher education [2].

2 Theory

2.1 Daily Smoking

Smoking is an essential determinant for CVD risk factors, incidence, and mortality in women (Fig. 1). Among women younger than 55 years, smoking is the single most important preventable cause of CVD, with sevenfold increased risk [3]. In younger ST-elevation myocardial infarction (STEMI) patients, one study found that smoking was the most prevalent modifiable risk factor. Smoking was five times more prevalent among 30–49-year-old patients with STEMI compared to patients 70 years and older and was more frequent among women; OR 9.88 (95% CI 6.94–14.08) compared to men; OR 3.78 (95% CI 3.12–4.58). In women under 50 years of age, smoking was reported in eight out of every 10 STEMI patients [4]. While smoking seems to be more harmful for young and middle-aged women compared to men, the gender contrast in risk is substantially reduced in smokers 75 years and above [5].

Smoking is an important risk factor for myocardial infarction (MI) and is more detrimental for women than men, as shown in many cohort studies [6, 7].When current smokers were compared to never smokers in 59 studies in a systematic review and meta-analysis with middle-aged and elderly women, the pooled relative risk for coronary heart disease (CHD) incidence was RR 3.12 (95% CI 2.15–4.52) for CHD incidence, 2.09 (95% CI 1.51–2.89) for stroke incidence and for CVD mortality the RR was 2.76 (95% CI 1.62–4.71) [8]. Daily smoking also doubles the risk of sudden cardiac death in women as shown in a systematic review and meta-analysis [9]. Smoking has an antiestrogenic effect, and low oestrogen levels could cause an adverse impact on lipid profile, with elevations in cholesterol and triglyceride levels and reductions in high-density lipoprotein cholesterol levels, leading to endothelium dysfunction and atherosclerotic plaque formation. Furthermore, studies have indicated that smoking could also trigger premature menopause which has been associated with increased risk of CHD. The risk of each of the three types of strokes has been shown to be higher among current female compared to male smokers in a meta-analysis, and the associations were dose dependent. The magnitude of smoking associated risk was greater for subarachnoid hemorrhage than for intracerebral hemorrhage and ischemic stroke [10].

Light or occasional smokers may think that this habit does not lead to any harm. However, for CHD and stroke, there exists no smoking level that is safe. A systematic review and meta-analysis which included 141 cohort studies worldwide showed that smoking only about one

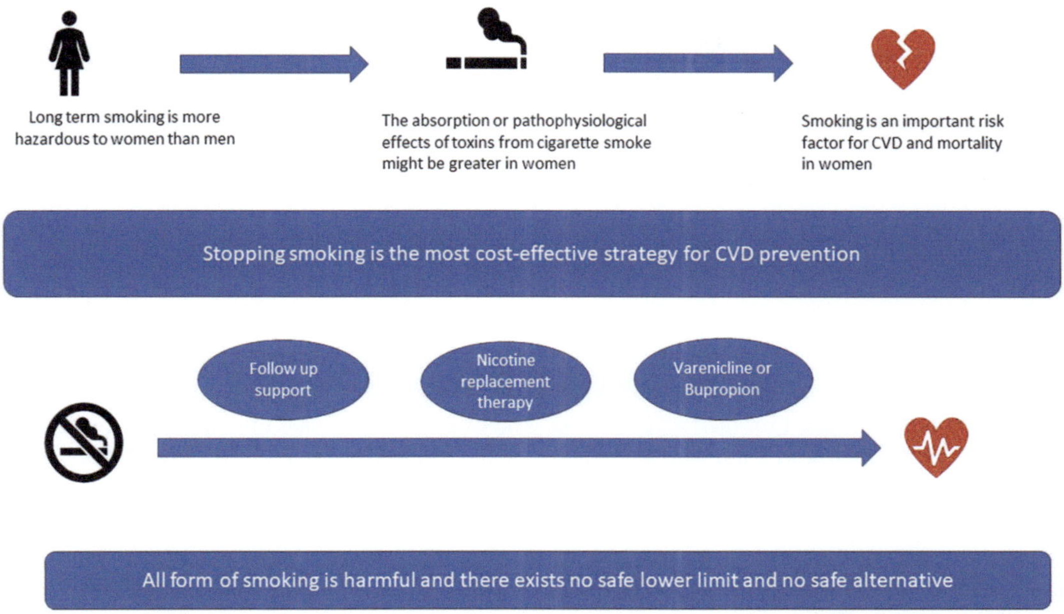

Fig. 1 Key issues for smoking cessation in women

to five cigarettes per day was associated with a risk of developing CHD and stroke that was much greater than expected and was about half that for those smoking 20 cigarettes per day. The relative risks of smoking were 25% higher for women than for men, independent of other risk factors. Men who smoke an average of one cigarette per day had a 48% and 25% greater risk of CHD and stroke, respectively compared to never smokers. In women, the estimates were higher: 57% for heart disease and 31% for stroke compared to never smokers [11]. Therefore, smokers should aim to quit smoking instead of cutting down to significantly reduce their risk of CVD (Fig. 1).

It is unclear if biological factors or differences in smoking behavior between men and women account for the sex difference in risk of CHD. Some authors speculate that the absorption or pathophysiological effects of toxins from cigarette smoke might be greater in women [12]. As populations that have so far been mostly unaffected by the smoking epidemic begin to smoke to an extent previously only seen in high-income nations, cigarette smoking will continue to be one of the leading causes of CHD globally. This is particularly true for young women in whom the popularity of smoking, particularly in some low-income and middle-income countries, seems to be on the rise. Tobacco-control programs should consider women, particularly in those countries where smoking among young women is increasing [13].

Reducing smoking use and inciting early cessation are crucial public health initiatives that should be tailored particularly for women's preferences, attitudes, and individual smoking patterns in order to avoid CVD and death [8]. Women and men should receive the same access to guideline based treatments and to resources to help them and stop smoking [7].

2.2 Occasional Smoking

In a large prospective cohort study, occasional smoking increased total mortality by 38% compared to never smokers. No sex difference was observed, and most deaths were due to cancer and AMI [14]. Another study showed that although the mortality risk for non-daily smokers were lower than for daily smokers, it was still substantial with about 55% increased risk for both sexes. Policies should be specifically directed at this growing group of occasional smokers [15].

2.3 Passive Smoking

Passive smoking is a risk factor for CHD on its own, but whereas the effect for men seemed to be explained by their own active smoking, the effect in females remained statistically significant even after adjusting for own active smoking. Approximately 20% of the incident cases of AMI in women could be attributed to passive smoking as shown in a large, prospective cohort study. This indicates a stronger effect for passive smoking in women than in men [6]. In addition, an estimated 6.77% (95% CI: 5.31–8.46%) of all CVD cases in men and 7.15% (95% CI: 5.62–8.93%) in women might be attributed to secondhand smoke exposure worldwide. Well enforced smoke-free laws could possibly reduce a substantial risk of CVD caused by secondhand smoke [16].

Husband smoking was associated with female hypertension prevalence in a dose–response pattern. Compared with never smokers, the risk was nearly doubled for females whose husbands were smoking. A family-based smoking restriction strategy may reduce smoking in males and improve hypertension control in females [17].

2.4 Snuffing (Smokeless Tobacco)

In a systematic review and meta-analysis, a significant positive association was detected between smokeless tobacco use and risk of fatal CHD, especially users consuming snus/snuff RR 1.30 (1.14–1.47). In view of the positive association even after strict adjustment for smoking, these results underscore the need for inclusion of cessation efforts for smokeless tobacco in addition to smoking for control of fatal CHD [18].

In a study including 26% women, discontinuation of snus use after an MI was associated with a nearly halved mortality risk, similar to the benefit associated with smoking cessation. These observations suggest that the use of snus after MI should be discouraged [19].

2.5 Electronic Cigarettes

Evidence shows that the rising use of e-cigarette use, especially among young people, may increase the likelihood of conventional smoking. Some studies have found e-cigarettes to cause harmful cardiovascular effects, but more studies focusing on long term effects of e-cigarettes on cardiovascular outcomes are needed. Currently, there is a lack of robust longitudinal data on the impact of e-cigarettes on smoking cessation, and more research is warranted. Nonetheless, health professionals should inform their patients and the general population about the possible cardiovascular risk of e-cigarette smoking. Continued monitoring and legislation to limit use is important [20].

3 Clinical Practice

3.1 Smoking Cessation

Stopping smoking is the most cost-effective strategy for CVD prevention (Fig. 1) [21]. A majority of smokers (70%) report that they want to quit smoking of which 50% tried quitting the previous year and 7% of those succeed [22]. Despite the guideline recommendations, assessment of CVD risk score (including smoking habits) in primary health care has been shown to be low in both sexes. Further, women were 32% less likely to be assessed for their smoking status than men [23]. Although it is certainly not the most significant cause, smoking cessation may contribute to an increase in obesity in the population. Public health interventions should continue to target smoking cessation in addition to obesity prevention [24]. It has been shown in a large cohort study that women in midlife who quit smoking and women who became physically active between 1986/87 and 1995/95 had higher survival when compared to those who continued to smoke and remained physically inactive. This study demonstrates the importance of having no or few risk factors in midlife with respect to longevity [25]. An article discusses a woman-centered approach to smoking cessation that could underpin initiatives in clinical, community or public health settings and could inform campaigns and messaging. Women-centered approaches that include motivational interviewing and trauma-informed elements are the new frontiers in interventions to encourage smoking cessation for women. The women who continue to smoke in high income countries, as well as the women who are taking up smoking cigarettes in low-income countries would all benefit from a clearer focus on equity, social context, and more nuanced responses to women's smoking than often exist in typical mainstream health care and health promotion. Giving women space to be heard about smoking may open up a process and conversation that ultimately leads to better health [26].

Very brief advice on smoking is a proven 30-s clinical intervention which identifies smokers, advises them on the best quitting method and supports subsequent quit attempts. There are three elements to very brief advice: ASK—establishing smoking status; ADVISE—advising on the best ways of stopping; ACT—offering help. Doctor's brief advice helps smokers to quit, and cessation increases [27].

More advice on motivational support is given in a recommended article and in the 2021 ESC Guidelines on Cardiovascular Disease Prevention in Clinical Practice [1, 28]. The personalized approach to motivate the patient for smoking cessation includes communication strategies such as motivational interviewing, consultation sessions, connection and focus, open-ended questions, affirmation, and reflecting listening. A clear benefit of mindfulness-based smoking cessation interventions for increasing smoking quit rates or changing mental health and well-being was not detected when compared with intensity-matched smoking cessation treatment, less intensive smoking cessation treatment, or no treatment. However, the evidence was of low and very low certainty due to risk of bias, inconsistency, and imprecision. This implies that the interpretation of these results may alter considering subsequent evidence in the future. Further randomized clinical trials of mindfulness-based interventions for smoking cessation compared with active comparators are needed. In addition, there is a need for more consistent reporting of mental health and well-being outcomes in studies of mindfulness-based interventions for smoking cessation [29].

According to a review including 54 reviews combined behavioral and pharmacotherapy interventions increased cessation by 82% compared with minimal intervention or usual care. Behavioral interventions increased smoking cessation at 6 months or more (physician advice had a pooled risk ratio RR 1.76 [95% CI, 1.58–1.96]). In addition, nicotine replacement therapy (RR, 1.60 [CI, 1.53–1.68]), bupropion (RR, 1.62 [CI, 1.49–1.76]), and varenicline (RR, 2.27 [CI, 2.02–2.55]) were also effective for smoking cessation. None of the drugs were associated with major cardiovascular adverse events [30].

The first day of a quit attempt has been shown to be more challenging for women than men in low- and middle-income countries. In addition to counseling and pharmacotherapy, tailored interventions including national policy may be crucial in helping women in these countries quit smoking during the initial abstinence phase [31]. Behavioral and pharmacotherapy interventions alone or combined for smoking cessation targeting women in low socio-economic status groups or women living in areas of disadvantage were effective in the short term. However, longer follow-up periods indicated reduced effectiveness. Future studies to explore ways to prevent smoking relapse in these populations are needed [32].

WHO Framework Convention on Tobacco Control (WHO FCTC) has introduced MPOWER measures to offer help to quit tobacco use [33]. The acronym MPOWER stands for M: monitor tobacco use and prevention policies; P: protect people from tobacco smoke; O: offer help to quit tobacco smoking; W: warn about the dangers of tobacco; E: enforce bans on tobacco advertising, promotion, and sponsorship; and R: raise taxes on tobacco. These measures are intended to assist in the country-level implementation of effective interventions to reduce the demand for tobacco. While many countries still have not fully implemented the core WHO FCTC measures, some are implementing more advanced measures such as plain packaging, banning of characterizing flavors from tobacco products, the licensing of tobacco retailers and extensions of smoking bans into places like cars, outdoor areas, and public streets. The necessity for monitoring data on tobacco and nicotine product usage across Europe, protecting tobacco control legislation from tobacco industry interference, and a lack of dedicated funding for scientific research are among the remaining challenges [34].

Currently, non-randomized observational studies with small sample numbers, average quality overall, and short-term follow-up comprise most of the indirect information that is available about the cardiovascular impact of e-cigarettes. According to a systematic review of 38 studies on the cardiovascular effect of e-cigarette use, most of the studies suggest potential cardiovascular harm from e-cigarettes through mechanisms that increase the risk of thrombosis and atherosclerosis. However, it is yet unclear if the indicated hemodynamic alterations are related to a clinical risk of CVD, and these findings should be interpreted cautiously. The existing evidence suggests that it should not be regarded as a cardiovascular safe product. Moreover, on a population level, it is anticipated that the potentially 'decreased' harm induced by e-cigarettes (versus conventional tobacco smoking) may in part be offset by its increased use, in more vulnerable populations such as the young. A non-linear dose–response relationship exists between smoking and the risk of CVD and mortality, wherein light smoking (less than three cigarettes per-day), is associated with elevated rates of adverse health outcomes. Hence, it is hypothesized that increased e-cigarette use may ultimately not result in proportional harm reduction of cardiovascular mortality. At the population level, such adverse health effects are expected to increase by the widespread adoption of e-cigarettes for both active smoking and smoking cessation [20]. Health professionals should therefore be cautious in recommending the use of e-cigarettes to their patients and the general public for smoking cessation as: (a) mounting evidence suggests that e-cigarettes are harmful to health, including to the heart; (b) smokers might end up using e-cigarettes as a supplement to smoking without cutting back their tobacco consumption; (c) there is a lack of robust evidence that e-cigarettes are effective as a smoking cessation tool; (d) e-cigarettes seem to be used instead of evidence-based smoking cessation products and smoking cessation clinics. E-cigarette should only be considered for very short-term use to aid tobacco cessation alongside a formal tobacco cessation program [20].

4 Conclusions

Cigarette smoking is more harmful for women than for men and is responsible for 50% of all preventable deaths in smokers, with CVD accounting for 50% of these deaths. More research is needed into the mechanisms that contribute to this elevated risk and to the possible sex differences. There are effective smoking cessation methods on patient and population levels.

Key Issues

- All use of tobacco should be stopped, as tobacco use is an independent cause of CVD.
- All smoking is harmful, there is no safe lower limit.
- Occasional smoking is not a safe smoking alternative.
- In smokers, offering follow-up support, nicotine replacement therapy, varenicline, and bupropion individually or in combination should be considered.
- Smoking cessation is recommended regard-

less of weight gain, as weight gain does not lessen the CVD benefits of cessation.

- Use of e-cigarettes for smoking cessation is generally not recommended.

Questions and Answers

1. What could be the reason for smoking being more detrimental in women?
   (A) Difference in absorption or pathophysiological effects
   (B) Frequency of smoking higher in women
   (C) There are no sex differences related to smoking effects
   (D) Due to difference in other lifestyle habits
   Comments: The best answer is A. Some authors speculate that the absorption or pathophysiological effects of toxins from cigarette smoke might be greater in women. Smoking has an antiestrogenic effect in smokers, low estrogen levels could cause an adverse impact on lipid profile, with elevations in cholesterol and triglyceride levels and reductions in high-density lipoprotein cholesterol levels, leading to endothelium dysfunction and atherosclerotic plaque formation. Furthermore, studies have indicated that smoking could also trigger premature menopause which has been associated with increased risk of CHD. However, more research is needed into the mechanisms that contribute to this elevated risk and to the possible sex differences.
2. Is there a safe lower limit for smoking in women with regards to risk of CVD?
   (A) Yes, less than 3 per day
   (B) Yes, less than 8 per day
   (C) Yes, less than 20 per month
   (D) No
   Comment: The best answer is D. All smoking is harmful, there is no safe lower limit. A non-linear dose–response relationship exists between smoking and the risk of CVD and mortality. Occasional smoking is not a safe smoking alternative. Light or occasional smokers may think that this habit does not lead to any harm. However, for CHD and stroke, there exists no smoking level that is safe.
3. Which methods for smoking cessation is considered most effective?
   (A) Switching to e-cigarettes
   (B) Follow-up support
   (C) Nicotine replacement therapy
   (D) Varenicline or bupropion
   (E) All of the above
   Comment: The best answer is E. Stopping smoking is the most cost-effective strategy for CVD prevention. In smokers, offering follow-up support, nicotine replacement therapy, varenicline, and bupropion individually or in combination should be considered as most effective smoking cessation method. Some studies have found e-cigarettes to cause harmful cardiovascular effects, but more studies focusing on long term effects of e-cigarettes on cardiovascular outcomes are needed. E-cigarettes should only be considered to aid tobacco cessation alongside a formal tobacco cessation program on very rare occasions.

References

1. Visseren FLJ, Mach F, Smulders YM, Carballo D, Koskinas KC, Bäck M, et al. 2021 ESC Guidelines on cardiovascular disease prevention in clinical practice. Eur Heart J. 2021;42(34):3227–337.
2. Statistics Norway. Tobacco, alcohol and other drugs. 2022. https://www.ssb.no/en/statbank/table/11426.
3. Mulvagh SL, Mullen KA, Nerenberg KA, Kirkham AA, Green CR, Dhukai AR, et al. The Canadian Women's Heart Health Alliance Atlas on the epidemiology, diagnosis, and management of cardiovascular disease in women - chapter 4: sex- and gender-unique disparities: CVD across the lifespan of a woman. CJC Open. 2022;4(2):115–32.
4. Gleerup HB, Dahm CC, Thim T, Jensen SE, Jensen LO, Kristensen SD, et al. Smoking is the dominating modifiable risk factor in younger patients with STEMI. Eur Heart J Acute Cardiovasc Care. 2020;9(1):70–5.
5. Albrektsen G, Heuch I, Løchen ML, Thelle DS, Wilsgaard T, Njølstad I, et al. Risk of incident myocardial infarction by gender: interactions with serum lipids, blood pressure and smoking. The Tromsø Study 1979-2012. Atherosclerosis. 2017;261:52–9.
6. Iversen B, Jacobsen BK, Løchen ML. Active and passive smoking and the risk of myocardial infarction in 24,968 men and women during 11 year of

follow-up: the Tromsø Study. Eur J Epidemiol. 2013;28(8):659–67.
7. Millett ERC, Peters SAE, Woodward M. Sex differences in risk factors for myocardial infarction: cohort study of UK Biobank participants. BMJ. 2018;363:4247.
8. Colpani V, Baena CP, Jaspers L, van Dijk GM, Farajzadegan Z, Dhana K, et al. Lifestyle factors, cardiovascular disease and all-cause mortality in middle-aged and elderly women: a systematic review and meta-analysis. Eur J Epidemiol. 2018;33(9):831–45.
9. Aune D, Schlesinger S, Norat T, Riboli E. Tobacco smoking and the risk of sudden cardiac death: a systematic review and meta-analysis of prospective studies. Eur J Epidemiol. 2018;33(6):509–21.
10. Price AJ, Wright FL, Green J, Balkwill A, Kan SW, Yang TO, et al. Differences in risk factors for 3 types of stroke: UK prospective study and meta-analyses. Neurology. 2018;90(4):e298–306.
11. Hackshaw A, Morris JK, Boniface S, Tang JL, Milenković D. Low cigarette consumption and risk of coronary heart disease and stroke: meta-analysis of 141 cohort studies in 55 study reports. BMJ. 2018;360:j5855.
12. King A. Cigarette smoking increases the risk of coronary heart disease in women more than in men. Nat Rev Cardiol. 2011;8(11):612.
13. Huxley RR, Woodward M. Cigarette smoking as a risk factor for coronary heart disease in women compared with men: a systematic review and meta-analysis of prospective cohort studies. Lancet. 2011;378(9799):1297–305.
14. Løchen ML, Gram IT, Mannsverk J, Mathiesen EB, Njølstad I, Schirmer H, et al. Association of occasional smoking with total mortality in the population-based Tromsø study, 2001-2015. BMJ Open. 2017;7(12):e019107.
15. Inoue-Choi M, McNeel TS, Hartge P, Caporaso NE, Graubard BI, Freedman ND. Non-daily cigarette smokers: mortality risks in the U.S. Am J Prev Med. 2019;56(1):27–37.
16. Zhang D, Liu Y, Cheng C, Wang Y, Xue Y, Li W, et al. Dose-related effect of secondhand smoke on cardiovascular disease in nonsmokers: systematic review and meta-analysis. Int J Hyg Environ Health. 2020;228:113546.
17. Yang Y, Liu F, Wang L, Li Q, Wang X, Chen JC, et al. Association of husband smoking with wife's hypertension status in over 5 million Chinese females aged 20 to 49 years. J Am Heart Assoc. 2017;6(3):e004924.
18. Gupta R, Gupta S, Sharma S, Sinha DN, Mehrotra R. Risk of coronary heart disease among smokeless tobacco users: results of systematic review and meta-analysis of global data. Nicotine Tob Res. 2019;21(1):25–31.
19. Arefalk G, Hambraeus K, Lind L, Michaëlsson K, Lindahl B, Sundström J. Discontinuation of smokeless tobacco and mortality risk after myocardial infarction. Circulation. 2014;130(4):325–32.
20. Kavousi M, Pisinger C, Barthelemy JC, De Smedt D, Koskinas K, Marques-Vidal P, et al. Electronic cigarettes and health with special focus on cardiovascular effects: position paper of the European Association of Preventive Cardiology (EAPC). Eur J Prev Cardiol. 2021;28(14):1552–66.
21. Rigotti NA. Pharmacotherapy for smoking cessation in adults: UpToDate; 2023. https://www.uptodate.com/contents/pharmacotherapy-for-smoking-cessation-in-adults.
22. MD Anderson Cancer Center. What's the best way to quit smoking? 2019. https://www.mdanderson.org/publications/focused-on-health/what-s-the-best-way-to-quit-smoking-.h18-1592991.html.
23. Hyun KK, Millett ER, Redfern J, Brieger D, Peters SA, Woodward M. Sex differences in the assessment of cardiovascular risk in primary health care: a systematic review. Heart Lung Circ. 2019;28(10):1535–48.
24. Løvsletten O, Njølstad I, Wilsgaard T, Hopstock LA, Jacobsen BK, Bønaa KH, et al. Is the ongoing obesity epidemic partly explained by concurrent decline in cigarette smoking? Insights from a longitudinal population study. The Tromsø Study 1994-2016. Prev Med. 2021;147:106533.
25. Løvsletten O, Brenn T. Healthy choices in midlife predict survival to age 85 in women: the Tromsø study 1979-2019. Int J Environ Res Public Health. 2022;19(9):5219.
26. Greaves L. The meanings of smoking to women and their implications for cessation. Int J Environ Res Public Health. 2015;12(2):1449–65.
27. Stead LF, Buitrago D, Preciado N, Sanchez G, Hartmann-Boyce J, Lancaster T. Physician advice for smoking cessation. Cochrane Database Syst Rev. 2013;5:CD000165.
28. Tonstad S. Smoking cessation: how to advise the patient. Heart. 2009;95(19):1635–40.
29. Jackson S, Brown J, Norris E, Livingstone-Banks J, Hayes E, Lindson N. Mindfulness for smoking cessation. Cochrane Database Syst Rev. 2022;4(4):Cd013696.
30. Patnode CD, Henderson JT, Thompson JH, Senger CA, Fortmann SP, Whitlock EP. Behavioral counseling and pharmacotherapy interventions for tobacco cessation in adults, including pregnant women: a

review of reviews for the U.S. Preventive Services Task Force. Ann Intern Med. 2015;163(8):608–21.
31. Castaldelli-Maia JM, Nesoff ED, Lima DR, Sanchez ZM, Martins SS. The first day of smoking abstinence is more challenging for women than men: a meta-analysis and meta-regression across 12 low- and middle-income countries. Addict Behav. 2022;128:107234.
32. O'Connell N, Burke E, Dobbie F, Dougall N, Mockler D, Darker C, et al. The effectiveness of smoking cessation interventions for socio-economically disadvantaged women: a systematic review and meta-analysis. Syst Rev. 2022;11(1):111.
33. World Health Organization. WHO framework convention on tobacco control; 2023. https://fctc.who.int/who-fctc/overview.
34. Willemsen MC, Mons U, Fernández E. Tobacco control in Europe: progress and key challenges. Tob Control. 2022;31(2):160–3.

Nutrition, Exercise and Alcohol Use

Johanna M. Geleijnse

Abstract

Healthy nutrition and regular exercise are crucial for the prevention and treatment of cardiovascular disease (CVD), on top of cardiovascular medication. Lifestyle interventions should be based on evidence-based guidelines by independent health authorities. Nutrition and exercise differ from targeted drug treatment because of relatively small effects on a wide range of health outcomes, accumulating over an extended period of time. Long-term commitment to lifestyle changes is therefore important. The patient's social context and self-management skills should be considered when implementing lifestyle interventions. Cardiac rehabilitation and approved lifestyle intervention programs, with support from dieticians, physiotherapists, and psychologists, are recommended. CVD patients should aim at moving towards a more plant-based diet while reducing added sugars and salt. Intake of red and processed meat, sugar-sweetened beverages and highly refined grain products should be limited, amongst others. Deviating from evidence-based dietary guidelines may lead to nutrient deficiencies and adverse long-term health effects. Adequate calcium and vitamin D intake are vital for bone health, particularly post-menopause. Dietary supplements are not needed with a diverse dietary pattern, except when recommended by health authorities or in case of extreme diets. Regular aerobic exercise, strength training and breaking up sedentary time are important for cardiovascular health. Alcohol should be abstained from or limited to a maximum of one glass per day, for overall health benefits.

Keywords

Lifestyle · Evidence-based nutrition
Exercise · Alcohol · Dietary supplements

J. M. Geleijnse (✉)
Division of Human Nutrition and Health,
Wageningen University,
Wageningen, The Netherlands
e-mail: marianne.geleijnse@wur.nl

A. H.E.M. Maas, E. Gerdts (eds.), *Manual of Cardiovascular Disease in Women*,
https://doi.org/10.1007/978-3-031-65952-2_4

Test your learning and check your understanding of this book's contents: use the "Springer Nature Flashcards" app to access questions using ▶ https://sn.pub/51ny7m
To use the app, please follow the instructions in chapter 1.

1 Introduction

This chapter highlights the important role of lifestyle modification in preventing and treating cardiovascular disease (CVD), in particular nutrition, exercise, and alcohol use. Smoking, stress, and sleep are also important lifestyle factors, but outside the scope of this chapter. Patients may obtain information from social media or other popular sources and adopt lifestyle practices that do not offer optimal protection for their health. Evidence-based advice on a heart-healthy lifestyle is provided in this chapter, based on recommendations by health authorities such as the Health Council of the Netherlands [1–7], European Society of Cardiology [8, 9], American Heart Association [10–13], and other scientific bodies [13–20]. The evidence is translated to clinical practice and tailored to women's health, whenever possible.

2 Lifestyle in the Clinic

Lifestyle modification is an integral part of cardiovascular risk management [8, 11, 13]. In academic training for medical doctors, however, less than 5% of education is spent on nutrition and exercise. This section provides a general overview of the importance of lifestyle in CVD, addressing potential hurdles from the doctor's and patient's perspectives.

2.1 Lifestyle and CVD: A Multifaceted Approach

Healthy nutrition and regular exercise are not only important for body weight control. A heart-healthy lifestyle favorably impacts all major risk factors for CVD, including blood pressure, blood lipids and insulin sensitivity [8, 11, 20]. It has beneficial effects on underlying disease pathways, including atherosclerosis, liver steatosis, low-grade inflammation, vascular dysfunction and kidney damage. The role of lifestyle in CVD is complex, with generally small health effects that only become visible after an extended period, affecting multiple organs and disease pathways simultaneously ('pleiotropic effect'). This contrasts with cardiovascular medication, which targets specific risk factors and has a more substantial impact within a relatively short timeframe.

Nutrition and exercise impact the entire body, and lifestyle interventions should be valued also for effects on non-visible health outcomes (e.g. vascular function, mental well-being), beyond weight reduction and long-term disease risk. A healthy lifestyle also positively influences muscle strength, bone health, bowel function, and vitality. Doctors should have that broad perspective in mind when encouraging lifestyle changes. For instance, in managing blood glucose for diabetic patients through dietary advice, the doctor could also consider the diet's impact on quality of life and reduced risks of gastrointestinal cancers, stroke and kidney disease. A heart-healthy lifestyle forms the cornerstone of CVD prevention and treatment, also for patients using medication for CVD, diabetes or weight loss.

2.2 The Role of the Medical Doctor

Prescribing a healthy diet and lifestyle is not a straightforward task for a medical specialist. It asks for personalized behavioral guidance considering a patient's food and health literacy, self-management skills, and social environment. The difficulty of accurately measuring habitual diet and exercise levels hinders effective feedback and monitoring of changes over time. Given limited training and time constraints, medical doctors could primarily raise awareness about the importance of a healthy lifestyle rather than assuming the role of knowledge experts in the field of nutrition and exercise.

Many patients consider their doctor as trustworthy source of information. Doctors can serve as ambassadors of a healthy lifestyle by setting an example and through educational materials in their clinics. Medical specialists should proactively refer patients for lifestyle coaching to cardiac rehabilitation and combined lifestyle intervention programs [17, 21]. Dieticians, physiotherapists, and psychologists play crucial roles in supporting patients as they implement lifestyle changes. Regular clinic visits offer opportunities for doctors to reiterate the importance of a healthy lifestyle, preferably involving the patient's social network. Effective collaboration across the entire care chain, such as between medical specialists and general practitioners, is vital for lifestyle medicine.

2.3 Lifestyle from the Patient's Perspective

Following a diagnosis of CVD, diabetes or risk factors like hypertension or hypercholesterolemia, patients initially show increased motivation for healthier lifestyles. However, as time progresses, many of them return to previous habits. Lifestyle choices are not solely driven by health. Major drivers are taste and price of food, social and cultural norms and the 'obesogenic' living environment with abundance of unhealthy food [10], promoting also a sedentary lifestyle. Lifestyle modification can be challenging and emotionally demanding. This asks for shared decision-making and small-step approaches with realistic goals, supported also by the patient's social environment.

A broad view on health, as reflected in the "Positive Health" concept [22], is relevant in this context, also for women. This includes the patient's ability to deal with physical, emotional and social challenges, beyond the biomedical perspective. Patients may also need proper education about lifestyle and health, along with help in identifying their personal drivers for lifestyle behaviours. Addressing mental or psychosocial barriers (e.g., poverty, substance abuse, or unsafe living conditions) may be necessary and could involve collaboration with social workers or psychologists.

3 Healthy Nutrition

3.1 Healthy Nutrition: An Integrated Approach

The human diet is complex and difficult to measure and monitor. Dimensions of healthy and sustainable nutrition include energy balance, nutrient requirements, food-based dietary guidelines, food safety and environmental sustainability, as explained in Table 1. These dimensions all need to be integrated for the best possible dietary advice, by an impartial organization that is free of commercial interests. In the Netherlands, the Nutrition Centre achieves this through its "Wheel of Five" [23–25], based on multidisciplinary and independent advisory reports by the Health Council [1–7]. Dieticians can tailor this evidence-based advice to the individual patient. Patients can also gain insight into their diet via an online application by the Nutrition Centre ("Eetmeter"), which provides tailored feedback [26].

Table 1 Multiple dimensions of healthy, sustainable nutrition

1.	Energy balance	Daily caloric intake should align with energy expenditure resulting from metabolic processes and physical activity [1, 23]. Pregnant and lactating women have higher energy needs. Older women generally need less calories due to declining muscle mass and metabolic rate. A positive energy balance leads to weight gain and associated health risks. Visceral (or central) adiposity with excess fat in the abdomen is more detrimental than peripheral obesity
2.	Nutrient requirements	An adequate intake of energy and macro- and micronutrients (i.e., vitamins, minerals) is essential for growth and development, physical functioning, and well-being. Recommendations for the intake of specific nutrients (i.e., dietary reference values; DRVs) have been formulated by health authorities [7, 14, 24]. DRVs may depend on age, sex, pregnancy and lactation
3.	Food-based dietary guidelines	Foods, beverages and overall dietary patterns impact the risk of CVD, diabetes, various cancers and osteoporosis. Health authorities, including the Health Council of the Netherlands, have developed food-based dietary guidelines for mitigating the burden of chronic diseases [1–4, 11]
4.	Food safety	Good hygiene while handling and preparing food lowers the risk of foodborne illnesses [23]. Minimizing the intake of toxins and chemical contaminants is also important to prevent cancers, liver damage, and developmental disorders. Food safety is vital for pregnant and lactating women, protecting their offspring, and for vulnerable patients with a compromised immune system
5.	Environmental sustainability	Climate change has raised interest in the environmental impact of our diet and food production systems [5]. Excessive caloric consumption and diets that emphasize animal-based protein sources (especially red meat) are less sustainable because they lead to more greenhouse-gas emissions and land use. Fish consumption is affected by the pressure on marine ecosystems

3.2 Dietary Guidelines

Dietary guidelines for the general population are also a solid basis for dietary advice to patients with atherosclerotic CVD and type 2 diabetes [3, 4]. According to recent guidelines, patients are recommended to move towards a more plant-based diet [1–5, 8, 10, 11, 23]. Such a diet is rich in fibre and healthy nutrients, and helps maintain a normal body weight. The focus should not only be on calories and macronutrients, for lowering body weight and diabetes risk, but also on minerals and bioactive substances in plant foods to improve vascular health, kidney function and cardiac function. Supplemental intake of nutrients is not needed in case of a varied diet, except for some target groups (described elsewhere in this chapter). Specific recommendations for food and beverage intakes are outlined in Table 2.

3.3 Functional Foods

Functional foods containing phytosterols (plant sterols and stanols) may lower LDL-cholesterol levels by approximately 10% when consumed in amounts of 2 g/day [3, 8]. Red yeast rice supplements that contain monacolin K are not recommended because of interactions with statin use and possible adverse side-effects [3, 8]. Liquorice root contains glycyrrhizin, which may interfere with hormonal systems and fluid balance. Caution is needed regarding black liquorice or certain herbal teas, especially in CVD patients with hypertension [16, 27]. Dark chocolate (>70% of cocoa) is rich in cocoa polyphenols, which may improve blood pressure and vascular health [28]. Because of saturated fat and sugar, however, chocolate intake should be limited [23].

Table 2 Dietary guidelines for CVD patients

Guideline[a]	Comments
Consume at least 200 g of vegetables and at least 200 g of fruit daily	• Fruits and vegetables provide dietary fibre, potassium, essential nutrients (e.g. vitamins and minerals) and phytonutrients that benefit cardiometabolic health • Fresh or minimally processed fruits and vegetables are preferred, or frozen products that contain less salt and sugar than canned products • The nutritional value of organic produce is not higher than that of regular produce • Fruit juices have less nutritional value compared to fresh fruit, and may be high in sugar
Consume at least 90 g of whole grain bread or other whole grain products daily Replace refined grain products with whole grain products	• Whole-grain bread and cereals (e.g. brown rice, rye) are rich in fibre, micronutrients and phytonutrients that benefit cardiometabolic health • Beta-glucans, e.g. in oat meal, lower LDL-cholesterol • Highly processed grain products (e.g. white bread, pastries, sugary breakfast cereals) with little nutritional value should be avoided
Consume legumes weekly	• Legumes are rich in fibre, essential amino acids, iron and other micronutrients that benefit cardiometabolic health • Legumes include soybeans, kidney beans, other beans, lentils and peas • Soy-based products and other legumes are a healthy alternative to meat, because of their amino acid profile
Consume at least 15 g of unsalted nuts per day	• The ESC recommends 30 grams of unsalted nuts per day [8] • Nuts contain alpha-linolenic acid, a plant-based omega-3 fatty acid, dietary fibre and other micronutrients that benefit cardiometabolic health • While technically a legume, unsalted peanuts (more affordable) may also be considered as nuts • Intakes higher than 30 grams per day offer no additional health benefit and should be avoided because of calories and environmental sustainability
Consume a few servings of dairy per day, including milk or yogurt	• Dairy is a main source of calcium and other minerals, including potassium and magnesium • Calcium from dairy is important for the efficacy of vitamin D supplementation and bone health • Full-fat products can be replaced by (semi)skimmed products for management of body weight • Avoid dairy foods and beverages with added sugar • Cheese is rich in salt, saturated fat and calories, and should be limited; fresh cheese (e.g. cottage cheese) provides a good alternative
Consume fish 1–2 times per week	• Fish is the major source of long-chain omega-3 fatty acids (eicosapentaenoic acid [EPA] and docosahexaenoic acid [DHA]); it also contains other important nutrients, such as protein, B-vitamins, vitamin D, iodine and selenium • The recommendation includes both fatty and lean fish. Examples of fatty fish species are herring, salmon and mackerel; examples of lean fish are pollock, cod, plaice, and pangasius • Higher fish intake than recommended is not needed for health and should be avoided because of salt or contaminants in some fish, and environmental sustainability
Replace butter and other solid (baking) fats with soft margarines and vegetable oils	• Replacing saturated fatty acids and trans fatty acids (solid fats) by poly- and monounsaturated fatty acids (oils) lowers blood LDL-cholesterol and CVD risk • Saturated fatty acids remain solid at room temperature, while (poly) unsaturated fats remain liquid because of a lower melting point • Trans fatty acids are partially hydrogenated oils, e.g. in industrially processed foods, which raise LDL-cholesterol • Olive oil, soybean oil, plant seed oils (e.g. sunflower, rapeseed) and soft margarines are good choices; tropical oils (e.g. coconut, palm) are rich in saturated fatty acids and not preferred

(continued)

Table 2 (continued)

Guideline[a]	Comments
Drink three cups of black or green tea daily	• Tea is beneficial for blood pressure and vascular function, possibly due to polyphenols • Herbal and "rooibos" teas do not contain polyphenols
Replace unfiltered coffee with filtered coffee	• Unfiltered coffee contains diterpenes (cafestol, kahweol) that raise blood cholesterol • Diterpenes are present in boiled coffee, cafetiere coffee, French pressed coffee, Turkish coffee and (to a lesser extent) in espresso • No quantitative dietary guideline for coffee exists, but intakes up to 6 cups per day spread over the day are unlikely to cause problems for CVD patients • Unhealthy additives (sugar, syrups, creamers) in coffee should be avoided • There is growing evidence for a beneficial effect of coffee (caffeinated or decaf) on cardiometabolic health • Caffeinated coffee in the evening may adversely affect sleep • Limit caffeine intake if pregnant or lactating
Limit the consumption of red meat, particularly processed meat	• The ESC recommends that red meat should be reduced to a maximum of 350–500 g a week and limitation of processed meat in particular [8] • Red meat includes for example beef, pig and lamb; white meat is mainly poultry • Red and/or processed meat increase the risk of cardiometabolic diseases and various cancers, including colorectal cancer • Reducing meat consumption and replacing red meat with white meat contribute to environmental sustainability [5] • Healthy meat replacers include soy-based products (tofu, tempeh), legumes (e.g., beans, chickpeas), mushrooms, nuts and seeds
Minimize the intake of sugar-sweetened beverages (SSBs)	• SSBs include carbonated and uncarbonated soft drinks (e.g. cola), sweetened dairy drinks and fruit juices (especially if industrially processed) • Liquid calories lead to a high energy intake rate, which strongly promotes weight gain • Health effects of artificially sweetened beverages are not yet clear. SSB may best be replaced by water, tea or filtered coffee
Limit the intake of salt to a maximum of 6 grams per day	• The ESC recommends less than 5 grams per day [8], as does the World Health Organization • Sodium increases blood pressure and CVD risk, and causes kidney damage • People in western societies consume around 9 grams of salt per day, and industrially processed and take-away foods are major contributors to salt intake • Home cooking using fresh ingredients, avoidance of the salt shaker, and reading labels on food products are relevant measures for controlling salt intake

ESC European Society of Cardiology

[a] Based on the 2023 advisory report by the Health Council of the Netherlands [3]

4 Dietary Supplementation

The safety and efficacy of dietary supplements are often unknown. Patients with a diverse diet generally do not need vitamin or mineral supplements. Use of dietary and botanical supplements may have serious adverse health effects and interact with medication [14–16, 29]. For adults, the Health Council only recommends supplementation for vitamin D and folic acid (vitamin B11) for specific target groups [1, 7], as described below.

4.1 Vitamin D

Vitamin D, together with calcium, is important for bone health. It is produced in the skin, after daylight exposure. For an adequate vitamin D status, the Health Council recommends spending 15–30 min outdoors daily between 11:00 am and 3:00 pm from March to November, with the head and hands exposed [7]. Dietary sources of vitamin D include fatty fish, liver, meat, eggs, mushrooms, dairy and (fortified) margarines and baking fats. Circulating calcidiol (25OHD), a biomarker of vitamin D status, fluctuates throughout the year with lowest values after the winter. The Health Council defines vitamin D deficiency as 25OHD below 30 nmol/L for individuals below 70 and below 50 nmol/L for those over age 70 [7]. Postmenopausal women, at risk of osteoporosis, particularly benefit from an adequate vitamin D status and sufficient calcium intake (e.g. from dairy foods). Vitamin D deficiency is hard to correct by diet. Therefore, the Health Council recommends vitamin D supplementation with a dosage of 10 μg/day for women aged 50–70 and pregnant women, 20 μg/day for women over age 70, and 10 μg/day for women below age 50 when they have a dark skin or little daylight exposure [7]. Vitamin D supplementation is unlikely to reduce CVD or diabetes risk. Potential interactions of vitamin D supplements with medication, including statins and thiazide diuretics, have been described [16].

4.2 Folic Acid

According to the Health Council, women who want to become pregnant are advised to take folic acid supplements of 400 μg/day, starting at least 4 weeks prior to conception, to prevent neural tube defects in the offspring. This is also advised to pregnant women until 10 weeks of pregnancy [7]. Folic acid supplementation is not recommended for CVD [16].

4.3 Other Supplements

Fish oil supplementation with doses of omega-3 fatty acids in the dietary range (<1 g/day of EPA + DHA) are not recommended for CVD patients by the Health Council, based on lack of scientific evidence [3]. If supplements are used, fish oil rich in EPA and DHA are advised, rather than fish liver oil. High-dose supplementation with purified EPA and/or DHA is considered as pharmacological treatment, and outside the scope of this chapter.

Vitamin or mineral supplements may be considered for elderly people with low food intake and people with a poor diet (e.g. problem drinkers or extreme dieters). Iron supplementation may be considered for anaemia, e.g. in women experiencing heavy menstrual bleeding. Vegans (see below), pregnant or lactating women may also benefit from low-dose supplementation of specific nutrients [24].

Patients should check labels for over-the-counter supplements, as excessive intakes (e.g. vitamin A, D, E, B-vitamins) can pose health risks. As a rule of thumb, dosages of individual vitamins and minerals from supplements should not exceed 100% of the recommended daily allowance (RDA). RDAs and upper levels are available from the Nutrition Center [24] and European Food and Safety Authority [14].

5 Diets and Eating Habits

This section provides information on dietary patterns for CVD patients and diets that are popular especially amongst women. Also, dietary aspects related to menopause are discussed.

5.1 Heart-Healthy Diets

Cardioprotective diets emphasize fruits, vegetables, legumes, whole grains, and lean protein sources, while limiting added sugar, salt, saturated and trans-fatty acids and sugar sweetened beverages. The European Society of Cardiology supports the Mediterranean diet for CVD patients, with extra-virgin olive oil and nuts, based on clinical trial evidence [8]. The Health Council concluded that the Dutch dietary guidelines are a solid basis also for CVD patients [3]. Olive oil may be exchanged for other vegetable oils that are cheaper. Compared to the Mediterranean diet, the Dutch guidelines put more emphasis on (whole-grain) bread, less salt, adequate amounts of dairy and choice of beverages (e.g. tea, filtered coffee, no alcohol). Other examples of heart-healthy diets include the DASH diet and various dietary patterns that emphasize plant foods [1–3, 8, 11].

5.2 Weight Loss Diets

Weight loss results from a negative energy balance, when calories burned exceed calories consumed, regardless of specific macronutrients (fat, protein, carbohydrate) involved. Fast energy intake, like from sugar-sweetened beverages and highly processed foods, strongly promotes weight gain. Numerous dietary supplements and botanicals are promoted for weight loss [16], for which efficacy lacks conclusive evidence, apart from costs and health risks. An effective and sustainable weight loss approach involves a (supervised) healthy eating plan, with reduced caloric intake and increased physical activity. Psychosocial or emotional issues may contribute to overeating and obesity, requiring psychological support. The Nutrition Centre provides information on healthy dieting [23], and patients benefit from evidence-based, combined lifestyle interventions [17].

5.3 Intermittent Fasting

Intermittent fasting can lead to weight loss by limiting the eating window, providing a straightforward approach for patients to manage caloric intake. Examples include the 16/8 method (16 h of daily fasting) and the 5:2 method (two non-consecutive days of reduced caloric intake a week) [23]. Beneficial effects on body weight and cardiometabolic outcomes may occur. Intermittent fasting is not primarily focused on changing food choice or enhancing overall diet quality, so patients may not achieve optimal health benefits. The long-term effects of intermittent fasting are not scientifically clear.

5.4 Low-Carb and Ketogenic Diets

Reduced carbohydrate diets are increasingly popular for weight loss and glucose control. Dutch people obtain around 45% of their energy from carbohydrates, equivalent to 200–350 g/day for a 2000-kcal diet. A diet with 50–130 g of carbohydrates per day is commonly labeled as 'low-carb' [4]. The ketogenic diet is characterized by a very low carb intake (<50 g/day) and an increased fat and protein intake. Lowering the intake of simple carbohydrates, such as added sugars and SSBs, is beneficial for cardiometabolic health and aligns with evidence-based dietary guidelines. The intake of complex carbohydrates (e.g. from fruit, vegetables and whole-grain products), on the other hand, should be increased rather than decreased [1–4]. Low-carb diets that exclude bread and cereals may lead to a higher consumption of animal-based foods, which adversely affects long-term health and is not environmentally sustainable [5]. Low-carb diets have been shown to lower weight and blood glucose after 3–6 months, but this cannot be disentangled from caloric restriction as such. The Health Council concludes that there is lack of scientific evidence for long-term (>1 year) benefits of low-carb diets compared to other diets on these outcomes [4].

5.5 Vegetarian and Vegan Diets

Cardiovascular patients, particularly women, may opt for a vegetarian or vegan diet for planetary health or other reasons. The vegetarian diet excludes meat but generally includes eggs, dairy, and sometimes fish. This diet can align well with evidence-based dietary guidelines, especially when fish is included [5]. The vegan diet excludes all animal-based products. Dietetic support is advisable, since vegans may need to increase their protein intake for essential amino acids, and they are at risk of nutrient deficiencies. Intake of iron, calcium, iodine, fish fatty acids and vitamins B1, B2, and B12 are generally lower in vegans, which may require supplementation [24].

5.6 Eating After Menopause

Postmenopausal women may experience muscle loss and abdominal weight gain. For weight management, women should consume the right amount of food for their age, as outlined in the "Wheel of Five" by the Nutrition Centre [25]. Osteoporosis risk also increases after menopause. This asks for an adequate calcium intake (e.g. from dairy), coupled with vitamin D supplementation and exercise. Full-fat dairy can be replaced with (semi)skimmed variants for lowering the intake of calories and saturated fat. No specific diet is needed during or after menopause. Soy products with phytoestrogens (specifically isoflavones) have been suggested to alleviate menopausal symptoms and to lower chronic disease risk (e.g. CVD, breast cancer, osteoporosis). Research on these beneficial effects of soy products, however, is not conclusive [14, 23]. Menopausal women may report complaints when consuming (caffeinated) coffee, tea, alcohol or spicy food, although this is not substantiated by science. Scientific evidence for effective diets that mitigate menstrual complaints, endometriosis or polycystic ovary syndrome is also lacking [23].

6 Exercise

Regular exercise offers major health benefits, beyond weight control [6, 8, 9, 12]. It reduces the risk of CVD, type 2 diabetes, cancers and osteoporosis, while improving vital capacity, cardiac function, muscle and bone health and body balance. Beneficial effects also include improved mental health and sleep quality. Outdoor activities with exposure to daylight helps maintain an optimal vitamin D status. Guidelines for physical activity in CVD patients are summarized in Table 3. Various types of exercise include:

1. Aerobic exercise (cardiorespiratory training), which includes activities like running, swimming, cycling, and dancing.
2. Resistance exercise (strength training), which involves working with weights to build and tone muscles.
3. Flexibility and stability training, which improves balance, helps prevent falling and injuries and relieves stress.

Regular household activities are important for the prevention of a sedentary lifestyle, as are other daily routines like taking the stairs, going out for grocery shopping and walking the dog. Low-impact activities may be considered such as walking and swimming, putting less stress on the joints. Weight bearing exercise is important for postmenopausal women who are at risk of osteoporosis. Strength training can make use of the patient's own body weight or resistance bands, instead of heavy weights. Chair exercises focusing on leg lifts and marches are suitable for those with limited mobility. Flexibility exercises and balance training, such as supported one-legged stands, contribute to overall health and fall prevention. Older patients are advised to engage in multicomponent physical activity, combining aerobic, muscle-strengthening, and balance exercises to prevent falls [8]. Heart failure patients may also engage in physical activity, like walking, cycling, or swimming for 30 minutes twice a day, if not causing health problems [9]. CVD patients benefit from enrolment in a cardiac rehabilitation programme and supervision by a physiotherapist.

6.1 Barriers and Facilitators

Hurdles may be encountered when implementing exercise in the clinical care of CVD patients [21, 30]. Small-step approaches that align with the patient's personal preferences, including also rewards for progress, are vital for success. After shared goal setting, the patient can start exercise activities with short durations and low intensity, gradually increasing as their tolerance improves. Social support (e.g. workout buddy or group) and a pleasant and safe environment are important for developing an exercise routine. Psychological support may be necessary for issues like anxiety or body shame. Health issues, such as incontinence, gastrointestinal complaints, pelvic instability or menstrual problems in women could be

Table 3 Physical activity guidelines for CVD patients

Guideline[a]	Comments
Perform at least 150–300 min a week of moderate-intensity or 75–150 min a week of vigorous-intensity aerobic exercise	• Moderate intensity (3–5.9 MET) Walking at moderate or brisk pace (4.1–6.5 km/h), slow cycling (15 km/h), painting/decorating, vacuuming, gardening (mowing lawn), golf (pulling clubs in trolley), tennis (doubles), ballroom dancing, water aerobics • Vigorous intensity (≥6 MET) Race-walking, jogging, or running, cycling >15 km/h, heavy gardening (continuous digging or hoeing), swimming laps, tennis (singles)
Replace sedentary time by (light) activities throughout the day	• Light intensity (1.1–2.9 MET) Walking <4.7 km/h, light household work • For physically inactive (i.e., sedentary) adults, light-intensity physical activity, even as little as 15 min a day, is likely to produce benefits
Perform resistance training, in addition to aerobic exercise, for 2 or more days per week	• The recommended regimen involves 1–3 sets of 8–12 repetitions at 60–80% of the patient's 1 RM, at least twice a week with 8–10 different exercises targeting major muscle groups • Older and deconditioned patients could start with 1 set of 10–15 repetitions at 40–50% of 1 RM

MET is estimated as the energy cost of a given activity divided by resting energy expenditure: 1 MET = 3.5 mL oxygen kg^{-1} min^{-1} VO2

1 RM: One-repetition maximum, which is the maximum amount of weight that a person can possibly lift for one repetition

[a] Adopted from the 2021 guidelines by the European Society of Cardiology [8]

major barriers to engaging in exercise, and need to be also addressed.

Patients who are not used to exercising may misinterpret their body signals, such as changes in heart rate, breathing pattern, and energy levels, requiring extra coaching. Adequate warm-up and cool-down, and understanding the balance between activity and rest, is important for CVD patients. Monitoring devices and activity trackers (e.g., Fitbit) could be useful and rewarding, but guidance may be needed. For patients using beta-blocking agents, for example, heart rate may not be a reliable indicator for fitness and exercise load.

A (socially) safe exercise environment is important, especially for women. Some women may not want to share sporting facilities with men, for personal or religious reasons. Practical and financial constraints, such as the cost of sporting gear, club fees, and lack of transport can be major obstacles. Furthermore, some women may prioritize caregiving responsibilities over personal well-being or may not be able to leave the home environment. Medical doctors could refer these patients to societal organisations or municipal services for support.

7 Alcohol

Ethanol, the active ingredient in alcoholic beverages, is a potent substance that has a wide array of effects on the body. A standard glass of alcohol (e.g. 200 mL of beer or 100 mL of wine) contains roughly 10 g of ethanol. Alcohol metabolism differs between men and women due to body composition and hormonal factors. The higher amount of body fat and smaller water compartment in women affects the distribution and storage of alcohol. In the liver, alcohol dehydrogenase (ADH) breaks down alcohol into acetaldehyde. Men generally have higher levels of ADH and a more efficient breakdown. For the same dose of alcohol, women have higher and more prolonged levels of alcohol in the blood [31].

Epidemiological studies suggest lower CVD risks for light to moderate alcohol consumption, despite its adverse effect on blood pressure [32]. Higher intakes, however, have been associated with heart failure, cardiomyopathy, and atrial fibrillation. Alcohol poses risks for pre and post-menopausal breast cancer and gastrointestinal cancers [18]. While alcohol can induce temporary relaxation, it also impairs judgment, leading to potential negative outcomes such as violence, sexual risk behaviors and injuries. It adversely affects pregnancy outcomes and child development, also through breastfeeding. Prolonged and heavy alcohol use causes damage to the liver, brain and other parts of the nervous system.

Alcoholic beverages provide ethanol, while not having nutritional value. Drinks may be high in sugars (e.g. beer, cocktails). Concentrations of polyphenols in alcoholic beverages (e.g., resveratrol in red wine) are too low to exert a meaningful biological effect. Ethanol is potentially toxic and alcoholic beverages should not be viewed as a normal component of the diet. Lower inhibition due to ethanol can lead to food cravings and excessive caloric intake. Alcohol is often consumed with savory snacks, and in such settings, thirst from salt is quenched by beer or other unhealthy beverages. This common practice contributes to obesity and adverse effects on the cardiovascular system.

The European Society of Cardiology recommends alcohol restriction to a maximum of 100 g/week, regardless of sex [8]. This equals roughly 10 drinks per week, or 1–2 glasses/day [8]. The Health Council recommends abstinence or, for those who drink, a maximum of 1 glass/day both for male and female CVD patients [3]. Binge drinking, i.e., 4 or more glasses at a single occasion for women, should be avoided. Pregnant women should abstain from alcohol, and lactating women should not drink or ensure a time gap of >3 h between drinking and breastfeeding. Alcohol can interact with medication, including cardiovascular drugs [15]. This may, for example, result in large blood pressure drops and risk of falling, or extended bleeding time. How to deal with problematic alcohol use is beyond the scope of this chapter, and information can be found elsewhere [19].

Recommendations on alcohol use for CVD patients:

- Do not start drinking for heart health.
- Abstinence from alcohol helps prevent breast cancer, gastrointestinal cancers, liver damage, and adverse health outcomes related to risk behaviours.
- If drinking, limit to 1 glass/day or less both for men and women.
- Avoid binge drinking.
- Avoid alcoholic beverages with added sugar, such as cocktails and mixed drinks.
- Consider interactions of alcohol with medication.

Key Issues

- Healthy nutrition and exercise are crucial for CVD prevention and treatment.
- Lifestyle interventions should be based on evidence-based guidelines by independent health authorities.
- Nutrition and exercise affect the whole body, with relatively small effects on a wide range of health outcomes that accumulate over an extended period of time.
- A heart-healthy lifestyle is important on top of medication.
- The patient's social context and self-management skills should be considered when implementing lifestyle interventions.
- CVD patients benefit from cardiac rehabilitation and approved lifestyle intervention programs.
- CVD patients may need support from dieticians, physiotherapists and psychologists when implementing lifestyle changes.
- Moving towards a more plant-based diet, while reducing added sugars and salt, is important for CVD prevention and treatment.
- Diets that deviate from the dietary guidelines may lead to nutrient deficiencies and negative long-term effects on health.
- Sufficient calcium and vitamin D intake are important for bone health, especially after menopause.
- Dietary supplements are not needed when the patient has a diverse diet, except for specific recommendation (e.g. vitamin D) by health authorities.
- Regular aerobic exercise (e.g. brisk walking or cycling) for at least 150 minutes and strength training twice a week improve cardiovascular health.
- Abstinence from alcohol or limiting consumption to a maximum of one glass per day (if drinking) benefits overall health.

Questions and Answers

1. Why should the doctor have a broad view on health when implementing lifestyle interventions in cardiovascular risk management?

   Answer: Nutrition and exercise not only impact CVD, but also other chronic diseases such as cancers and osteoporosis, as well as mental health and quality of life. Lifestyle changes have relatively small effects in the short term, but major cumulative effects in the long term. Patients may have difficulty implementing lifestyle changes because of physical, emotional and social challenges, for which support from a dietician, physiotherapist or psychologist may be needed.
2. What are the dimensions of healthy and sustainable nutrition that should be integrated for the best possible dietary advice to patients?

   Answer: Dietary advice should be based on energy balance for body weight control, requirements of specific nutrients for optimal body functioning and food-based dietary guidelines for preventing recurrent CVD and other chronic diseases. Food safety aspects and environmental sustainability of the diet are also relevant dimensions to take into account.
3. Which are key components of a healthy diet for CVD patients?

   Answer: A heart-healthy diet emphasizes plant foods, with ample fruit and vegetables, whole grains, legumes, and nuts and seeds. It includes a few daily servings of dairy, and one or two weekly portions of fish. It is low in red and processed meats and solid fats are replaced by vegetable oils. Beverages include water, tea or filtered coffee, while sugar-sweetened beverages and alcohol are reduced. Salt intake is below 5-6 grams per day.
4. Do female cardiovascular patients need dietary supplements?

   Answer: Female cardiovascular patients do not need dietary supplements if they maintain a well-balanced and varied diet. Exceptions are vitamin D, if prone to deficiency, and folic acid around pregnancy. Patients who have vegan diets or extreme diets may also benefit from low-dose supplementation, in case of nutrient deficiencies.
5. Which are evidence-based recommendations for physical activity for CVD patients?

   Answer: Include at least 150–300 min/week of moderate-intensity aerobic exercise, such as brisk walking, cycling, or gardening. Additionally, incorporate vigorous-intensity activities, like jogging or swimming, for 75–150 min/week. Break up sedentary time with light activities, especially for those who are physically inactive. Include resistance training at least twice a week, targeting multiple muscle groups. Chair exercises are an alternative for patients who are immobile. Supervision by a physiotherapist, social support and a safe sporting environment should be considered when implementing an exercise routine.

Conflicts of Interest None.

References

1. Health Council of the Netherlands (Gezondheidsraad). Dutch dietary guidelines 2015. The Hague: Health Council of the Netherlands; 2015.
2. Kromhout D, Spaaij CJK, de Goede J, Weggemans R. The 2015 Dutch food-based dietary guidelines. Eur J Clin Nutr. 2016;70:869–78.
3. Health Council of the Netherlands (Gezondheidsraad). Dutch dietary guidelines for people with atherosclerotic cardiovascular disease. The Hague: Health Council of the Netherlands; 2023.
4. Health Council of the Netherlands (Gezondheidsraad). Dutch dietary guidelines for people with type 2 diabetes. The Hague: Health Council of the Netherlands; 2021.
5. Health Council of the Netherlands (Gezondheidsraad). A healthy protein transition. The Hague: Health Council of the Netherlands; 2023.
6. Health Council of the Netherlands (Gezondheidsraad). Dutch physical activity guidelines 2017. The Hague: Health Council of the Netherlands; 2017.
7. Health Council of the Netherlands (Gezondheidsraad). Dietary reference values for vitamins and minerals for adults. The Hague: Health Council of the Netherlands; 2018.
8. Visseren FLJ, Mach F, Smulders YM, Carballo D, Koskinas KC, Bäck M, Benetos A, et al. 2021 ESC guidelines on cardiovascular disease prevention in clinical practice. Eur Heart J. 2021;42:3227–337.
9. Pelliccia A, Sharma S, Gati S, Bäck M, Börjesson M, Caselli S, et al. 2020 ESC guidelines on sports car-

diology and exercise in patients with cardiovascular disease. Eur Heart J. 2021;42:17–96.
10. Lichtenstein AH, Appel LJ, Vadiveloo M, Hu FB, Kris-Etherton PM, Rebholz CM, et al. Dietary guidance to improve cardiovascular health: a scientific statement from the American Heart Association. Circulation. 2021;144:e472–87.
11. Lloyd-Jones DM, Allen NB, Anderson CAM, Black T, Brewer LC, Foraker RE, et al. Life's essential 8: updating and enhancing the American Heart Association's construct of cardiovascular health: a presidential advisory from the American Heart Association. Circulation. 2022;146:e18–43.
12. Paluch AE, Boyer WR, Franklin BA, Laddu D, Lobelo F, Lee DC, et al. Resistance exercise training in individuals with and without cardiovascular disease: 2023 update: a scientific statement from the American Heart Association. Circulation. 2024;149:e217–31.
13. Federation of Medical Specialists (Federatie van Medisch Specialisten). Richtlijnendatabase cardiovascular risk management (CVRM) [in Dutch]. 2024. https://richtlijnendatabase.nl/richtlijn/cardiovasculair_risicomanagement_cvrm/samenvatting_cvrm.html.
14. European Food Safety Authority (EFSA). Nutrition. 2024. https://www.efsa.europa.eu/en/topics/topic/nutrition.
15. Medicines Evaluation Board (College ter Beoordeling van Geneesmiddelen, CBG). Kruiden [in Dutch]. 2024. https://www.cbg-meb.nl/onderwerpen/medicijninformatie-kruiden.
16. National Institutes of Health – Office of Dietary Supplements (NIH/ODS). Dietary supplement fact sheets. 2024. https://ods.od.nih.gov/factsheets/list-all/.
17. National Institute for Public Health and the Environment (RIVM). Loket Gezond Leven. Bilthoven: RIVM; 2024. www.loketgezondleven.nl.
18. World Cancer Research Fund/American Institute for Cancer Research. Diet, nutrition, physical activity and cancer: a global perspective. 2018. Continuous update project expert report. 2024. https://www.wcrf.org/diet-activity-and-cancer/risk-factors.
19. Boomsma LJ, Drost IM, Larsen IM, Luijkx JJHM, Meerkerk GJ, et al. NHG-standaard M10: problematisch alcoholgebruik. 2024. https://richtlijnen.nhg.org/standaarden/problematisch-alcoholgebruik.
20. German CA, Baum SJ, Ferdinand KC, Gulati M, Polonsky TS, Toth PP, Shapiro MD. Defining preventive cardiology: a clinical practice statement from the American Society for Preventive Cardiology. Am J Prev Cardiol. 2022;12:100432.
21. Zurynski Y, Smith C, Siette J, NicGiolla Easpaig BNG, Simons M, Knaggs GT. Identifying enablers and barriers to referral, uptake and completion of lifestyle modification programmes: a rapid literature review. BMJ Open. 2021;11:e045094.
22. Institute for Positive Health. The wider benefits of positive health. 2024. www.iph.nl/en.
23. Netherlands Nutrition Centre (Voedingscentrum). Gezond, duurzaam en veilig eten. 2024. www.voedingscentrum.nl.
24. Netherlands Nutrition Centre (Voedingscentrum). Supplementen, vitamines en mineralen. 2024. https://www.voedingscentrum.nl/nl/thema/alles-over-supplementen.aspx.
25. Netherlands Nutrition Centre (Voedingscentrum). Schijf van Vijf. 2024. https://www.voedingscentrum.nl/nl/gezond-eten-met-de-schijf-van-vijf.aspx.
26. Netherlands Nutrition Centre (Voedingscentrum). Eetmeter. 2024. https://www.voedingscentrum.nl/nl/thema/apps-en-tools-voedingscentrum/mijn-eetmeter-app-online.aspx.
27. Penninkilampi R, Eslick EM, Eslick GD. The association between consistent licorice ingestion, hypertension and hypokalaemia: a systematic review and meta-analysis. J Hum Hypertens. 2017;31:699–707.
28. Hooper L, Kay C, Abdelhamid A, Kroon PA, Cohn JS, Rimm EB, Cassidy A. Effects of chocolate, cocoa, and flavan-3-ols on cardiovascular health: a systematic review and meta-analysis of randomized trials. Am J Clin Nutr. 2012;95:740–51.
29. Netherlands Food and Consumer Product Safety Authority (NVWA). Risico's gebruik voedingssupplementen. 2024. https://www.nvwa.nl/onderwerpen/voedingssupplementen/risico-s-voedingssupplementen.
30. Curran F, Davis ME, Murphy K, Tersigni N, King A, Ngo N, O'Donoghue G. Correlates of physical activity and sedentary behavior in adults living with overweight and obesity: a systematic review. Obes Rev. 2023;24:e13615.
31. Baraona E, Abittan CS, Dohmen K, Moretti M, Pozzato G, Chayes ZW, Schaefer C, Lieber CS. Gender differences in pharmacokinetics of alcohol. Alcohol Clin Exp Res. 2001;25:502–7.
32. Di Federico S, Filippini T, Whelton PK, Cecchini M, Iamandii I, Boriani G, Vinceti M. Alcohol intake and blood pressure levels: a dose-response meta-analysis of nonexperimental cohort studies. Hypertension. 2023;80:1961–9.

Dyslipidemia in Women

Jeanine E. Roeters van Lennep and Kirsten B. Holven

Abstract

Lipid levels of women show a distinct pattern during different stages of their lives. Differences between women and men in lipids and lipoproteins are observed in distribution and trajectory from infancy to adulthood. Transitional periods such as the menstrual cycle, pregnancy, breastfeeding, and menopause influence lipid metabolism. Women are equally affected by hereditary dyslipidemias. Women with Familial Hypercholesterolemia, characterized by increased LDL-cholesterol levels from birth onwards, have an increased risk of atherosclerotic cardiovascular disease compared to men, most likely because of delayed diagnosis, undertreatment and treatment interruptions because of pregnancy and lactation. Hyperlipoproteinemia(a) [Lp(a)] is an independent risk factor of atherosclerotic cardiovascular disease. AlthoughLlp(a) levels are mainly genetically determined and considered to be stable, Lp(a) levels increase in women after menopause. Despite evidence that lipid lowering treatment is equally effective in women and men, women are undertreated with a result not reaching their LDL-cholesterol targets. Women are less often prescribed statins and other lipid lowering medications, are less likely to be prescribed potent statins and combination lipid lowering therapy.

Keywords

Dyslipidemia · Cholesterol · Treatment · Risk factor

Test your learning and check your understanding of this book's contents: use the "Springer Nature Flashcards" app to access questions using ▶ https://sn.pub/51ny7m
To use the app, please follow the instructions in chapter 1.

J. E. Roeters van Lennep (✉)
Department of Internal Medicine, Erasmus MC, University Medical Center, Rotterdam, The Netherlands
e-mail: j.roetersvanlennep@erasmusmc.nl

K. B. Holven
Department of Nutrition, Institute for Basic Medical Science, University of Oslo and National Advisory Unit on FH, Oslo University Hospital, Oslo, Norway

A. H.E.M. Maas, E. Gerdts (eds.), *Manual of Cardiovascular Disease in Women*, https://doi.org/10.1007/978-3-031-65952-2_5

1 Introduction

The two main types of lipids in the body are triglycerides and cholesterol. The main function of triglycerides is energy storage, while cholesterol plays a crucial role as a component of plasma membranes and as a precursor for various substances like bile acids, oxysterols, and steroid hormones, including sex hormones. Since both triglycerides and cholesterol are hydrophobic, they require transportation in the bloodstream by lipoproteins, which are hydrophilic particles. Lipoproteins consist of a central hydrophobic core of non-polar lipids (primarily cholesterol esters and triglycerides) surrounded by phospholipids, apolipoproteins, and free cholesterol. Apolipoproteins facilitate the formation and function of lipoproteins. The synthesis and metabolism of lipoproteins occur through both the exogenous and endogenous pathways.

Plasma lipoproteins can be classified into different types based on their size, lipid composition, and apolipoprotein content. The largest triglyceride-rich lipoproteins are chylomicrons and very-low-density lipoproteins (VLDL), which cannot cross the endothelium and are considered non-atherogenic. However, chylomicrons- and VLDL-remnants, low-density lipoprotein (LDL) and lipoprotein(a) [Lp(a)]contribute to the development and progression of atherosclerosis and subsequent cardiovascular events. On the other hand, high-density lipoprotein (HDL) generally exhibits anti-atherosclerotic properties. However, HDL is a highly heterogeneous lipoprotein with effects extending beyond lipid metabolism, including involvement in wound healing, coagulation, and inflammation.

This chapter provides a comprehensive overview of lipids and their role in women's health, We will explore the variations in lipid levels of women during different stages of their lives. Specifically, we will discuss how transitional periods such as the menstrual cycle, pregnancy, breastfeeding, and menopause influence lipid metabolism. These periods are known to have significant impact on lipid profiles, and understanding these changes is crucial for comprehending the physiological and metabolic adaptations that occur in women.

We will also emphasize the importance of lipid-lowering treatments in women. Addressing dyslipidemia and effectively managing lipid levels in women is vital for reducing their risk of cardiovascular disease. We will review various treatment options and strategies that can effectively lower lipid levels and mitigate the associated cardiovascular risks. Furthermore, we will discuss the most significant inherited lipid disorders and their effects on women. These genetic conditions can disrupt lipid metabolism and result in substantial health implications. Understanding the specific challenges faced by women with inherited lipid disorders is essential to optimize management, and to provide personalized treatment. By examining lipid levels during different stages of a woman's life, understanding the importance of lipid-lowering treatments, and exploring the impact of inherited lipid disorders on women, we aim to enhance knowledge and promote targeted approaches to optimize lipid management and eventually improve cardiovascular health outcomes for women.

2 Epidemiology Lipids During Life Course

Differences between women and men in lipids and lipoproteins are observed in distribution and trajectory from infancy to adulthood (Fig. 1). Already in cord blood, the majority of studies find that the levels are higher in cord blood in female infants compared to male infants even though the levels of total cholesterol are very low (between 1.6 mmol/l and 2.0 mmol/l) [3–6]. Cholesterol levels increases rapidly during the first two years of life and remain relatively stable until puberty. During the entire childhood and adolescence, girls have higher total and LDL-cholesterol levels than boys [1, 7]. At onset of puberty, the cholesterol levels (total-, LDL- and non-HDL cholesterol) decline in both girls and boys. HDL-cholesterol declines only among the boys but remain stable in girls in this period.

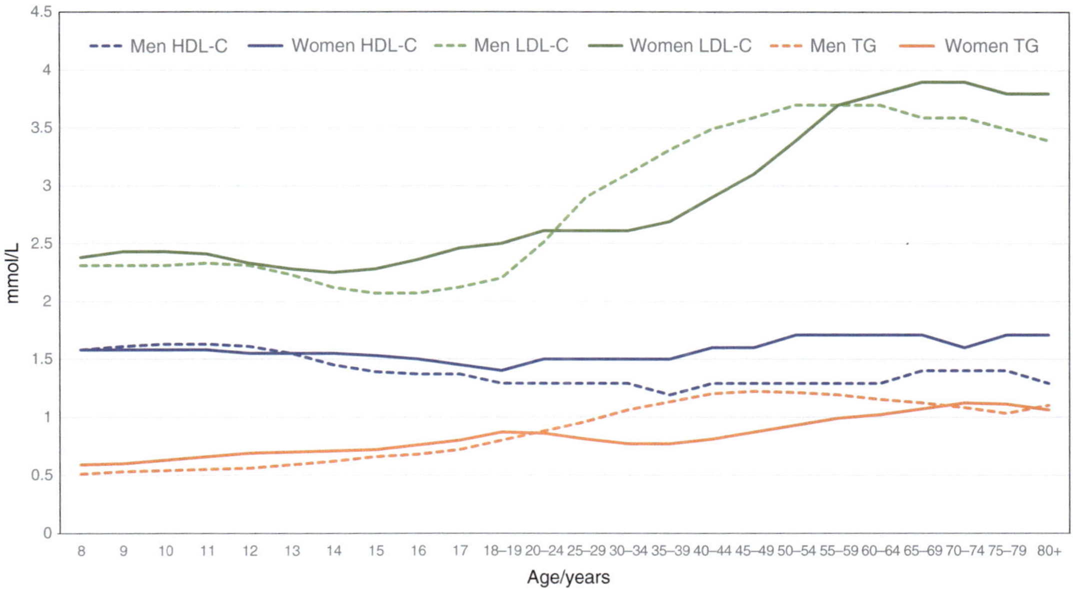

Fig. 1 LDL-cholesterol, HDL-cholesterol and triglyceride levels across the life course for women and men (source Balder et al. [1, 2])

Puberty is associated with an increase in triglycerides in both sexes [1, 8]. From the age of around 20 years, total and LDL -cholesterol levels increase more steeply among men and total and LDL-cholesterol levels exceed the levels of women until around early fifties where the levels in women again is higher than the men [2]. From the mid-fifties and up until old age, women have higher total and LDL-cholesterol levels than men. In men, triglyceride levels increase from the early twenties and remain higher than female levels, leading to an overall more adverse lipid profile from 20 to 55 year of age [2].

3 Women Specific Aspects of Dyslipidemia

3.1 Contraceptives

Both estrogen and progesterone have effects on lipid levels. Estrogen is associated with increases of triglycerides and HDL-cholesterol levels and a decrease in total cholesterol and LDL-cholesterol levels. This is due to the effect of estrogen increases the production of the VLDL—a triglyceride-rich liporoprotein—in the liver but also upregulating LDL-receptor expression enhancing hepatic uptake of LDL [9, 10]. Moreover, estrogen is associated with increased HDL-cholesterol levels which is attributed to augmentation of apolipoprotein A-I secretion, the major apolipoprotein of HDL [11]. Higher doses of estrogen cause more increase of triglycerides and HDL-cholesterol and more decrease in LDL-cholesterol levels [12]. The effect of the combination oral contraceptive pill on lipid levels depends on the dose of estrogen and type of progesterone. Depending on the type and androgenicity of the progesterone the positive lipid effects of estrogen are counteracted.

Overall, progesteron-only contraceptives, both oral and intra-uterine administration, are associated with no clinical significant effects on lipid levels [13, 14].

For Clinical Practice

It is important to discuss safe contraception timely in girls and women with dyslipidemia and/or who use lipid lowering therapy, based on the preferences of the patient in shared decision. There is no contraindication for girls and women with hypercholesterolemia to use the oral contraceptive pill. In women with hypertriglyceridemia, triglycerides should be monitored closely and if level increase, estrogen-free contraception should be considered.

3.2 Menstrual Cycle

Many—mostly small studies—assessed the effect of the menstrual cycle on serum lipids levels in healthy women with a regular cycle. Most studies observed that total cholesterol and LDL-cholesterol levels were highest in the follicular phase before ovulation, and lowest in the luteal phase after ovulation [15–22]. These changes were small: total cholesterol levels declined by on average 3% and LDL-cholesterol levels on average by 5%. HDL-cholesterol levels are highest during ovulation and remain relatively stable during the luteal phase. Even though in women with low to normal cholesterol levels the variation in lipid levels in modest, these can be aggravated in women with elevated cholesterol levels.

For Clinical Practice
Consider to measure lipid levels every time in the same phase of the menstrual cycle in women with hypercholesterolemia. Take into account that LDL-cholesterol levels are highest in the follicular phase before ovulation and lowest at the end of the luteal phase.

3.3 PolyCystic Ovarian Syndrome (PCOS)

Women with PCOS cluster components of the metabolic syndrome including obesity, insulin-resistance/diabetes type 2 and hypertension. Having PCOS is associated with an atherogenic lipid profile with low HDL cholesterol levels and elevate triglyceride levels and in some studies but not all, also increased LDL cholesterol levels [23, 24]. Most studies showed that even after adjustment for BMI, women with PCOS have a more adverse lipid profile compared to women without PCOS, especially those with hyperandrogenism [23, 25].

For Clinical Practice
Cardiovascular risk factor screening including assessment of dyslipidemia is warranted for women with PCOS [24]. *Lifestyle interventions in women with PCOS have a favorable effect on weight and lipids* [26]. *Therefore lifestyle intervention is recommended as first line-therapy for women with PCOS who are overweight or obese.*

3.4 Pregnancy and Breast Feeding

During pregnancy large physiological changes occur due to the increased fetal demands. There is a slight decrease in lipid levels very early in the pregnancy, however from 2 months into the pregnancy total-, LDL- and HDL-cholesterol as well as triglycerides levels increase considerably until delivery. Total and LDL-cholesterol levels increase approximately 40–60%, HDL cholesterol-with 20–40% and triglyceride levels increase more than 100% from conception to delivery [27]. Lipid levels then return to pre-pregnancy levels after a few months [27, 28]. In addition to the well-known beneficial effects from the infant, breastfeeding is related to favorable metabolic effects in the lactating woman such as positive effects on glucose metabolism, lipid profile, body weight and body composition [29]. Breastfeeding leads to an improved lipid profile with more reduction in LDL-cholesterol and triglycerides and less reduction of HDL-cholesterol compared with to women who did not breastfeed or breastfed for short duration [29].

Current guidelines recommend that statin therapy should be discontinued when planning pregnancy, during pregnancy and during the breastfeeding period [30]. Although recently, the US Food and Drug Administration (FDA) updated their guidance to allow for more flexible options for shared decision making in highest-risk women during pregnancy, the FDA also acknowledges the lack of data on the efficacy, risks, and benefits of statin therapy during pregnancy and the need for more research, both into safety for the fetus and adverse effect on high-risk women without effective lipid lowering therapy. The European Medicines Agency has so far not responded to the statement of the FDA. For now, therefore as yet the recommendation is to stop statin therapy during pregnancy and breastfeeding [31].

For Clinical Practice
It is important to counsel inform women of reproductive age who use statin therapy that they should stop treatment when they have a wish to conceive. Health care professionals should be aware of the physiological increase of lipid levels due to pregnancy. To acquire representative lipid levels, measure lipid levels >3 months after pregnancy. Stimulate breastfeeding and in addition to the positive health effects for the baby, mention the favorable metabolic effects for the mother.

3.5 Menopause and Hormone Replacement Therapy

The menopausal transition is associated with adverse metabolic characteristic including a more atherogenic lipid profile. It is still a scientific debate whether these changes are merely driven by chronological aging or menopause itself. The increase of cholesterol, LDL-cholesterol and apoB levels seem independent of age and independently driven by the menopausal transition per se [32]. A meta-analysis showed that compared to premenopausal women, postmenopausal women have 0.58 mmol/L higher total cholesterol and 0.45 mmol/L LDL-cholesterol levels [33]. Lipid changes occur primarily during the later phases of menopause. Although women who have a high BMI have higher lipid levels before the menopausal transition, women with normal BMI show the highest increase in lipid levels during menopausal transition [34].

Early menopause is a risk factor for cardiovascular disease, especially women who have premature ovarian failure and experience menopause <40 years [35]. The increase in lipid levels is likely one of the driving factors for this risk. Menopausal hormone therapy (MHT) -both oral and transdermal administrated- reduce LDL-cholesterol levels, but only oral MHT increase HDL-cholesterol and triglyceride levels [36].

For Clinical Practice
It is important to monitor lipid levels during the menopausal transition and assess the effect of MHT on lipid levels.

3.6 Inherited Dyslipidemia

The most common inherited dyslipidemias are Familial Hypercholesterolemia (FH) and elevated lipoproteinemia(a) (lp[a]). Both are associated with an increased risk of premature cardiovascular disease. The prevalence of inherited dyslipidemias is similar for women and men, however both sex and gender play a role in diagnosis, treatment and outcome of these conditions.

3.7 Familial Hypercholesterolemia (FH)

FH is an autosomal dominant disease leading to elevated total and LDL cholesterol levels from birth. As LDL-cholesterol is a causal risk factor of atherosclerotic cardiovascular disease (ASCVD), individuals with FH have a markedly increased risk of premature ASCVD [37]. The excess ASCVD risk in FH seems to be higher in female FH patients compared to male FH patients [37–39]. Possible reasons for this excess are later diagnosis, undertreatment with lipid lowering medication, and treatment interruptions because of pregnancy and breast-feeding [40, 41]. The levels of total and LDL-cholesterol are low at birth also in newborn children with FH, however still higher than in normal children [42]. The difference are, however not large enough to be diagnostic per se. After one year of age, the plasma levels of total and LDL-cholesterol are increased and reaching adult levels with levels of total and LDL-cholesterol ranging from 7–11 mmol/L and 5–9 mmol/L, respectively [42]. As in healthy children, girls have higher levels of total and LDL-cholesterol than boys during childhood and adolescence [43]. However, in contrast to healthy children the difference in cholesterol levels are considerable: with girls having approximate 0.5

mmol/L higher total cholesterol and 0.4 mmol/L higher LDL-cholesterol levels than boys [43], leading to an increased LDL-cholesterol burden in young women with FH compared to young men with FH [44].

During pregnancy women with FH show the same percentage increase in lipid levels as women without FH [45]. However due to the discontinuation of statin during pregnancy and the physiological increase, plasma levels of LDL-cholesterol are typically above 8 mmol/L from week 30 gestation until delivery [45].

Fewer women with FH breastfeed and they breastfeed for a shorter duration than women in the general population [41].

For Clinical Practice
Extra efforts should be made to diagnose and treat women with FH timely and that LDL-cholesterol targets are achieved. It is essential that women with FH are closely monitored before, during and after pregnancy to minimize time off statin treatment.

3.8 Lipoprotein (a)

Lipoprotein "little a" [Lp(a)] is an LDL-like particle covalently bound to plasminogen-like apolipoprotein(a). Epidemiological and genetic evidence show a causal association between elevated Lp(a) levels and cardiovascular disease independent of other risk factors [46]. Lp(a) is associated with calcification of the aortic valve and has proinflammatory and proatherogenic properties. The levels of Lp(a) are predominantly genetically determined with approximately 20% of the adult population having high levels (>42 mg/dL or >88 nmol/L).

Cord blood and neonatal levels of Lp(a) are very low but reaching adult levels at 15 months of age [47]. Generally, women have 5–10% higher Lp(a) levels than men. In women, the levels increase after menopause, whereas in men and the levels remain relatively stable throughout life [46]. Hormone replacement therapy improves lipid profile by reducing both Lp(a) levels and concentration of atherogenic lipoproteins [48].

In a recent consensus from the Eupopean Atherosclerosis Society (EAS), it is recommended to measure Lp(a) level once in all adults. At present, there are no specific Lp(a) lowering therapy available so early intensive risk factor management according to global ASCVD risk is recommended [46].

For Clinical Practice
Consider to remeasure Lp(a) level after the menopausal transition and/or after discontinuation of hormone replacement therapy.

4 Treatment

Although the inclusion of women in randomized controlled trials (RCTs) of lipid lowering therapies is increasing, women remain to be underrepresented in RCTs [49]. A meta-analysis showed that statin therapy is as effective in women as in men in lowering atherosclerotic cardiovascular disease risk [50]. However, women at high risk for ASCVD are less likely than men to be prescribed any statin therapy or to receive a statin at guideline-recommended intensity [51, 52], and more likely to refuse or discontinue statin treatment due to reported side effects [51, 53, 54]. Notably, women describe different side effects of statins compared to men [55]. Women more often report that their health care professional did not provide information about the risk of cardiovascular disease and the relation to cholesterol levels and are more often dissatisfied with the explanation about lipid lowering treatment [56]. This is especially important that a large proportion of the statin-attributed side effects are due to the nocebo effect [57, 58].

For Clinical Practice
It is essential to inform women about the relation between cholesterol and cardiovascular risk, the benefit of statin therapiy and the existence of the nocebo effect. Monitor women and up-titrate lipid lowering therapy until LDL-cholesterol targets are reached.

5 Conclusion

Sex and gender should be acknowledged as an integral part of lipid research as well as dyslipidemia management as both play a role in all aspects of dyslipidemia ranging from the effect of sex hormones on the lipid metabolism, to the attitude of women toward lipid lowering therapy. Currently knowledge which pathways within the lipid metabolism are influenced by sex hormones is incomplete. Therefore the effect of female specific conditions (such as pregnancy, menstrual cycle and menopause) on lipid levels is also not fully known, also because this has been a research area which was neglected for a long time. For optimal clinical management of dyslipidemia it is essential to increase the number of women participating in clinical trials for (new) lipid lowering medication to ensure optimal safety and efficacy of these drugs for women.

Key Issues

- Women are characterized by a more atherogenic lipid profile from infancy to early adulthood and from middle age to old age.
- Lipid levels are affected by specific transition periods in girls/women such as the menstrual cycle, pregnancy, breastfeeding and menopause.
- Dyslipidemia is a major cardiovascular risk factor for women, but many women are undertreated and do not reach target LDL-cholesterol levels

Questions and Answers

1. During early puberty, total- and LDL-cholesterol levels
   (A) Do not change
   (B) Increase in both sexes
   (C) Decline in both sexes
   (D) Increase only in women
   (E) Decline only in women
   Correct answer c)
2. What is the main determinant of Lp(a) in plasma?
   (A) Diet is the main regulator of Lp(a) levels
   (B) Exercise is the main regulator of Lp(a) levels
   (C) Lp(a) is primarily genetically determined
   (D) Sex is the main determinant of Lp(a)
   Correct answer c)
3. Why do women less often reach LDL-cholesterol targets?
   (A) Statins are less often prescribed
   (B) High potency statins are less often prescribed
   (C) Combination lipid lowering therapy is less often prescribed
   (D) All of the above
   Correct answer d)

References

1. Balder JW, Lansberg PJ, Hof MH, Wiegman A, Hutten BA, Kuivenhoven JA. Pediatric lipid reference values in the general population: The Dutch lifelines cohort study. J Clin Lipidol. 2018;12(5):1208–16.
2. Balder JW, de Vries JK, Nolte IM, Lansberg PJ, Kuivenhoven JA, Kamphuisen PW. Lipid and lipoprotein reference values from 133,450 Dutch Lifelines participants: age- and gender-specific baseline lipid values and percentiles. J Clin Lipidol. 2017;11(4):1055–64.
3. Khoury J, Henriksen T, Christophersen B, Tonstad S. Effect of a cholesterol-lowering diet on maternal, cord, and neonatal lipids, and pregnancy outcome: a randomized clinical trial. Am J Obstet Gynecol. 2005;193(4):1292–301.
4. Bastida S, Sanchez-Muniz FJ, Cuesta C, Perea S, Aragones A. Male and female cord blood lipoprotein profile differences throughout the term-period. J Perinat Med. 1997;25(2):184–91.
5. Felzer-Kim IT, Visker JR, Ferguson DP, Hauck JL. Infant blood lipids: a systematic review of predictive value and influential factors. Expert Rev Cardiovasc Ther. 2020;18(7):381–94.
6. Oyri LKL, Bogsrud MP, Christensen JJ, Ulven SM, Brantsaeter AL, Retterstol K, et al. Novel associations between parental and newborn cord blood metabolic profiles in the Norwegian Mother, Father and Child Cohort Study. BMC Med. 2021;19(1):91.
7. Dathan-Stumpf A, Vogel M, Hiemisch A, Thiery J, Burkhardt R, Kratzsch J, et al. Pediatric reference data of serum lipids and prevalence of dyslipidemia: results from a population-based cohort in Germany. Clin Biochem. 2016;49(10-11):740–9.
8. Berenson GS, Srinivasan SR, Cresanta JL, Foster TA, Webber LS. Dynamic changes of serum lipoproteins in children during adolescence and sexual maturation. Am J Epidemiol. 1981;113(2):157–70.

9. Inukai T, Takanashi K, Takebayashi K, Tayama K, Aso Y, Takiguchi Y, et al. Estrogen markedly increases LDL-receptor activity in hypercholesterolemic patients. J Med. 2000;31(5-6):247–61.
10. Schaefer EJ, Foster DM, Zech LA, Lindgren FT, Brewer HB Jr, Levy RI. The effects of estrogen administration on plasma lipoprotein metabolism in premenopausal females. J Clin Endocrinol Metab. 1983;57(2):262–7.
11. Lamon-Fava S, Ordovas JM, Schaefer EJ. Estrogen increases apolipoprotein (apo) A-I secretion in hep G2 cells by modulating transcription of the apo A-I gene promoter. Arterioscler Thromb Vasc Biol. 1999;19(12):2960–5.
12. Godsland IF, Crook D, Simpson R, Proudler T, Felton C, Lees B, et al. The effects of different formulations of oral contraceptive agents on lipid and carbohydrate metabolism. N Engl J Med. 1990;323(20):1375–81.
13. Palacios S, Colli E, Regidor PA. Metabolic and laboratory effects of a progestin-only pill containing drospirenone 4 mg in comparison to desogestrel 75 microg: a double-blind, double-dummy, prospective, randomised study. Eur J Contracept Reprod Health Care. 2021;26(6):454–61.
14. Ng YW, Liang S, Singh K. Effects of Mirena (levonorgestrel-releasing intrauterine system) and Ortho Gynae T380 intrauterine copper device on lipid metabolism–a randomized comparative study. Contraception. 2009;79(1):24–8.
15. Barnett JB, Woods MN, Lamon-Fava S, Schaefer EJ, McNamara JR, Spiegelman D, et al. Plasma lipid and lipoprotein levels during the follicular and luteal phases of the menstrual cycle. J Clin Endocrinol Metab. 2004;89(2):776–82.
16. Jones DY, Judd JT, Taylor PR, Campbell WS, Nair PP. Menstrual cycle effect on plasma lipids. Metabolism. 1988;37(1):1–2.
17. Lebech AM, Kjaer A. Lipid metabolism and coagulation during the normal menstrual cycle. Horm Metab Res. 1989;21(8):445–8.
18. Muesing RA, Forman MR, Graubard BI, Beecher GR, Lanza E, McAdam PA, et al. Cyclic changes in lipoprotein and apolipoprotein levels during the menstrual cycle in healthy premenopausal women on a controlled diet. J Clin Endocrinol Metab. 1996;81(10):3599–603.
19. Mumford SL, Schisterman EF, Siega-Riz AM, Browne RW, Gaskins AJ, Trevisan M, et al. A longitudinal study of serum lipoproteins in relation to endogenous reproductive hormones during the menstrual cycle: findings from the BioCycle study. J Clin Endocrinol Metab. 2010;95(9):E80–5.
20. Tonolo G, Ciccarese M, Brizzi P, Milia S, Dessole S, Puddu L, et al. Cyclical variation of plasma lipids, apolipoproteins, and lipoprotein(a) during menstrual cycle of normal women. Am J Phys. 1995;269(6 Pt 1):E1101–5.
21. Vashishta S, Gahlot S, Goyal R. Effect of menstrual cycle phases on plasma lipid and lipoprotein levels in regularly menstruating women. J Clin Diagn Res. 2017;11(5):CC5–7.
22. Woods M, Schaefer EJ, Morrill A, Goldin BR, Longcope C, Dwyer JD, et al. Effect of menstrual cycle phase on plasma lipids. J Clin Endocrinol Metab. 1987;65(2):321–3.
23. Wild RA, Rizzo M, Clifton S, Carmina E. Lipid levels in polycystic ovary syndrome: systematic review and meta-analysis. Fertil Steril. 2011;95(3):1073–9.
24. Wekker V, van Dammen L, Koning A, Heida KY, Painter RC, Limpens J, et al. Long-term cardiometabolic disease risk in women with PCOS: a systematic review and meta-analysis. Hum Reprod Update. 2020;26(6):942–60.
25. Krentowska A, Kowalska I. Metabolic syndrome and its components in different phenotypes of polycystic ovary syndrome. Diabetes Metab Res Rev. 2022;38(1):e3464.
26. Khatlani K, Njike V, Costales VC. Effect of lifestyle intervention on cardiometabolic risk factors in overweight and obese women with polycystic ovary syndrome: a systematic review and meta-analysis. Metab Syndr Relat Disord. 2019;17(10):473–85.
27. Wiznitzer A, Mayer A, Novack V, Sheiner E, Gilutz H, Malhotra A, et al. Association of lipid levels during gestation with preeclampsia and gestational diabetes mellitus: a population-based study. Am J Obstet Gynecol. 2009;201(5):482.
28. Wang Q, Wurtz P, Auro K, Makinen VP, Kangas AJ, Soininen P, et al. Metabolic profiling of pregnancy: cross-sectional and longitudinal evidence. BMC Med. 2016;14(1):205.
29. Gunderson EP, Lewis CE, Wei GS, Whitmer RA, Quesenberry CP, Sidney S. Lactation and changes in maternal metabolic risk factors. Obstet Gynecol. 2007;109(3):729–38.
30. Visseren FLJ, Mach F, Smulders YM, Carballo D, Koskinas KC, Back M, et al. 2021 ESC guidelines on cardiovascular disease prevention in clinical practice. Eur Heart J. 2021;42(34):3227–337.
31. https://www.fda.gov/drugs/drug-safety-and-availability/fda-requests-removal-strongest-warning-against-using-cholesterol-lowering-statins-during-pregnancy.
32. Matthews KA, Crawford SL, Chae CU, Everson-Rose SA, Sowers MF, Sternfeld B, et al. Are changes in cardiovascular disease risk factors in midlife women due to chronological aging or to the menopausal transition? J Am Coll Cardiol. 2009;54(25):2366–73.
33. Ambikairajah A, Walsh E, Cherbuin N. Lipid profile differences during menopause: a review with meta-analysis. Menopause. 2019;26(11):1327–33.
34. Derby CA, Crawford SL, Pasternak RC, Sowers M, Sternfeld B, Matthews KA. Lipid changes during the menopause transition in relation to age and weight: the Study of Women's Health Across the Nation. Am J Epidemiol. 2009;169(11):1352–61.
35. Roeters van Lennep JE, Heida KY, Bots ML, Hoek A, Dutch Multidisciplinary Guideline Development Group on Cardiovascular Risk Management after Reproductive D. Cardiovascular disease risk in women with premature ovarian insufficiency: a sys-

tematic review and meta-analysis. Eur J Prev Cardiol. 2016;23(2):178–86.
36. Goldstajn MS, Mikus M, Ferrari FA, Bosco M, Uccella S, Noventa M, et al. Effects of transdermal versus oral hormone replacement therapy in postmenopause: a systematic review. Arch Gynecol Obstet. 2022;307(6):1727–45.
37. Iyen B, Qureshi N, Weng S, Roderick P, Kai J, Capps N, et al. Sex differences in cardiovascular morbidity associated with familial hypercholesterolaemia: a retrospective cohort study of the UK Simon Broome register linked to national hospital records. Atherosclerosis. 2020;315:131–7.
38. Ahmad Z, Li X, Wosik J, Mani P, Petr J, McLeod G, et al. Premature coronary heart disease and autosomal dominant hypercholesterolemia: increased risk in women with LDLR mutations. J Clin Lipidol. 2016;10(1):101–8.
39. Mundal L, Sarancic M, Ose L, Iversen PO, Borgan JK, Veierod MB, et al. Mortality among patients with familial hypercholesterolemia: a registry-based study in Norway, 1992-2010. J Am Heart Assoc. 2014;3(6):e001236.
40. Collaboration EASFHS. Global perspective of familial hypercholesterolaemia: a cross-sectional study from the EAS Familial Hypercholesterolaemia Studies Collaboration (FHSC). Lancet. 2021;398(10312):1713–25.
41. Klevmoen M, Bogsrud MP, Retterstol K, Svilaas T, Vesterbekkmo EK, Hovland A, et al. Loss of statin treatment years during pregnancy and breastfeeding periods in women with familial hypercholesterolemia. Atherosclerosis. 2021;335:8–15.
42. Vuorio AF, Miettinen TA, Turtola H, Oksanen H, Gylling H. Cholesterol metabolism in normal and heterozygous familial hypercholesterolemic newborns. J Lab Clin Med. 2002;140(1):35–42.
43. Holven KB, Narverud I, van Lennep JR, Versmissen J, Oyri LKL, Galema-Boers A, et al. Sex differences in cholesterol levels from birth to 19 years of age may lead to increased cholesterol burden in females with FH. J Clin Lipidol. 2018;12(3):748–55.
44. Johansen AK, Bogsrud MP, Christensen JJ, Narverud I, Langslet G, Retterstol K, et al. Young women with familial hypercholesterolemia have higher LDL-cholesterol burden than men: Novel data using repeated measurements during 12-years follow-up. Atherosclerosis Plus. 2023;51:28–34.
45. Amundsen AL, Khoury J, Iversen PO, Bergei C, Ose L, Tonstad S, et al. Marked changes in plasma lipids and lipoproteins during pregnancy in women with familial hypercholesterolemia. Atherosclerosis. 2006;189(2):451–7.
46. Kronenberg F, Mora S, Stroes ESG, Ference BA, Arsenault BJ, Berglund L, et al. Lipoprotein(a) in atherosclerotic cardiovascular disease and aortic stenosis: a European Atherosclerosis Society consensus statement. Eur Heart J. 2022;43(39):3925–46.
47. Strandkjaer N, Hansen MK, Nielsen ST, Frikke-Schmidt R, Tybjaerg-Hansen A, Nordestgaard BG, et al. Lipoprotein(a) levels at birth and in early childhood: the COMPARE study. J Clin Endocrinol Metab. 2022;107(2):324–35.
48. Gregersen I, Hoibraaten E, Holven KB, Lovdahl L, Ueland T, Mowinckel MC, et al. Effect of hormone replacement therapy on atherogenic lipid profile in postmenopausal women. Thromb Res. 2019;184:1–7.
49. Khan SU, Khan MZ, Raghu Subramanian C, Riaz H, Khan MU, Lone AN, et al. Participation of women and older participants in randomized clinical trials of lipid-lowering therapies: a systematic review. JAMA Netw Open. 2020;3(5):e205202.
50. Cholesterol Treatment Trialists C, Fulcher J, O'Connell R, Voysey M, Emberson J, Blackwell L, et al. Efficacy and safety of LDL-lowering therapy among men and women: meta-analysis of individual data from 174,000 participants in 27 randomised trials. Lancet. 2015;385(9976):1397–405.
51. Nanna MG, Wang TY, Xiang Q, Goldberg AC, Robinson JG, Roger VL, et al. Sex differences in the use of statins in community practice. Circ Cardiovasc Qual Outcomes. 2019;12(8):e005562.
52. Schreuder MM, Hamkour S, Siegers KE, Holven KB, Johansen AK, van de Ree MA, et al. LDL cholesterol targets rarely achieved in familial hypercholesterolemia patients: a sex and gender-specific analysis. Atherosclerosis. 2023;384:117117.
53. Bradley CK, Wang TY, Li S, Robinson JG, Roger VL, Goldberg AC, et al. Patient-reported reasons for declining or discontinuing statin therapy: insights from the PALM registry. J Am Heart Assoc. 2019;8(7):e011765.
54. Navar AM, Peterson ED, Li S, Robinson JG, Roger VL, Goldberg AC, et al. Prevalence and management of symptoms associated with statin therapy in community practice: insights from the PALM (patient and provider assessment of lipid management) registry. Circ Cardiovasc Qual Outcomes. 2018;11(3):e004249.
55. de Vries ST, Denig P, Ekhart C, Burgers JS, Kleefstra N, Mol PGM, et al. Sex differences in adverse drug reactions reported to the National Pharmacovigilance Centre in the Netherlands: an explorative observational study. Br J Clin Pharmacol. 2019;85(7):1507–15.
56. Karalis DG, Wild RA, Maki KC, Gaskins R, Jacobson TA, Sponseller CA, et al. Gender differences in side effects and attitudes regarding statin use in the understanding statin use in America and gaps in patient education (USAGE) study. J Clin Lipidol. 2016;10(4):833–41.
57. Herrett E, Williamson E, Brack K, Perkins A, Thayne A, Shakur-Still H, et al. The effect of statins on muscle symptoms in primary care: the StatinWISE series of 200 N-of-1 RCTs. Health Technol Assess. 2021;25(16):1–62.
58. Wood FA, Howard JP, Finegold JA, Nowbar AN, Thompson DM, Arnold AD, et al. N-of-1 trial of a statin, placebo, or no treatment to assess side effects. N Engl J Med. 2020;383(22):2182–4.

Diabetes in Women

Carola Deischinger, Jürgen Harreiter, and Alexandra Kautzky-Willer

Abstract

Diabetes mellitus does not only double the risk to develop a cardiovascular disease (CVD) but also leads to a relative risk increase in coronary heart disease in females compared to males. Moreover, females with diabetes mellitus are more affected by cardiovascular diseases in terms of mortality and hospitalization rate than males.

Although the increased risk for females with diabetes mellitus to develop cardiovascular diseases is more and more commonly known amongst healthcare personnel, studies show that females were less likely to receive statins, aspirin, and beta blockers. Consequently, females had higher blood pressure, low density lipoprotein cholesterol, and glucose levels than males despite a higher prevalence of stroke and heart failure history. As a result, fewer females with type 2 diabetes mellitus were treated according to guidelines compared to males. Moreover, cardioprotective glucose-lowering drugs like SGLT-2 inhibitors or GLP-1 receptor agonists are less often prescribed for females with type 2 diabetes mellitus and CVD than for males.

Females with type 2 diabetes mellitus are currently less likely to receive guideline-recommended treatment and CVD risk reduction compared to males. Both males and females with type 2 diabetes mellitus require intensified efforts to screen for glucose metabolism disorders and other cardiovascular risk factors, as well as the early implementation of preventive measures and aggressive risk management strategies.

Keywords

Cardiovascular diseases · Diabetes mellitus Females · Sex differences · Gender differences

C. Deischinger · J. Harreiter
Department of Internal Medicine III, Clinical Division of Endocrinology and Metabolism, Gender Medicine Unit, Medical University of Vienna, Vienna, Austria
e-mail: carola.deischinger@meduniwien.ac.at; juergen.harreiter@meduniwien.ac.at

A. Kautzky-Willer (✉)
Department of Internal Medicine III, Clinical Division of Endocrinology and Metabolism, Gender Medicine Unit, Medical University of Vienna, Vienna, Austria

Gender Institute, Gars am Kamp, Austria
e-mail: alexandra.kautzky-willer@meduniwien.ac.at

A. H.E.M. Maas, E. Gerdts (eds.), *Manual of Cardiovascular Disease in Women*,
https://doi.org/10.1007/978-3-031-65952-2_6

Test your learning and check your understanding of this book's contents: use the "Springer Nature Flashcards" app to access questions using ▶ https://sn.pub/51ny7m To use the app, please follow the instructions in chapter 1.

1 Introduction

Type 2 diabetes mellitus is a non-communicable, chronic disease of hyperglycemia currently affecting over 8% of the world's population. Diabetes mellitus is associated with a vast array of micro- and macrovascular complications such as an increased risk to develop cardiovascular diseases (CVD) [1]. In coronary heart disease and stroke, diabetes mellitus is even a more potent risk factor in females than in males [2–4]. Diabetes mellitus does not only double the risk to develop a cardiovascular disease but also increases the risk in females by an additional 25–50% [5, 6]. Moreover, females with diabetes mellitus are more affected by cardiovascular diseases in terms of mortality and hospitalization rate than males [7, 8].The cardiovascular disease risk increase in females might be caused by a combination of behavioral, environmental and biological factors, the exact pathophysiology still remaining unclear at this point [6].

In order to mitigate cardiovascular disease risk in females, prevention and treatment of diabetes mellitus should be the focus of personalized medicine approaches. Not only do females report more adverse drug reactions (ADR) than males for medications such as metformin, glucagon like peptide 1 (GLP-1) receptor agonists and sodium glucose transporter 2 (SGLT 2) inhibitors [9–11] but also the efficacy differs between the sexes for some drugs [12].

The following book chapter aims at giving an overview of sex and gender differences in type 1 and type 2 diabetes mellitus, associated macrovascular complications as well as prevention and treatment strategies in order to further personalized, sex and gender specific medicine.

2 Theory

2.1 Sex and Gender Differences in Risk, Pathophysiology of Diabetes Mellitus

The development and pathophysiology of type 1 and type 2 diabetes mellitus exhibit several sex differences [6]. Type 1 diabetes mellitus is more prevalent in children, accounting for nearly 90% of childhood diabetes cases and 10–15% of all diabetes mellitus patients [13]. Both genetic and environmental factors contribute to the risk of developing type 1 diabetes mellitus [14]. While females are generally more prone to autoimmune diseases, type 1 diabetes mellitus rates are about 1.7 times higher in males aged 15–40 years in Europe [15, 16]. Sex hormones may play a significant role in the development of type 1 diabetes mellitus, as the sex ratio shifts from 1:1 in childhood to 1.7:1 males to females over the age of 15 years [15, 16].

Type 2 diabetes mellitus is more common in males, who are diagnosed at a younger age and lower body mass index than females [6, 17]. However, in their teenage years, females are more likely to be diagnosed with type 2 diabetes mellitus than males, with the trend gradually reversing towards a male predominance in middle age [18–20]. The origin of the sexual dimorphism in diabetes mellitus remains unclear [21].

Estrogen is believed to have a protective effect on pancreatic beta cells in both type 1 and type 2 diabetes mellitus [16]. The potential beneficial effects of estrogens on beta cells may explain the higher rates of both types of diabetes mellitus in males after puberty [22]. A potentially protective effect of estrogen is further supported by the higher incidence of type 2 diabetes mellitus in females during pre-menopause, menopause, or with premature ovarian insufficiency, and the reduced risk of diabetes mellitus in menopausal females undergoing estrogen-based hormone replacement therapy [23, 24]. Normoglycemic females show greater insulin secretion and sensitivity in oral glucose tolerance tests than males [25]. These sex-specific advantages in insulin secretion and sensitivity disappear in individuals with type 2 diabetes mellitus [26]. The increased insulin secretion might be explained by a 6% higher level of beta cells in female pancreatic biopsies compared to male pancreases [27]. Additionally, normoglycemic females exhibit a 20% increased glucagon-like-peptide 1 secretion after an oral glucose tolerance test compared to males, a sex difference that vanishes in individuals with diabetes mellitus or prediabetes [28]. Experimental studies suggest that insulin resistance/sensitivity may be influenced by estrogenic activation of the estrogen receptor alpha (ERα) pathway in insulin-sensitive tissues such as skeletal muscle, adipose tissue, and pancreatic beta cells [29, 30]. Estrogen might stimulate the synthesis and secretion of insulin and exert protective effects on pancreatic islet cells in females [31].

Other sex-specific risk factors for type 2 diabetes mellitus include polycystic ovary syndrome and gestational diabetes mellitus in females, and erectile dysfunction or low testosterone levels in males [6].

Gestational diabetes mellitus (GDM) is the most significant independent risk factor for type 2 diabetes mellitus progression in females [32]. A recent meta-analysis revealed that females with GDM had a relative risk of type 2 diabetes mellitus of 8.3 (95% confidence interval (CI) 6.5–10.6) [33]. Androgens have been linked to increased metabolic risks, primarily in the context of a balanced ratio between estrogen and androgen [34]. Low testosterone levels are also associated with an increased risk of metabolic diseases, and its supplementation can improve glucose tolerance [34]. Females and males exhibit differences in prediabetes as well [35, 36]. Females are more likely to have impaired glucose tolerance, which reflects insulin resistance after a meal, while males are more prone to impaired fasting glucose, which reflects insulin resistance in a fasted state [35, 36].

Despite exhibiting higher adiposity levels at a given BMI, younger females face lower cardiometabolic risks than males of a similar age [6, 37, 38]. Females have a greater capacity for adipose tissue expansion in gluteofemoral and subcutaneous fat, which results in better metabolic health [6, 37, 38]. While males are often diagnosed with type 2 diabetes mellitus at lower BMIs than females, the associations between obesity indices, including BMI and type 2 diabetes mellitus risk, are generally stronger in females [6, 16, 39]. Post-menopause, the fat distribution in females shifts from a gynoid to an android pattern, leading to an increased cardiometabolic risk [6, 37, 38].

High work demands and generally active jobs appear to be stronger protective factors for men, while low decision latitude is more strongly associated with type 2 diabetes mellitus development in women [6, 40]. Sedentary time is closely linked to anxiety, depressive symptoms, higher perceived interference, and lower self-efficacy, with more pronounced effects in women with type 2 diabetes mellitus [41]. Prolonged night work was associated with increased type 2 diabetes mellitus risk only in women (hazard ratio (HR) 1.46) [42], and similar results have been reported for shift work in women [43]. In conclusion, psychosocial risk factors have a more significant impact on type 2 diabetes mellitus development in women than in men.

While depression and diabetes distress are interconnected, studies have indicated that diabetes distress is considerably more common in patients with diabetes mellitus, affecting an estimated 36% of patients [44, 45]. Diabetes distress encompasses feelings of being overwhelmed by disease self-management, medications, doctor appointments, multiple medications, and concerns about potential future health issues [46, 47]. Overall, diabetes distress is prevalent among patients with type 2 diabetes mellitus (approximately 36%) and is strongly associated with comorbid depressive symptoms, anxiety, and female gender [45].

In contrast to type 1 diabetes mellitus, preventive actions can alter or even reverse the progression of type 2 diabetes mellitus [6]. Lifestyle interventions or surgery can prevent the development of type 2 diabetes mellitus and other metabolic diseases in high-risk populations [6]. Most studies do not provide data on sex differences in the effectiveness of these interventions [6]. Guidelines for treating type 2 diabetes mellitus increasingly emphasize personalized medicine, however, the patient's sex is often not considered in clinical decisions [11]. Females generally undergo bariatric surgery more often and at a lower body mass index (BMI) and younger age than males, with body image concerns being their primary motivation [48, 49]. In contrast, males cite health issues as their main reason for bariatric surgery [48, 49]. Post-surgery outcomes are comparable between sexes, but male patients experience higher morbidity and mortality rates, likely due to their older age and higher BMI at the time of surgery [50].

A systematic review and meta-analysis showed that lifestyle interventions are equally effective in both sexes, with a 40% reduction in diabetes risk and significant weight loss after 3 years [51]. However, males experienced greater improvements in specific parameters such as insulin resistance, hemoglobin A1c (HbA1c), triglycerides, and glucose tolerance in the Diabetes Prevention Program [52, 53]. A meta-analysis of 13 trials demonstrated similar weight loss percentages between sexes in weight management programs, with males losing more weight on low-fat diets and physical activity or exercise programs [54, 55]. Oral or subcutaneous pharmacological interventions like Orlistat or glucagon-like-peptide 1 (GLP-1) receptor agonists are more effective in females regarding weight reduction [54, 56].

2.2 Sex and Gender Differences in Prevention and Therapy of Diabetes Mellitus

Treatment choices should take sex differences in adverse drug reactions (ADRs) and effectiveness into account. A dramatic example includes the withdrawal of Rosiglitazone in some European countries due to increased rates of edema resulting in heart failure [57]. When taking thiazolidinediones, adverse events such as the development of edema were reported more often by females than males [58].

Females also report more ADRs with metformin, primarily gastrointestinal side effects, resulting in lower prescribed dosages [9]. Gastrointestinal side effects are more likely to be reported by females taking GLP-1 receptor agonists [10], and sodium glucose transporter 2 (SGLT2) inhibitors are associated with an increased risk of urinary tract infections, particularly in females [11].

Regarding sex differences in efficacy, males experience a greater HbA1c reduction with sulfonylureas, while females have better blood sugar control with thiazolidinediones. This effect has been demonstrated in large-scale studies such as ADOPT (a diabetes outcome progression trial) and RECORD (rosiglitazone evaluated for cardiac outcomes and regulation of glycaemia in diabetes) [58–60]. Metformin can reduce the risk of several gastrointestinal cancers, particularly colorectal cancer in females and hepatocellular cancer in males [61]. For newer oral glucose lowering therapies, a large Canadian study found greater cardiovascular effects in females using GLP-1 receptor agonists, while a meta-analysis on cardiovascular outcome trials reported similar reductions in major adverse cardiac events (MACE) for GLP-1 receptor agonists but a significantly lower reduction in MACE for females compared to males taking SGLT2 inhibitors [12, 62]. Other meta-analyses found a similar risk reduction in MACE for females and males taking SGLT2 inhibitors putting a clear emphasis on the efficacy of SGLT2 inhibitors in both sexes [63, 64]. Whether the found sex differences are due to an underrepresentation of females in cardiovascular outcome trials or can be attributed to a true sex difference remains unclear [62]. Females tend to lose more weight and experience a more pronounced reduction in fasting glucose levels and blood pressure when using GLP-1 receptor agonists [10]. Insulin therapy also exhibits sex differences, with females showing less improvement in HbA1c levels despite being more likely to experience hypoglycemic events and taking higher insulin dosages [65]. Overall, females display worse blood sugar control across various studies regardless of the type of diabetes treatment they received [65–68]. The reasons for these sex differences are unclear and vary significantly between studied populations. Potential explanations range from a higher percentage of females being illiterate, females suffering more from ADRs to a lack of health insurance and unknown factors [65–68]. In summary, diabetes mellitus therapy should be highly personalized based on sex, lifestyle, and each patient's unique set of comorbidities.

2.3 Sex and Gender Aspects in Diabetes Mellitus and Cardiovascular Diseases (CVD)

Diabetes mellitus complications can affect males and females differently. Females with diabetes report more physical and cognitive limitations and associated comorbidities than males with the condition [69]. One of the most important differences is that diabetes mellitus is a greater risk factor for non-fatal coronary heart disease and stroke in females than in males [2–4]. Females with diabetes mellitus and comorbid cardiovascular disease (CVD) experience higher mortality and hospitalization rates than males with diabetes, particularly if their diabetes mellitus was diagnosed late (at least one diabetic complication at time of diagnosis of diabetes mellitus) [7, 8].

In the general population, the risk to develop CVD is higher in males than females, especially before menopause. This "female protection" is lost though amongst females with insulin-treated diabetes mellitus [70]. In patients with type 1 diabetes mellitus, the female to male ratio for incident coronary heart disease was 2.54 [3]. Females with type 2 diabetes mellitus displayed a 25–50% greater excess risk of coronary heart disease compared to males with the same condition, although this difference has not been seen consistently in other large studies [71, 72]. Besides diabetes mellitus, risk factors for myocardial infarction such as hypertension, low physical activity, and alcohol intake display a stronger association with myocardial infarction in females than in males [73].

Although not yet diagnosed with cardiovascular disease, newly diagnosed diabetes patients already exhibit signs of atherosclerosis and increased intima-media thickness [74]. Carotid atherosclerosis is more prevalent in females with newly-diagnosed diabetes than in healthy female controls, suggesting that diabetes may reduce the protective effect of pre-menopausal females against cardiovascular disease [74]. This protective effect is partially attributed to sex hormones, but the underlying pathophysiological processes remain unclear [75]. Potential explanations include higher nitric oxide (NO) production levels in females, leading to more robust endothelium-dependent vasodilation and favorable atherosclerotic profiles [76]. Diabetes mellitus/hyperglycemia may impair endothelial function in pre-menopausal females, leading to endothelial dysfunction typically seen in males with the condition [76]. Diabetes mellitus seems to attenuate the protective effect of female sex hormones, although the exact reasons for this loss of protection still require further investigation [76]. The increased risk may be due to a combination of behavioral, environmental, and biological factors [6]. Biological causes include hyperglycemia-induced oxidative stress and elevated endothelin-1 levels, which impair vessel relaxation through vasoconstriction and platelet aggregation [77], as well as reduced NO production due to impaired insulin signaling [78]. Hyperglycemia may also modulate estrogen receptor activity [78], inhibiting estrogen's antiproliferative effects on vascular smooth muscle cells via selective estrogen receptor activation [79]. Additionally, hyperglycemia can promote the formation of advanced glycation end products (AGE) [80], which, when interacting with their receptors (RAGE), can contribute to oxidative stress, a proinflammatory environment, and accelerated atherosclerotic processes [81], ultimately leading to a loss of protective estrogen effects in females with diabetes mellitus [76, 79].

Among patients with type 2 diabetes mellitus, females also have a higher relative risk of heart failure and hospitalization due to heart failure than males [82, 83]. Hypertension is a major contributor to heart failure progression, particularly in females with hypertension compared to females without hypertension (threefold increase in risk for females vs twofold for males) [84]. Type 2 diabetes mellitus has a more significant impact on heart failure progression in females (females: 5-fold vs males: 2.4-fold risk) [85]. Females are more prone to diastolic dysfunction due to hypertension, insulin resistance, and obesity, leading to a higher frequency of heart failure with preserved ejection fraction (HFpEF) [86]. The detrimental effect of diabetes mellitus on CVD risk is especially prominent in young patients diagnosed with type 2 diabetes mellitus under the age of 40 years. These young patients have the highest excess risk for all-cause mortality, cardiovascular mortality, heart failure and CHD amongst those with diabetes mellitus. The effect is even more pronounced in young females with type 2 diabetes mellitus suggesting a heightened need for CVD risk prevention and therapy in this patient collective [87–89].

3 Clinical Practice

As a result of the ongoing rise in obesity, there has been a global surge in the number of patients with type 2 diabetes mellitus. Early detection of type 2 diabetes mellitus and accompanying cardiovascular risk factors is vital for preventing CVD events. Differences exist between males and females regarding type 2 diabetes mellitus and other cardiovascular risk factors in terms of comorbidities, complication manifestations, and initiation of and adherence to treatment.

Since females with type 2 diabetes mellitus have a higher relative risk of CVD, clinicians need to focus on more intense treatment of risk factors to reduce vascular comorbidities. For instance, greater attention should be given to blood pressure management, especially for females with obesity and type 2 diabetes mellitus, who exhibit higher cardiovascular risk at a young age. Lower treatment thresholds in females could help decrease CVD, but this requires evidence from clinical studies and follow-up. Currently, aggressive multifactorial treatment following existing guidelines is essential and must be provided to all individuals with type 2 diabetes mellitus, regardless of sex, age, or ethnicity.

Although it is well-known that females are almost similarly affected by coronary heart disease as males and the risk to develop coronary heart disease is even greater in females than males with diabetes mellitus, health professionals seem to underestimate CVD risk in females with type 2 diabetes mellitus [89]. This ultimately leads to less usage of CVD protective medications and insufficient management of CVD risk factors, which should begin as early as possible. Medication adherence and prescriptions for addressing multiple CVD risk factors are lower in females than males with type 2 diabetes mellitus. In cardiovascular outcome trials, females with type 2 diabetes mellitus were found to use statins, aspirin, and beta blockers less frequently, despite a higher prevalence of stroke and heart failure history [90]. Consequently, females had higher blood pressure, low density lipoprotein (LDL)-cholesterol, and glucose levels than males. As a result, regardless of their comorbidities, fewer females with type 2 diabetes mellitus were treated according to guidelines compared to males [90]. In a recent EUROASPIRE survey, females with type 2 diabetes mellitus or impaired glucose tolerance (IGT) were older and less likely to achieve recommended targets for physical activity, blood pressure, or LDL-cholesterol than males, possibly contributing to their higher CVD risk [91]. Furthermore, a Danish cohort study reported that cardioprotective glucose-lowering drugs like SGLT-2 inhibitors or GLP-1 receptor agonists were prescribed less often for females with type 2 diabetes mellitus and CVD [92].

Moreover, depression and diabetes distress significantly undermine diabetes management and self-care activities, especially among females. Increased awareness, better screening tools, psychological support, and research are necessary to address these gender gaps. Additionally, educational initiatives for physicians and the general public can help raise awareness of type 2 diabetes mellitus and its consequences in both males and females.

4 Conclusion

Females with diabetes mellitus lose their premenopausal "female protection" against CVD. Diabetes mellitus does not only double CVD risk but rather adds an additional 25–50% risk to females compared to males. Although guidelines for treating type 2 diabetes mellitus increasingly emphasize personalized medicine, the patient's sex is often not considered in clinical decisions. Young females with type 2 diabetes mellitus are currently less likely to receive guideline-recommended treatment and CVD risk reduction compared to males. Present medical recommendations do not offer insights on sex-specific or gender-sensitive prevention strategies and management. Consequently, additional research on sex differences, including underlying mechanisms, is necessary to strengthen future evidence. Weight management, combined with the use of effective new drugs offering cardiorenal benefits and personalized lifestyle intervention approaches, is critical for type 2 diabetes mellitus prevention and treatment in females. Nonetheless, both males and females at increased risk of type 2 diabetes mellitus still require intensified efforts to screen for glucose metabolism disorders and other cardiovascular risk factors, as well as the early implementation of preventive measures and aggressive risk management strategies.

Key Issues

- Females with diabetes mellitus lose their premenopausal "female protection" against CVD.
- Diabetes mellitus does not only double CVD risk but rather adds an additional 25–50% risk to females compared to males.
- Females report more adverse drug reactions when taking oral antidiabetic medications.
- Young females with type 2 diabetes mellitus are currently less likely to receive guideline-recommended treatment and CVD risk reduction compared to males.

Questions and Answers

1. In how far does diabetes mellitus influence the cardiovascular risk profile in females?
   (A) Females with diabetes mellitus appear to lose their "female protection" against CVD. Diabetes mellitus does not only double CVD risk but rather adds an additional 25 to 50% risk to females compared to males.
2. Please describe 2 classes of antidiabetic drugs with sex specific adverse drug reactions.
   (A) females report more ADRs than males for metformin: usually gastrointestinal side effects
   (B) more gastrointestinal side effects in females in GLP-1 agonists
   (C) increased risk to develop urinary tract infections in females when taking SGLT2 inhibitors
3. Please describe a possible prevention strategy to mitigate the increased cardiovascular risk of females with diabetes mellitus.

References

1. WHO. Global Rep Diabetes. 2016;978:6–86. https://www.who.int/publications/i/item/9789241565257.
2. Peters SAE, Huxley RR, Woodward M. Diabetes as risk factor for incident coronary heart disease in women compared with men: a systematic review and meta-analysis of 64 cohorts including 858,507 individuals and 28,203 coronary events. Diabetologia. 2014;57(8):1542–51. https://doi.org/10.1007/s00125-014-3260-6.
3. Huxley RR, Peters SAE, Mishra GD, Woodward M. Risk of all-cause mortality and vascular events in women versus men with type 1 diabetes: a systematic review and meta-analysis. Lancet Diabetes Endocrinol. 2015;3(3):198–206. https://doi.org/10.1016/S2213-8587(14)70248-7.

4. Peters SAE, Huxley RR, Woodward M. Diabetes as a risk factor for stroke in women compared with men: a systematic review and meta-analysis of 64 cohorts, including 775,385 individuals and 12 539 strokes. Lancet. 2014;383(9933):1973–80. https://doi.org/10.1016/S0140-6736(14)60040-4.
5. Woodward M, Peters SA, Huxley RR. Diabetes and the female disadvantage. Womens Health. 2015;11(6):833–9.
6. Kautzky-Willer A, Harreiter J, Pacini G. Sex and gender differences in risk, pathophysiology and complications of type 2 diabetes mellitus. Endocr Rev. 2016;37(3):278–316.
7. The DECODE Study Group. Gender difference in all-cause and cardiovascular mortality related to hyperglycaemia and newly-diagnosed diabetes. Diabetologia. 2003;46(5):608–17.
8. Roche MM, Wang PP. Sex differences in all-cause and cardiovascular mortality, hospitalization for individuals with and without diabetes, and patients with diabetes diagnosed early and late. Diabetes Care. 2013;36(9):2582–90.
9. de Vries ST, Denig P, Ekhart C, Mol PGM, van Puijenbroek EP. Sex differences in adverse drug reactions of metformin: a longitudinal survey study. Drug Saf. 2020;43(5):489–95. https://doi.org/10.1007/s40264-020-00913-8.
10. Pencek R, Blickensderfer A, Li Y, Brunell SC, Chen S. Exenatide once weekly for the treatment of type 2 diabetes: effectiveness and tolerability in patient subpopulations. Int J Clin Pract. 2012;66(11):1021–32.
11. Kautzky-Willer A, Harreiter J. Sex and gender differences in therapy of type 2 diabetes. Diabetes Res Clin Pract. 2017;131:230–41.
12. Raparelli V, Elharram M, Moura CS, Abrahamowicz M, Bernatsky S, Behlouli H, et al. Sex differences in cardiovascular effectiveness of newer glucose-lowering drugs added to metformin in type 2 diabetes mellitus. J Am Heart Assoc. 2020;9(1):e012940.
13. Katsarou A, Gudbjörnsdottir S, Rawshani A, Dabelea D, Bonifacio E, Anderson BJ, et al. Type 1 diabetes mellitus. Nat Rev Dis Prim. 2017;3:1–18. https://doi.org/10.1038/nrdp.2017.16.
14. Bilous R, Donnelly R, Idris I. Handbook of diabetes. 5th ed. Hoboken: Wiley; 2021.
15. Östman J, Lönnberg G, Arnqvist HJ, Blohme G, Bolinder J, Ekbom Schnell A, et al. Gender differences and temporal variation in the incidence of type 1 diabetes: results of 8012 cases in the nationwide Diabetes Incidence Study in Sweden. J Intern Med. 2008;263:386–94.
16. Tramunt B, Smati S, Grandgeorge N, Lenfant F, Arnal J. Sex differences in metabolic regulation and diabetes susceptibility. Diabetologia. 2020;63:453–61.
17. World Health Organization. Global status report on noncommunicable diseases 2014 - global target 7: halt the rise in diabetes and obesity; 2014, p. 78–93. Available from: http://www.who.int/nmh/publications/ncd-status-report-2014/en/.
18. Mayer-Davis EJ, Lawrence JM, Dabelea D, Divers J, Isom S, Dolan L, et al. Incidence trends of type 1 and type 2 diabetes among youths, 2002–2012. N Engl J Med. 2017;376(15):1419–29.
19. Sattar N. Gender aspects in type 2 diabetes mellitus and cardiometabolic risk. Best Pract Res Clin Endocrinol Metab. 2013;27(4):501–7.
20. Lipscombe LL, Hux JE. Trends in diabetes prevalence, incidence, and mortality in Ontario, Canada 1995-2005: a population-based study. Lancet. 2007;369(9563):750–6.
21. Williams JM, Poudel B, Shields CA. Chapter 15 - Sex differences in autoimmune type-1 diabetes. In: LaMarca B, Alexander SD, editors. Sex differences in cardiovascular physiology and pathophysiology. Academic: New York; 2019. p. 239–49. https://www.sciencedirect.com/science/article/pii/B9780128131978000154.
22. Gale EAM, Gillespie KM. Diabetes and gender. Diabetologia. 2001;44:3–15.
23. Anagnostis P, Christou K, Artzouchaltzi A, Gkekas NK. Early menopause and premature ovarian insufficiency are associated with increased risk of type 2 diabetes: a systematic review and meta-analysis. Eur J Endocrinol. 2019;180:41–50.
24. Kanaya AM, Herrington D, Vittinghoff E, Lin F, Grady D, Bittner V, et al. Glycemic effects of postmenopausal hormone therapy: the heart and estrogen/progestin replacement study: a randomized, double-blind, placebo-controlled trial. Ann Intern Med. 2003;138(1):1–9. https://doi.org/10.7326/0003-4819-138-1-200301070-00005.
25. Kautzky-Willer A, Brazzale AR, Moro E, Vrbíková J, Bendlova B, Sbrignadello S, et al. Influence of increasing BMI on insulin sensitivity and secretion in normotolerant men and women of a wide age span. Obesity. 2012;20:1966–73.
26. Tura A, Pacini G, Moro E, Vrbíková J, Bendlová B, Kautzky-Willer A. Sex- and age-related differences of metabolic parameters in impaired glucose metabolism and type 2 diabetes compared to normal glucose tolerance. Diabetes Res Clin Pract. 2018;146:67–75. https://doi.org/10.1016/j.diabres.2018.09.019.
27. Marchese E, Rodeghier C, Monson RS, Mccracken B, Shi T, Schrock W, et al. Enumerating B-cells in whole human islets: sex differences and associations with clinical outcomes after islet transplantation. Diabetes Care. 2015;38(April):176–7.
28. Færch K, Torekov SS, Vistisen D, Johansen NB, Witte DR, Jonsson A, et al. GLP-1 response to oral glucose is reduced in prediabetes, screen-detected type 2 diabetes, and obesity and influenced by sex: the ADDITION-PRO study. Diabetes. 2015;64(July):2513–25.
29. Handgraaf S, Riant E, Fabre A, Waget A, Burcelin R, Lière P, et al. Prevention of obesity and insulin resistance by estrogens requires ER a activation function-2 (ER a AF-2), whereas ER a AF-1 is dispensable. Diabetes. 2013;63:4098–108.

30. Riant E, Gourdy P. Estrogens protect against high-fat diet-induced insulin resistance and glucose intolerance in mice. Endocrinology. 2009;150:2109–17.
31. Mauvais-Jarvis F. Role of sex steroids in beta cell function, growth, and survival. Trends Endocrinol Metab. 2016;27(12):844–55. https://doi.org/10.1016/j.tem.2016.08.008.
32. McIntyre HD, Catalano P, Zhang C, Desoye G, Mathiesen ER, Damm P. Gestational diabetes mellitus. Nat Rev Dis Prim. 2019;5(1):47. https://doi.org/10.1038/s41572-019-0098-8.
33. Dennison RA, Chen ES, Green ME, Legard C, Kotecha D, Farmer G, et al. The absolute and relative risk of type 2 diabetes after gestational diabetes: a systematic review and meta-analysis of 129 studies. Diabetes Res Clin Pract. 2021;171:108625. https://doi.org/10.1016/j.diabres.2020.108625.
34. Yassin A, Haider A, Haider KS, Caliber M, Doros G, Saad F. Testosterone therapy in men with hypogonadism prevents progression from prediabetes to type 2 diabetes: eight-year data from a registry study. Diabetes Care. 2019;42(June):1104–11.
35. Mauvais-Jarvis F. Gender differences in glucose homeostasis and diabetes. Physiol Behav. 2018;187:20–3.
36. Glumer C, Jorgensen T, Borch-Johnsen K. Prevalence of diabetes and impaired glucose regulation in a Danish population. Diabetes Care. 2003;26(8):2335–40.
37. Kautzky-Willer A, Leutner M, Harreiter J. Sex differences in type 2 diabetes. Diabetologia. 2023;66(6):986–1002.
38. Goossens GH, Jocken JWE, Blaak EE. Sexual dimorphism in cardiometabolic health: the role of adipose tissue, muscle and liver. Nat Rev Endocrinol. 2021;17(1):47–66. https://doi.org/10.1038/s41574-020-00431-8.
39. Lee DH, Keum NN, Hu FB, Orav EJ, Rimm EB, Willett WC, et al. Comparison of the association of predicted fat mass, body mass index, and other obesity indicators with type 2 diabetes risk: two large prospective studies in US men and women. Eur J Epidemiol. 2018;33(11):1113–23. https://doi.org/10.1007/s10654-018-0433-5.
40. Eriksson AK, Van Den Donk M, Hilding A, Östenson CG. Work stress, sense of coherence, and risk of type 2 diabetes in a prospective study of middle-aged Swedish men and women. Diabetes Care. 2013;36(9):2683–9.
41. Indelicato L, Dauriz M, Bacchi E, Donà S, Santi L, Negri C, et al. Sex differences in the association of psychological status with measures of physical activity and sedentary behaviour in adults with type 2 diabetes. Acta Diabetol. 2018;55(6):627–35. https://doi.org/10.1007/s00592-018-1132-0.
42. Silva-Costa A, Rotenberg L, Toivanen S, Nobre AA, Barreto SM, Schmidt MI, et al. Lifetime night work exposure and the risk of type 2 diabetes: results from the longitudinal study of adult health (ELSA-Brasil). Chronobiol Int. 2020;37(9-10):1344–7. https://doi.org/10.1080/07420528.2020.1804923.
43. Gao Y, Gan T, Jiang L, Yu L, Tang D, Wang Y, et al. Association between shift work and risk of type 2 diabetes mellitus: a systematic review and dose-response meta-analysis of observational studies. Chronobiol Int. 2020;37(1):29–46. https://doi.org/10.1080/07420528.2019.1683570.
44. Fisher L, Mullan JT, Skaff MM, Glasgow RE, Arean P, Hessler D. Predicting diabetes distress in patients with type 2 diabetes mellitus: a longitudinal study. Diabet Med. 2009;26(6):622–7.
45. Perrin NE, Davies MJ, Robertson N, Snoek FJ, Khunti K. The prevalence of diabetes-specific emotional distress in people with Type 2 diabetes: a systematic review and meta-analysis. Diabet Med. 2017;34(11):1508–20.
46. Adriaanse MC, Pouwer F, Dekker JM, Nijpels G, Stehouwer CD, Heine RJ, et al. Diabetes-related symptom distress in association with glucose metabolism and comorbidity. Diabetes Care. 2008;31(12):2268–70.
47. Pouwer F. Should we screen for emotional distress in type 2 diabetes mellitus? Nat Rev Endocrinol. 2009;5(12):665–71.
48. Libeton M, Dixon JB, Laurie C, O'Brien PE. Patient motivation for bariatric surgery: characteristics and impact on outcomes. Obes Surg. 2004;14(3):392–8.
49. Stroh C, Weiner R, Wolff S, Knoll C, Manger T. Are there gender-specific aspects in obesity and metabolic surgery? Data analysis from the German bariatric surgery registry. Visz Gastrointest Med Surg. 2014;30(2):125–32.
50. Harreiter J, Kautzky-Willer A. Sex and gender differences in prevention of type 2 diabetes. Front Endocrinol. 2018;9:1–15.
51. Glechner A, Harreiter J, Gartlehner G, Rohleder S, Kautzky A, Tuomilehto J, et al. Sex-specific differences in diabetes prevention: a systematic review and meta-analysis. Diabetologia. 2015;58(2):242–54.
52. Kautzky-Willer A, Harreiter J, Abrahamian H, Weitgasser R, Fasching P, Hoppichler F, et al. Sex and gender-specific aspects in prediabetes and diabetes mellitus—clinical recommendations (update 2019). Wien Klin Wochenschr. 2019;131:221–8.
53. Perreault L, Yong M, Dagogo-Jack S, Horton E, Marrero D, Crandall J, et al. Sex differences in diabetes risk and the effect of intensive lifestyle modification in the diabetes prevention program. Diabetes Care. 2008;31(7):1416–21.
54. Robertson C, Avenell A, Boachie C, Stewart F, Archibald D, Douglas F, et al. Should weight loss and maintenance programmes be designed differently for men? A systematic review of long-term randomised controlled trials presenting data for men and women: the ROMEO project. Obes Res Clin Pract. 2016;10(1):70–84. https://doi.org/10.1016/j.orcp.2015.04.005.
55. Svetkey LP, Ard JD, Stevens VJ, Loria CM, Young DY, Hollis JF, et al. Predictors of long-term weight loss in adults with modest initial weight loss, by sex

and race. Obesity. 2012;20(9):1820–8. https://doi.org/10.1038/oby.2011.88/nature06264.
56. Buysschaert M, Preumont V, Oriot PR, Paris I, Ponchon M, Scarnière D, et al. Évolution métabolique après un an de patients diabétiques de type 2 traités par exénatide et suivis en routine clinique. Diabetes Metab. 2010;36(5):381–8. https://doi.org/10.1016/j.diabet.2010.03.009.
57. Wallach JD, Wang K, Zhang AD, Cheng D, Grossetta Nardini HK, Lin H, et al. Updating insights into rosiglitazone and cardiovascular risk through shared data: individual patient and summary level meta-analyses. BMJ. 2020;368:l7078.
58. Dennis JM, Henley WE, Weedon MN, Lonergan M, Rodgers LR, Jones AG, et al. Sex and BMI alter the benefits and risks of sulfonylureas and thiazolidinediones in type 2 diabetes: a framework for evaluating stratification using routine clinical and individual trial data. Diabetes Care. 2018;41(9):1844–53.
59. Viberti G, Lachin J, Holman R, Zinman B, Haffner S, Kravitz B, et al. A diabetes outcome progression trial (ADOPT). Diabetes Care. 2002;25(10):1737–43.
60. Home PD, Pocock SJ, Beck-Nielsen H, Gomis R, Hanefeld M, Dargie H, et al. Rosiglitazone evaluated for cardiac outcomes and regulation of glycaemia in diabetes (RECORD): study design and protocol. Diabetologia. 2005;48(9):1726–35.
61. Lee MS, Hsu CC, Wahlqvist ML, Tsai HN, Chang YH, Huang YC. Type 2 diabetes increases and metformin reduces total, colorectal, liver and pancreatic cancer incidences in Taiwanese: a representative population prospective cohort study of 800,000 individuals. BMC Cancer. 2011;11:20.
62. Singh AK, Singh R. Gender difference in cardiovascular outcomes with SGLT-2 inhibitors and GLP-1 receptor agonist in type 2 diabetes: a systematic review and meta-analysis of cardio-vascular outcome trials. Diabetes Metab Syndr Clin Res Rev. 2020;14(3):181–7.
63. Diallo A, Carlos-Bolumbu M, Galtier F. Age, sex, race, BMI, and duration of diabetes differences in cardiovascular outcomes with glucose lowering drugs in type 2 diabetes: a systematic review and meta-analysis. eClinicalMedicine. 2022;54:101697. https://doi.org/10.1016/j.eclinm.2022.101697.
64. Bhattarai M, Salih M, Regmi M, Al-Akchar M, Deshpande R, Niaz Z, et al. Association of sodium-glucose cotransporter 2 inhibitors with cardiovascular outcomes in patients with type 2 diabetes and other risk factors for cardiovascular disease: a meta-analysis. JAMA Netw Open. 2022;5(1):e2142078.
65. McGill JB, Vlajnic A, Knutsen PG, Recklein C, Rimler M, Fisher SJ. Effect of gender on treatment outcomes in type 2 diabetes mellitus. Diabetes Res Clin Pract. 2013;102(3):167–74. https://doi.org/10.1016/j.diabres.2013.10.001.
66. Kamuhabwa AR, Charles E. Predictors of poor glycemic control in type 2 diabetic patients attending public hospitals in Dar es Salaam. Drug Healthc Patient Saf. 2014;6:155–65.
67. Wexler DJ, Grant RW, Meigs JB, Nathan DM, Cagliero E. Sex disparities in treatment of cardiac risk factors in patients with type 2 diabetes. Diabetes Care. 2005;28(3):514–20.
68. Hawthorne K, Tomlinson S. Pakistani moslems with type 2 diabetes mellitus: Effect of sex, literacy skills, known diabetic complications and place of care on diabetic knowledge, reported self-monitoring management and glycaemic control. Diabet Med. 1999;16(7):591–7.
69. McCollum M, Hansen LS, Lu L, Sullivan PW. Gender differences in diabetes mellitus and effects on self-care activity. Gend Med. 2005;2(4):246–54.
70. Garcia MJ, McNamara PM, Gordon T, Kannell WB. Morbidity and mortality in diabetics in the Framingham population. Sixteen year follow up study. Diabetes. 1974;23(2):105–11.
71. Huebschmann AG, Huxley RR, Kohrt WM, Zeitler P, Regensteiner G, Reusch JEB, et al. Sex differences in the burden of type 2 diabetes and cardiovascular risk across the life course. Diabetologia. 2019;62(10):1761–72.
72. Wang Y, O'Neil A, Jiao Y, Wang L, Huang J, Lan Y, et al. Sex differences in the association between diabetes and risk of cardiovascular disease, cancer, and all-cause and cause-specific mortality: a systematic review and meta-analysis of 5,162,654 participants. BMC Med. 2019;17(1):136.
73. Rosengren A, Hawken S, Ôunpuu S, Sliwa PK, Zubaid M, Almahmeed WA, et al. Association of psychosocial risk factors with risk of acute myocardial infarction in 11,119 cases and 13,648 controls from 52 countries (the INTERHEART study): case-control study. Lancet. 2004;364(9438):953–62.
74. Catalan M, Herreras Z, Pinyol M, Sala-Vila A, Amor AJ, de Groot E, et al. Prevalence by sex of preclinical carotid atherosclerosis in newly diagnosed type 2 diabetes. Nutr Metab Cardiovasc Dis. 2015;25(8):742–8. https://doi.org/10.1016/j.numecd.2015.04.009.
75. Regitz-Zagrosek V. Therapeutic implications of the gender-specific aspects of cardiovascular disease. Nat Rev Drug Discov. 2006;5(5):425–39.
76. Steinberg HO, Paradisi G, Cronin J, Crowde K, Hempfling A, Hook G, et al. Type II diabetes abrogates sex differences in endothelial function in premenopausal women. Circulation. 2000;101(17):2040–6.
77. Cardillo C, Campia U, Bryant MB, Panza JA. Increased activity of endogenous endothelin in patients with type II diabetes mellitus. Circulation. 2002;106(14):1783–7.
78. Dantas APV, Fortes ZB, De Carvalho MHC. Vascular disease in diabetic women: why do they miss the female protection? Exp Diabetes Res. 2012;2012:570598.
79. Ortmann J, Veit M, Zingg S, Di Santo S, Traupe T, Yang Z, et al. Estrogen receptor-α but not -β or GPER inhibits high glucose-induced human VSMC proliferation: potential role of ROS and ERK. J Clin Endocrinol Metab. 2011;96(1):220–8.
80. Yamagishi S, Maeda S, Matsui T, Ueda S, Fukami K, Okuda S. Role of advanced glycation end prod-

ucts (AGEs) and oxidative stress in vascular complications in diabetes. Biochim Biophys Acta. 2012;1820(5):663–71.
81. Farmer DGS, Kennedy S. RAGE, vascular tone and vascular disease. Pharmacol Ther. 2009;124(2):185–94. https://doi.org/10.1016/j.pharmthera.2009.06.013.
82. Fujita Y, Morimoto T, Tokushige A, Ikeda M, Shimabukuro M, Node K, et al. Women with type 2 diabetes and coronary artery disease have a higher risk of heart failure than men, with a significant gender interaction between heart failure risk and risk factor management: a retrospective registry study. BMJ Open Diabetes Res Care. 2022;10(2):e002707.
83. Ohkuma T, Komorita Y, Peters SAE, Woodward M. Diabetes as a risk factor for heart failure in women and men: a systematic review and meta-analysis of 47 cohorts including 12 million individuals. Diabetologia. 2019;62(9):1550–60.
84. Levy D, Larson MG, Vasan RS, Kannel WB, Ho KKL. The progression from hypertension to congestive heart failure. JAMA. 1996;275(20):1557–62. https://doi.org/10.1001/jama.1996.03530440037034.
85. Beale AL, Meyer PMD, Marwick TH, Lam CSP, Kaye DM. Sex differences in cardiovascular pathophysiology why women are overrepresented in heart failure with preserved ejection fraction. Circulation. 2018;138(2):198–205.
86. Gerdts E, Regitz-Zagrosek V. Sex differences in cardiometabolic disorders. Nat Med. 2019;25(11):1657–66. https://doi.org/10.1038/s41591-019-0643-8.
87. Malmborg M, Schmiegelow MDS, Nørgaard CH, Munch A, Gerds T, Schou M, et al. Does type 2 diabetes confer higher relative rates of cardiovascular events in women compared with men? Eur Heart J. 2020;41(13):1346–53.
88. Sattar N, Rawshani A, Franzén S, Rawshani A, Svensson AM, Rosengren A, et al. Age at diagnosis of type 2 diabetes mellitus and associations with cardiovascular and mortality risks: findings from the swedish national diabetes registry. Circulation. 2019;139(19):2228–37.
89. Harreiter J, Fadl H, Kautzky-Willer A, Simmons D. Do women with diabetes need more intensive action for cardiovascular reduction than men with diabetes? Curr Diab Rep. 2020;20:11.
90. Clemens KK, Woodward M, Neal B, Zinman B. Sex disparities in cardiovascular outcome trials of populations with diabetes: a systematic review and meta-analysis. Diabetes Care. 2020;43(5):1157–63.
91. Ferrannini G, De Bacquer D, Vynckier P, De Backer G, Gyberg V, Kotseva K, et al. Gender differences in screening for glucose perturbations, cardiovascular risk factor management and prognosis in patients with dysglycaemia and coronary artery disease: results from the ESC-EORP EUROASPIRE surveys. Cardiovasc Diabetol. 2021;20(1):1–12. https://doi.org/10.1186/s12933-021-01233-6.
92. Funck KL, Bjerg L, Isaksen AA, Sandbæk A, Grove EL. Gender disparities in time-to-initiation of cardioprotective glucose-lowering drugs in patients with type 2 diabetes and cardiovascular disease: a Danish nationwide cohort study. Cardiovasc Diabetol. 2022;21(1):1–11. https://doi.org/10.1186/s12933-022-01713-3.

Hypertension Along Women's Life Course

Ester A. Kringeland and Eva Gerdts

Abstract

Hypertension is the most common risk factor for cardiovascular diseases (CVD) and mortality in women. In young adults, women have a lower blood pressure (BP) than men, and hypertension is uncommon. Hypertensive pregnancy complications and several fertility related factors are associated with development of hypertension in young women. From the third decade onwards BP increases more steeply in women than men. Older women have a higher BP than men at similar age, and hypertension is found in >60%. Obesity, autoimmune disorders and reduced renal function are common co-morbidities in these women. Menopausal transition results in clustering of metabolic risk factors and a transformation from low to high CVD risk in many women. Salt sensitive hypertension is particularly common in post-menopausal women. The risk for CVD increases at a lower BP level in women than in men. Although the effect of antihypertensive treatment on reduction of CVD was the same in women as in men in a meta-analysis of clinical trials, adverse antihypertensive drug effects are more prevalent among women, and BP control declines with aging in women. Taken together, women should regularly measure their BP from age 40 years onward to avoid delayed diagnosis of hypertension. Women with hypertensive pregnancy complications should thereafter measure their BP annually. Future research should document whether lower BP threshold values and treatment targets may further improve CVD prevention in women.

Keywords

Hypertension · Blood pressure regulators
Blood pressure measurement
Antihypertensive treatment

E. A. Kringeland (✉)
Department of Heart Disease, Haukeland University Hospital, Bergen, Norway

Department of Health Registry Research and Development, Norwegian Institute of Public Health, Bergen, Norway
e-mail: ester.kringeland@uib.no

E. Gerdts
Department of Clinical Science, University of Bergen, Bergen, Norway
e-mail: eva.gerdts@uib.no

A. H.E.M. Maas, E. Gerdts (eds.), *Manual of Cardiovascular Disease in Women*,
https://doi.org/10.1007/978-3-031-65952-2_7

Test your learning and check your understanding of this book's contents: use the "Springer Nature Flashcards" app to access questions using ▶ https://sn.pub/51ny7m
To use the app, please follow the instructions in chapter 1.

1 Introduction

High blood pressure (hypertension) is the most common modifiable risk factor for cardiovascular disease (CVD) in women and the leading cause of death in women worldwide [1]. The World Health Organization has defined hypertension as presence of a systolic blood pressure (BP) ≥140 mmHg or a diastolic BP ≥90 mmHg both in women and men. Hypertension is a stronger risk factor for development of cardiac organ damage like left ventricular hypertrophy and CVD like myocardial infarction, heart failure and atrial fibrillation in women than in men [2, 3].

Worldwide, the age standardized prevalence of hypertension was 32% in women and 34% in men aged 30–79 years in 2019 [4]. Although this prevalence has remained stable over the past two decades, the number of women with hypertension has more than doubled over this period as a consequence of population increase, aging and longevity. Over the past 20 years a reduction in hypertension prevalence in high income countries has been paralleled by a comparable increase in hypertension prevalence in low-income countries [4]. Nowadays, an estimated 600 million women have hypertension worldwide [4].

Worldwide treatment and control rates of hypertension have increased during the last 20 years but are still suboptimal [4]. In a global overview, rates of diagnosis, treatment and control of hypertension in women were 59%, 47% and 23%, respectively. Of note, both diagnosis and treatment rates of hypertension were lower in women aged 30–44 years compared to older women [4]. Women of African ancestry had the highest prevalence and the lowest control rates of hypertension [5]. A recent report from the Canadian Health Measures Survey, reported worsening of awareness, treatment and control of hypertension in women from 2007 onwards [6]. This chapter gives an overview of current knowledge on epidemiology, pathophysiology, risk factors, comorbidities, cardiovascular consequences and management of hypertension in women.

2 Theory

2.1 Epidemiology

The prevalence of hypertension in women differs by age, ethnicity and geographic region [5]. In 2019, the age-standardized prevalence of hypertension was lowest for women in Canada, Peru, and in some countries in Western Europe, but hypertension was still found in around 25% of women in these countries. The highest prevalence of hypertension in women was found in Central and Eastern Europe, Central Asia, Oceania, Sub-Saharan Africa, and in some countries in Latin America and the Caribbean [4]. In general, BP increases with age both in women and men. Among individuals younger than 40 years, BP is on average considerably lower in women compared to men, and hypertension is uncommon, and even more uncommon in young women than in young men [7, 8]. Only 5.6% of US women aged 18–39 years had hypertension in the 2015–2016 National Health and Nutrition Examination Survey (NHANES), compared to 9.2% of men of similar age [8]. In contrast, in individuals older than 65 years, hypertension is very common, found in more than 60%, and even more common in women than in men, found in 67% vs. in 59% of men in this age group in NHANES [8]. In the Hordaland Health Study, a stronger association of high-normal BP in early midlife with incident hypertension 26 years later was demonstrated in women than in men [9].

Traditionally, the more pronounced age-associated increase in BP in women has been attributed to menopausal transition. However, analysis of pooled BP data from four longitudinal population-based cohorts in the Unites States of America (US) demonstrated that BP increases more steeply in women starting already from the third decade of life, i.e. 20 years prior to menopause in most women [7]. This exaggerated BP increase concerns all components of the BP, i.e., includes systolic and diastolic BP, mean BP and pulse pressure [7], and the underlying pathophysiology remains incompletely understood [5].

2.2 Pathophysiology

The same mechanisms of BP regulation are present in women and men, but these systems are shifted towards cardioprotective pathways in premenopausal women [10]. Women generally have shorter stature, which influences pulse wave reflection in the central aorta [11], and smaller sizes of arteries and the heart. Blood pressure development in women is influenced by biological effects of genes on the X chromosome, sex hormones and reproductive factors [3, 12]. Recent research has demonstrated that autosomal-like loci on *the X chromosome* affect phenotypic sex differences in many organ systems and associated diseases, including CVD, and metabolic and immune disorders [13]. Inactivation of the second X chromosome in women is often partial, and up to 20% of genes escape the inactivation, which may contribute to a stronger influence of X chromosome related factors in women than in men [13].

Differences between women and men in major regulators of BP like *the autonomic nervous system* and *the renin-angiotensin-aldosterone system* (RAAS) [14], but also related to bradykinin, endothelin, nitric oxide and brain natriuretic peptides are documented [3]. Healthy young women have lower baroreceptor reflex sensitivity and lower heart rate variability compared to men at similar age [15]. With aging and obesity women have a larger increase in sympathetic nervous activity compared to men. Postmenopausal women with hypertension have impaired autonomous function compared to both normotensive women and hypertensive men of the same age [16], and the sympathetic nervous system is upregulated.

The ovarian hormones oestrogen and progesterone have major roles in BP regulation in women [10, 17]. *Oestrogen* modulates BP directly through effects on calcium pathways in renal, cardiac, and vascular cells, and through genes controlling the RAAS and endothelin system. In particular, oestrogen reduces plasma renin and angiotensin-converting enzyme (ACE) activity, and up-regulate angiotensinogen expression, leading to increased levels of angiotensin and aldosterone, and to sodium retention [3, 18]. *Progesterone* is a mineralocorticoid receptor antagonist, blocking aldosterone effects, and counteracting the sodium-retaining effect of oestrogen [19]. Additionally, enhanced activation of the endothelial cell mineralocorticoid receptor which promotes vascular dysfunction, has been demonstrated both in rodent and human studies [20]. Taken together, when ovarian hormone production declines, the RAAS and the endothelin system are upregulated, and endothelial nitric oxide bioavailability declines, promoting endothelial and cardiovascular dysfunction and sodium retention.

The Intersalt study in >10,000 women and men aged 20–59 years across the world, demonstrated that high dietary sodium intake promotes BP increase with aging [21]. In particular, women with obesity, women of African ancestry and women with high dietary sodium ingestion are prone to develop salt sensitive hypertension [19, 20]. The combination of obesity and excess dietary sodium intake is a damaging duo [22]. Sodium sensitivity also contributes to increased risk of CVD independent of BP through activation of the immune system and promotes CV organ damage and vascular dysfunction [23].

2.3 Risk Factors for Hypertension in Women

Both traditional and women-specific risk factors for hypertension may impact BP in different parts of women's life course (Fig. 1).

2.3.1 Traditional Risk Factors for Hypertension in Women

Among traditional risk factors, obesity, diabetes, physical inactivity and unhealthy diet (including low consumption of fruits and vegetables, and high intake of sodium and alcohol), are prevalent in women and associated with increased risk for hypertension [3]. Although higher body mass index (BMI) is associated with higher BP in both sexes, obesity has emerged as a particularly strong risk factor for hypertension in women [24, 25]. In post-menopausal women, a shift from subcutaneous to visceral storage of excess fat is observed. Visceral fat tissue is more metabolically active and contributes to risk of hypertension through production of several paracrine and inflammatory substances that influence BP regulation [26].

Women more often than men suffer from *chronic inflammatory and autoimmune disorders* that are associated with increased risk of hypertension [27]. Also in persons without autoimmune disorders, a recent study found a stronger association of inflammation with BP increase and new onset hypertension in young women compared to men [28]. Cardiovascular organ damage like arterial stiffness, left ventricular hypertrophy and left ventricular dysfunction are prevalent in women with autoimmune disorders [29, 30], and particularly when concomitant hypertension is present [31].

2.3.2 Women-Specific Risk Factors for Hypertension

Women-specific risk factors for hypertension include several factors related to reproduction and infertility [5, 12] (Fig. 1). *Adverse pregnancy outcomes* (e.g. hypertensive disorders of pregnancy, gestational diabetes, preterm delivery, and intrauterine growth restriction) are all associated with increased risk for hypertension and CVD [5, 32]. Several of these factors have been associated with inducing an unhealthy

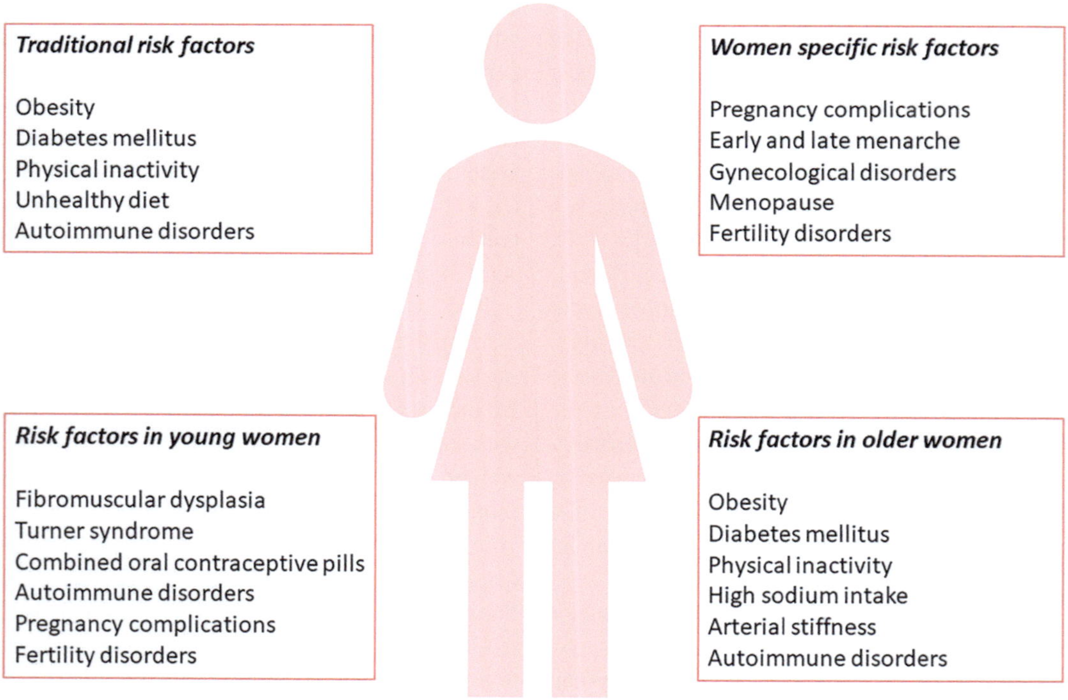

Fig. 1 Traditional and women specific risk factors for hypertension in young and older women

immune response promoting systemic inflammation, hypertension and CVD in early age [12, 33, 34]. *Hypertensive pregnancy disorders* complicate 5–10% of all pregnancies and are accountable for 14% of all maternal deaths worldwide [35]. Hypertensive disorders in pregnancy increase the risk of future hypertension and CVD, in particular in younger women (<55 years) [36, 37] Among 45–55 years old women, hypertension was found in 60% of women with a history of preeclampsia, compared to 26% in the control group [38]. In the same study, 30% of women with former preeclampsia had coronary artery calcification, compared to 18% in the control group, reflecting that preeclampsia often induces a chronic inflammatory state in the maternal cardiovascular system that does not terminate with the delivery and promotes arterial damage [33, 34, 39]. This may explain why cardiovascular risk after hypertensive pregnancy disorders are largely, but not entirely mediated by development of chronic hypertension [40].

Both *early and late menarche* have been linked to increased risk of metabolic risk factors, including hypertension [41]. Around 2–10% of women in the reproductive age have *endometriosis*, which is characterized by the presence of non-malignant endometrium-like tissue outside of the uterus [42]. Endometriosis is associated with chronic inflammation, pelvic pain and increased risk of hypertension, infertility and hypertensive pregnancy complications [43]. In addition, women with other menstrual disorders and uterine fibroids have increased risk of future hypertension [5].

Oral contraceptive pills containing high dose ethinyl estradiol are associated with increased BP [36]. Potential causes include RAAS stimulation and sodium retention [44]. Furthermore, use of combined oral contraceptive pills increases the risk of venous thrombosis, myocardial infarction, and stroke. The dose and type of oestrogen in the combined pill may change the strength of these associations. However, use of combined oral contraceptive pills is not recommended in women older than 35 years who smoke, and in women with severe dyslipidemia, obesity or uncontrolled hypertension [45]. Progestin only contraceptives are associated with little or no increased CVD risk.

The association between *assisted reproductive therapies* and risk of CVD is still debated, but several registry studies have documented an increased risk for hypertension. In the Nurses' Health Study II, an increased risk for hypertension was found in women with tubal disease, but not in women with other causes of infertility [46]. In an analysis based on Swedish National Registries, in vitro fertilization (IVF) was associated with 27% higher risk of incident hypertension over 8 years, compared to natural conception [47]. A retrospective longitudinal cohort study of more than 1 million hospital births in Quebec during the years 2008–2019, found that IVF was associated with increased risk of hypertension both in fathers and offspring compared with natural conception during 11 years of follow-up, while no post-delivery association with hypertension was found for mothers [48].

Polycystic ovary syndrome (PCOS) is the most common endocrine disorder in women of reproductive age, characterized by amenorrhea or oligomenorrhea, hyperandrogenism and polycystic ovaries, and associated with endothelial dysfunction and clustering of metabolic risk factors, including hypertension [49, 50]. PCOS affects 6–16% of all women. In a cross-sectional study from the Netherlands, middle-aged women with PCOS had twice the risk of hypertension compared to healthy age matched women [49].

Menopause is associated with adverse changes in metabolic risk factors and BP regulating systems, including upregulation of the RAAS, endothelin and the sympathetic nervous system, and increase in visceral adipose tissue, as depicted above [3, 10, 17]. As a consequence, the cardiometabolic health declines in many women during menopausal transition [36]. While young women have much lower risk of CVD than men at the same age, from age 55 years onwards, the lifetime risk of CVD is the same in women and men [51]. From the US Study across the nation including serial BP measurements over 10 years before and after menopausal transition in 3302 multiethnic women, a diversity in BP development during the study period was reported [52]. An accelerated BP increase after menopause was found in 35% of women [52], and increase in BP was particularly associated with early menopause, vasomotor symptoms, and weight increase. Furthermore, increase in BMI was the main factor associated with incident hypertension in the perimenopausal period in a population-based study in Prague [53]. Many women that develop hypertension during menopause report symptoms as palpitations, hot flushes, headache, chest pain, tiredness and sleeping disturbances, which are often attributed to menopause [36]. Thus, it is important to measure BP in perimenopausal women that report such symptoms to avoid delay in the diagnosis of hypertension.

2.4 Causes of Secondary Hypertension in Women

About 90% of women diagnosed with hypertension have essential hypertension, i.e., not caused by an underlying disorder or disease [54]. However, in young women who develop hypertension, secondary causes should always be suspected, particularly in women without obesity or with an abnormal reproductive history (Fig. 1). *Fibromuscular dysplasia* is a non-atherosclerotic vascular disease that may lead to renal artery obstruction. More than 90% of patients with fibromuscular dysplasia are women [44]. Presence of fibromuscular dysplasia has also been associated with risk of spontaneous coronary artery dissection, which is the underlying cause of up to 35% of myocardial infarction in women younger than 50 years, and a causal role of hypertension was recently suggested by a genome wide association meta-analysis [55].

Other causes of secondary hypertension in young women include primary aldosteronism, renal parenchymal diseases, autoimmune thyroid disease, coarctation of the aorta, illicit drug use, and high intake of licorice or other dietary factors [44]. The most common genetic abnormality of young women, *Turner syndrome*, is a risk factor for both hypertension and CVD [56].

3 Clinical Practice

3.1 Diagnosis of Hypertension in Women

The World Health Organization defines hypertension as a systolic BP ≥140 mmHg or a diastolic BP ≥90 mmHg in both women and men. This definition is consistently used in European guidelines on the management of systemic arterial hypertension [45, 54]. In contrast, the American guidelines on systemic arterial hypertension from 2018 lowered the BP threshold for identification of hypertension in both genders, and identifies Stage 1 hypertension as BP 130–139/80–89 mmHg and Stage 2 hypertension as BP ≥140/90 mmHg [57]. Of note, isolated systolic hypertension (combined systolic BP ≥140 mmHg and diastolic BP <90 mmHg) is more common in older women, and isolated diastolic hypertension (combined systolic BP <140 mmHg and diastolic BP ≥90 mmHg) is less common in young women compared to men at similar age. In women with diabetes and women older than 70 years, BP should also be measured in the upright position to identify orthostatic hypotension that may influence BP management. Details on measurement and management of hypertension is given in current guidelines [45, 54].

For accurate diagnosis of hypertension, confirmation of an elevated office BP by ambulatory BP measurement is recommended [45, 54]. Using 24-h ambulatory BP measurement, an average BP through the 24-h period <130 mmHg systolic and <80 mmHg diastolic is considered normal. Women are at increased risk for white coat hypertension, i.e. elevated office BP, but normal 24-h ambulatory BP (Fig. 2) [58]. This has been attributed to stronger BP response to stress in women [59], and to higher prevalences of anxiety and metabolic syndrome in older women. In contrast, the prevalence of masked hypertension (i.e. a normal office BP, but elevated 24-h ambulatory BP) is 50% lower in women compared to men [58]. However, the prevalence of masked hypertension in women increases with higher BMI and alcohol intake.

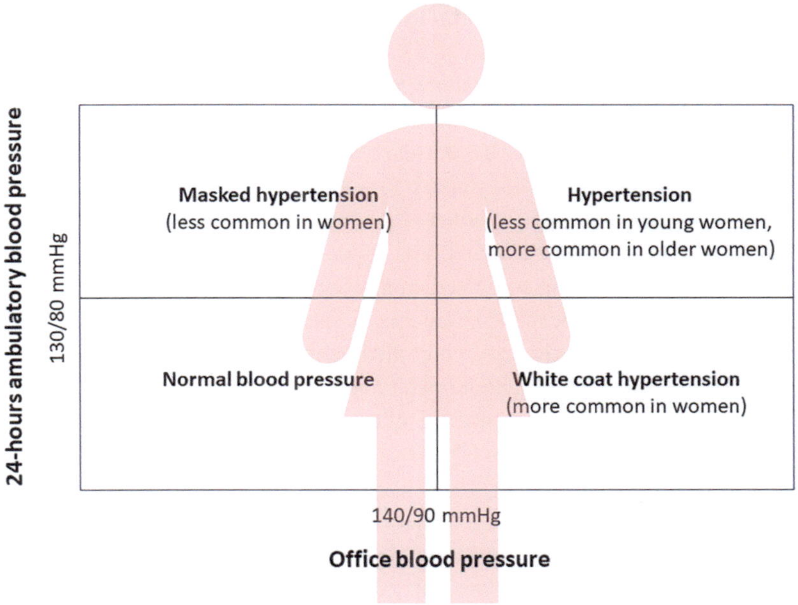

Fig. 2 Identification of hypertension, masked hypertension and white coat hypertension in women from combining office and 24-h ambulatory BP

3.2 Treatment of Hypertension in Women

Recent publications have demonstrated that the risk of CVD increases at a lower BP level in women than in men [60, 61]. In the Hordaland health Study, including >12,300 women and men aged 41 years, women with a systolic of BP 130–139 mmHg or a diastolic BP 80–89 mmHg (reflecting stage 1 hypertension in American guidelines and high-normal BP in European guidelines) had a twofold increased risk of hospitalization and death from acute coronary syndromes compared to women with normal BP, while this BP level was not associated with increased risk in men [60]. Of note, these findings were not explained by higher burden of traditional CVD risk factors in women or use of contraceptive pills. In a pooled analysis of data from four US longitudinal population-based cohorts including >27,000 women and men, risk of CVD, myocardial infarction, stroke and heart failure all increased at a lower BP level in women compared to men [61]. However, few clinical studies have tested the effect of lower vs. standard BP targets [62, 63]. The SPRINT (systolic blood pressure intervention trial) compared the effect of antihypertensive treatment to systolic BP <120 mmHg vs. standard target (systolic BP <140 mmHg) [62]. Unfortunately, too few women were included to document the benefit of the lower target in women, while this was highly significant in men. The STEP (Strategy of Blood Pressure Intervention in the Elderly Hypertensive Patients) trial further documented that intensive BP reduction to a systolic BP 110–129 mmHg was associated with lower incidence of CVD in 60–80 years old patients with hypertension compared to a target of 130–149 mmHg [64]. Despite including 8511 patients, of whom 53.5% were women, the STEP trial has so far not reported sex specific results. In the HOT [63] study, [63] the effect of three different targets of diastolic BP (80 vs. 85 vs. 90 mmHg) was compared among 18,790 persons with treated hypertension. The lowest BP target was associated with lower incidence of myocardial infarction in women [63]. Thus, the potential benefit in women from using lower BP levels for diagnosis of hypertension and treatment target needs further research.

Few clinical trials in hypertension have reported pre-specified sex-specific results [65, 66]. In the VALUE (Valsartan Antihypertensive Long-term Use Evaluation) trial which compared valsartan-based to amlodipine-based treatment, women randomized to amlodipine-based treatment had a lower incidence of combined CVD morbidity and mortality [65]. Furthermore, in the LIFE (Losartan Intervention For Endpoint reduction in hypertension) study 9193 women and men with hypertension and left ventricular hypertrophy on the electrocardiogram were randomized to losartan-based versus atenolol-based treatment [66]. In LIFE women, losartan-based treatment was associated with a larger reduction in combined cardiovascular death, stroke and myocardial infarction. A recent meta-analysis of 51 randomized controlled trials in hypertension involving individual participant-level data from >358,000 participants, the effect of a 5 mmHg BP reduction on risk of CVD was similar in women and men [67].

Current guidelines on management of hypertension recommend the same treatment algorithm in women and men [45, 54]. Personalized lifestyle intervention is recommended to all women including smoking cessation, limit alcohol intake, weight reduction/normalization, daily physical activity, stress management and healthy diet. A healthy dietary approach associated with BP reduction is the combination of low-sodium intake and the DASH (dietary approach to stop hypertension) diet, rich in fruits, vegetables, and low-fat dairy products [68]. Healthy lifestyle can augment the BP lowering effect of antihypertensive drug treatment and reduce the number of drugs needed for BP control [45]. The majority of women with hypertension will need antihypertensive drug treatment to achieve the treatment target of BP [54].

Antihypertensive drug treatment should be initiated in all women when BP≥140/90 mmHg is confirmed [69]. Single-pill combinations of ACE inhibitor/angiotensin receptor blocker with either hydrochlorothiazide or calcium channel blocker is recommended as the initial treatment step in most patients [54]. This strategy facilitates improved persistence to medication and subsequent lower CVD events and mortality [70]. The treatment target in most women should be a BP 120–129/70–79 mmHg, and up-titration should follow the detailed recommendations in current guidelines. In very old women, and in women with symptomatic orthostatic hypotension, a higher BP target level must be accepted. Antihypertensive drug treatment should also be considered in women with BP 130–139/80–89 mmHg that have high CV risk when traditional and female-specific CV risk factors are carefully assessed [69].

Of note, several of the recommended antihypertensive drug classes are not safe in pregnancy. Thus, women of reproductive age must be informed about potential harm to the fetus when these drug classes are used, so that treatment preferably may be adjusted before conception, or as soon as possible after the pregnancy is known [36, 71].

3.3 Antihypertensive Drug Use, Adverse Events and BP Control

Despite the guideline recommendations for using the same treatment algorithm in both genders, differences in drug prescription of antihypertensive treatment have been documented from real world practice. Based on prescription drugs in >292,000 persons with hypertension in the Stockholm Regional Healthcare Data Warehouse, the number of dispensed drugs was lower in women, and women more often than men used diuretics and beta blockers [72]. In particular, more elderly women were treated with diuretics and beta blockers. This may be related to the better BP response in women from diuretics, beta blockers, and ACE inhibitors [44]. Of note, women more often experience adverse events related to treatment with diuretics, beta blocker, calcium channel blockers and ACE inhibitors than men (Fig. 3) [73]. In particular, women are more likely to experience hyponatremia and hypokalemia with diuretics, ankle edema from dihydropyridine calcium channel blockers, and dry cough from ACE inhibitors.

3.4 BP Control in Women

Uncontrolled BP is defined as an office BP >140 mmHg systolic or >90 mmHg diastolic despite antihypertensive treatment. The Canadian Health Measure Survey found lower rates of BP control in women than men, and a worsening trend from 2007 onwards [6]. Among >229,000 persons

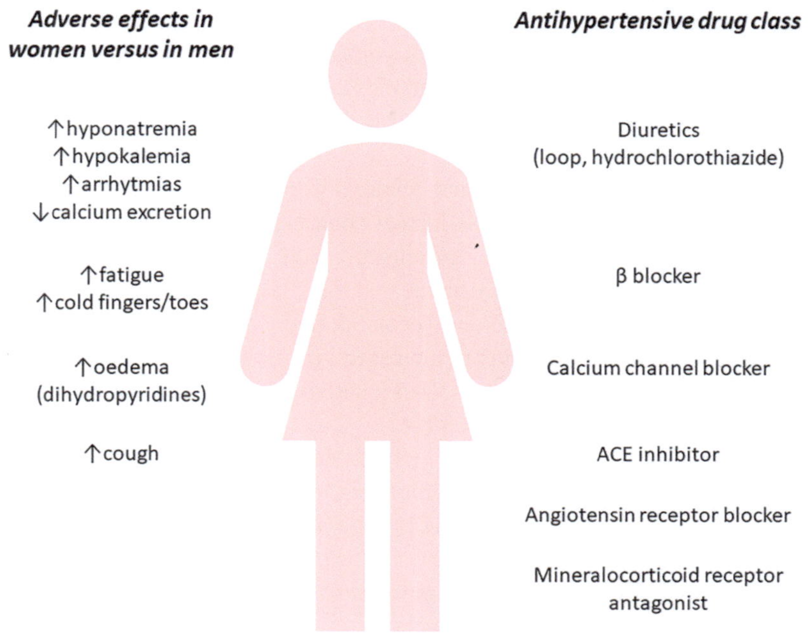

Fig. 3 Adverse effects with higher prevalences in women in relation to the different antihypertensive drug classes

treated for hypertension in the Swedish region of Västra Götaland, BP control declined with increasing age in women, while the opposite was found in men [74]. It is not known whether this is due to differences in drug adherence or adverse drug effects between women and men, or disparity in physician inertia when managing female and male patients [74]. Among older women participating in a cohort study in Louisiana, USA, particular barriers to antihypertensive drug adherence included depression and dissatisfaction with communication with the health care provider [75]. In a national study of uncontrolled hypertension in Norway, including >1100 persons who had uncontrolled office BP despite being prescribed at least two antihypertensive agents, 50% had controlled BP when ambulatory BP measurement was performed [76]. Furthermore, experimental evidence indicates that women with combined obesity and hypertension may particularly benefit from treatment with mineralocorticoid receptor antagonists [77]. From this, using 24-h ambulatory BP recording for more accurate identification of uncontrolled BP, and adding an mineralocorticoid receptor antagonist to the drug treatment regimen seem the first steps in management of uncontrolled BP in women.

4 Conclusions

Hypertension is the number one cause of death and reduced quality of life in women worldwide, and therefore a major determinant of women's health. Obesity and high intake of sodium and alcohol are prevalent traditional risk factors for hypertension in women. In addition, the higher burden of autoimmune disorders and female-specific risk factors related to pregnancy, infertility and menopause contribute to the risk of hypertension in women. Around 50% of hypertension in women originates during the perimenopausal period. Women should therefore measure their BP annually starting from the age of 40 years to facilitate early detection and management of hypertension. Ambulatory BP measurements are useful to demask the white coat effect which is prevalent in women and ensure good BP control. The same treatment algorithm for hypertension is recommended for both genders by current guidelines, but adverse drug effects are more common in women. It is important to improve adverse lifestyle factors and manage co-morbidities to facilitate BP control.

Key Issues

- Women have less hypertension at young age and more at older age compared to men due to a steeper increase in BP from the 3rd decade of life.
- Women specific risk factors and gender differences in traditional CVD risk factors contribute to the CVD risk associated with hypertension in individual women.
- Decline in ovarian hormone levels during menopause transition leads to increased sympathetic nervous system and RAAS activity, and to a more sodium sensitive BP.
- Women report more adverse effects from treatment with diuretics, beta blockers, calcium channel blockers and ACE inhibitors than men.
- BP control declines with aging in women.

Questions and Answers

1. What are the most important risk factors for hypertension in young women (<50 years)?
   (A) Polycystic ovary syndrome
   (B) Weight gain and obesity
   (C) Pregnancy complications
   (D) Fibromuscular dysplasia and other causes of secondary hypertension

   Comment: Answer C) is the best answer. In young healthy women, the BP is lower than BP both in men and in older women. Thus, hypertension is uncommon. Pregnancy complications occurs in around 10% of women and are the most important risk factors for hypertension in young women. When young women are diagnosed with hypertension, secondary causes of hypertension should always be suspected, and particularly in normal weight women without an abnormal reproduction history.
2. What are the most important risk factors for hypertension in older women (>65 years)?
   (A) Weight gain and obesity
   (B) Menopausal transition
   (C) Autoimmune disorders
   (D) High dietary sodium intake

   Comment: Answer A) is the best answer. After the age of 60 years hypertension is more common in women than in men, and at least 60% of women have hypertension. Midlife weight gain and obesity are associated with increased prevalence of hypertension in older women, but also metabolic syndrome and diabetes mellitus contribute. During menopausal transition, weight gain, visceral fat deposition and vasomotor symptoms have been identified as important predictors of hypertension in older women. However, most of the menopausal effect on BP is mediated through an increase in obesity. Many autoimmune diseases are more common in women and associated with chronic cardiovascular inflammation that promotes development of arterial stiffening and hypertension. Furthermore, salt sensitivity contributes to the predisposition for hypertension in post-menopausal women with obesity or high dietary sodium intake.
3. What is the recommended first step in medical treatment of hypertension in women?
   (A) Hydrochlorothiazide as monotherapy
   (B) Single-pill combinations of a beta blockers with either hydrochlorothiazide or calcium channel blocker
   (C) Single-pill combinations of an ACE inhibitor/angiotensin receptor blocker with either a hydrochlorothiazide or calcium channel blocker
   (D) A mineralocorticoid receptor antagonist as monotherapy

   Comment: Answer C) is the best answer. Current European guidelines on management of hypertension recommend the same treatment algorithm in women and men. Single-pill combinations of ACE inhibitor/angiotensin receptor blocker with either a hydrochlorothiazide or a calcium channel blocker is recommended as the initial treatment step in most patients. Importantly, in women who are frail or very old (>80 years) using monotherapy as first step should be considered. Lifestyle intervention is recommended to all, but most women with hypertension will need drug treatment to achieve the recommended BP targets. After menopause, women often have salt sensitive hypertension, and postmenopausal women with hypertension are often obese. In these groups, adding a mineralocorticoid receptor

antagonist to the antihypertensive therapy may promote better BP control. However, a mineralocorticoid receptor antagonist as monotherapy is not recommended as the first step of treatment.

References

1. Collaborators GBDRF. Global burden of 87 risk factors in 204 countries and territories, 1990-2019: a systematic analysis for the Global Burden of Disease Study 2019. Lancet. 2020;396(10258):1223–49.
2. Gerdts E, Regitz-Zagrosek V. Sex differences in cardiometabolic disorders. Nat Med. 2019;25(11):1657–66.
3. Gerdts E, Sudano I, Brouwers S, Borghi C, Bruno RM, Ceconi C, et al. Sex differences in arterial hypertension. Eur Heart J. 2022;43(46):4777–88.
4. NCD Risk Factor Collaboration (NCD-RisC). Worldwide trends in hypertension prevalence and progress in treatment and control from 1990 to 2019: a pooled analysis of 1201 population-representative studies with 104 million participants. Lancet. 2021;398(10304):957–80.
5. Chapman N, Ching SM, Konradi AO, Nuyt AM, Khan T, Twumasi-Ankrah B, et al. Arterial hypertension in women: state of the art and knowledge gaps. Hypertension. 2023;80(6):1140–9.
6. Leung AA, Williams JVA, McAlister FA, Campbell NRC, Padwal RS, et al. Worsening hypertension awareness, treatment, and control rates in Canadian women between 2007 and 2017. Can J Cardiol. 2020;36(5):732–9.
7. Ji H, Kim A, Ebinger JE, Niiranen TJ, Claggett BL, Bairey Merz CN, et al. Sex differences in blood pressure trajectories over the life course. JAMA Cardiol. 2020;5(3):19–26.
8. Fryar CD, Ostchega Y, Hales CM, Zhang G, Kruszon-Moran D. Hypertension prevalence and control among adults: United States, 2015-2016. NCHS Data Brief. 2017;289:1–8.
9. Ohldieck AE, Kringeland E, Midtbo H, Tell GS, Gerdts E. High-normal blood pressure in midlife is a stronger risk factor for incident hypertension 26 years later in women than men: the Hordaland Health Study. Blood Press. 2023;32(1):2179337.
10. Colafella KMM, Denton KM. Sex-specific differences in hypertension and associated cardiovascular disease. Nat Rev Nephrol. 2018;14(3):185–201.
11. McEniery CM, Yasmin, Hall IR, Qasem A, Wilkinson IB, Cockcroft JR, et al. Normal vascular aging: differential effects on wave reflection and aortic pulse wave velocity: the Anglo-Cardiff Collaborative Trial (ACCT). J Am Coll Cardiol. 2005;46(9):1753–60.
12. Jeong SM, Jeon KH, Jung W, Yoo JE, Yoo J, Han K, et al. Association of reproductive factors with cardiovascular disease risk in pre-menopausal women: nationwide population-based cohort study. Eur J Prev Cardiol. 2023;30(3):264–73.
13. Bartz D, Chitnis T, Kaiser UB, Rich-Edwards JW, Rexrode KM, Pennell PB, et al. Clinical advances in sex- and gender-informed medicine to improve the health of all: a review. JAMA Intern Med. 2020;180(4):574–83.
14. Nwia SM, Leite APO, Li XC, Zhuo JL. Sex differences in the renin-angiotensin-aldosterone system and its roles in hypertension, cardiovascular, and kidney diseases. Front Cardiovasc Med. 2023;10:1198090.
15. Philbois SV, Facioli TP, Gastaldi AC, Rodrigues JAL, Tank J, Fares TH, et al. Important differences between hypertensive middle-aged women and men in cardiovascular autonomic control-a critical appraisal. Biol Sex Differ. 2021;12(1):11.
16. Sevre K, Lefrandt JD, Nordby G, Os I, Mulder M, Gans RO, et al. Autonomic function in hypertensive and normotensive subjects: the importance of gender. Hypertension. 2001;37(6):1351–6.
17. Reckelhoff JF. Gender differences in the regulation of blood pressure. Hypertension. 2001;37(5):1199–208.
18. Oparil S, Miller AP. Gender and blood pressure. J Clin Hypertens. 2005;7(5):300–9.
19. Mallareddy M, Hanes V, White WB. Drospirenone, a new progestogen, for postmenopausal women with hypertension. Drugs Aging. 2007;24(6):453–66.
20. Barris CT, Faulkner JL, Belin de Chantemele EJ. Salt sensitivity of blood pressure in women. Hypertension. 2023;80(2):268–78.
21. Intersalt Cooperative Research Group. Results for 24 hour urinary sodium and potassium excretion. BMJ. 1988;297(6644):319–28.
22. Watso JC, Fancher IS, Gomez DH, Hutchison ZJ, Gutierrez OM, Robinson AT. The damaging duo: obesity and excess dietary salt contribute to hypertension and cardiovascular disease. Obes Rev. 2023;24(8):e13589.
23. Weinberger MH, Fineberg NS, Fineberg SE, Weinberger M. Salt sensitivity, pulse pressure, and death in normal and hypertensive humans. Hypertension. 2001;37(2):429–32.
24. Kringeland E, Tell GS, Midtbo H, Haugsgjerd TR, Igland J, Gerdts E. Factors associated with increase in blood pressure and incident hypertension in early midlife: the Hordaland Health Study. Blood Press. 2020;29(5):267–75.
25. Sharabi Y, Grotto I, Huerta M, Grossman E. Susceptibility of the influence of weight on blood pressure in men versus women: lessons from a large-scale study of young adults. Am J Hypertens. 2004;17(5):404–8.
26. Lyon CJ, Law RE, Hsueh WA. Minireview: adiposity, inflammation, and atherogenesis. Endocrinology. 2003;144(6):2195–200.
27. Han C, Robinson DW Jr, Hackett MV, Paramore LC, Fraeman KH, Bala MV. Cardiovascular disease and risk factors in patients with rheumatoid arthritis, psoriatic arthritis, and ankylosing spondylitis. J Rheumatol. 2006;33(11):2167–72.

28. Kringeland E, Gerdts E, Ulvik A, Tell GS, Igland J, Haugsgjerd TR, et al. Inflammation, sex, blood pressure changes and hypertension in midlife: the Hordaland Health Study. J Hum Hypertens. 2023;37(8):718–25.
29. Midtbo H, Gerdts E, Kvien TK, Olsen IC, Hirth A, Davidsen ES, et al. Disease activity and left ventricular structure in patients with rheumatoid arthritis. Rheumatology. 2015;54(3):511–9.
30. Midtbo H, Semb AG, Matre K, Kvien TK, Gerdts E. Disease activity is associated with reduced left ventricular systolic myocardial function in patients with rheumatoid arthritis. Ann Rheum Dis. 2017;76(2):371–6.
31. Midtbo H, Gerdts E, Kvien TK, Olsen IC, Lonnebakken MT, Davidsen ES, et al. The association of hypertension with asymptomatic cardiovascular organ damage in rheumatoid arthritis. Blood Press. 2016;25(5):298–304.
32. O'Kelly AC, Michos ED, Shufelt CL, Vermunt JV, Minissian MB, Quesada O, et al. Pregnancy and reproductive risk factors for cardiovascular disease in women. Circ Res. 2022;130(4):652–72.
33. Sondergaard MM, Hlatky MA, Stefanick ML, Vittinghoff E, Nah G, Allison M, et al. Association of adverse pregnancy outcomes with risk of atherosclerotic cardiovascular disease in postmenopausal women. JAMA Cardiol. 2020;5(12):1390–8.
34. Khosla K, Heimberger S, Nieman KM, Tung A, Shahul S, et al. Long-term cardiovascular disease risk in women after hypertensive disorders of pregnancy: recent advances in hypertension. Hypertension. 2021;78(4):927–35.
35. Dimitriadis E, Rolnik DL, Zhou W, Estrada-Gutierrez G, Koga K, Francisco RPV, et al. Pre-eclampsia. Nat Rev Dis Primers. 2023;9(1):8.
36. Maas A, Rosano G, Cifkova R, Chieffo A, van Dijken D, Hamoda H, et al. Cardiovascular health after menopause transition, pregnancy disorders, and other gynaecologic conditions: a consensus document from European cardiologists, gynaecologists, and endocrinologists. Eur Heart J. 2021;42(10):967–84.
37. Magee LA, Nicolaides KH, von Dadelszen P. Preeclampsia. N Engl J Med. 2022;386(19):1817–32.
38. Zoet GA, Benschop L, Boersma E, Budde RPJ, Fauser B, van der Graaf Y, et al. Prevalence of subclinical coronary artery disease assessed by coronary computed tomography angiography in 45- to 55-year-old women with a history of preeclampsia. Circulation. 2018;137(8):877–9.
39. Redman CW, Staff AC. IFPA award in placentology lecture: preeclampsia, the decidual battleground and future maternal cardiovascular disease. Placenta. 2014;35(Suppl):S26–31.
40. Riise HKR, Sulo G, Tell GS, Igland J, Egeland G, Nygard O, et al. Hypertensive pregnancy disorders increase the risk of maternal cardiovascular disease after adjustment for cardiovascular risk factors. Int J Cardiol. 2019;282:81–7.
41. Lakshman R, Forouhi NG, Sharp SJ, Luben R, Bingham SA, Khaw KT, et al. Early age at menarche associated with cardiovascular disease and mortality. J Clin Endocrinol Metab. 2009;94(12):4953–60.
42. Becker CM, Bokor A, Heikinheimo O, Horne A, Jansen F, Kiesel L, et al. ESHRE guideline: endometriosis. Hum Reprod Open. 2022;2022(2):9.
43. Mu F, Rich-Edwards J, Rimm EB, Spiegelman D, Forman JP, Missmer SA. Association between endometriosis and hypercholesterolemia or hypertension. Hypertension. 2017;70(1):59–65.
44. Wenger NK, Arnold A, Bairey Merz CN, Cooper-DeHoff RM, Ferdinand KC, Fleg JL, et al. Hypertension across a woman's life cycle. J Am Coll Cardiol. 2018;71(16):1797–813.
45. Mancia G, Kreutz R, Brunstrom M, Burnier M, Grassi G, Januszewicz A, et al. 2023 ESH guidelines for the management of arterial hypertension The Task Force for the management of arterial hypertension of the European Society of Hypertension Endorsed by the International Society of Hypertension (ISH) and the European Renal Association (ERA). J Hypertens. 2023;41(12):1874–2071.
46. Farland LV, Grodstein F, Srouji SS, Forman JP, Rich-Edwards J, Chavarro JE, et al. Infertility, fertility treatment, and risk of hypertension. Fertil Steril. 2015;104(2):391–7.
47. Westerlund E, Brandt L, Hovatta O, Wallen H, Ekbom A, Henriksson P. Incidence of hypertension, stroke, coronary heart disease, and diabetes in women who have delivered after in vitro fertilization: a population-based cohort study from Sweden. Fertil Steril. 2014;102(4):1096–102.
48. Wei SQ, Paradis G, Ayoub A, Lewin A, Auger N. Assisted reproductive technology and cardiovascular outcomes in parents and offspring. Can J Cardiol. 2023;40:130–7.
49. Meun C, Gunning MN, Louwers YV, Peters H, Roos-Hesselink J, Roeters van Lennep J, et al. The cardiovascular risk profile of middle-aged women with polycystic ovary syndrome. Clin Endocrinol. 2020;92(2):150–8.
50. Amiri M, Ramezani Tehrani F, Behboudi-Gandevani S, Bidhendi-Yarandi R, Carmina E. Risk of hypertension in women with polycystic ovary syndrome: a systematic review, meta-analysis and meta-regression. Reprod Biol Endocrinol. 2020;18(1):23.
51. Leening MJ, Ferket BS, Steyerberg EW, Kavousi M, Deckers JW, Nieboer D, et al. Sex differences in lifetime risk and first manifestation of cardiovascular disease: prospective population based cohort study. BMJ. 2014;349:5992.
52. Samargandy S, Matthews KA, Brooks MM, Barinas-Mitchell E, Magnani JW, Thurston RC, et al. Trajectories of blood pressure in midlife women: does menopause matter? Circ Res. 2022;130(3):312–22.
53. Cifkova R, Pitha J, Lejskova M, Lanska V, Zecova S. Blood pressure around the menopause: a population study. J Hypertens. 2008;26(10):1976–82.

54. Williams B, Mancia G, Spiering W, Agabiti Rosei E, Azizi M, Burnier M, et al. 2018 ESC/ESH guidelines for the management of arterial hypertension. Eur Heart J. 2018;39(33):3021–104.
55. Adlam D, Berrandou TE, Georges A, Nelson CP, Giannoulatou E, Henry J, et al. Genome-wide association meta-analysis of spontaneous coronary artery dissection identifies risk variants and genes related to artery integrity and tissue-mediated coagulation. Nat Genet. 2023;55(6):964–72.
56. Mavinkurve M, O'Gorman CS. Cardiometabolic and vascular risks in young and adolescent girls with Turner syndrome. BBA Clin. 2015;3:304–9.
57. Whelton PK, Carey RM, Aronow WS, Casey DE Jr, Collins KJ, Dennison Himmelfarb C, et al. 2017 ACC/AHA/AAPA/ABC/ACPM/AGS/APhA/ASH/ASPC/NMA/PCNA guideline for the prevention, detection, evaluation, and management of high blood pressure in adults: a report of the American College of Cardiology/American Heart Association Task Force on clinical practice guidelines. Hypertension. 2018;71(6):e13–5.
58. Ahmad A, Oparil S. Hypertension in women: recent advances and lingering questions. Hypertension. 2017;70(1):19–26.
59. Rossi A, Mikail N, Bengs S, Haider A, Treyer V, Buechel RR, et al. Heart-brain interactions in cardiac and brain diseases: why sex matters. Eur Heart J. 2022;43(39):3971–80.
60. Kringeland E, Tell GS, Midtbo H, Igland J, Haugsgjerd TR, Gerdts E. Stage 1 hypertension, sex, and acute coronary syndromes during midlife: the Hordaland Health Study. Eur J Prev Cardiol. 2022;29(1):147–54.
61. Ji H, Niiranen TJ, Rader F, Henglin M, Kim A, Ebinger JE, et al. Sex differences in blood pressure associations with cardiovascular outcomes. Circulation. 2021;143(7):761–3.
62. Wright JT, Williamson JD, Whelton PK, Snyder JK, Sink KM, et al. A randomized trial of intensive versus standard blood-pressure control. N Engl J Med. 2015;373(22):2103–16.
63. Kjeldsen SE, Warnold I, Hansson L, HOTSGHOTS. Influence of gender on prevention of myocardial infarction by antihypertensives and acetylsalicylic acid: the HOT study. J Gend Specif Med. 2000;3(8):35–8.
64. Zhang W, Zhang S, Deng Y, Wu S, Ren J, Sun G, et al. Trial of intensive blood-pressure control in older patients with hypertension. N Engl J Med. 2021;385(14):1268–79.
65. Zanchetti A, Julius S, Kjeldsen S, McInnes GT, Hua T, Weber M, et al. Outcomes in subgroups of hypertensive patients treated with regimens based on valsartan and amlodipine: an analysis of findings from the VALUE trial. J Hypertens. 2006;24(11):2163–8.
66. Os I, Franco V, Kjeldsen SE, Manhem K, Devereux RB, Gerdts E, et al. Effects of losartan in women with hypertension and left ventricular hypertrophy: results from the Losartan Intervention for Endpoint Reduction in Hypertension Study. Hypertension. 2008;51(4):1103–8.
67. Bidel Z, Nazarzadeh M, Canoy D, Copland E, Gerdts E, Woodward M, et al. Sex-specific effects of blood pressure lowering pharmacotherapy for the prevention of cardiovascular disease: an individual participant-level data meta-analysis. Hypertension. 2023;80:21496.
68. Sacks FM, Svetkey LP, Vollmer WM, Appel LJ, Bray GA, Harsha D, et al. Effects on blood pressure of reduced dietary sodium and the dietary approaches to stop hypertension (DASH) diet. DASH-Sodium Collaborative Research Group. N Engl J Med. 2001;344(1):3–10.
69. McEvoy JW, McCarthy CP, Bruno RM, Brouwers S, Canavan MD, Ceconi C, et al. 2024 ESC Guidelines for the management of elevated blood pressure and hypertension. Eur Heart J. 2024:ehae178. PMID: 39210715.
70. Schmieder RE, Wassmann S, Predel HG, Weisser B, Blettenberg J, Gillessen A, et al. Improved persistence to medication, decreased cardiovascular events and reduced all-cause mortality in hypertensive patients with use of single-pill combinations: results from the START-study. Hypertension. 2023;80(5):1127–35.
71. Cifkova R. Hypertension in pregnancy: a diagnostic and therapeutic overview. High Blood Press Cardiovasc Prev. 2023;30(4):289–303.
72. Wallentin F, Wettermark B, Kahan T. Drug treatment of hypertension in Sweden in relation to sex, age, and comorbidity. J Clin Hypertens. 2018;20(1):106–14.
73. Tamargo J, Rosano G, Walther T, Duarte J, Niessner A, Kaski JC, et al. Gender differences in the effects of cardiovascular drugs. Eur Heart J Cardiovasc Pharmacother. 2017;3(3):163–82.
74. Bager JE, Manhem K, Andersson T, Hjerpe P, Bengtsson-Bostrom K, Ljungman C, et al. Hypertension: sex-related differences in drug treatment, prevalence and blood pressure control in primary care. J Hum Hypertens. 2023;37(8):662–70.
75. Holt E, Joyce C, Dornelles A, Morisky D, Webber LS, Muntner P, et al. Sex differences in barriers to antihypertensive medication adherence: findings from the cohort study of medication adherence among older adults. J Am Geriatr Soc. 2013;61(4):558–64.
76. Bergland OU, Halvorsen LV, Soraas CL, Hjornholm U, Kjaer VN, Rognstad S, et al. Detection of nonadherence to antihypertensive treatment by measurements of serum drug concentrations. Hypertension. 2021;78(3):617–28.
77. Faulkner JL, Belin de Chantemele EJ. Sex differences in mechanisms of hypertension associated with obesity. Hypertension. 2018;71(1):15–21.

Hypertensive Cardiovascular Organ Damage

Costantino Mancusi and Eva Gerdts

Abstract

Hypertension leads to development of structural and function changes in the heart and arteries which may be assessed by cardiovascular imaging. These changes are collectively termed hypertension associated organ damage and are in fact the preclinical stages of cardiovascular disease. In the heart, women with hypertension more often develop left ventricular (LV) hypertrophy, concentric LV geometry, left atrial enlargement and LV diastolic dysfunction, while LV ejection fraction most often is normal. LV hypertrophy is less modifiable by antihypertensive drug treatment in women and increases the risk of clinical cardiovascular events relatively more in women than men. Women also more often develop new-onset LV hypertrophy during antihypertensive drug treatment. Large artery stiffness increases steeper with aging in women. Increased arterial stiffness carries a higher risk of cardiovascular events in women than men. Women with hypertension have more positive remodeling and less plaque calcifications in the carotid arteries. Similarly, women have a lower coronary artery calcium (CAC) score by computed tomography. Young women may have extensive coronary artery disease even when the CAC score is zero. Early onset of coronary calcification is found in women who develop hypertension early in life due to autoimmune disorders or a history of preeclampsia. Taken together, use of multimodality cardiovascular imaging and sex specific reference values are needed for accurate identification of cardiovascular organ damage in women.

Keywords

Left ventricular hypertrophy · Left atrial enlargement · Arterial stiffness · Coronary artery calcium score · Carotid atherosclerosis

C. Mancusi
Department of Advanced Biomedical Science, Federico II University, Naples, Italy
e-mail: costantino.mancusi@unina.it

E. Gerdts (✉)
Department of Clinical Science, University of Bergen, Bergen, Norway
e-mail: eva.gerdts@uib.no

A. H.E.M. Maas, E. Gerdts (eds.), *Manual of Cardiovascular Disease in Women*,
https://doi.org/10.1007/978-3-031-65952-2_8

Test your learning and check your understanding of this book's contents: use the "Springer Nature Flashcards" app to access questions using ▶ https://sn.pub/51ny7m
To use the app, please follow the instructions in chapter 1.

1 Introduction

Hypertension leads to structural and functional changes of small and large arteries and of the end-organs (the heart, brain, eyes and kidneys) [1], collectively named organ damage [2, 3]. The presence of such organ damage actually reflects cardiovascular disease (CVD) in the preclinical stage, and is associated with high risk of clinical CVD events (Fig. 1) [4]. Active search for cardiovascular organ damage is therefore recommended by the European guidelines on management of hypertension as a tool for identification of women with high risk for CVD [3, 4]. Research over the past two decades has demonstrated gender differences related to hypertension associated cardiovascular organ damage, including prevalence, clinical manifestation and modification by antihypertensive treatment [5, 6]. Diversity in presence of cardiovascular organ damage has been linked to smaller dimension of arteries and the heart in women, differences in body composition and co-morbidities, and differences in arterial aging and blood pressure (BP) development over the life course in women compared to men [5, 6]. However, the underlying mechanisms for the observed gender differences in cardiovascular organ damage in hypertension are still incompletely understood. This chapter will give an overview of current knowledge on diagnosis and management of arterial and cardiac organ damage in women with hypertension.

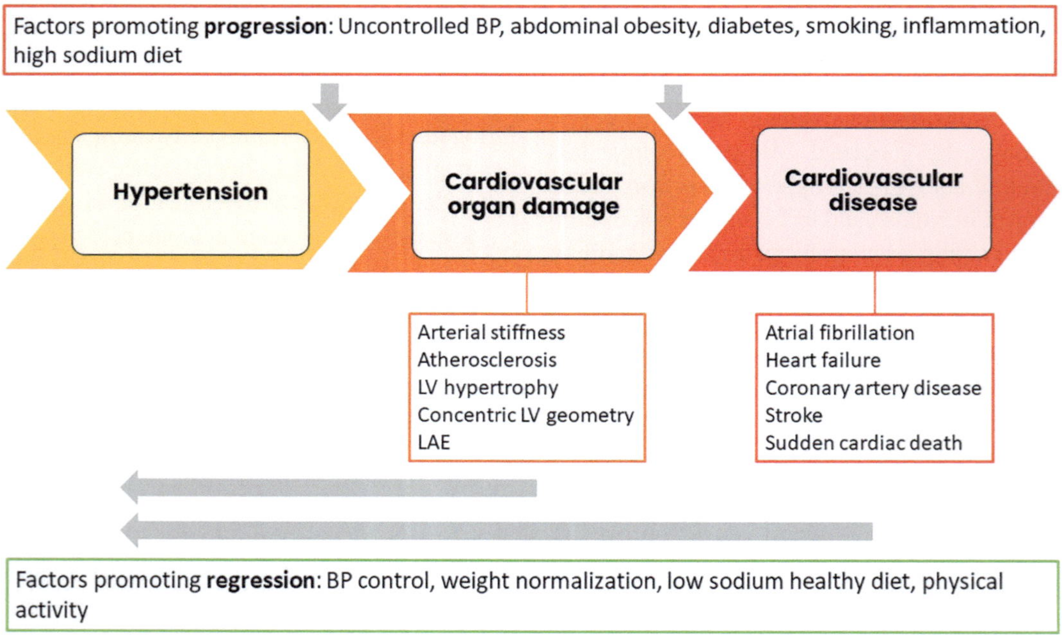

Fig. 1 The progression from hypertension to organ damage and clinical cardiovascular disease

2 Theory

2.1 Hypertensive Organ Damage in the Arteries

Conduit and resistance vessels of women are smaller in diameter and have a higher basal tonus compared to men, even after normalization to body weight, body height, body mass index, or heart weight [7]. Arterial organ damage in hypertension develops as a consequence of both arteriosclerosis, reflecting proliferation of smooth muscle cells and connective tissue in media leading to thickening and stiffening of the artery, and of atherosclerosis, reflecting lipid deposition and plaque development in intima [8]. Arteriosclerosis and atherosclerosis are pathologically distinct processes, that often co-exist in both women and men with hypertension [8].

Gender differences in both micro- and macrovascular structure and function have been documented [1, 9, 10]. In women, arterial function is influenced by the life course changes in oestrogen. Oestrogen depletion leads to impaired endothelial dependent vasodilation secondary to reduced nitric oxide production, contributing to arterial dysfunction in post-menopausal women, including impaired coronary flow reserve, and a more pronounced increase in arterial stiffness with aging [9, 11]. Hypertension associated damage in small arteries may be diagnosed by lumen-media ratio and by flow-mediated vasodilatation [7, 12]. Hypertension associated remodelling in large arteries may be diagnosed by ultrasound, and increased arterial stiffness by carotid-femoral pulse wave velocity (PWV) [13, 14]. Hypertension associated calcification and plaque may be diagnosed by vascular ultrasound or coronary computed tomography [15, 16].

2.1.1 Carotid Intima Media Thickness and Plaque

In the population based Tromsø study from Norway, a more pronounced positive remodelling in the carotid arteries was found by ultrasound in women compared to men, whereas the burden of atherosclerotic plaque was more pronounced in men [17]. In the Italian Campania Salute Network project, a prospective study of women and men treated for hypertension, presence of carotid plaque in participants without known CVD increased with age, was less prevalent in women, and was associated with a higher brachial pulse pressure, and presence of uncontrolled hypertension independent of antihypertensive and statin treatment [18]. A recent systematic review and meta-analysis of 42 publication in women and men with carotid atherosclerosis, all plaque features, including plaque size, composition, and morphology, were smaller or less common in women than in men [19]. Women less often had plaque with calcifications, lipid-rich necrotic core or intraplaque haemorrhage, reflecting vulnerable plaque characteristics. Gender differences in carotid atherosclerosis were also identified by proteomic analysis of carotid endarterectomy samples from 320 patients, in particular related to proteins associated with plaque calcification and inflammation [20]. Increased proteoglycan content in plaques in post-menopausal women was particularly associated with worse outcome over 2 years of follow-up [20]. Taken together, future integration of clinical, imaging and omics data may advance current understanding of the gender differences in atherosclerosis.

2.1.2 Arterial Stiffness

Stiffening of large arteries is one of the hallmarks of hypertension associated organ damage. Increased arterial stiffness in not only found in postmenopausal women, but also found in women with autoimmune disorders, polycystic ovary syndrome, endometriosis and previous hypertensive pregnancy complications or pre-eclampsia, probably reflecting that these disorders induce chronic arterial inflammation in these women [9]. New insights in longitudinal development of BP components and arterial stiffness in women was recently published based on observations in the Framingham Heart Study [21]. Pulse pressure, a measure of aortic flow pulsatility, was lower in young women and increased more with aging in women [21]. Development of a wide pulse pressure (brachial pulse pressure >60 mmHg) was strongly associated with proximal aortic stiffening, a higher characteristic impedance of the aorta and a larger forward wave amplitude in women [21]. In the longitudinal Study in Women Across the Nation (SWAN) including 339 women, a significant increase in carotid-femoral PWV was found around the 1-year period surrounding the final menstrual period during perimenopause, and typically associated with increases in BP and waist circumference [22]. The increase in carotid-femoral PWV was larger and initiated earlier in Black women in SWAN [22]. Aging, CVD risk factors including hypertension, hyperlipidaemia and central obesity and menopause may promote arterial stiffness through increased collagen deposition, inflammation and loss of arterial elasticity. When arterial stiffness was assessed by brachial-ankle PWV in >11,700 South Korean women and men with hypertension, diabetes, dyslipidemia and stable coronary artery disease, an increase in arterial stiffness carried higher risk for CVD events and death in women than men [23]. Arterial stiffness has also been associated with more prominent cardiac remodelling and changes in left ventricular-vascular interaction in women which in turn predispose to development of heart failure with preserved ejection fraction [24]. Furthermore, increased arterial stiffness has been associated with higher burden of coronary artery plaque and calcification in women [1].

2.1.3 Coronary Atherosclerosis

It has been increasingly common to assess subclinical atherosclerosis by cardiac computed tonometry angiography (CCTA) imaging, reporting coronary artery calcium (CAC) score or coronary artery plaque presence and volume, as part of screening for CV organ damage in hypertension [15, 16]. The CAC Consortium including more than 63,000 asymptomatic women and men who underwent CCTA, documented sex differences in CAC, plaque composition and prevalence of non-obstructive coronary artery disease [25]. Women have lower CAC than men at similar age, and age and sex-specific threshold values for CAC score is therefore recommended for diagnosis and interpretation of the findings [25]. In persons without CAC, the risk of CV death is equally low in women and men [26]. However, when CAC is present, women have a 30% higher risk of CV death compared to men with similar CAC score [25, 26]. In the Multi-Ethnic Study of Atherosclerosis (MESA), women classified as low CVD risk by the Framingham Risk Score that had a CAC >0, experienced a 6.5-fold increased risk of myocardial infarction over the following 4 years compared with women without detectable CAC [27]. Women with a history of pre-eclampsia, have a twofold higher risk of a positive CAC score at age 50 years compared to women with normotensive pregnancies [28]. Early onset of CAC in women with a history of preeclampsia and with autoimmune disorders is well documented [28, 29], in line with the increased risk of CVD later in life in these women. Many of these CVD events occur already in midlife.

2.2 Hypertensive Heart Disease

Chronic hypertension leads to structural and functional changes of the myocardium, including left ventricular (LV) hypertrophy, left atrial enlargement (LAE), abnormal LV geometry, or reduced LV systolic or diastolic function [30]. Presence of such cardiac organ damage is collectively termed hypertensive heart disease which is associate with high or very high risk of subsequent CVD events [3, 4] (Fig. 1). Co-presence of other metabolic comorbidities like obesity, diabetes mellitus or reduced renal function, potentiate the risk of cardiac organ damage in hypertension, particularly in women [31].

2.2.1 Left Ventricular Hypertrophy

In studies using echocardiography and sex-specific threshold values to identify LV hypertrophy, women are documented to have higher prevalence of LV hypertrophy than men [32–34]. In the population-based Framingham Heart Study, including participants aged 17–90 years, LV hypertrophy was on average found in 19% of women and in 16% of men, and increased more with age in women [32]. In the age-group >70 years, 49% of women and 33% of men had LV hypertrophy [32]. In the Campania Salute Network registry, LV hypertrophy was found at baseline in 43% of women and 32% of men with treated hypertension [33]. The difference was not explained by older age or higher prevalence of obesity in women. However, in both the Framingham Heart Study and in the Campania Salute Network registry, co-presence of obesity was an important independent confounder. In the Losartan Intervention for Endpoint reduction in hypertension (LIFE) study, a randomized clinical trial comparing the effect of losartan versus atenolol-based treatment on LV hypertrophy regression in women and men with signs of LV hypertrophy on the electrocardiogram (ECG), women had higher prevalence of LV hypertrophy by echocardiography both at baseline (80 vs. 70%) and after 5-years systematic antihypertensive treatment (47 vs. 32%). This may have contributed to the higher occurrence of hospitalization for angina pectoris in women than men during follow-up in that study [35]. Concentric LV hypertrophy may lead to arterial-muscle mismatch and myocardial ischemia, particularly in the endocardial part of the myocardium. Presence of myocardial ischemia in this setting may be diagnosed using myocardial contrast enhance echocardiography at rest or during stress [36]. Less regression of LV hypertrophy in women was also documented in the Campania Salute Network registry [33]. Furthermore, data from this registry also demonstrated that the regression of LV hypertrophy in clinical practice was much less than what had been documented from clinical trials, and only observed in 14% of participants [37]. Female sex was the strongest predictor of persistent LV hypertrophy, independent of BP control and obesity [37]. Among native North-American Indians with treated hypertension participating in the Strong Heart Study, LV hypertrophy was found in 36% of women and 23% of men at baseline, and regression of LV hypertrophy over 4 years was only observed in 3% women and in 10% of men [38]. The main confounders of lack of LV hypertrophy regression were female sex, and concomitant obesity or albuminuria [38]. Finally, among patients without LV hypertrophy at baseline, participating in the Campania Salute Network registry, 21% developed LV hypertrophy during 16 years follow-up, despite systematic antihypertensive therapy [39]. Women with obesity had the highest risk of developing LV hypertrophy, but also normal-weight women had twice the risk compared to that of obese men [39].

2.2.2 Left Ventricular Geometry

LV hypertrophy may be further divided into eccentric and concentric LV hypertrophy based upon the LV posterior wall to LV internal diameter at end-diastole. If this ratio, referred to as relative wall thickness, is ≥ 0.43, the LV hypertrophy is considered concentric. Traditionally, LV geometry is divided into four geometric types in hypertension, based upon LV hypertrophy and the LV posterior wall to LV internal diameter at end-diastole normal (relative wall thickness, RWT) [40]. These different geometric types are characterized by clusters of clinical risk factors and co-morbidities (Fig. 2). It is well demonstrated that the concentric LV geometry carries the highest risk of CVD in hypertension [41]. In the LIFE study, LV concentric remodelling and LV concentric hypertrophy were both associated with a twofold higher risk of combined CV death, myocardial infarction and stroke over 4.8-years follow up [41]. In morbidly obese women participating in the Norwegian FATWEST study, including 57% with treated hypertension, LV hypertrophy was reduced by 46% in women within 1-year after undergoing bariatric surgery, and treated hypertension by 55% [42]. However, women more often remained with concentric LV remodelling rather than normal LV geometry, and with reduced LV midwall function, despite improvements in LV hypertrophy and LV long axis function by global longitudinal strain (GLS). Taken together, this points to the difficulties in preventing and treating LV hypertrophy in women with hypertension if metabolic co-morbidities are not managed. In the Vobarno cohort from Northern Italy, concentric LV hypertrophy was also associated with presence of increased carotid intima-media thickness and plaques, probably contributing to the worsened prognosis in these patients [43].

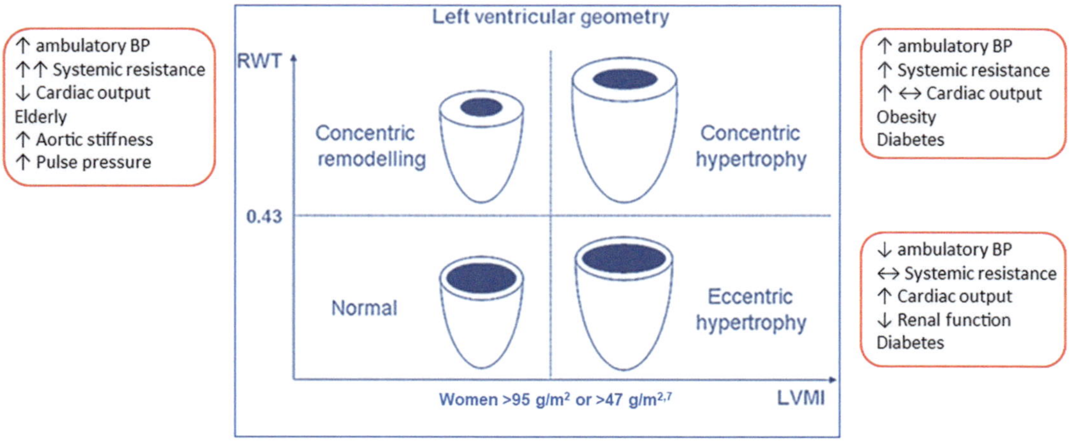

RWT, relative wall thickness; LVMI, left ventricular mass index; BP, blood pressure

Fig. 2 Clinical and hemodynamic characteristics of different LV geometric patterns in hypertension using echocardiography

2.2.3 Left Atrial Enlargement

Although LV hypertrophy is the cardinal sign of cardiac organ damage in hypertension, LAE is another highly prevalent type of cardiac organ damage that is particularly associated with risk of atrial fibrillation and heart failure with preserved ejection fraction in women. Many clinical studies have found LAE to be more common in women than in men when left atrium volume is indexed to body height squared, rather than to body surface area [44–46]. This may reflect that overadjustment occurs when body surface area is used as indexation in obese subjects [44]. In an Italian multicentre study, LAE was found in 59% of women compared to in 43% of men. The prevalence of LAE also increased in parallel with increasing body mass index. In the Norwegian FATCOR (FAT-associated CardiOvasculaR dysfunction) study in obese subjects, 74% of women versus 56% of men had LAE [46]. Finally, in the LIFE study, 56% of women and 38% of men had LAE [45, 47]. Thus, co-presence of obesity is an important confounder for development of LAE in hypertension. As demonstrated in the LIFE study, little reduction in LAE occurred during 4.8-years of antihypertensive therapy, and patients remaining with LAE had an increased risk of combined myocardial infarction, ischemic stroke and CV death, and of atrial fibrillation [45, 48]. Important confounders of LAE were female gender, independent of older age, presence of LV hypertrophy, mitral regurgitation or history of atrial fibrillation [47]. In the Norwegian Tromsø Study, physical activity attenuated the risk of atrial fibrillation with LAE in both women and men [49].

2.2.4 LV Systolic and Diastolic Dysfunction

LV systolic function is normal in most women with hypertension, but reduced LV ejection fraction or reduced myocardial function by LV midwall shortening or LV global longitudinal strain (GLS) may be present [50, 51]. Measures of systolic function all vary in relation to the LV geometry [52]. All measures of LV systolic function are higher in women compared to men. In the Strong Heart Study, women had a 3% higher LV ejection fraction and a 2.7% greater stress-corrected LV midwall shortening [53]. In the LIFE study, women had a 2% higher LV ejection fraction and stress-corrected LV midwall shortening, and these indices of LV systolic function were particularly higher in women with LV hypertrophy [52].

Few studies have reported gender-specific thresholds for GLS. Compared to women with normotension, GLS is worse in women with hypertension, and if concentric geometry or LV concentric LV hypertrophy is present. Several studies have found that women have better (more negative) GLS than men [51, 54, 55]. In obese women in the FATCOR study, low GLS was particularly associated with presence of higher arterial stiffness, abdominal obesity and lower LV ejection fraction [55]. Furthermore, co-presence of hypertension was associated with reduced GLS [55, 56]. In the Copenhagen City Heart Study, less decline in GLS with aging was found in women and in normotensive individuals [57]. In the same cohort, LV mass index and GLS improved identification of high risk individuals beyond clinical CVD risk factors in individuals with hypertension [58]. Lower GLS was a weaker prognostic marker for risk of heart failure, myocardial infarction and CV death in women than in men [59]. In a much smaller, retrospective study in patients with treated hypertension, GLS added some prognostic information to that of clinical risk factors and presence of concentric LV hypertrophy [60], but sex specific results were not presented. Thus, we still lack information about how to best identify and use low GLS as a risk marker in women with hypertension.

Hypertension is associated with reduced early (E) and increased atrial trans-mitral blood velocity, increased atrial filling fraction and prolonged E deceleration time and isovolumic relaxation time. LV diastolic dysfunction is common in individuals with hypertension, and more complex to assess than LV systolic dysfunction, even using recent joint European and American guidelines [61]. The prevalence of LV diastolic dysfunction increases with age and is higher in women than in men at older age [31, 62]. The higher prevalence in women has been attributed to higher arterial stiffness, differences in central aortic wave reflection, and clustering of metabolic and inflammatory co-morbidities. Most women with LV hypertrophy have LV diastolic dysfunction. In the Atherosclerosis Risk in Communities (ARIC) study, women had lower early myocardial relaxation velocity (e′), but better GLS than men [63]. In the MESA study, magnetic resonance T1 mapping demonstrated that interstitial fibrosis was associated with lower early diastolic strain rate and preserved LV ejection fraction in women [64]. Taken together, these findings reflect that women develop greater myocardial stiffness and more often LV diastolic dysfunction with aging than men.

3 Clinical Practice

3.1 Diagnosis of Hypertensive Organ Damage in the Arteries

Sex- and age-specific threshold values for diagnosis of arterial organ damage in large arteries by arterial stiffness and intima-media thickness, and in small arteries by lumen-media ratio and flow-mediated vasodilatation have been published [7, 12–14, 65]. Current guidelines on hypertension recommend that diagnosis of arterial organ damage is done by ultrasound of the carotid arteries to measure intima-media thickness and identify presence of atherosclerotic plaques, by using aplanation tonometry to measure arterial stiffness, and by using CT for assessment of coronary atherosclerosis by CAC score [3, 4] (Table 1).

3.1.1 Carotid Atherosclerosis

A carotid intima media thickness (cIMT) >0.9 mm is considered abnormal, but the upper limit of normality varies with age. The presence of a carotid plaque can be identified by a cIMT ≥1.5 mm, or by a focal increase in thickness of 0.5 mm or more than 50% of the surrounding cIMT value. The cIMT is lower in women than in men and increases less with aging in women [10, 65]. In parallel, the prevalence of asymptomatic carotid stenosis increases with age in both women and men, but is lower in women at all ages. Still, the recommended thresholds for identification of increased cIMT and carotid plaque in clinical practice are the same in both genders [3, 4].

3.1.2 Large Artery Stiffness

Arterial stiffness can be estimated from the brachial pulse pressure, the ratio of pulse pressure to stroke volume index combining brachial blood pressure measurement and echocardiography, or more directly from measurement of carotid-femoral or brachial-ankle PWV. A brachial pulse pressure >60 mmHg is considered a marker of increased arterial stiffness in the absence of

Table 1 Prognostically validated markers of cardiovascular organ damage in women with hypertension

Method	Marker	Organ damage threshold in women
Arterial organ damage		
BP	Brachial pulse pressure	>60 mmHg
Ultrasound	Carotid IMT	>0.9 mm
	Carotid plaque	≥1.5 mm
Aplanation tonometry	Carotid-femoral PWV	>10 m/s if <60 years
	Brachial-ankle PWV	>18 m/s if >60 years
Cardiac organ damage		
ECG	Rhythm	Atrial fibrillation
	LV hypertrophy	Sokolow-Lyon voltage >38 mm
		Cornell product >2440 mm x ms
Echocardiography	LV hypertrophy	>47 g/body height in $m^{2.7}$ if overweight
		>95 g/body surface area if normal weight
	LV relative wall thickness	>0.42
	LAE	>16.5 ml/body height^2
	LV ejection fraction	<54%
Coronary CT	Coronary calcium score	>reference for age

hemodynamic significant aortic valve regurgitation, and has been associated with presence of CV organ damage in several studies [66, 67]. Women normally have a higher brachial pulse pressure than men. In primary health care, a pulse pressure >60 mmHg may serve as an indicator for arterial organ damage and high CV risk in hypertension. A carotid-femoral PWV >10 m/s is considered a sign of increased arterial stiffness, reflecting arterial organ damage in both women and men, particularly in individuals younger than 60 years [3]. The brachial-ankle PWV has so far primarily been explored in Asian populations. Brachial-ankle PWV increases with age in both genders, is lower in women than men up to age 58 years, thereafter it increases steeper in women. A brachial-ankle PWV >18 m/s is considered a sign of increased arterial stiffness in both women and men older than 60 years [4, 68, 69]. (Table 1) Despite the documented gender differences in longitudinal increase in pulse pressure and arterial stiffness with aging, and the stronger association between arterial stiffness and all-cause mortality in women [9], gender-specific threshold values for detection of arterial organ damage by the above markers have not been well enough documented to be included in current European guidelines [3, 4, 70]. Serial assessments of carotid-femoral PWV in follow-up of ischemic stroke survivors found a similar increase in PWV in both genders, and higher age and BP and lack of antihypertensive drug treatment were the main confounders of progressive arterial stiffening [71]. From this, early and accurate identification of hypertension and normalization of BP by drug treatment is suggested to reduce hypertension-associated increase in PWV.

3.1.3 Coronary Computed Tomography Calcium Score and Angiography

Current European guidelines on CVD prevention recommend the use of CAC score for more accurate atherosclerotic CVD risk assessment in women with a calculated risk from SCORE2 around the decision threshold, and when the result is likely to change management of the patient [70]. If CAC is detected, its extent should be interpreted using sex and age-specific thresholds. Higher-than-expected CAC score will increase the CVD risk and lower-than-expected CAC score will decrease the CVD risk in the individual person. In women, this is particularly relevant when chronic inflammatory disorders or female specific CVD risk factors, like premature menopause (i.e. before age 40 years) and pregnancy complications are present, or when clinical risk assessment is low or intermediate when using 10-year risk scores like the Framingham Risk Score or the SCORE2 [29]. In women with intermediate CVD risk, CAC score may also be used when there is uncertainty about the safety of menopausal hormone therapy [72].

Of note, women may have coronary plaques and significant stenoses despite no detectable CAC. In a pooled analysis of two clinical trials of women with chest pain diagnosed with non-obstructive CAD diagnosed by CCTA, presence of non-obstructive CAD was associated with future CVD, while CAC score was not, suggesting that CAC scoring is a better prognosticator in men than in women with chest pain [73]. In the CONFIRM (Coronary CT Angiography Evaluation for Clinical Outcomes: An International Multicentre) registry, presence of hypertension or diabetes did not worsen prognosis in patients with normal CCTA, while it did in patients with non-obstructive CAD [74]. It should also be noted that the diagnostic value of a CAC score of 0 to rule out CAD in women with clinical risk factors is less effective in women younger than 60 years who may have obstructive CAD and increased risk of myocardial infarction and death despite a CAC score of 0, pointing to the added value of performing combined CAC score and CCTA in these women [75].

3.2 Diagnosis of Hypertensive Heart Disease

In clinical practice, ECG and echocardiography remain the main methods for diagnosis of cardiac organ damage in women with hypertension. Although LV hypertrophy may be diagnosed by both ECG and by echocardiography, the latter is preferred due to higher sensitivity and information about functional consequences and additional cardiac disease. LV hypertrophy may also be diagnosed by cardiac CT or magnetic resonance imaging; however, these methods are less available and more costly. In clinical practice, taking an ECG at initial diagnosis of hypertension and at annual BP controls is advised.

3.2.1 ECG

ECG is primarily used for detection of atrial fibrillation or LV hypertrophy in hypertension, but P wave analysis may also indicate LAE. Presence of atrial fibrillation in women with hypertension reflects presence of cardiac organ damage. Performance of commonly used ECG criteria for diagnosis of LV hypertrophy vary by gender [76]. Women have shorter QRS duration and lower QRS voltage with consequent parallel gender differences in ECG criteria for LV hypertrophy. Furthermore, gender differences in body size, obesity and LV mass may contribute to these diagnostic differences. The Sokolow Lyon voltage criterion is more often false negative in women, probably reflecting that the same threshold value ($S_{V1} + R_{V5}$ >38 mm) is recommended in both women and men [3, 4]. In contrast, the Cornell product ($R_{AVL} + S_{V3}$ [+ 6 mm added in women] multiplied by QRS duration >2440 ms mm) performs better in women and in obese individuals [77] (Table 1). Combination of more than one ECG criterion is recommended for better identification of LV hypertrophy by ECG [78].

3.2.2 Echocardiography

Ideally, echocardiography should be performed in all patients with hypertension, irrespective of the severity of hypertension and presence of symptoms, given the documented high prevalence of cardiac organ damage like LV hypertrophy and LAE particularly in women even in asymptomatic mild-moderate hypertension [5]. Standard echocardiography includes reporting of left atrial volume and LV mass. Current guidelines recommend identification of LV hypertrophy from LV mass indexed to height$^{2.7}$ in women with overweight or obesity, while indexation to body surface area may be used in the minority of normal weight women with hypertension [3]. Prognostically validated sex specific threshold values for identification of LV hypertrophy should always be applied (Table 1). In parallel, identification of LAE should be based on left atrial volume indexed to height^2, and gender specific threshold values (Table 1). LV concentric remodelling is diagnosed as the ratio between LV posterior wall thickness × 2 and internal chamber diameter at end-diastole ≥0.43 in both women and men (Table 1).

Given the known higher indices of LV systolic function in women compared to men, low LV systolic function should be identified by gender specific thresholds whenever possible [50]. In women, LV ejection is considered low if <54%, while <52% is used as threshold for low LV ejection fraction in men [50]. Low LV midwall shortening is considered present if <16% in women and <14% in men (Table 1). Gender specific thresholds for low GLS are not well established. In healthy individuals, Kokabay et al. suggested GLS >18.5% in women and >16.9% in men as threshold values for low GLS [51]. In the population-based Tromsø Study, low GLS was identified as >17.8% in women and >15.9% in men [54]. Current guidelines in hypertension suggest GLS<20% as normal both for women and men [4]. Of note, it is common to find reduced LV midwall shortening or GLS despite a normal LV ejection fraction in women with hypertension when LV hypertrophy or concentric LV remodelling is present, reflecting the increased myocardial fibrosis associated with concentric LV geometry [79].

Reduced LV diastolic function is common in women with hypertension and may be present also in absence of LV hypertrophy. Detailed algorithms for diagnosis of LV diastolic dysfunction by echocardiography are provided in the joint European and American guidelines [61]. These guidelines use the same diagnostic algorithm for women and men and recommend assessing LV diastolic function from a combination of four variables: left atrial volume/body surface area >34 ml/m^2, mitral annular e′ velocity <7 cm/s septal or <10 cm/s lateral, mitral E/e′ ratio >14, and peak tricuspid valve regurgitation jet velocity >2.8 m/s [61]. In a sub study of the ASCOT (Anglo-Scandinavian Cardiac Outcomes Trial) in hypertension, the E/e′ ratio independently predicted increased risk of myocardial infarction [80]. Based on this, an average E/e′ ratio >14 and low e′ has been suggested as markers of cardiac organ damage in hypertension in recent guidelines [4]. However, prognostic validation of gender specific thresholds for e′ or E/e′ ratio in hypertension have not been published. Taken together, diagnosis of LV diastolic dysfunction as markers of hypertensive heart disease remains less established compared to LV hypertrophy and LAE. It also remains difficult to differentiate between LV diastolic dysfunction as part of hypertensive heart disease and versus heart failure with preserved ejection fraction in clinical practice, in particular in women with hypertension who report dyspnoea. Measurement of N-terminal pro-brain natriuretic peptide (NTproBNP) and use of the Heart Failure Association PEFF score may be helpful in making this differential diagnosis [81].

3.3 Management of Cardiovascular Organ Damage

Women diagnosed with any type of cardiovascular organ damage have CVD in its preclinical phase, and thorough CVD risk factors exploration and intervention is recommended to reduce progression to clinical CVD. In particular smoking cessation and treatment of hypertension, diabetes and obesity to recommended targets should be implemented in the individual woman [3, 82].

In women with asymptomatic carotid atherosclerosis, the European Society for Vascular Surgery guidelines recommend thorough risk factor management, including smoking cessation, and management of obesity, hypertension and diabetes [82]. Treatment with statins and antihypertensive drugs to targets and optimal glycaemic control are recommended (class I) to reduce the risk of stroke, and antiplatelet therapy with aspirin or clopidogrel may be considered (class IIA) mainly to reduce risk of other CVD [82]. The European Lacidipine Study on Atherosclerosis (ELSA) in asymptomatic patients with hypertension and increased cIMT demonstrated that lacidipine-based treatment reduced progression of carotid atherosclerosis better than atenolol-based treatment independent of BP reduction [83]. Serial assessment using carotid ultrasound is in general not recommended, since it will not change the clinical management.

Many women with hypertension report exertional dyspnoea, particularly when LV hypertrophy is present, and referral to CCTA to rule out significant CAD in these women is advisable. If non-obstructive CAD or a higher-than-expected CAC score for age is detected in asymptomatic women undergoing CCTA, this reflects preclinical CAD, and intensive lifestyle and pharmacological therapies should be implemented to lower risk of clinical CVD. In particular, statin therapy and antihypertensive drug therapy to achieve recommended targets should be used as prevention of clinical CVD in these women.

In general, early detection of hypertension is suggested to reduce hypertensive heart disease, although this is not well documented from clinical trials [3, 4] (Fig. 1). Opportunistic BP screening may help early detection of hypertension, as will more widely use of out-of-office measurement of BP, either home BP or 24-h ambulatory BP measurements [3, 4]. In women diagnosed with cardiac organ damage, antihypertensive drug treatment shoudl be considered when BP >130/80 mmHg [84]. Treatment to recommended BP target 120–129/70–79 mmHg is important. Angiotensin receptor blocker-based treatment is recommended as first choice in combination with a calcium channel blocker or a hydrochlorothiazide, preferably in a single pill combination [4]. Among these women, a focus on comorbidities like obesity and diabetes is also of utmost important, since reduction of LV hypertrophy seldom will occur if these metabolic CVD risk factors are not all controlled. Furthermore, referral to hypertension specialists may be important to exclude secondary causes of hypertension or drug non-adherence in those women that do not obtain a normal BP after prescription of a combination of three drugs including a diuretic in maximal tolerable dosages [4]. Finally, doctor inertia remains an important cause of undiagnosed and uncontrolled hypertension even in areas with modern healthcare systems. Women themselves should therefore be informed about the high risk of organ damage in hypertension and get actively involved in early diagnosis and optimalization of their hypertension management.

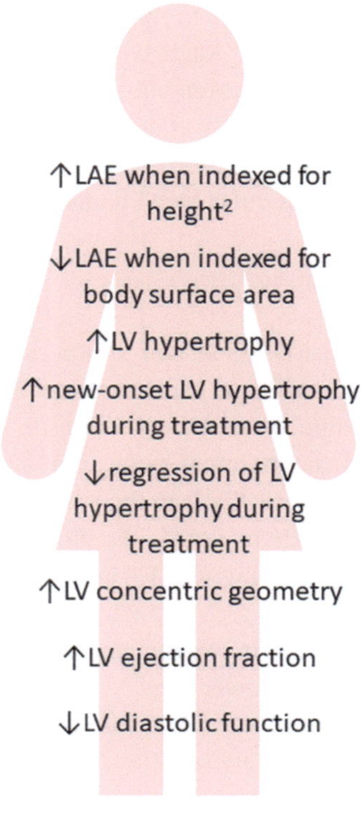

Fig. 3 Characteristics of hypertensive heart disease in women

4 Conclusions

Cardiovascular organ damage differs by gender in hypertension (Fig. 3). Arterial stiffness increases steeper in women than men with aging, and high arterial stiffness carries higher risk of CVD in women. Women have less CAC, but presence of significant CAD and risk of myocardial infarction and death may be high despite undetectable CAC, in particular in women <60 years of age. Women with hypertension are more prone to develop cardiac organ damage like LV hypertrophy and LAE but retain higher LV ejection fraction and other indices of LV systolic function, and more often reduced LV diastolic function. Sex specific thresholds are recommended for accurate diagnosis of LV hypertrophy, LAE and LV ejection fraction, while gender specific thresholds for identification of high arterial stiffness, low GLS and LV diastolic dysfunction are still not firmly established. When hypertension is complicated by LV hypertrophy, the risk of CVD increases relatively more in women and becomes similar to that of men. Antihypertensive drug therapy is less effective in inducing regression of LV hypertrophy in women. Women also more often develop new-onset LV hypertrophy during antihypertensive treatment. The underlying mechanisms for these gender differences remain unknown, pointing to the need for more research on CV organ damage in women with hypertension. Aggressive antihypertensive treatment and management of other important risk factors like obesity and atherosclerosis is recommended to induce regression or slow progression of cardiovascular organ damage into clinical CVD.

Key Issues

- Hypertension associated structural and functional changes in the heart are collectively termed hypertensive heart disease
- Cardiovascular organ damage in the heart and arteries reflects CVD in the preclinical state
- Women with hypertension more often have LV hypertrophy, LAE and LV diastolic dysfunction
- PWV is lower in women, and the risk of CVD increases at a lower level
- Women have lower CAC than men, and severe CAD may be present despite no detectable CAC in women
- Combined CAC and CCTA is recommended in high-risk or symptomatic women with hypertension for accurate identification of significant CAD

Questions and Answers

1. What does the term hypertensive heart disease mean?
   (A) Structural changes in the heart caused by hypertension
   (B) Presence of LV hypertrophy
   (C) Asymptomatic LV diastolic dysfunction in hypertension
   (D) Structural and functional changes in the heart in hypertension
   Comment: Answer D) is the best answer. Hypertensive heart disease is a term used for different structural and functional changes in the heart that develop as a consequence of chronic hypertension. Types of hypertensive heart disease includes LV hypertrophy, LAE, reduced LV systolic or diastolic function.
2. Which factor is the most important for development of LV hypertrophy in women with hypertension?
   (A) Older age
   (B) Concomitant obesity
   (C) Menopause
   (D) Concomitant diabetes
   Comment: Answer B) is the best answer. Obesity was a key confounder of new-onset LV hypertrophy during antihypertensive treatment in the Campania Salute Network registry. Persistent obesity is also a main obstacle to regression of LV hypertrophy during antihypertensive drug treatment, as demonstrated both in clinical trials and in prospective cohort studies. Although prevalence of LV hypertrophy increases with aging, higher prevalence of LV hypertrophy in women compared to men has been demonstrated both in pre- and postmenopausal women. In the LIFE study, obesity was a stronger confounder of LV hypertrophy than diabetes mellitus.
3. A 56 years-old woman complaints about exertional dyspnea that has evolved over the past 6 months. She was diagnosed with hypertension four years ago, around the time of menopause, and is treated with a single pill combination of an angiotensin receptor blocker and hydrochlorothiazide. She had a hypertensive pregnancy complication 20 years ago and has been obese most of her adult life. She is a never smoker. At the primary care physician's office her BP is 140/90 mmHg, the BMI is 35 kg/m^2, and the ECG is normal. What additional testing would you perform?
   (A) Echocardiography
   (B) None
   (C) CCTA
   (D) NT-proBNP
   Comment: Answer A) is the best. You would start by referring to an echocardiography to evaluate the cardiac structure and function for diagnosis of hypertensive heart disease. The patient has increased risk of premature CAD beyond what is captured by SCORE2. To rule out significant CAD, a CCTA should also be performed. In clinical practice, NT-proBNP may be measured to rule out heart failure as the cause of dyspnea. At the same time, analysis of hemoglobin, renal function and thyroid function should be performed to rule out other common causes of dyspnea. If all tests turn out to be normal, a chest X-ray and lung function testing should be performed. However,

obesity is also a well-known cause of reduced physical capacity and exertional dyspnea.

4. You referred a 75 years-old woman with hypertension to echocardiography due to a routine ECG demonstrating LV hypertrophy. She is taking a hydrochlorothiazide diuretic as monotherapy. At the office, her seated BP is 150/70 mmHg and the heart rate is 64 and regular. Her BP is 160/70 mmHg in the upright position. She does not have any complaints. Her renal function and serum electrolytes are normal. The echocardiogram demonstrated combined LAE and concentric LV remodeling. How would you manage this patient?
   (A) Continue the drug treatment unchanged
   (B) Add low-dose aspirin
   (C) Switch to a single pill combination of angiotensin receptor blocker and hydrochlorothiazide
   (D) Add an angiotensin receptor blocker

   Comment: Answer C) is the best. This patient has asymptomatic hypertensive heart disease. Combination therapy with an angiotensin receptor blocker and a calcium channel blocker or a hydrochlorothiazide in a single pill is recommended as the initial treatment of hypertension in most women. The LIFE study demonstrated that reduction in LAE was somewhat better in response to losartan-based compared to atenolol-based therapy and gave a larger reduction in risk of stroke and atrial fibrillation. Therefore, switching to a single pill combination of angiotensin receptor blocker and hydrochlorothiazide to improve systolic BP control and reduce risk of stroke and atrial fibrillation is suggested.

References

1. Coutinho T, Yam Y, Chow BJW, Dwivedi G, Inacio J. Sex differences in associations of arterial compliance with coronary artery plaque and calcification burden. J Am Heart Assoc. 2017;6(8):e006079.
2. Devereux RB, Alderman MH. Role of preclinical cardiovascular disease in the evolution from risk factor exposure to development of morbid events. Circulation. 1993;88(4):1444–55.
3. Williams B, Mancia G, Spiering W, Agabiti Rosei E, Azizi M, Burnier M, et al. 2018 ESC/ESH guidelines for the management of arterial hypertension. Eur Heart J. 2018;39(33):3021–104.
4. Mancia G, Kreutz R, Brunstrom M, Burnier M, Grassi G, Januszewicz A, et al. 2023 ESH guidelines for the management of arterial hypertension the task force for the management of arterial hypertension of the European Society of Hypertension Endorsed by the International Society of Hypertension (ISH) and the European Renal Association (ERA). J Hypertens. 2023;41:1874–2071.
5. Gerdts E, Sudano I, Brouwers S, Borghi C, Bruno RM, Ceconi C, et al. Sex differences in arterial hypertension. Eur Heart J. 2022;43(46):4777–88.
6. Gerdts E, Regitz-Zagrosek V. Sex differences in cardiometabolic disorders. Nat Med. 2019;25(11):1657–66.
7. Bruno RM, Grassi G, Seravalle G, Savoia C, Rizzoni D, Virdis A, et al. Age- and sex-specific reference values for media/lumen ratio in small arteries and relationship with risk factors. Hypertension. 2018;71(6):1193–200.
8. Vasan RS, Pan S, Larson MG, Mitchell GF, Xanthakis V. Arteriosclerosis, atherosclerosis, and cardiovascular health: joint relations to the incidence of cardiovascular disease. Hypertension. 2021;78(5):1232–40.
9. DuPont JJ, Kenney RM, Patel AR, Jaffe IZ. Sex differences in mechanisms of arterial stiffness. Br J Pharmacol. 2019;176(21):4208–25.
10. Karikkineth AC, AlGhatrif M, Oberdier MT, Morrell C, Palchamy E, Strait JB, et al. Sex differences in longitudinal determinants of carotid intima medial thickening with aging in a community-dwelling population: the Baltimore longitudinal study on aging. J Am Heart Assoc. 2020;9(22):e015396.
11. Vaccarino V, Badimon L, Corti R, de Wit C, Dorobantu M, Hall A, et al. Ischaemic heart disease in women: are there sex differences in pathophysiology and risk factors? Position paper from the working group on coronary pathophysiology and microcirculation of the European Society of Cardiology. Cardiovasc Res. 2011;90(1):9–17.
12. Holder SM, Bruno RM, Shkredova DA, Dawson EA, Jones H, Hopkins ND, et al. Reference intervals for brachial artery flow-mediated dilation and the relation with cardiovascular risk factors. Hypertension. 2021;77(5):1469–80.
13. Van Bortel LM, Laurent S, Boutouyrie P, Chowienczyk P, Cruickshank JK, De Backer T, et al. Expert consensus document on the measurement of aortic stiffness in daily practice using carotid-femoral pulse wave velocity. J Hypertens. 2012;30(3):445–8.
14. McEniery CM, Yasmin, Hall IR, Qasem A, Wilkinson IB, Cockcroft JR, et al. Normal vascular aging: differential effects on wave reflection and aortic pulse wave velocity: the Anglo-Cardiff Collaborative Trial (ACCT). J Am Coll Cardiol. 2005;46(9):1753–60.
15. Greenland P, Blaha MJ, Budoff MJ, Erbel R, Watson KE. Coronary calcium score and cardiovascular risk. J Am Coll Cardiol. 2018;72(4):434–47.

16. Uddin SMI, Mirbolouk M, Kianoush S, Orimoloye OA, Dardari Z, Whelton SP, et al. Role of coronary artery calcium for stratifying cardiovascular risk in adults with hypertension. Hypertension. 2019;73(5):983–9.
17. Joakimsen O, Bonaa KH, Stensland-Bugge E, Jacobsen BK. Age and sex differences in the distribution and ultrasound morphology of carotid atherosclerosis: the Tromso Study. Arterioscler Thromb Vasc Biol. 1999;19(12):3007–13.
18. Mancusi C, Manzi MV, de Simone G, Morisco C, Lembo M, Pilato E, et al. Carotid atherosclerosis predicts blood pressure control in patients with hypertension: the campania salute network registry. J Am Heart Assoc. 2022;11(5):e022345.
19. van Dam-Nolen DHK, van Egmond NCM, Koudstaal PJ, van der Lugt A, Bos D. Sex differences in carotid atherosclerosis: a systematic review and meta-analysis. Stroke. 2023;54(2):315–26.
20. Theofilatos K, Stojkovic S, Hasman M, van der Laan SW, Baig F, Barallobre-Barreiro J, et al. Proteomic atlas of atherosclerosis: the contribution of proteoglycans to sex differences, plaque phenotypes, and outcomes. Circ Res. 2023;133(7):542–58.
21. Mitchell GF, Rong J, Larson MG, Cooper LL, Xanthakis V, Benjamin EJ, et al. Longitudinal hemodynamic correlates of and sex differences in the evolution of blood pressure across the adult lifespan: the framingham heart study. J Am Heart Assoc. 2023;12(12):e027329.
22. Samargandy S, Matthews KA, Brooks MM, Barinas-Mitchell E, Magnani JW, Janssen I, et al. Arterial stiffness accelerates within 1 year of the final menstrual period: the SWAN heart study. Arterioscler Thromb Vasc Biol. 2020;40(4):1001–8.
23. Kwak S, Kim HL, Lim WH, Seo JB, Kim SH, Zo JH, et al. Sex-specific associations of brachial-ankle pulse wave velocity with adverse cardiac remodeling and long-term cardiovascular outcome. J Hypertens. 2022;40(2):364–73.
24. Scantlebury DC, Borlaug BA. Why are women more likely than men to develop heart failure with preserved ejection fraction? Curr Opin Cardiol. 2011;26(6):562–8.
25. Shaw LJ, Min JK, Nasir K, Xie JX, Berman DS, Miedema MD, et al. Sex differences in calcified plaque and long-term cardiovascular mortality: observations from the CAC Consortium. Eur Heart J. 2018;39(41):3727–35.
26. Dzaye O, Al Rifai M, Dardari Z, Shaw LJ, Al-Mallah MH, Handy Marshall C, et al. Coronary artery calcium as a synergistic tool for the age- and sex-specific risk of cardiovascular and cancer mortality: the coronary artery calcium consortium. J Am Heart Assoc. 2020;9(8):e015306.
27. Lakoski SG, Greenland P, Wong ND, Schreiner PJ, Herrington DM, Kronmal RA, et al. Coronary artery calcium scores and risk for cardiovascular events in women classified as "low risk" based on Framingham risk score: the multi-ethnic study of atherosclerosis (MESA). Arch Intern Med. 2007;167(22):2437–42.
28. Benschop L, Brouwers L, Zoet GA, Meun C, Boersma E, Budde RPJ, et al. Early onset of coronary artery calcification in women with previous preeclampsia. Circ Cardiovasc Imaging. 2020;13(11):e010340.
29. Dzaye O, Dudum R, Reiter-Brennan C, Kianoush S, Tota-Maharaj R, Cainzos-Achirica M, et al. Coronary artery calcium scoring for individualized cardiovascular risk estimation in important patient subpopulations after the 2019 AHA/ACC primary prevention guidelines. Prog Cardiovasc Dis. 2019;62(5):423–30.
30. Newby DE, Mannucci PM, Tell GS, Baccarelli AA, Brook RD, Donaldson K, et al. Expert position paper on air pollution and cardiovascular disease. Eur Heart J. 2015;36(2):83–93.
31. Muiesan ML, Paini A, Aggiusti C, Bertacchini F, Rosei CA, Salvetti M. Hypertension and organ damage in women. High Blood Press Cardiovasc Prev. 2018;25(3):245–52.
32. Levy D, Anderson KM, Savage DD, Kannel WB, Christiansen JC, Castelli WP. Echocardiographically detected left ventricular hypertrophy: prevalence and risk factors. The Framingham Heart Study. Ann Intern Med. 1988;108(1):7–13.
33. Gerdts E, Izzo R, Mancusi C, Losi MA, Manzi MV, Canciello G, et al. Left ventricular hypertrophy offsets the sex difference in cardiovascular risk (the campania salute network). Int J Cardiol. 2018;258:257–61.
34. Gerdts E, Okin PM, de Simone G, Cramariuc D, Wachtell K, Boman K, et al. Gender differences in left ventricular structure and function during antihypertensive treatment: the losartan intervention for endpoint reduction in hypertension study. Hypertension. 2008;51(4):1109–14.
35. Os I, Franco V, Kjeldsen SE, Manhem K, Devereux RB, Gerdts E, et al. Effects of losartan in women with hypertension and left ventricular hypertrophy: results from the losartan intervention for endpoint reduction in hypertension study. Hypertension. 2008;51(4):1103–8.
36. Lonnebakken MT, Rieck AE, Gerdts E. Contrast stress echocardiography in hypertensive heart disease. Cardiovasc Ultrasound. 2011;9:33.
37. Lonnebakken MT, Izzo R, Mancusi C, Gerdts E, Losi MA, Canciello G, et al. Left ventricular hypertrophy regression during antihypertensive treatment in an outpatient clinic (the campania salute network). J Am Heart Assoc. 2017;6(3):e004152.
38. de Simone G, Devereux RB, Izzo R, Girfoglio D, Lee ET, Howard BV, et al. Lack of reduction of left ventricular mass in treated hypertension: the strong heart study. J Am Heart Assoc. 2013;2(3):e000144.
39. Izzo R, Losi MA, Stabile E, Lonnebakken MT, Canciello G, Esposito G, et al. Development of left ventricular hypertrophy in treated hypertensive outpatients: the campania salute network. Hypertension. 2017;69(1):136–42.
40. Koren MJ, Devereux RB, Casale PN, Savage DD, Laragh JH. Relation of left ventricular mass and geometry to morbidity and mortality in uncomplicated essential hypertension. Ann Intern Med. 1991;114(5):345–52.

41. Gerdts E, Cramariuc D, de Simone G, Wachtell K, Dahlof B, Devereux RB. Impact of left ventricular geometry on prognosis in hypertensive patients with left ventricular hypertrophy (the LIFE study). Eur J Echocardiogr. 2008;9(6):809–15.
42. Grymyr LMD, Nadirpour S, Gerdts E, Nedrebo BG, Hjertaas JJ, Matre K, et al. One-year impact of bariatric surgery on left ventricular mechanics: results from the prospective FatWest study. Eur Heart J Open. 2021;1(2):oeab024.
43. Muiesan ML, Salvetti M, Zulli R, Pasini GF, Bettoni G, Monteduro C, et al. Structural association between the carotid artery and the left ventricle in a general population in Northern Italy: the Vobarno study. J Hypertens. 1998;16(12):1805–12.
44. Airale L, Paini A, Ianniello E, Mancusi C, Moreo A, Vaudo G, et al. Left atrial volume indexed for height(2) is a new sensitive marker for subclinical cardiac organ damage in female hypertensive patients. Hypertens Res. 2021;44(6):692–9.
45. Gerdts E, Wachtell K, Omvik P, Otterstad JE, Oikarinen L, Boman K, et al. Left atrial size and risk of major cardiovascular events during antihypertensive treatment: losartan intervention for endpoint reduction in hypertension trial. Hypertension. 2007;49(2):311–6.
46. Halland H, Lonnebakken MT, Pristaj N, Saeed S, Midtbo H, Einarsen E, et al. Sex differences in subclinical cardiac disease in overweight and obesity (the FATCOR study). Nutr Metab Cardiovasc Dis. 2018;28(10):1054–60.
47. Gerdts E, Oikarinen L, Palmieri V, Otterstad JE, Wachtell K, Boman K, et al. Correlates of left atrial size in hypertensive patients with left ventricular hypertrophy: the losartan intervention for endpoint reduction in hypertension (LIFE) Study. Hypertension. 2002;39(3):739–43.
48. Wachtell K, Gerdts E, Aurigemma GP, Boman K, Dahlof B, Nieminen MS, et al. In-treatment reduced left atrial diameter during antihypertensive treatment is associated with reduced new-onset atrial fibrillation in hypertensive patients with left ventricular hypertrophy: the LIFE study. Blood Press. 2010;19(3):169–75.
49. Heitmann KA, Lochen ML, Stylidis M, Hopstock LA, Schirmer H, Morseth B. Associations between physical activity, left atrial size and incident atrial fibrillation: the Tromso Study 1994-2016. Open Heart. 2022;9(1):e001823.
50. Lang RM, Badano LP, Mor-Avi V, Afilalo J, Armstrong A, Ernande L, et al. Recommendations for cardiac chamber quantification by echocardiography in adults: an update from the American Society of Echocardiography and the European Association of Cardiovascular Imaging. Eur Heart J Cardiovasc Imaging. 2015;16(3):233–70.
51. Kocabay G, Muraru D, Peluso D, Cucchini U, Mihaila S, Padayattil-Jose S, et al. Normal left ventricular mechanics by two-dimensional speckle-tracking echocardiography. Reference values in healthy adults. Rev Esp Cardiol. 2014;67(8):651–8.
52. Gerdts E, Zabalgoitia M, Bjornstad H, Svendsen TL, Devereux RB. Gender differences in systolic left ventricular function in hypertensive patients with electrocardiographic left ventricular hypertrophy (the LIFE study). Am J Cardiol. 2001;87(8):980–3.
53. Bella JN, Palmieri V, Roman MJ, Paranicas MF, Welty TK, Lee ET, et al. Gender differences in left ventricular systolic function in American Indians (from the Strong Heart Study). Am J Cardiol. 2006;98(6):834–7.
54. Stylidis M, Leon DA, Rösner A, Schirmer H. Global myocardial longitudinal strain in a general population-associations with blood pressure and subclinical heart failure: the tromso study. Int J Cardiovasc Imaging. 2020;36(3):459–70.
55. Pristaj N, Saeed S, Midtbo H, Halland H, Matre K, Gerdts E. Covariables of myocardial function in women and men with increased body mass index. High Blood Press Cardiovasc Prev. 2020;27(6):579–86.
56. Herfindal B, Gerdts E, Kringeland EA, Saeed S, Midtbo H, Halland H. Concomitant hypertension is associated with abnormal left ventricular geometry and lower systolic myocardial function in overweight participants: the FAT associated CardiOvasculaR dysfunction study. J Hypertens. 2020;38(6):1158–64.
57. Skaarup KG, Lassen MCH, Marott JL, Biering-Sorensen SR, Jorgensen PG, Appleyard M, et al. The impact of cardiovascular risk factors on global longitudinal strain over a decade in the general population: the copenhagen city heart study. Int J Cardiovasc Imaging. 2020;36(10):1907–16.
58. Modin D, Biering-Sorensen SR, Mogelvang R, Landler N, Jensen JS, Biering-Sorensen T. Prognostic value of echocardiography in hypertensive versus nonhypertensive participants from the general population. Hypertension. 2018;71(4):742–51.
59. Biering-Sorensen T, Biering-Sorensen SR, Olsen FJ, Sengelov M, Jorgensen PG, Mogelvang R, et al. Global longitudinal strain by echocardiography predicts long-term risk of cardiovascular morbidity and mortality in a low-risk general population: the Copenhagen city heart study. Circ Cardiovasc Imaging. 2017;10(3):e005521.
60. Saito M, Khan F, Stoklosa T, Iannaccone A, Negishi K, Marwick TH. Prognostic implications of LV strain risk score in asymptomatic patients with hypertensive heart disease. JACC Cardiovasc Imaging. 2016;9(8):911–21.
61. Nagueh SF, Smiseth OA, Appleton CP, Byrd BF, Dokainish H, Edvardsen T, et al. Recommendations for the evaluation of left ventricular diastolic function by echocardiography: an update from the American Society of Echocardiography and the European Association of Cardiovascular Imaging. Eur Heart J Cardiovasc Imaging. 2016;17(12):1321–60.
62. Sotomi Y, Hikoso S, Nakatani D, Mizuno H, Okada K, Dohi T, et al. Sex differences in heart failure with preserved ejection fraction. J Am Heart Assoc. 2021;10(5):e018574.
63. Hung CL, Goncalves A, Shah AM, Cheng S, Kitzman D, Solomon SD. Age- and sex-related influences on

left ventricular mechanics in elderly individuals free of prevalent heart failure: the ARIC study (atherosclerosis risk in communities). Circ Cardiovasc Imaging. 2017;10(1):e004510.
64. Donekal S, Venkatesh BA, Liu YC, Liu CY, Yoneyama K, Wu CO, et al. Interstitial fibrosis, left ventricular remodeling, and myocardial mechanical behavior in a population-based multiethnic cohort: the Multi-Ethnic Study of Atherosclerosis (MESA) study. Circ Cardiovasc Imaging. 2014;7(2):292–302.
65. Engelen L, Ferreira I, Stehouwer CD, Boutouyrie P, Laurent S. Reference intervals for common carotid intima-media thickness measured with echotracking: relation with risk factors. Eur Heart J. 2013;34(30):2368–80.
66. Mancusi C, Losi MA, Izzo R, Canciello G, Carlino MV, Albano G, et al. Higher pulse pressure and risk for cardiovascular events in patients with essential hypertension: The Campania Salute Network. Eur J Prev Cardiol. 2018;25(3):235–43.
67. Glasser SP, Krasikov T, Devereux RB, Oberman A, Patki A, Kitzman DW, et al. Subclinical, hemodynamic, and echocardiographic abnormalities of high pulse pressure in hypertensive and non-hypertensive adults. Am J Cardiovasc Dis. 2012;2(4): 309–17.
68. Yiming G, Zhou X, Lv W, Peng Y, Zhang W, Cheng X, et al. Reference values of brachial-ankle pulse wave velocity according to age and blood pressure in a central Asia population. PLoS One. 2017;12(4):e0171737.
69. Lu Y, Pechlaner R, Cai J, Yuan H, Huang Z, Yang G, et al. Trajectories of age-related arterial stiffness in Chinese men and women. J Am Coll Cardiol. 2020;75(8):870–80.
70. Visseren FLJ, Mach F, Smulders YM, Carballo D, Koskinas KC, Back M, et al. 2021 ESC Guidelines on cardiovascular disease prevention in clinical practice. Eur Heart J. 2021;42(34):3227–337.
71. Webb AJS, Lawson A, Wartolowska K, Mazzucco S, Rothwell PM, Cohort OS. Aortic stiffness, pulse pressure, and cerebral pulsatility progress despite best medical management: the OXVASC cohort. Stroke. 2022;53(4):1310–7.
72. Maas A. Cardiovascular risk assessment in women: which women are suited for menopausal hormone therapy? Climacteric. 2023;27(1):89–92.
73. Mansour M, Radaideh Q, Alaiwah MN, Alnimer Y, Devabhaktuni SR, Dhar G, et al. Major adverse cardiac events in symptomatic women with non-obstructive CAD on coronary CTA: pooled analysis from PROMISE and SCOT-HEART. Int J Cardiovasc Imaging. 2022;38(3):683–93.
74. van Rosendael AR, Bax AM, Smit JM, van den Hoogen IJ, Ma X, Al'Aref S, et al. Clinical risk factors and atherosclerotic plaque extent to define risk for major events in patients without obstructive coronary artery disease: the long-term coronary computed tomography angiography CONFIRM registry. Eur Heart J Cardiovasc Imaging. 2020;21(5):479–88.
75. Mortensen MB, Gaur S, Frimmer A, Botker HE, Sorensen HT, Kragholm KH, et al. Association of age with the diagnostic value of coronary artery calcium score for ruling out coronary stenosis in symptomatic patients. JAMA Cardiol. 2022;7(1):36–44.
76. Okin PM, Gerdts E, Kjeldsen SE, Julius S, Edelman JM, Dahlof B, et al. Gender differences in regression of electrocardiographic left ventricular hypertrophy during antihypertensive therapy. Hypertension. 2008;52(1):100–6.
77. Okin PM, Roman MJ, Devereux RB, Kligfield P. Electrocardiographic identification of left ventricular hypertrophy: test performance in relation to definition of hypertrophy and presence of obesity. J Am Coll Cardiol. 1996;27(1):124–31.
78. Okin PM, Roman MJ, Devereux RB, Kligfield P. Electrocardiographic identification of increased left ventricular mass by simple voltage-duration products. J Am Coll Cardiol. 1995;25(2):417–23.
79. Marwick TH, Gillebert TC, Aurigemma G, Chirinos J, Derumeaux G, Galderisi M, et al. Recommendations on the use of echocardiography in adult hypertension: a report from the European Association of Cardiovascular Imaging (EACVI) and the American Society of Echocardiography (ASE) dagger. Eur Heart J Cardiovasc Imaging. 2015;16(6):577–605.
80. Sharp AS, Tapp RJ, Thom SA, Francis DP, Hughes AD, Stanton AV, et al. Tissue Doppler E/E′ ratio is a powerful predictor of primary cardiac events in a hypertensive population: an ASCOT substudy. Eur Heart J. 2010;31(6):747–52.
81. Pieske B, Tschope C, de Boer RA, Fraser AG, Anker SD, Donal E, et al. How to diagnose heart failure with preserved ejection fraction: the HFA-PEFF diagnostic algorithm: a consensus recommendation from the Heart Failure Association (HFA) of the European Society of Cardiology (ESC). Eur Heart J. 2019;40(40):3297–317.
82. Naylor R, Rantner B, Ancetti S, de Borst GJ, De Carlo M, Halliday A, et al. Editor's choice - European Society for Vascular Surgery (ESVS) 2023 clinical practice guidelines on the management of atherosclerotic carotid and vertebral artery disease. Eur J Vasc Endovasc Surg. 2023;65(1):7–111.
83. Zanchetti A, Bond MG, Hennig M, Neiss A, Mancia G, Dal Palu C, et al. Calcium antagonist lacidipine slows down progression of asymptomatic carotid atherosclerosis: principal results of the European Lacidipine Study on Atherosclerosis (ELSA), a randomized, double-blind, long-term trial. Circulation. 2002;106(19):2422–7.
84. McEvoy JW, McCarthy CP, Bruno RM, Brouwers S, Canavan MD, Ceconi C, et al. 2024 ESC Guidelines for the management of elevated blood pressure and hypertension. Eur Heart J. 2024:ehae178. PMID: 39210715.

Part II

Non-traditional CVD Risk Factors in Women

Cycle Abnormalities and Cardiometabolic Health

M. P. Nadine Daan, Angela H.E.M. Maas, and Bart C. J. M. Fauser

Abstract

Cycle abnormalities are predominantly known to affect women's reproductive health due to irregular or absent menstrual bleeding and anovulation. However, a women's future cardiometabolic health may also be affected by ovarian dysfunction.

The polycystic ovary syndrome (PCOS) constitutes the most common form of chronic ovulatory dysfunction in women of reproductive age. PCOS is often associated with hyperandrogenism, insulin resistance and cardiometabolic abnormalities, affecting women's health during various life stages including peri- and postmenopause. Moreover, pregnancy complications and the health of offspring may be compromised.

Ovulatory dysfunction due to premature menopause or the occurrence of hypothalamic amenorrhea in female athletes, is often associated with an extended hypoestrogenic state. Next to increased chances for osteoporosis and associated bone fractures, this prolonged state of hypoestrogenism impairs cardiometabolic health and is associated with an increase in cardiovascular disease and mortality. Furthermore premature menopause is associated with a decrease in circulating androgen concentrations, which may influence cognition, sexual health, general wellbeing along with cardiometabolic health.

Thus, cardiometabolic health in women with cycle abnormalities is characterized by a complex interaction between hormonal changes, specific patient features such as age and BMI, underlying genetic traits and different environmental factors.

Keywords

Anovulation · Hyperandrogenism
Hypoestrogenism · Cardiometabolic risk
Cardiovascular disease

M. P. Nadine Daan (✉)
Department of Gynaecology, University Utrecht, Utrecht, The Netherlands
e-mail: nadinedaan86@gmail.com

A. H.E.M. Maas
Department of Cardiology, route 616, Radboud University Medical Center, Nijmegen, The Netherlands
e-mail: angela.maas@radboudumc.nl

B. C. J. M. Fauser
Department of Gynaecology, University of Utrecht and University Medical Center Utrecht, Utrecht, The Netherlands

A. H.E.M. Maas, E. Gerdts (eds.), *Manual of Cardiovascular Disease in Women*,
https://doi.org/10.1007/978-3-031-65952-2_9

Test your learning and check your understanding of this book's contents: use the "Springer Nature Flashcards" app to access questions using ▶ https://sn.pub/51ny7m
To use the app, please follow the instructions in chapter 1.

1 Introduction

Ovulatory dysfunction is known to affect women's health. Next to reproductive health issues like prolonged time to conception or even infertility, anovulation disorders are associated with psychological, endocrine and cardiometabolic health associated health risks.

Ovulation disorders are common amongst women of reproductive age, with a prevalence up to 13% dependent on age and different definitions applied [1]. Irregular menstrual cycles are highly common in adolescents, especially in the first 3 years after menarche [1]. Thereafter, an ovulatory menstrual cycle is defined as cycle lasting between 21–35 days. Oligomenorrhea is defined as a menstrual cycle anywhere between 35 days and 6 months duration, resulting in less than 8 ovulations per year. The absence of menses after 6 months is commonly referred to as amenorrhea [2].

Over fifty years ago, the World Health Organization (WHO) first classified anovulation disorders into three categories based on serum measurements of follicle stimulating hormone (FSH), luteinizing hormone (LH) and oestradiol (E_2) levels [3].

Over the years some modifications in this classification has been proposed. This classification system remains under debate since it was adopted whilst lacking a thorough scientific foundation [2]. Recently, the FIGO has proposed a new classification system for ovulatory disorders based on the presumed primary origin of the ovulation disorder (hypothalamic, pituitary, ovarian or other) [4]. Although an etiology based classification system appears logical, it remains unclear whether this is actually possible based on current evidence and whether it would indeed improve the diagnosis and/or treatment of women with anovulation compared to the WHO classification which has been proven useful in clinical practice over the past decades [5].

The WHO classification for anovulation disorders amounts to:

- Women classified as WHO class 1 anovulation present with low FSH/LH levels, and low E_2 levels.
- Women classified as WHO 2 anovulation present with normal FSH and normal to high LH levels, and normal E_2 levels. Women in this category may demonstrate increased serum androgen levels.
- Women classified as WHO 3 anovulation present with high FSH levels and low E2 levels.

Women with ovulatory dysfunction are mostly classified in the WHO 2 category (~85%), followed by WHO 1 (~10%) and ultimately WHO 3 anovulation (~5%).

Hyperprolactinemia, either physiological, pathological, or idiopathic of origin, may also lead to anovulation. Increased prolactin levels inhibit gonadotropin secretion and impair LH responses to gonadotropin-releasing hormone (GnRH). Serum FSH and E2 levels are generally slightly decreased or in the normal range. Anovulation due to hyperprolactinemia is considered a separate entity in the spectrum of ovulation disorders. A general history assessment in these women includes information on previous pregnancies, medication use, metabolic disorders such as kidney/liver/thyroid disease, and (iatrogenic) damage to the pituitary. Diagnostic assessment of hyperprolactinemia encompasses an endocrinological screening of all pituitary hormonal axes. In the suspicion of a prolactinoma, a magnetic resonance imaging scan of the brain is performed. In general, ovulation can be effectively restored through the administration of oral dopamine agonists in the case of isolated hyperprolactinemia.

To better understand the short and long term health effects of ovulatory dysfunction, we will first discuss the different background and mechanisms of each form of WHO ovulatory dysfunction. Thereafter we will discuss the cardiometabolic health risks associated with these endocrine disorders in more detail.

2 Categories and Underlying Mechanisms of Ovulatory Dysfunction

2.1 Hypogonadotropic Hypoestrogenic Anovulation (WHO I Anovulation)

Hypogonadotropic hypoestrogenic anovulation is caused by inhibition of the hypothalamic-pituitary-ovarian (HPO) axis. WHO type 1 anovulation can be categorized in hypogonadotrophic hypogonadism, hypopituitarism and hypothalamic amenorrhoea [6].

In clinical practice WHO 1 anovulation is most commonly caused by a form of functional hypothalamic amenorrhea which is either weight loss-related, stress-related, and/or exercise-related [7].

Substantial (>10% of body mass) and rapid weight loss results in an internal energy deficiency. This leads to suppression of the pulsatile release of GnRH from the hypothalamus, resulting in a decreased production of FSH and LH within the pituitary [7]. The mechanisms of folliculogenesis, ovulation, and estrogen production are consequently disrupted.

Furthermore, weight loss affects the distribution of adipose tissue. Adipose tissue is known to play an important role in reproduction. Especially through the actions of adipocytokines, of which leptin and adiponectin are probably the most well-known [8]. Leptin directly acts on GnRH secreting neurons in the hypothalamus in response to nutritional and energy expenditure changes. A decrease in adiposity results in low leptin levels, which may interfere with the process of ovulation [8]. Leptin is known to be essential in the induction of puberty and further reproductive maturation. Adiponectin, the most ample adipokine, affects the hypothalamic gonadal axis on numerous levels. Adiponectin receptors are present throughout the entire reproductive pathway. Adiponectin directly inhibits the secretion of GnRH and, insulin sensitivity through IGF-1 production. This leads to an increases of steroidogenesis in granulosa cells in the ovaries [8].

Finally, stress of any kind results in the activation of the hypothalamic-pituitary-adrenal axis. This results in an increase of circulating corticotrophin-releasing hormone (CRH), acetylcholine (ACTH) and cortisol levels, which inhibit GnRH secretion [9]. Women with energy deprived conditions such as anorexia nervosa, chronic disease and athletes indeed demonstrate increased CRH, ACTH and cortisol levels and low leptin levels, often resulting in hypothalamic amenorrhea [9].

2.2 Normogonadotropic Normoestrogenic Anovulation (WHO II Anovulation)

The polycystic ovary syndrome (PCOS) is the most common form of WHO II anovulation, and is prevalent in up to 13% of women of reproductive age [1]. WHO II anovulation is categorized in WHO II PCOS and non-PCOS, with PCOS comprising up to 90% of women with WHO II anovulation. The diagnosis of PCOS is made in presence of two or more of the following symptoms: oligo- or anovulation, polycystic ovarian morphology on ultrasound and hyperandrogenism (clinical and/or biochemical) [1, 10].

PCOS is a complex heterogenous endocrine disorder, characterized by anovulation, hyperandrogenism, obesity and cardiometabolic dysfunction. Asides fertility problems, these women exhibit increased cardiometabolic and cardiovascular risk factors at a young age [11]. A pivotal feature in the pathophysiology of PCOS is insulin resistance. In general, 75% of lean women and 95% of obese women with PCOS are found to be insulin resistant [12]. Insulin resistance and compensatory hyperinsulinemia act on the pituitary, ovaries and liver leading to an increase in androgen production, a decrease in sex hormone binding globulin (SHBG) production and an arrest in follicular development. A decline in SHBG levels results in a higher circulation of free androgens attributing to the severity of PCOS symptoms. Obesity further increases insulin resistance and attributes to this vicious cycle of PCOS symptoms. Approximately half of the women with PCOS are obese [12]. Together, obesity and insulin resistance significantly worsen cardiometabolic risk in women with PCOS. However there is no evidence that PCOS is caused by obesity. Previous studies in women with PCOS demonstrated an intrinsic insulin resistance, independent of weight [13].

2.3 Hypergonadotropic Hypoestrogenic Anovulation (WHO III Anovulation)

Hypergonadotropic hypoestrogenic anovulation is indicative of an advanced depletion of the ovarian follicle pool, eventually resulting in menopause. Menopause is defined by the permanent cessation of menses after a period of 12 months of amenorrhea. The average global age at menopause is 51 years. However in 1–2% of women menopause occurs prior to the age of 40 years and is referred to as premature ovarian insufficiency (POI) [14]

The etiology of POI can be iatrogenic, for instance after chemotherapy or surgery. It can be genetic, due to mutations in the FMR 1 gene or mosaic Turner syndrome. Furthermore POI can occur as a genetic familial trait, and POI can be caused by auto-immune disorders. However, in the vast majority (85%) of women the cause of POI remains unknown.

The physical and psychological health burden associated with POI is enormous. POI reduces a woman's lifetime chance of spontaneous conception to 2–10%. Artificial reproductive techniques such as in vitro fertilization are proven ineffective in these women, unless women have access to donor oocytes [14].

3 Cardiometabolic Implications of Ovulatory Dysfunction

3.1 Hyperandrogenism and Cardiometabolic Risk

PCOS is by far the most common form of ovulatory dysfunction, and as mentioned previously affects up to 13% of women in the general population [1]. In early life, PCOS is already associated with an unfavorable cardiometabolic risk profile [11]. Especially women with PCOS and hyperandrogenism exhibit cardiometabolic derangements, due to the catalyzing pathophysiological actions of androgens on insulin resistance and chronic low grade inflammation [15, 16].

Furthermore, body mass index and circulating androgen levels are strongly associated with unfavorable changes in leptin and adiponectin expression [17]. Disruption in adipocytokine expression may impair the vascular endothelium by stimulating migration of monocytes into the vessel wall, and inducing the conversion of monocytes into macrophages. These macrophages phagocytize LDL cholesterol to form fatty streak formation in the vessel walls, ultimately resulting in atherosclerotic plaque formation [17].

Various meta-analyses have indeed shown that women with PCOS of reproductive age exhibit a marked increased risk of hypertension (risk ratio (RR): 1.75, 95% CI 1.42–2.15), type 2 diabetes (RR: 3.00, 95% CI 2.56–3.51), dyslipidemia (higher serum concentration of triglycerides (mean difference (MD): 7.14 95% CI 1.58–12.70 mg/dl), a lower serum concentration of HDL-Cholesterol (MD: −2.45 95% CI −4.51 to −0.38 mg/dl) when compared to women without PCOS [12, 13, 18].

These associations remain significant after adjusting for confounders such as age and BMI. The metabolic syndrome was found to be more prevalent in overweight or obese women with PCOS (odd ratio (OR) 1.88, 95% 1.16, 3.04) but not in lean women with PCOS (OR 1.45, 95% CI 0.35, 6.12) [12].

These cardiometabolic risk factors in women with PCOS of reproductive age may result in complications during pregnancy and delivery for both mother and child. A meta-analysis of data unadjusted for weight demonstrated a three- to fourfold increased risk of pregnancy-induced hypertension and pre-eclampsia, a threefold increased risk of gestational diabetes and twofold higher chance for premature delivery in women with PCOS compared to controls [19]. Data corrected for confounders, such as BMI and age and smoking, showed a marked persistent increased risk of gestational diabetes in women with PCOS compared to controls, with an adjusted OR of 4.15 (95% CI 2.07–8.33) [20]. Apart from dyslipidemia, obesity and onset of type 2 diabetes mellitus, androgens are thought to influence cardiovascular health in later life.

Several studies have reported vascular dysfunction in women with PCOS compared to controls. A recent meta-analysis on functional and structural markers of subclinical atherosclerosis as measured by carotid intima-media thickness (cIMT), flow-mediated vasodilation (FMD), nitroglycerin-mediated vasodilation (NMD), pulse wave velocity (PWV), and coronary artery calcium (CAC) involving 5550 PCOS patients and 5974 controls demonstrated that women with PCOS showed significantly thicker cIMT (SMD (95% CI) = 0.587 (0.398, 0.776), $P < 0.001$), lower FMD (SMD (95% CI) = −0.649 (−0.946, −0.353), $P < 0.001$) and NMD (SMD (95% CI) = −0.502 (−0.686, −0.317), $P < 0.001$), as well as higher PWV (SMD (95% CI) = 0.382 (0.019, 0.746), $P = 0.039$), and increased CAC incidence (OR (95% CI) = 2.204 (1.687, 2.879), $P < 0.001$) compared to controls. When analyzing subgroups by age and body mass index (BMI), results were still significant ($P < 0.05$) except for PWV in the BMI subgroup [21].

However, data on long term cardiovascular outcomes in women with PCOS are inconsistent. Result of meta-analyses on this matter should be interpreted with caution due to a general lack of prospective studies with sufficient follow up, small sample sizes and substantial study population heterogeneity. In a large recent meta-analysis PCOS was reportedly associated with an increased risks of non-fatal cerebrovascular disease events (RR: 1.41, 95% CI 1.02–1.94), and not associated with a significant increased risk for coronary disease events (RR: 1.78, 95% CI 0.99–3.23) [13, 22]. In contrast, another recent large follow up study on the risk for atherosclerosis and CVD in hyperandrogenic women 20 years after menopause, found no association between high androgen levels and atherosclerosis, incident stroke, coronary heart disease, or CVD. The authors concluded that high androgen levels in the post menopause, were not associated with an elevated risk for CVD [23].

The association between androgen levels and cardiovascular disease and mortality turns out be complex. Cardiovascular health in women with PCOS might even be better than anticipated based on the presence of cardiometabolic riskfactors in their reproductive years [23]. Furthermore, women with PCOS enter menopause at a later age compared to controls, which might exert a preventive effect on the development of cardiovascular disease [23].

What happens to women with PCOS after menopause and their cardiovascular health risk in later life remains to be elucidated in more detail. In the meanwhile, the international guideline by the European Society for Human Reproduction and Embryology (ESHRE) and the American Society of Reproductive Medicine (ASRM) advises health care professionals to screen women with PCOS for the presence of cardiovascular risk factors on a yearly base, to prevent potential deterioration of cardiovascular health in these women [1]. Furthermore, health care providers are strongly advised to offer life style intervention therapy since this has been shown to alleviate the severity of metabolic, reproductive and psychological features of PCOS [1, 24].

3.2 Hypoestrogenism, Hypoandrogenism and Cardiometabolic Risk

Hypoestrogenism is present in both women with WHO I and women with WHO III anovulation disorders, and this condition is associated with increased cardiometabolic risks. It is widely known that in premenopausal women estrogens exert a protective effect on the cardiovascular system. It mediates anti-inflammation, decreases oxidative stress, increases endothelial-cell growth and inhibits smooth muscle cell proliferation [25]. Furthermore hypoestrogenism is associated with impaired lipid profiles with increased serum total cholesterol, low density lipoprotein cholesterol and triglyceride levels [6].

Between the two categories of hypoestrogenic anovulation, WHO I is more prevalent (respectively 10% versus WHO III 5% prevalent in women with anovulation disorders). As mentioned previously, WHO 1 anovulation is generally caused by a form of functional hypothalamic amenorrhea due to excessive weight loss, stress, and/or exercise [7].

WHO 1 hypothalamic amenorrhea may exert negative effects on reproductive, bone, psychological and cardiometabolic health. The coinciding activation of the hypothalamic-pituitary-adrenal stress system in these women may further undermine their cardiometabolic health. Health sequelae in women with WHO 1 hypoestrogenism are largely determined by the duration and underlying cause of this condition. Women with prolonged hypoestrogenism are at risk for the development of osteopenia and osteoporosis and ultimately osteoporotic bone fractures. Especially women with eating disorders missing various other nutrients (for instance calcium and vitamin D) demonstrate a decreased bone health [26]. Long term follow up on cardiovascular disease in women with chronic WHO I anovulation is lacking.

Several small sample sized studies have reported endothelial dysfunction in amenorrheic athletes [27–30]. Endothelium-dependent vasodilation was diminished in these women, suggesting that hypoestrogenic athletes with amenorrhea may be exposed to increased cardiovascular risk.

Treatment of WHO I anovulation is primarily aimed on treatment of the underlying condition. For instance in hypothalamic amenorrhea by altering diet and/or exercise regimes and offering psychotherapy. Although hypothalamic amenorrhea is a reversable state, alleviating this medical condition may proof to be challenging. Whilst attempting to treat the cause of WHO I anovulation, hormone suppletion therapy is generally advised for the restoration of estrogen levels to minimize short and long term health sequelae.

The effects of hypoestrogenism on women's health are better known for women with WHO III anovulation. Women with premature ovarian insufficiency (POI) experience menopause before the age of 40 years, and are therefore subject to a longer period of hypoestrogenism compared to women in the general population with an average age at menopause of 51 years.

POI is associated with serious adverse effects on women's health. Asides the well-known association with decreased bone mineral density, middle aged women with POI demonstrate an unfavorable cardiovascular risk profile compared to healthy controls after correcting for confounders such as BMI and use of hormone suppletion therapy. This includes dyslipidemia and increased abdominal fat, hypertension, and elevated chronic inflammatory factors although no significant associations were found for carotid intima media thickness or coronary artery calcium scores [31–33]. Even more importantly, untreated POI is associated with a reduced life expectancy, largely due to cardiovascular disease [14].

Previous meta-analyses consistently demonstrate that women with early menopause exhibit a higher risk of coronary heart disease and overall cardiovascular disease mortality [22, 34, 35]. After controlling for confounders such as BMI and age, postmenopausal status and early menopause prove to be independent risk factors for cardiovascular disease, which is especially profound in women after early surgical menopause [36]. Data on stroke risk in women with POI are more inconsistent. Some studies report an increased stroke risk in women with early menopause, and others found no significant association between the two [22, 35, 37].

This increased CVD risk may be caused by the decrease in endogenous estrogen synthesis after menopause. Estrogens attribute to the relaxation and expansion of blood vessels, stimulating blood flow and elasticity within in healthy blood vessels [34]. Therefore, decreased estrogen levels may impair vascular health. Indeed, a large meta-analysis demonstrated that early menopause is associated with an increased risk of arterial hypertension [38]. This association was not affected by potential confounding factors, such as age, BMI, and smoking. A proposed pathogenetic mechanism in this process is that the decline in estrogen after menopause, activates the production of vasoconstrictive factors, such as endothelin and angiotensinogen. This may result in upregulation of the renin-angiotensin system, renal sodium reabsorption and vasoconstriction, endothelial dysfunction, inflammation, and immune dysfunction [38]. These processes are associated with obesity, diabetes, and hypertension [34].

Asides hypoestrogenism, postmenopausal women demonstrate a gradual decrease in circulating androgen levels with advancing age. Several studies have shown that women with POI may also exhibit hypoandrogenism at an earlier age [39–41]. Various observational studies have proposed that hypoandrogenism in postmenopausal women may be associated with a greater risk of all-cause mortality and cardiovascular events [42, 43]. These observations together with the findings of impaired cardiometabolic health in hyperandrogenic women, suggests a complex and potential U shaped association between androgens and cardiometabolic risk. Furthermore this association is influenced by many other factors such as estrogen and sex hormone globulin hormone concentrations, BMI and age [40, 44].

The association between menopause and CVD risk seems to be multifactorial and comprises more than the cause and effect of hormonal changes. Interestingly it appears that age at menopause shares a mutual genetic background with the risk of CVD. A large meta-analysis of 22 genome wide association studies examining age at menopause identified several shared loci between age at menopause and CVD, which are involved in DNA repair and inflammatory response and oxidative stress [45]. Furthermore various corresponding environmental factors, dietary factors and life style factors are known to attribute to the risk of entering menopause early and developing cardiovascular disease [46–48].

Women who experience menopause at an early age are internationally advised to start hormone suppletion therapy to treat bothersome climacteric symptoms and to reduce long term effects on morbidity and mortality. It is advised to at least continue this medication until an average age at menopause is reached. Thereafter the need for additional hormone suppletion therapy is further individualized and primarily continued in the presence of bothersome menopausal complaints [14].

Key Issues

- Anovulation in women of reproductive age is associated with increased cardiometabolic risk.
- Androgens and estrogens are important denominators in cardiometabolic health.
- The effect of anovulation disorders on the final development of actual cardiovascular disease appears multifactorial and complex.

Questions and Answers

1. Which anovulation disorder is most prevalent among the general population?
   (A) Answer: The polycystic ovary syndrome (PCOS)
2. Name a singular hormonal finding in these women which greatly affects their cardiometabolic health?
   (A) Answer: hyperandrogenism
3. What is the name of the medical condition for women who enter menopause prior to the age of 40 years?
   (A) Answer: Premature ovarian insufficiency
4. What is the essential treatment in these women to improve their short and long term health?
   (A) Answer: hormone suppletion therapy

References

1. Teede HJ, Misso ML, Costello MF, et al. Recommendations from the international evidence-based guideline for the assessment and management of polycystic ovary syndrome. Hum Reprod. 2018;33(9):1602–18. https://doi.org/10.1093/humrep/dey256.
2. Rowe PJ, Comhaire FH, Hargreave TB, Mellows HJ. WHO manual for the standardized investigation of the infertile couple. Cambridge: Cambridge University Press; 1993.
3. WHO-Scientific-Group. Agents stimulating gonadal function in the human; 1973.
4. Munro MG, Balen AH, Cho S, et al. The FIGO ovulatory disorders classification system. Fertil Steril. 2022;118(4):768–86. https://doi.org/10.1016/j.fertnstert.2022.07.009.
5. Balen AH, Munro MG, O'Neill HC, Lunenfeld B, Fauser BCJM. The new international federation of gynecology and obstetrics (FIGO) ovulatory disorder classification: PRO and CON. Fertil Steril. 2023;119(4):562–9. https://doi.org/10.1016/j.fertnstert.2023.01.043.
6. Vikram T, Ephia Y. WHO type 1 anovulation: an update on diagnosis, management and implications for long-term health. TOG. 2020;22:178–90. https://doi.org/10.1111/tog.12665.
7. Morrison AE, Fleming S, Levy MJ. A review of the pathophysiology of functional hypothalamic amenorrhoea in women subject to psychological stress, disordered eating, excessive exercise or a combination of these factors. Clin Endocrinol. 2021;95(2):229–38. https://doi.org/10.1111/cen.14399.
8. Mathew H, Castracane VD, Mantzoros C. Adipose tissue and reproductive health. Metabolism. 2018;86:18–32. https://doi.org/10.1016/j.metabol.2017.11.006.
9. Valsamakis G, Chrousos G, Mastorakos G. Stress, female reproduction and pregnancy. Psychoneuroendocrinology. 2019;100:48–57. https://doi.org/10.1016/j.psyneuen.2018.09.031.
10. Rotterdam ESHRE/ASRM-Sponsored PCOS Consensus Workshop Group. Revised 2003 consensus on diagnostic criteria and long-term health risks related to polycystic ovary syndrome (PCOS). Hum Reprod. 2004;19(1):41–7. https://doi.org/10.1093/humrep/deh098.
11. Gunning MN, Fauser BCJM. Are women with polycystic ovary syndrome at increased cardiovascular disease risk later in life? Climacteric. 2017;20(3):222–7. https://doi.org/10.1080/13697137.2017.1316256.
12. Lim SS, Kakoly NS, Tan JWJ, et al. Metabolic syndrome in polycystic ovary syndrome: a systematic review, meta-analysis and meta-regression. Obes Rev. 2019;20(2):339–52. https://doi.org/10.1111/obr.12762.
13. Wekker V, van Dammen L, Koning A, et al. Long-term cardiometabolic disease risk in women with PCOS: a systematic review and meta-analysis. Hum Reprod Update. 2020;26(6):942–60. https://doi.org/10.1093/humupd/dmaa029.
14. Webber L, Davies M, et al. ESHRE guideline: management of women with premature ovarian insufficiency. Hum Reprod. 2016;31(5):926–37. https://doi.org/10.1093/humrep/dew027.
15. Daan NMP, Louwers YV, Koster MPH, et al. Cardiovascular and metabolic profiles amongst different polycystic ovary syndrome phenotypes: who is really at risk? Fertil Steril. 2014;102(5):1444–51. https://doi.org/10.1016/j.fertnstert.2014.08.001.
16. Meun C, Gunning MN, Louwers YV, et al. The cardiovascular risk profile of middle-aged women with polycystic ovary syndrome. Clin Endocrinol. 2020;92(2):150–8. https://doi.org/10.1111/cen.14117.
17. Daan NMP, Koster MPH, de Wilde MA, et al. Biomarker profiles in women with PCOS and PCOS offspring; a pilot study. PLoS One. 2016;11(11):e0165033. https://doi.org/10.1371/journal.pone.0165033.
18. Wild RA, Rizzo M, Clifton S, Carmina E. Lipid levels in polycystic ovary syndrome: systematic review and meta-analysis. Fertil Steril. 2011;95(3):1073–11. https://doi.org/10.1016/j.fertnstert.2010.12.027.
19. Palomba S, de Wilde MA, Falbo A, Koster MPH, La Sala GB, Fauser BC. Pregnancy complications in women with polycystic ovary syndrome. Hum Reprod Update. 2015;21(5):575–92. https://doi.org/10.1093/humupd/dmv029.
20. de Wilde MA, Lamain-de Ruiter M, Veltman-Verhulst SM, et al. Increased rates of complications in singleton pregnancies of women previously diagnosed with polycystic ovary syndrome predominantly in the hyperandrogenic phenotype. Fertil Steril. 2017;108(2):333–40. https://doi.org/10.1016/j.fertnstert.2017.06.015.
21. Sun D, Wu Y, Ding M, Zhu F. Comprehensive meta-analysis of functional and structural markers of subclinical atherosclerosis in women with polycystic ovary syndrome. Angiology. 2022;73(7):622–34. https://doi.org/10.1177/00033197211072598.
22. Roeters van Lennep JE, Heida KY, Bots ML, Hoek A. Cardiovascular disease risk in women with premature ovarian insufficiency: a systematic review and meta-analysis. Eur. J Prev Cardiol. 2016;23(2):178–86. https://doi.org/10.1177/2047487314556004.
23. Meun C, Franco OH, Dhana K, et al. High androgens in postmenopausal women and the risk for atherosclerosis and cardiovascular disease: the Rotterdam study. J Clin Endocrinol Metab. 2018;103(4):1622–30. https://doi.org/10.1210/jc.2017-02421.
24. Lim SS, Hutchison SK, Van Ryswyk E, Norman RJ, Teede HJ, Moran LJ. Lifestyle changes in women with polycystic ovary syndrome. Cochrane Database Syst Rev. 2019;3(3):CD007506. https://doi.org/10.1002/14651858.CD007506.pub4.
25. Roberts RE, Farahani L, Webber L, Jayasena C. Current understanding of hypothalamic amenorrhoea. Ther

Adv Endocrinol Metab. 2020;11:2042018820945854. https://doi.org/10.1177/2042018820945854.
26. Shufelt CL, Torbati T, Dutra E. Hypothalamic amenorrhea and the long-term health consequences. Semin Reprod Med. 2017;35(3):256–62. https://doi.org/10.1055/s-0037-1603581.
27. Grosman-Rimon L, Wright E, Freedman D, et al. Can improvement in hormonal and energy balance reverse cardiovascular risk factors in athletes with amenorrhea? Am J Physiol Heart Circ Physiol. 2019;317(3):H487–95. https://doi.org/10.1152/ajpheart.00242.2019.
28. Rickenlund A, Eriksson MJ, Schenck-Gustafsson K, Hirschberg AL. Amenorrhea in female athletes is associated with endothelial dysfunction and unfavorable lipid profile. J Clin Endocrinol Metab. 2005;90(3):1354–9. https://doi.org/10.1210/jc.2004-1286.
29. Zeni Hoch A, Dempsey RL, Carrera GF, et al. Is there an association between athletic amenorrhea and endothelial cell dysfunction? Med Sci Sports Exerc. 2003;35(3):377–83. https://doi.org/10.1249/01.MSS.0000053661.27992.75.
30. Hoch AZ, Papanek P, Szabo A, Widlansky ME, Schimke JE, Gutterman DD. Association between the female athlete triad and endothelial dysfunction in dancers. Clin J Sport Med. 2011;21(2):119–25. https://doi.org/10.1097/JSM.0b013e3182042a9a.
31. Daan NMP, Muka T, Koster MPH, et al. Cardiovascular risk in women with premature ovarian insufficiency compared to premenopausal women at middle age. J Clin Endocrinol Metab. 2016;101(9):3306–15. https://doi.org/10.1210/jc.2016-1141.
32. Huang L, Wang H, Shi M, Kong W, Jiang M. Lipid profile in patients with primary ovarian insufficiency: a systematic review and meta-analysis. Front Endocrinol. 2022;13:876775. https://doi.org/10.3389/fendo.2022.876775.
33. Gunning MN, Meun C, van Rijn BB, et al. Coronary artery calcification in middle-aged women with premature ovarian insufficiency. Clin Endocrinol. 2019;91(2):314–22. https://doi.org/10.1111/cen.14003.
34. Muka T, Oliver-Williams C, Kunutsor S, et al. Association of age at onset of menopause and time since onset of menopause with cardiovascular outcomes, intermediate vascular traits, and all-cause mortality: a systematic review and meta-analysis. JAMA Cardiol. 2016;1(7):767–76. https://doi.org/10.1001/jamacardio.2016.2415.
35. Tao X, Zuo A, Wang J, Tao F. Effect of primary ovarian insufficiency and early natural menopause on mortality: a meta-analysis. Climacteric. 2016;19(1):27–36. https://doi.org/10.3109/13697137.2015.1094784.
36. Atsma F, Bartelink MEL, Grobbee DE, van der Schouw YT. Postmenopausal status and early menopause as independent risk factors for cardiovascular disease: a meta-analysis. Menopause. 2006;13(2):265–79. https://doi.org/10.1097/01.gme.0000218683.97338.ea.
37. Mishra SR, Chung H, Waller M, Mishra GD. Duration of estrogen exposure during reproductive years, age at menarche and age at menopause, and risk of cardiovascular disease events, all-cause and cardiovascular mortality: a systematic review and meta-analysis. BJOG. 2021;128(5):809–21. https://doi.org/10.1111/1471-0528.16524.
38. Anagnostis P, Theocharis P, Lallas K, et al. Early menopause is associated with increased risk of arterial hypertension: a systematic review and meta-analysis. Maturitas. 2020;135:74–9. https://doi.org/10.1016/j.maturitas.2020.03.006.
39. Janse F, Tanahatoe SJ, Eijkemans MJC, Fauser BC. Testosterone concentrations, using different assays, in different types of ovarian insufficiency: a systematic review and meta-analysis. Hum Reprod Update. 2012;18(4):405–19. https://doi.org/10.1093/humupd/dms013.
40. Daan NMP, Jaspers L, Koster MPH, et al. Androgen levels in women with various forms of ovarian dysfunction: associations with cardiometabolic features. Hum Reprod. 2015;30(10):2376–86. https://doi.org/10.1093/humrep/dev195.
41. Soman M, Huang L, Cai W, et al. Serum androgen profiles in women with premature ovarian insufficiency: a systematic review and meta-analysis. Menopause. 2019;26(1):78–93. https://doi.org/10.1097/GME.0000000000001161.
42. Sievers C, Klotsche J, Pieper L, et al. Low testosterone levels predict all-cause mortality and cardiovascular events in women: a prospective cohort study in German primary care patients. Eur J Endocrinol. 2010;163(4):699–708. https://doi.org/10.1530/EJE-10-0307.
43. Davis SR. Androgens in premenopausal women and women with premature ovarian insufficiency. Climacteric. 2021;24(5):459–65. https://doi.org/10.1080/13697137.2020.1866530.
44. Aribas E, Roeters van Lennep JE, De Rijke YB, et al. Sex steroids and sex steroid-binding globulin levels amongst middle-aged and elderly men and women from general population. Eur J Clin Investig. 2022;52(12):e13866. https://doi.org/10.1111/eci.13866.
45. Stolk L, Perry JRB, Chasman DI, et al. Meta-analyses identify 13 loci associated with age at menopause and highlight DNA repair and immune pathways. Nat Genet. 2012;44(3):260–8. https://doi.org/10.1038/ng.1051.
46. Grisotto G, Farago JS, Taneri PE, et al. Dietary factors and onset of natural menopause: a systematic review and meta-analysis. Maturitas. 2022;159:15–32. https://doi.org/10.1016/j.maturitas.2021.12.008.
47. Taneri PE, Kiefte-de Jong JC, Bramer WM, Daan NMP, Franco OH, Muka T. Association of alcohol consumption with the onset of natural menopause: a systematic review and meta-analysis. Hum Reprod Update. 2016;22(4):516–28. https://doi.org/10.1093/humupd/dmw013.

48. Colpani V, Baena CP, Jaspers L, et al. Lifestyle factors, cardiovascular disease and all-cause mortality in middle-aged and elderly women: a systematic review and meta-analysis. Eur J Epidemiol. 2018;33(9):831–45. https://doi.org/10.1007/s10654-018-0374-z.

Hypertensive Disorders of Pregnancy and Cardiovascular Disease Risk

Anne Cathrine Staff, Ralf Dechend, and Daniel Pitz Jacobsen

Abstract

Pregnancy impacts health over decades and across generations. Epidemiological population-based studies over the last two decades show a strong association between future female cardiovascular disease and pregnancy complications. The association is especially strong for women with previous hypertensive disorders of pregnancy, in particular early-onset preeclampsia combined with a growth restricted offspring and following repeated preeclampsia. We describe hypertensive pregnancy disorders and their pathophysiology and summarize their associations to a wide range of cardiovascular diseases. We present established as well as novel hypotheses that may explain the mechanisms for these associations. Despite the knowledge of hypertensive pregnancy complications predicting premature cardiovascular disease, few women are today offered systematic cardio-preventive follow-up after such pregnancies. These women typically seek help from the health system at first clinical symptom of cardiovascular disease, by which time morbidity is significant. They will have missed preventive opportunities, as prevention of cardiovascular disease is most effective when started at preclinical stages. We and others argue that pregnancy is an underexploited sex-specific vascular stress test and an opportunity to initiate prevention of cardiovascular disease following delivery, when they are still at a young age. We present simple clinical follow-up suggestions after a hypertensive disorder of pregnancy, which could be amended according to local resources, health systems and the individual woman's risk factors. A more proactive approach postpartum than today may have large effects on women's cardiovascular health and quality of life, with positive effects also for her family, the health system expenses and would promote healthier societies.

Keywords

Cardiovascular disease · Gestational hypertension · Hypertensive disorders of pregnancy Maternal risk of cardiovascular disease · Preeclampsia

A. Cathrine Staff (✉) · D. P. Jacobsen
Faculty of Medicine, University of Oslo, Oslo, Norway

Division of Obstetrics and Gynaecology, Oslo University Hospital, Oslo, Norway
e-mail: uxnnaf@ous-hf.no; a.c.staff@medisin.uio.no

R. Dechend
HELIOS Clinic, Berlin, Germany

Experimental and Clinical Research Center, Charité Medical Faculty and Max-Delbrueck Center for Molecular Medicine, and HELIOS Clinic, Berlin, Germany

A. H.E.M. Maas, E. Gerdts (eds.), *Manual of Cardiovascular Disease in Women*,
https://doi.org/10.1007/978-3-031-65952-2_10

Test your learning and check your understanding of this book's contents: use the "Springer Nature Flashcards" app to access questions using ▶ https://sn.pub/51ny7m To use the app, please follow the instructions in chapter 1.

1 Introduction

Hypertensive disorders of pregnancy complicate a high rate of pregnancies world-wide. They encompass clinically defined categories with heterogeneous short-term outcomes for mother and offspring, as well as heterogeneous long-term outcomes for the survivors. Hypertension in pregnancy is defined as a systolic blood pressure (BP) 140 mmHg and/or diastolic BP ≥90 mmHg, based on an average of at least two measurement, and measured with a validated device for pregnancy [1].

Obstetric guidelines categorize hypertension discovered pre-pregnancy or the first 20 weeks of pregnancy as chronic hypertension [1], which will not be covered in this chapter further. Hypertensive disorders of pregnancy include de novo hypertension discovered from week 20 of pregnancy and is divided into 3 categories: Gestational hypertension, Preeclampsia or Superimposed preeclampsia. **Gestational hypertension is defined by** de novo hypertension at ≥20 weeks' gestation, but where there is no proteinuria or other preeclampsia-associated findings. **Preeclampsia** is defined by new-onset hypertension (Gestational hypertension) and proteinuria and/or at least one other preeclampsia-associated signs of organ dysfunction, after gestational week 20 [1]. Such new-onset organ dysfunction signs include (but are not restricted to) proteinuria, neurological complications (e.g., eclampsia), pulmonary oedema, haematological complications (e.g., platelet count <150,000/μL, haemolysis), acute kidney injury, liver involvement or signs of uteroplacental dysfunction. Uteroplacental dysfunction is now exemplified as placental abruption, angiogenic protein imbalance in maternal blood, fetal growth restriction, abnormal umbilical artery Doppler waveform analysis, or intrauterine fetal death) [1]. **Superimposed preeclampsia** is defined as development of new proteinuria (or another maternal organ dysfunction(s) sign), and/or evidence of uteroplacental dysfunction (as above), in women with chronic hypertension (as defined above).

Preeclampsia is a complex multisystem disease, with heterogeneous outcomes [2–5]. The rates of preeclampsia vary, usually affecting 3–5% of pregnancies. It is the most important antenatal complication of pregnancy, in terms of its incidence and combined short- and long-term effects on maternal and offspring health [6]. The maternal mortality rates are still high, especially in low-income countries, with >70,000 deaths annually [1, 7]. Perinatal death (estimated >500,000 annually) and maternal morbidity, including maternal hemorrhagic stroke due to malignant hypertensive development, remain a major challenge worldwide [1].

Preeclampsia is clinically often divided into early-onset and late-onset preeclampsia, commonly dichotomized as delivery prior to, or from, 34 weeks' gestation [8]. Early-onset preeclampsia is often accompanied by fetal growth restriction with low birthweight percentiles, whereas late-onset preeclampsia is not [9], highlighting the heterogeneous nature of the preeclampsia syndrome. The original two-stage model of preeclampsia was published by Redman in 1991 [10], and has been more recently updated in collaboration with Staff, explaining how both early-onset and late-onset preeclampsia result from placental syncytiotrophoblast stress [3, 11–13], but that the causes and timing of placental malperfusion differ [3, 11, 13]. Our proposed unifying concept of placental malperfusion and syncytiotrophoblast stress [12] as a common pathophysiological pathway in both early- and late-onset preeclampsia is also advocated in a recent review

[5]. Our model fits well with the clinical heterogeneity of preeclampsia and gestational hypertension, the increased risk of hypertensive disorders of pregnancy following chronic diseases (e.g., diabetes and obesity), and also with the different maternal angiogenic pattern of early- and late-onset preeclampsia in the first trimester of pregnancy [3, 11–13].

In our two-stage model of preeclampsia, stage 1 is defined by placental cellular stress. Inflammatory signaling molecules and dysregulated placenta-produced angiogenic factors (e.g. high level of fms-like tyrosine kinase-1 (sFlt-1) and low level of placenta growth factor (PlGF)) [14] from the dysfunctional placenta mediate stage 2 preeclampsia, defined by the maternal vascular responses and clinical signs of preeclampsia, including new-onset hypertension [13, 15]. This two-stage model of preeclampsia incorporates the epidemiological risk factors for preeclampsia, such as nulliparity [16], which is likely due to both immunological and anatomical factors related to uteroplacental artery remodeling and other placentation processes [3]. The known risk factors for preeclampsia (including increasing maternal age, pre-gestational diabetes mellitus, chronic hypertension, antiphospholipid syndrome, assisted reproduction, multiple pregnancy and obesity) are explained by affecting placentation processes, placental function, and/or the maternal vascular response to placenta-shed proinflammatory factors, as further detailed by Staff [3]. A combination of maternal KIR (killer-cell immunoglobulin-like receptor) genotype and fetal HLA-C genotype likely increases the risk of preeclampsia development due to shallow trophoblast invasion, followed by poor uteroplacental spiral artery remodeling and placental dysfunction [17]. The "smoking paradox" of preeclampsia, where there is an epidemiological "beneficial" risk reduction for preeclampsia in smokers, is not a straight-forward association, nor present in all populations today [18, 19]. The "protective" effect of smoking is suggested to be mediated by a modulatory effect of carbon monoxide on placental production of angiogenic factors [20, 21].

Some researchers challenge the concept of preeclampsia as a placenta-mediated disorder, but rather argue that preeclampsia has a cardiovascular etiology. According to this concept, suboptimal maternal cardiovascular performance results in uteroplacental hypoperfusion and causes a secondary placental dysfunction in preeclampsia [22]. However, a heart model for preeclampsia is inconsistent with many preeclampsia risk factors, including young age, primiparity and change of partner. These risk factors fit better with inappropriate placentation due to anatomical and immunological tolerization aspects [3]. Moreover, whatever model for preeclampsia and other hypertensive disorders of pregnancy, the placenta is the mandatory prerequisite for preeclampsia, as no man nor any non-pregnant woman ever develops preeclampsia, even if he or she suffers from clinical cardiovascular disease.

Approximately 20–25% of women first presenting with a diagnosis of gestational hypertension will later in pregnancy develop proteinuria [1], and thereby be diagnosed with preeclampsia, exemplifying that hypertensive disorders of pregnancy represent overlapping syndromes. The final clinical hypertensive pregnancy diagnosis likely depends on the sum of many factors, including degree of placentation and placental dysfunction problems, as well as variations in prepregnancy maternal vascular inflammation and thereby the maternal cardiovasculature's responsiveness to inflammatory factors shed from the increasingly dysfunctional placenta as pregnancy progresses [3].

Treatment of preeclampsia is today limited to target hypertension (to reduce maternal risk of cerebral hemorrhage) and seizures (using Magnesium sulphate to treat and prevent eclampsia), but the only "cure" today is removal of the dysfunctional placenta, and thereby also delivery of the baby [1, 3–5]. The last decade has however provided solid evidence for performing screening for women at high risk for early-onset disease, identified in the first trimester by screening for clinical risk factors, and dysregulated placental function biomarkers [7, 23]. These women are offered low-dose aspirin, which is effective in reducing the risk of early-onset preeclampsia [1, 4, 5]. The exact mechanisms by which low-dose aspirin reduces the risk, is still not clear [24], but a recent study supports an effect on reducing placental ageing [25], which may be due to a positive effect on trophoblast function and placenta development processes.

Pregnancy in itself poses large alterations in cardiovascular function and structure [26], in order to ensure adequate uteroplacental blood flow, as well as fetal nutrition and oxygenation. This includes striking physiological cardiovascular changes as well as metabolic changes, including insulin resistance. As reviewed recently [27], these complex physiological pathways of pregnancy include early pregnancy vasodilatation, with reduced total vascular resistance, accommodating greater intravascular volume, stroke volume and heart rate without increasing mean arterial pressure. In the second half of the first trimester, retrograde trophoblast invasion into the spiral artery is followed by comprehensive interaction with maternal immune cells and remodeling processes [28]. This remodeling ensures a good uteroplacental blood flow and is one of the reasons for increased uteroplacental vascular compliance. In most cases of early-onset preeclampsia, as well as in fetal growth restriction and other major obstetric syndromes, this remodeling process is suboptimal [28]. The latter half of the pregnancy is associated with insulin resistance, dyslipidemia and excessive vascular inflammation.

Excessive cardiovascular responses and remodeling processes, as compared to the normal physiology of pregnancy, are observed during and after preeclampsia [27, 29–31]. These alterations include increased endothelial dysfunction, arterial stiffness, left atrial remodeling, biventricular hypertrophy with impaired myocardial contractility and relaxation, inappropriate left ventricular mass and left ventricular myocardial fibrosis, both during and many years after the index pregnancy [31]. Importantly, women who have undergone a pregnancy complicated by fetal growth restriction, but that remained normotensive, also seem to have similar persistent cardiovascular alteration, with abnormal myocardial function [32], as those seen in many women after preeclampsia.

Historically, the remote cardiovascular prognosis of women after a hypertensive disorder of pregnancy was controversial, despite important published observations from US and UK in 1976 regarding increased rates of myocardial infarction, premature mortality and diabetes following eclampsia/preeclampsia [33, 34]. However, the last two decades have provided solid epidemiological population-based evidence for these associations, based on data predominantly from high-income countries and regions [35–39]. The following chapter is dedicated to the long-term maternal cardiovascular health effects and the utility of pregnancy as a stress test for cardiovascular disease later in life, representing an often-missed opportunity for screening, prevention and intervention [40–44].

2 Theory

2.1 The Epidemiological Data for the Associations Between Hypertensive Disorders of Pregnancy and Cardiovascular Disease

There is today solid support for an increased risk of premature maternal cardiovascular disease after a range of adverse pregnancy outcomes [43]. These adverse pregnancy outcomes are not restricted to hypertensive disorders of pregnancy (gestational hypertension and preeclampsia), but also encompass other obstetric syndromes linked to placental dysfunction and malperfusion, including fetal growth restriction, spontaneous preterm delivery and gestational diabetes mellitus [3, 13, 45].

A pivotal population-based study from Norway [35], including all primiparous women giving birth in 1967–1992, was important in establishing a clear epidemiological association between preeclampsia and preterm death of cardiovascular cause. The study included 600,000 first deliveries. The poorest survival rate was seen in women with preterm delivered preeclampsia, followed by preterm delivery without preeclampsia, whereas term delivery without preeclampsia had the best survival. Several other large population-based studies have confirmed these associations [35–39, 46], supporting a higher risk of a broad range of maternal cardiovascular diseases with more severe hypertensive disorders of pregnancy forms, particularly when complicated by fetal growth restriction [46], as well as with recurrent preeclampsia [47, 48], as reviewed previously [43].

Most studies estimate that women with prior late-onset preeclampsia or gestational hypertension have approximately a twofold increased risk of experiencing a cardiovascular adverse event later in life [39, 49], when compared to women with prior normotensive pregnancies, also after adjustment for known cardiovascular risk factors [50]. For pregnancies with more severe placental dysfunction, e.g. preterm preeclampsia and fetal growth restriction, the epidemiological cardiovascular disease risk is increased seven to eightfold [39]. Such a "dose-response" effect of hypertensive disorders of pregnancy on cardiovascular morbidity and mortality is also reflected in the epidemiological data demonstrating that women with previous gestational hypertension or late-onset preeclampsia are at lower risk for cardiovascular disease than after early-onset preeclampsia [39, 46, 51–53]. Accordingly, the highest risk for major coronary and cardiovascular events is among women with preeclampsia and a premature delivery of a small for gestational age offspring [46], and in women with repeated preeclampsia, the latter group also showing significantly shorter time to first cardiovascular event [47].

Available systematic reviews since 2007 conclude similarly [39, 54–56], namely that women with a history of hypertensive disorders of pregnancy (gestational hypertension or preeclampsia), gestational diabetes mellitus, placental abruption, preterm birth, and stillbirth are at increased risk of subsequent cardiovascular disease. One such review and meta-analysis from 2007 suggested that the absolute risk of a cardiovascular event for a women with a history of preeclampsia would be 18% in the age group of 50–59 and 31% in the age group of 60–69 years, which is much higher than the absolute risk among women not having experienced preeclampsia (8% and 14%, respectively) [39].

More recent population-based studies, likely including older and more obese mothers than previously, confirm the associations summarized above. As an example, a study based on electronic health records from 1997 to 2016 in the UK showed in adjusted analyses an increased cardiovascular risk after preeclampsia as well as after gestational hypertension, with a trend towards more risk after preterm preeclampsia [44]. The hazard ratios for stroke, myocardial infarction, heart failure, and cardiovascular death were approximately 2, and the hazard ratio for chronic hypertension was 4.5 [44], comparable to earlier reports. A systematic review and meta-analysis, including published studies between 2005 and 2015, confirmed that a history of preeclampsia was associated with an increased risk of future coronary heart disease, heart failure and stroke, after adjusting for age, body mass index and diabetes mellitus (RR 3–4) [49].

A recent UK study indicated that as many as 71% of women with a previous late preterm preeclampsia (34–37 weeks' gestation) [57] remained hypertensive at 6 months postpartum [58]. This is in striking contrast to our follow-up 1 year after a hypertensive disorder of pregnancy in Norway, where only 3.4% of women with early-onset preeclampsia, and 1.9% with previous late-onset preeclampsia had hypertension [59]. On the other hand, as many as 13.8% and 19.2% of these groups had prehypertension, respectively (diastolic BP of 120–139 and/or a systolic BP of 80–89 mmHg) [59]. The highest rate of hypertension and prehypertension in this Norwegian study was among women with a diagnosis of gestational hypertension (5.8% and 45.7%, respectively) [59]. This is in line with the rate of hypertension in a nationwide Danish study being less than 5% at 1 year since first birth with a hypertensive disorder pregnancy [60]. This

Danish study found the increased risk for hypertension within 10 years after a hypertensive disorder of pregnancy, to persist even after adjustment for other risk factors [60]. Another population-based study from Norway confirmed that adjustment for pre- and postpartum risk factors for hypertension (including breast feeding) did not alter the increased risk for postpartum hypertension after adverse pregnancy outcomes [61]. A recent coronary computer tomography angiography screening from Sweden found that in women aged 50–65 years, a history of hypertensive disorder of pregnancy (in particular preeclampsia) was associated with increased risk of image-identified coronary artery disease, even in women estimated to be at low risk of cardiovascular disease [62].

A recent report also supports preeclampsia being associated with subsequent higher risk of microvascular pathology, with reduced retinal vascular density, after adjustment for known risk factors [63]. Accordingly, a study measuring microvascular reactivity in the forearm demonstrated that preeclampsia is associated with heightened postpartum microvascular endothelium-dependent and endothelium-independent vasoreactivity [64]. Another study supports a microvascular involvement, as differences in cardiac structure and geometry, as well as microvascular rarefaction (assessed by finger capillaroscopy), are evident 5–10 years after a hypertensive pregnancy, independent of blood pressure [65].

Preeclampsia is not only linked to atherosclerotic events, but to a plethora of cardiovascular diseases [66], and premature cardiovascular events [47]. This includes subsequent development of cardiomyopathy [67], heart failure [68–70], and cardiac valvular pathology [68]. Recent studies have further analyzed types of heart failure. Heart failure with preserved ejection fraction (HFpEF) is more common in women than men and is associated with high rates of microvascular inflammation and vasculopathy, morbidity and mortality [71, 72]. It is argued that HFpEF is currently the largest unmet clinical need in cardiology, particularly regarding women's health worldwide [73]. Interestingly, the risk of developing hypertension and HFpEF is reported to be increased fourfold after preeclampsia, relative to prior uncomplicated pregnancies [43, 49, 74]. Another recent study showed that, even after adjustment for traditional HFpEF risk factors, women with previous preeclampsia or eclampsia had a twofold increased risk for hospitalization for HFpEF over the subsequent decade [75].

It is well known that women with hypertensive orders of pregnancy have an increased risk for heart failure due to peripartum cardiomyopathy, that develops in the last month of pregnancy or up to 5 months after delivery [76]. Gene variants known to be associated with idiopathic and peripartum cardiomyopathy have been shown to be associated with preeclampsia [77].

Also, preeclampsia increases the risk of end-stage renal disease, as shown in a Norwegian population-based registry study [78], which again impacts the risk of cardiovascular disease. A recent meta-analysis (including over 5.7 million pregnancies) concluded that a history of any of the large groups of adverse pregnancy outcomes (hypertensive disorders of pregnancy, gestational diabetes, and preterm delivery) increased the risk for maternal chronic kidney disease and end-stage kidney disease. The highest risk was for preeclampsia, especially preterm [79], again demonstrating a "dose-response" effect.

Preeclampsia is also linked to a twofold increased risk of diabetes development [43, 80], another important risk factor for premature cardiovascular disease. A recent meta-analysis concluded likewise, including over 3 million women from 16 studies, mostly from Europe, but also from North America, Asia and Australia [81].

The larger epidemiological studies from Northern Europe (e.g. Norway, Scotland and Denmark) [35, 36, 50, 82] and Israel [83] have low degree of ethnic diversity, whereas publications from the US demonstrate large variations in the epidemiology of both hypertensive disorders of pregnancy [84, 85] and long-term cardiovascular health effect of these complications among Black and White (non-Hispanic) women in general [86, 87]. This ethnic heterogeneity is supported by recent studies from California regarding heart failure [70], coronary heart disease, incident stroke and all-cause mortality within 5 years of delivery [88]. Another recent US study demonstrated higher stroke risks in Black and Hispanic women, compared to non-Hispanic White women, following a new-onset hypertension pregnancy, as well as following a pregnancy complicated by chronic hypertension [89].

The relative risks of cardiovascular events associated with hypertensive disorders of pregnancy (HDP) seem to persist until 65 years of age, at which time women without a history of HDP "catch up" with those with HDP history. It has been observed that the relative risk of risk factors [90] and cardiovascular events [91, 92] associated with HDP seem to fade with time since pregnancy and age. It has been suggested that as the excess risk diminishes after menopause due to a depletion of the susceptible population [93].

2.2 The Mechanisms: Why Are Hypertensive Pregnancy Disorders Associated with Increased Risk for Cardiovascular Disease?

2.2.1 Two Main Hypotheses for the Association Between Hypertensive Disorders of Pregnancy and Future Maternal CVD

The associations between having undergone preeclampsia or gestational hypertension to experiencing later cardiovascular disease are likely complex and multifactorial, and the strength of the associations likely differ between heterogeneous populations and over time. Shared risk factors and conference of risk during pregnancy are two main hypotheses for the mechanisms behind the associations that are not mutually exclusive [43, 94]. The two pathways are likely synergistic.

Both preeclampsia and atherosclerosis arise from vascular inflammation with its associated endothelial dysfunction [43]. As illustrated in Fig. 1, hypertensive disorders of pregnancy and cardiovascular disease share many risk factors [43]. Longitudinal population-based studies from Norway support that maternal predisposing factors prior to a hypertensive pregnancy (such as obesity, blood pressure and dyslipidemia) could be important mediators for the subsequent increased risk for cardiovascular disease [95–97]. However, even after adjusting for these risk factors prior to and after pregnancy, there was still a remaining association between a hypertensive disorder of pregnancy and cardiovascular disease [95], suggesting that the pregnancy complication per se also may contribute to the association. Two more recent studies from Norway confirmed that the association between hypertensive disorders of pregnancy and cardiovascular disease remained after statistical adjustment strategies, and that the risk is partly attributable to modifiable cardiovascular disease risk factors [50, 92].

An alternative pathway, as argued by us, and not excluding the first [43], suggests that pregnancy in general, and preeclampsia (and other placental dysfunction disorders) in particular, worsen pre-existing, subclinical cardiovascular disease risk factors or even induce de novo risk [43]. In this model, a long-term cardiovascular effect is driven by placental dysfunction and the subsequent release of anti-angiogenic signaling molecules and inflammatory factors, culminating in systemic endothelial dysfunction [43]. Preeclampsia and placental dysfunction include excessive hyperlipidemia and inflammation, angiogenic imbalances, and metabolic and vascular (mal)adaptation [43]. Increased angiotensin II sensitivity and sFlt-1 response to angiotensin II infusion in women with previous preeclampsia has been reported, supporting lasting dysfunctional angiogenic responses [98]. The hypertension, dyslipidemia and worsened insulin resistance typically seen in preeclampsia, together with a dysregulated angiotensin system [99], could possibly accelerate vascular progression towards premature clinical and more advanced atherosclerotic lesions and hypertension [100, 101].

Hypertension likely contributes strongly to the cardiovascular clinical events seen after these pregnancy complications. Mediation analyses

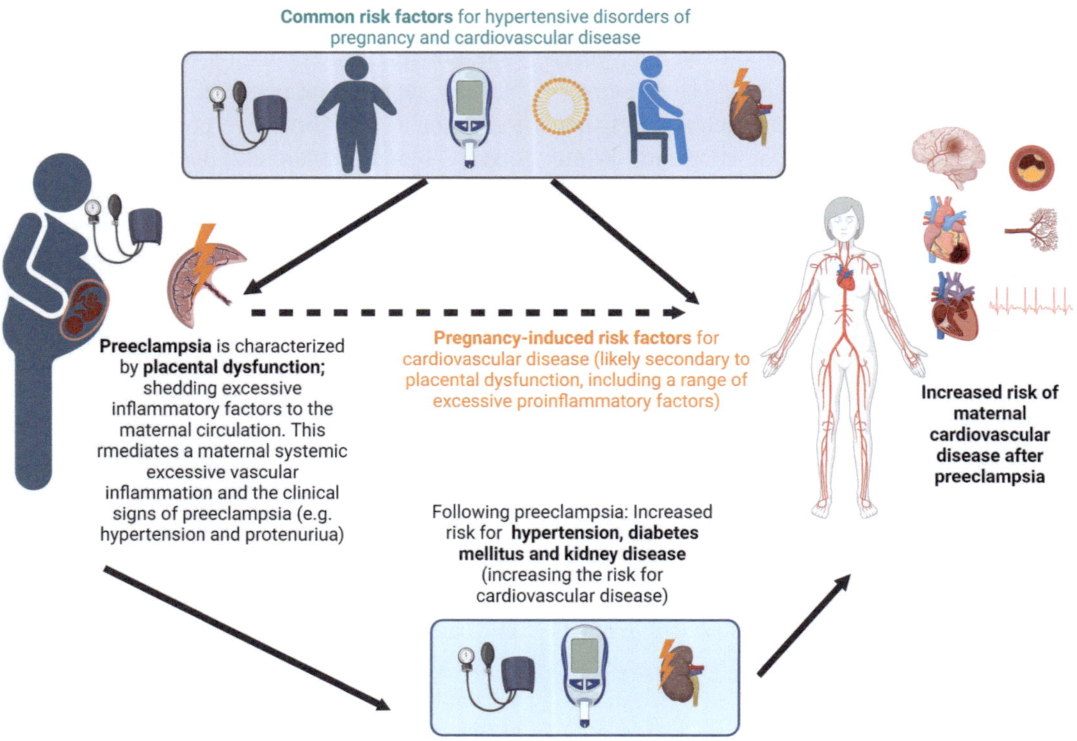

Fig. 1 Two main hypotheses for the association between hypertensive disorders of pregnancy and future maternal cardiovascular disease. A widely held hypothesis focuses on common risk factors, including hypertension, obesity, diabetes mellitus, insulin resistance and hyperglycemia, dyslipidemia, renal disease, a family history of cardiovascular disease, and the metabolic syndrome. An alternative hypothesis, not excluding the first, suggests that pregnancy in general, and preeclampsia (and other placental disorders) in particular, worsen preexisting, subclinical cardiovascular disease risk factors or even induce de novo risk [43]. Preeclampsia and other placenta dysfunction syndromes (including fetal growth restriction) involves (as compared to normotensive uncomplicated pregnancies) excessive hyperlipidemia and inflammation, angiogenic imbalance (maternal circulating low PlGF, high sFlt1), metabolic and vascular as well as cardiac tissue maladaptation. Also, women with hypertensive pregnancy disorders have increased postpartum risk of diabetes and kidney disease, that will further increase the risk for premature cardiovascular disease. Created in BioRender, with permission to publish

indicate however that chronic hypertension only explains one-half of the association between hypertensive disorders of pregnancy and heart failure [67, 68]. Other hypothesized mechanisms of heart failure predilection after preeclampsia have included oxidative stress, inflammation, senescence, persistent endothelial dysfunction, and coronary microvascular dysfunction [31, 66], all features relevant for the preeclampsia pathophysiology.

We propose that the many long-term effects of hypertensive pregnancy disorders on maternal cardiovascular health are likely synergistic, including mediated by their associations to increased postpartum risk of diabetes and kidney disease, as reviewed above. As an example, the higher risk for remote hypertension also alters the cerebral circulation, both in small and large vessels. This will negatively impact the pathophysiology of an ischemic stroke, which these women are also predisposed for, and thereby predispose to early cognitive impairment [102].

2.2.2 Duration of Preeclampsia and Risk for CVD

Some studies have indicated that the duration of preeclampsia before delivery is important for the long-tern maternal cardiovascular risk [103, 104]. The recent Phoenix randomized control trial investigated the obstetric and fetal outcomes according to prompt or delayed delivery [57]., and prompted an opportunity to study this intervention effect on maternal cardiovascular health [105]. The subsequent short, follow-up study (the Phoebe trial) [58] showed however no difference in cardiovascular outcomes according to prompt or delayed delivery in preeclampsia, but recognized that the majority of women with early-onset preeclampsia suffered from hypertension a short time after pregnancy, and left ventricular systolic dysfunction was found in 10%. This study should however reassure women in that “prolongation of a pregnancy affected by preterm pre-eclampsia will not further worsen their cardiovascular health” [58].

2.2.3 Is HFpEF Particularly Linked to Hypertensive Disorders of Pregnancy?

Recent theories pose that HFpEF originates from microvascular coronary alterations due to oxidative stress and chronic inflammation, sprouting from cardiovascular risk factors and comorbidities [73]. Thus, common pathophysiological pathways may be linking preeclampsia and HFpEF [31], including endothelial dysfunction, microvascular ischemia, inflammation, and increases in serum biomarkers [106]. Especially preterm preeclampsia is associated with left ventricular remodeling and diastolic dysfunction both acutely and in the years following delivery [29, 30], which are known precursors to clinical HFpEF [106]. A recent longitudinal eccocardiography study by Giorgione et al. suggests that women with persistent hypertension after hypertensive disorders of pregnancy are more at risk for persistent abnormal cardiac findings in the peripartum period, further accelerating a progress towards heart failure [107].

Interestingly, women are in general more prone to microvascular dysfunction than men and respond differently to cardiovascular stressors [108]. Sex hormones and sex-specific mechanisms influence glucose and lipid metabolism, as well as cardiac energy metabolism and function [109]. Also, obesity may represent a common pathway, as obesity seems to represent a particularly important risk factor for premature-onset HFpEF in the younger part of the population [110], similarly to its impact on hypertensive disorders of pregnancy as well as for atherosclerotic cardiovascular disease.

Sciatti et al. have suggested a model with documented cardiovascular findings following preeclampsia and growth restriction (e.g. systemic endothelial dysfunction, arterial stiffness, reduced coronary flow reserve, cardiac hypertrophy and interstitial fibrosis, reduced contractility and diastolic function), that may represent important pathophysiological pathways linking these adverse pregnancy outcomes to the increased risk of cardiovascular events (including HFpEF) [31]. His model, in line with ours [43], suggests that the “initiating” stressors, traditional risk factors as well as pregnancy-specific risk factors, combine their effects on the cascade of cardiovascular events starting with increased inflammation and oxidative stress [31].

2.3 Ethnic and Racial Disparities

A recent study from the UK suggested that many prior studies on the observed higher risk of preeclampsia in Black women may have been biased. The authors’ own adjusted analyses from routine screening for preeclampsia with ultrasound examination at 11–13 weeks of pregnancy, including more than 168 thousand women with singleton pregnancies, showed a relative twofold increased risk for preterm preeclampsia and 2.5-fold for total preeclampsia in Black women. The risk for gestational hypertension was 25% higher [111].

A recent US paper calls, however, for caution in using race as a proxy for biologically inherent (i.e., genetic) differences between races, as studies using geographic or cultural origin identifies large preeclampsia disparities within racial groups [85]. This paper summarizes that sub-Saharan African immigrants tend to have a higher risk of preeclampsia than US-born White populations but a lower risk than US-born Black women [85]. Sub-Saharan immigrants also had a higher risk of hypertensive disorders of pregnancy in our recent population-based study from Norway, but after adjustment for other covariates these women had a similar risk as Norwegian-born women [16], again illustrating the need for caution when suggesting causal pathways for any observed racial disparities.

The mechanisms for racial disparity in the risk for hypertensive disorders of pregnancy and their associations to short- and long-term health effects on maternal cardiovascular health are likely multifactorial [112], and likely not the same in all societies and countries. Other comorbidities such as higher rates of obesity, chronic hypertension and prepregnancy diabetes is more frequent among Black women in the US [86], but the risk of new-onset hypertension in pregnancy was still increased in Black women after adjustment for such preexisting risk factors [113]. Socioeconomic differences, reduced access to healthcare, lower quality of care, lack of appropriate health awareness and education in health providers and patients, as well as provider implicit bias and systemic racism may all contribute to the racial disparities seen in hypertensive disorders of pregnancy [86]. Socioeconomic status is also relevant in the development of HFpEF following preeclampsia. Williams et al identified in a US study that Black race, low income and rural locality were independent risk factors for HFpEF, suggesting that poor access to care likely contributes to cardiovascular risk factor modification and higher prevalence of HFpEF [75, 106].

3 Clinical Practice

3.1 How Can We Translate the Epidemiological Knowledge Into Clinical Practice?

The American Heart Association acknowledged in 2011 that adverse pregnancy outcome may predict cardiovascular disease [114], followed by recognition from a spectrum of cardiology communities [31, 66, 73, 115–118] and obstetric and cardiology joint forces [119]. Despite this, few women are today offered systematic cardiopreventive follow-up after hypertensive disorders of pregnancy, and evidence-based specific preventive programs are lacking.

All fertile women should ideally prior to any pregnancy reduce their risk for developing hypertensive pregnancy complications and placental dysfunction [120]. This includes obtaining a healthy weight and a healthy lifestyle before conception and reducing the burden of any chronic diseases (e.g. hypertension and diabetes mellitus). In general, it is recommended that following pregnancy, women with pre-existing renal or cardiac complications or suffering from diabetes mellitus, should be offered appropriate specialist follow-up to assess cardiovascular disease risk and optimize treatment and follow-up. The advice for clinical follow-up of an otherwise healthy woman following complication in pregnancy associated with higher cardiovascular disease risk is however fragmentary, without global consensus [43].

3.2 Prevention Initiation Already from the Postpartum Period

Women are at high risk for developing chronic hypertension the years following a hypertensive disorder of pregnancy. Hypertension may in fact represents a more important risk factor for cardiovascular disease in women than in men, supporting that early detection and treatment of elevated blood pressure may be especially important in women. The population-based Tromsø study in Norway showed that systolic blood pressure elevation is important for permanent atrial fibrillation complications in women, but not in men [121]. The main causal and modifiable atherosclerotic cardiovascular disease risk factors in both sexes are hypertension, dyslipidemia, adiposity, cigarette smoking, physical inactivity and diabetes mellitus [122] all of which should be assessed in postpartum follow-up in women at increased risk for cardiovascular disease. Of note, women exhibit a more accelerated rise in blood pressure than men already from their 30s [123], two decades before menopause, at which point women catch up with men in hypertension rates. Furthermore, women's increased risk for cardiovascular disease starts with elevations from lower systolic blood pressures than in men, possibly due to smaller arterial diameter relative to body size [124]. These observations point to blood pressure as an important risk factor to screen for following a pregnancy complication linked to increased cardiovascular disease risk, in order to treat any detected hypertension timely and appropriately.

The risk of cardiovascular diseases following a hypertensive pregnancy is high already from young ages. The focus for preventing strategies must therefore be applied as early as possible. Another worrying factor is that many health providers seem unaware of the associations between pregnancy complications and the increased risk for future maternal cardiovascular disease [125, 126]. Likewise, affected women themselves also often lack this knowledge [127, 128] and are therefore unlikely to act on their increased epidemiological risk. Importantly, these women seem motivated to be educated and participate in follow-up trials [127–129]. Lifestyle intervention seems to be well received [129–132], and has the potential for being put into preventive health strategies at a more systematic population level. Home monitoring of blood pressure may be an option for some women, as tested in a hospital postpartum clinic setting [133] and in a pilot study [129].

All current risk calculators are unsuitable for evaluating cardiovascular risk in most young women after pregnancy complications, as they neglect the impact of pregnancy complications and often are not applicable to populations below 40 years of age [59]. Similar conclusions were found in 3 other studies from US, Sweden and Norway, testing other risk models [134–136]. In older women, risk calculators provide more adequate cardiovascular disease risk scoring [137], but with advanced age, preventive strategies are likely less effective [138], and the potential mortality and morbidity gain from such effort is lower. Population-based studies from Denmark [60] and Norway [61] have shown that one third of women develop hypertension within 10 years of experiencing hypertensive disorders of pregnancy. A recent nation-wide study from France, including more than 2.2 million women (without prior hypertension) delivering in 2008–2010, showed that the risks of cardiovascular and cerebrovascular outcomes were the highest in the first year after a birth complicated by hypertensive disorders of pregnancy. The risk of chronic hypertension was 18 times higher in the first year and was "only" 5 times higher at 5-10 years after birth [53]. Middle age is therefore in our opinion far too late to start intensified follow-up for optimal prevention of cardiovascular disease.

Several studies have shown that risk factors and preclinical markers for cardiovascular disease are present in many women during and soon after hypertensive pregnancy complications [29, 30, 53, 58–60, 107, 139, 140], supporting the need for early intervention and follow-up strategies, not postponing these till after menopause or to the first clinical sign of cardiovascular disease emerges.

Pregnancy represents a life-changing event where women are particularly interested in their own and their offspring's health. This postpartum setting may therefore represent the optimal time point to empower women to improve their own cardiovascular health for life [40–43, 107]. We argue that a system for postpartum follow-up enables stratification of women according to cardiovascular risk, thereby offering appropriate follow-up level, for example at specialist versus community health service level, reducing a risk of overexploitation of an already critical specialist health system even in high-income countries.

3.3 Suggestions for Follow-Up Guidelines after Hypertensive Disorders of Pregnancy

Guidelines were prior to 2016 lacking any practical follow-up suggestions after hypertensive disorders of pregnancy, as revised by us (Supplemental material 1) [43] A UK guideline advised health carers to tell women about their increased risk of hypertension and its complications later in life, and advise on diet and weight before a next pregnancy [141].

As a response to the obvious gap in global maternal healthcare systems, we suggested in 2016 a first practical screening flow chart following delivery of any of the obstetric syndromes that was known to be associated with cardiovascular disease (including preeclampsia, gestational hypertension, fetal growth restriction and gestational diabetes mellitus) [43]. We suggested that further follow-up (in specialist or community health system) would be adapted to identified risk factors, and that the community health follow-up could be integrated with other potential screening programs (e.g. cervical cancer screening) [43]. We have since further detailed the risk assessments after these pregnancy complications [142], and adapted it to Norwegian guidelines for lifestyle support for prevention of cardiovascular disease and integrated it with the existing obstetric national guideline for hypertensive disorders of pregnancy, including a patient brochure [142]. Our thinking was that this guideline could be adapted to other countries, local guidelines and resources, as illustrated in Fig. 2, from Chesley's hypertensive disorders in pregnancy (5th edition) [94]. Here, we implemented the American lifestyle guidelines. Lately, we have made a simple infographic for a follow-up that may be easily accessible to all women and health carers worldwide [112].

We suggest as a minimum a "fourth trimester" follow-up, namely a basic cardiovascular screening withing the first 12 weeks following delivery. At 1 year postpartum, a cardiovascular screening, that also includes screening for dyslipidemia and diabetes, would stratify women for annual or less frequent follow-up. Less frequent follow-ups would be applicable for women without detected risk factors through this first one-year postpartum screening, and a community health follow-up of such women could be integrated into other potential screening programs (e.g. cervical cancer screening) [43, 142]. In contrast, women diagnosed with established risk factors (e.g. hypertension, obesity or smoking) likely benefit from more frequent controls [112], thus individualizing follow-up according to individual patient risk.

Long-term follow-up approaches after hypertensive disorders of pregnancy are today also recommended by international society guidelines (e.g. FIGO; The International Federation of Gynecology and Obstetrics and ISSHP; The International Society for the Study of Hypertension on Pregnancy) [1, 143], and national guidelines, such as in Norway [142]. In the national obstetric guidelines of Norway, we have also suggested implementing a similar follow-up system for women after gestational diabetes mellitus, and such screening and follow-up is also referred to in the chapters on preterm birth and fetal growth restriction.

Updated guidelines from the European Society of Cardiology suggest likewise an individualized

Fig. 2 A suggestion for postpartum follow-up and primary prevention of cardiovascular disease after hypertensive disorders of pregnancy, in otherwise healthy women. This flow chart is based on our first follow-up proposal from 2016 [43], further simplified for a Norwegian Obstetrical guideline and patient brochures in 2020 [142]. The flow chart below by us is adapted to US general health guidelines in 2022, and reprinted with permission [94]. This screening starts at the delivery ward during the hospital stay, where women with established cardiovascular or renal disease would continue follow-up at a specialist level (e.g. internist, cardiologist, nephrologist). Women with residual hypertension, proteinuria or hyperglycemia at hospital discharge, or with severe forms of pregnancy complications (e.g. HELLP, eclampsia, preterm delivery prior to week 34) would be followed through a specialist maternity health follow-up system that also would include a cardiovascular risk assessment at 2–3 months postpartum. Those without any such clinical features at discharge, as illustrated in the figure, are offered a simple cardiovascular assessment at 6–12 weeks in the community health system, which represents a common postpartum consultation time point in many countries. This assessment would include blood pressure, urine and body mass evaluations, investigating family history of cardiovascular disease and smoking as well as screening for diabetes (e.g. as HbA_{1c} analysis). We suggested that further follow-up (in specialist or community health system) would be adapted to identified risk factors, and that the community health follow-up could be integrated with other potential screening programs (e.g. cervical cancer screening). The follow-up intervals (more frequent or less frequent than annually), facility level (specialist or general health care) and content (e.g. diabetes screening, blood lipids and blood pressure measurements, cardiovascular imaging) need to be individualized by clinical findings, available resources, in a shared decision making with the woman. Drug therapy would be offered according to guidelines, and lifestyle advice and support would be important through the entire follow-up

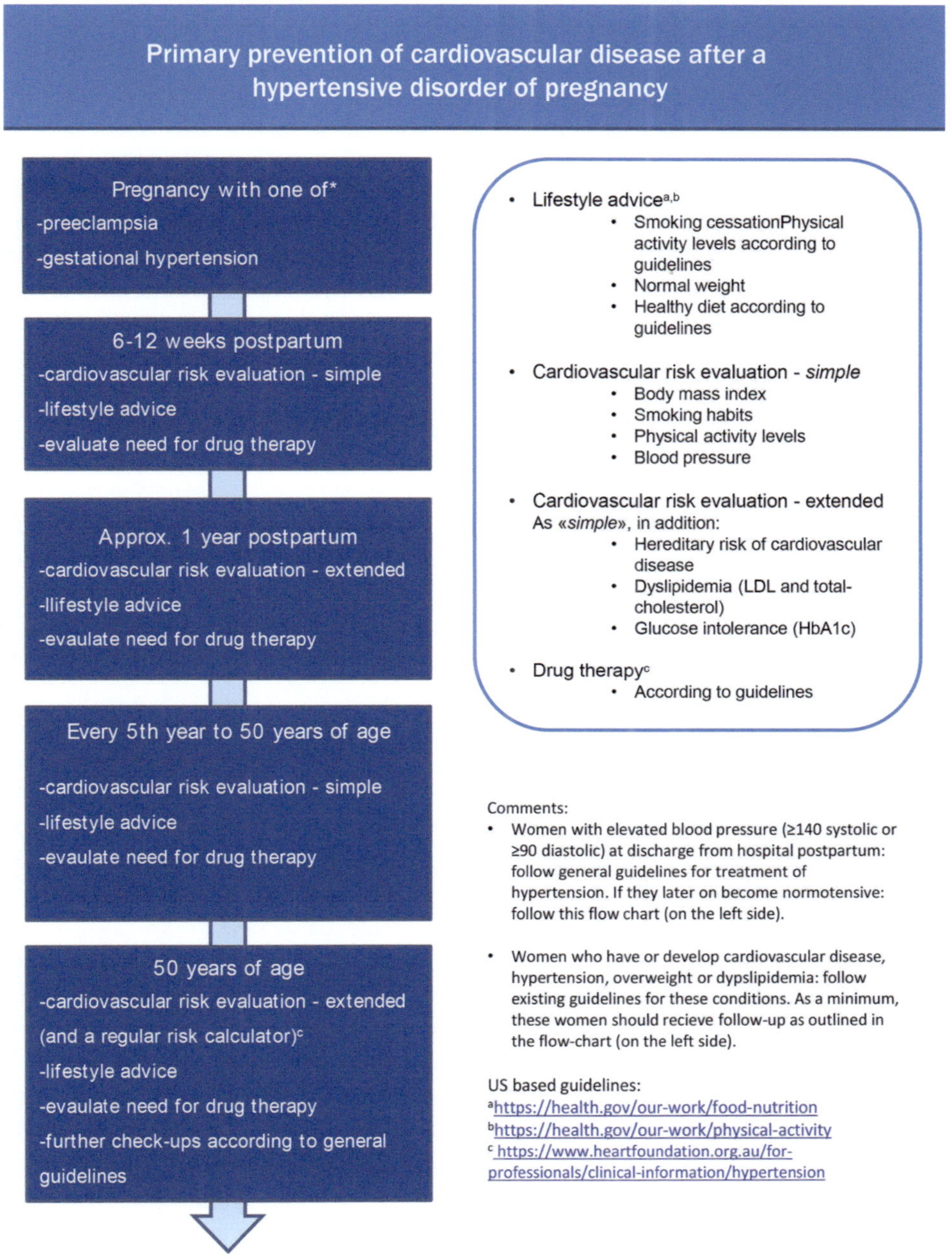
Primary prevention of cardiovascular disease after a hypertensive disorder of pregnancy
Pregnancy with one of*
-preeclampsia
-gestational hypertension
6-12 weeks postpartum
-cardiovascular risk evaluation - simple
-lifestyle advice
-evaluate need for drug therapy
Approx. 1 year postpartum
-cardiovascular risk evaluation - extended
-llifestyle advice
-evaulate need for drug therapy
Every 5th year to 50 years of age
-cardiovascular risk evaluation - simple
-lifestyle advice
-evaulate need for drug therapy
50 years of age
-cardiovascular risk evaluation - extended
(and a regular risk calculator)[c]
-lifestyle advice
-evaulate need for drug therapy
-further check-ups according to general guidelines
• Lifestyle advice[a,b]
• Smoking cessationPhysical activity levels according to guidelines
• Normal weight
• Healthy diet according to guidelines
• Cardiovascular risk evaluation - *simple*
• Body mass index
• Smoking habits
• Physical activity levels
• Blood pressure
• Cardiovascular risk evaluation - extended
As «*simple*», in addition:
• Hereditary risk of cardiovascular disease
• Dyslipidemia (LDL and total-cholesterol)
• Glucose intolerance (HbA1c)
• Drug therapy[c]
• According to guidelines
Comments:
• Women with elevated blood pressure (≥140 systolic or ≥90 diastolic) at discharge from hospital postpartum: follow general guidelines for treatment of hypertension. If they later on become normotensive: follow this flow chart (on the left side).
• Women who have or develop cardiovascular disease, hypertension, overweight or dypslipidemia: follow existing guidelines for these conditions. As a minimum, these women should recieve follow-up as outlined in the flow-chart (on the left side).
US based guidelines:
[a]https://health.gov/our-work/food-nutrition
[b]https://health.gov/our-work/physical-activity
[c] https://www.heartfoundation.org.au/for-professionals/clinical-information/hypertension

cardiopreventive approach, mentioning that "periodic screening for hypertension and diabetes mellitus should be considered" following preeclampsia and gestational diabetes mellitus [122].

3.4 Need for Better Stratification of Women at Highest Risk Following Hypertensive Disorders of Pregnancy: Biomarkers to Assist Personalized Follow-Up?

Even though survival following a cardiovascular event, such as myocardial infarction, is much improved today, it is alarming that the incidence of cardiovascular disease among young females is on the rise in some countries [144], most likely due to increases in adverse and modifiable life style factors such as obesity. Furthermore, most people below 45 years of age with an acute myocardial infarction are at a high risk of experiencing a new cardiovascular event or death within the next 10 years [145]. Understanding the risk factors is therefore key for optimizing prevention and health outcomes. To this end, biomarkers may be investigated to further target women at highest risk and for personalizing follow-up.

We suggested in our review in 2016 that maternal circulating placenta-associated angiogenic factors during pregnancy, reflecting placental function, could be explored as biomarker predictors for long-term risk of cardiovascular disease [43]. In line with our proposed concept [43], a Dutch study showed that low mid-pregnancy maternal PlGF levels predicted cardiac structural changes and elevated systolic blood pressure 6–9 years later, independent of hypertensive pregnancy disease [146]. Outside pregnancy, a high circulating PlGF (mostly endothelial-derived and representing a marker of vascular inflammation) is related to an increase in future cardiovascular disease events, when investigated in elderly persons (including women) with a previous acute coronary syndrome event [147].

We have explored other circulating cardiovascular biomarkers both during and following hypertensive pregnancies and other adverse pregnancy outcomes related to placental dysfunction. Although their final predictive value on hard cardiovascular endpoints have not been assessed, we propose them as promising and easily accessible potential predictive biomarkers for those in highest need for follow-up. We recently reported correlation prior to delivery between the cardiovascular markers cTnT (cardiac-specific high sensitive Troponin T) and NT-proBNP (N-terminal pro b-type natriuretic peptide) with two clinical proxies of placental dysfunction, namely antiangiogenic ratio (sFlt-1/PlGF ratio) and lower birthweight percentiles [148]. We also found dysregulated GDF-15 (Growth differentiation factor 15) to be elevated during pregnancy in all groups of women with hypertensive disorder of pregnancy [149], whereas it was elevated 1–3 year postpartum only in the group with previous early-onset preeclampsia [148]. These findings in a clinically healthy population, with low rate of overweight and hypertension, illustrate the short- and long-term cardiovascular burden of hypertensive disorders of pregnancy and the crosstalk with placental function [148]. We have suggested that GDF-15 may be explored for targeting postpartum women with most to gain from intensified preventive follow-up for cardiovascular disease.

We have previously suggested that uteroplacental acute atherosis, an arterial wall foam lesion often present in preeclampsia and resembling early stages of atherosclerosis, may be used as a marker to identify women at particularly high risk of atherosclerosis development [28, 150–152]. Our studies have supported this concept, in that circulating cardiovascular-related biomarkers in pregnancy differ according to acute atherosis, as well as according to fetal growth restriction and early- and late-onset preeclampsia [153]. Also, we have found that dyslipidemia associated with increased cardiovascular risk is a feature of uteroplacental acute atherosis in the older age group of pregnant women [154]. Other researchers have also followed this line of thinking, demonstrating increased cardiovascular risk factors in women with previous preeclampsia and evidence of decidual vasculopathy [155].

3.5 Anti-Inflammatory Pharmaceutical Preventive Strategies?

Large efforts are made today to improve the prediction and prevention of preeclampsia during pregnancy, including offering women screened at high risk for preeclampsia a daily low-dose aspirin from gestational week 11–14 [1, 4, 5, 23]. Aspirin antenatally is also suggested to have a cardioprotective effect [156], but randomized controlled trials with this as a primary endpoint are lacking.

It is possible that prompt postpartum pharmacological intervention (for example with statins, metformin, platelet inhibitors/anti-inflammatory drugs such as low dose aspirin, angiotensin-converting-enzyme inhibitors or angiotensin receptor blockers) could reduce future cardiovascular disease risk, as early stages of atherosclerosis are reversible [43]. Currently there is no available evidence in favor of any such intervention for the highest risk groups or more widely applied after hypertensive disorders of pregnancy, and long-term clinical studies are needed.

Ormesher et al. recently tested [157] in a double-blind placebo controlled randomized trial whether a pharmacological intervention for 6 months postpartum with an ACE (angiotensin-converting enzyme) inhibitor (enalapril) improved a negative trajectory towards cardiovascular disease after a pregnancy with preeclampsia. ACE inhibitors provide cardioprotection through a variety of mechanisms, including anti-inflammatory effects, increased nitrogen monoxide bioavailability and diminished fibrosis, which also are pathways affected in preeclampsia. The study found no difference in the primary clinical outcome (altered total vascular resistance), but significant differences were observed in secondary clinical outcomes related to cardiac remodeling and diastolic dysfunction. Larger multicenter studies are needed to confirm whether postpartum treatment with enalapril could reduce the prevalence of left ventricular diastolic function and remodeling [157].

4 Conclusions

The association between hypertensive disorders of pregnancy and future maternal cardiovascular disease is well documented, but there is still some controversy whether this association mostly or merely reflects common underlying risks for these hypertensive disorders and cardiovascular disease. Alternatively, these complications linked to placental dysfunction with ensuing maternal excessive systemic vascular inflammation may modify future cardiovascular risk across a wide spectrum, including atherosclerosis, microvascular disease, atrial fibrillation, stroke and heart failure. We argue that the analyses seeking to adjust for pre-pregnancy and postpartum risk factors support that both mechanisms may be at play.

As risk factors vary between populations and by socioeconomic factors, it is possible that the causative pathways for the associations differ between cohorts. The pattern of a dose-response relationship between degree of placental dysfunction and severity of hypertensive disorders being linked to the degree of risk of cardiovascular disease, persist across most published studies so far, even in studies that have adjusted for known cardiovascular risk factors.

Hypertension is identified as an important, but not the only, mediator for the associations, and appropriate screening and follow-up with early identification of hypertension after a hypertensive disorder of pregnancy is important, already from the early postpartum days. Hopefully, optimal treatment of risk factors will reduce the long-term cardiovascular disease rates, including the emerging heart failure problems.

Whatever the mechanisms for the associations between a hypertensive disorder of pregnancy and cardiovascular disease, we argue that pregnancy is an underexploited opportunity to initiate early targeting and primary prevention in women at increased risk of cardiovascular disease. As several studies identify hypertension and cardiovascular dysfunction early in the postpartum period, we argue that a systematic approach to screening and prevention of long-term clinical cardiovascular disease should start as soon as possible after delivery. We have suggested some simple follow-up programs after pregnancy complications associated with increased cardiovascular risk, which could be adapted according to local health resources and personal risk identification.

Cardiovascular disease prevention is a priority as incidence and costs are rising [158]. Women are more prone to microvascular dysfunction and respond differently to cardiovascular stressors [108]. Sex hormones and sex-specific mechanisms influence glucose and lipid metabolism, as well as cardiac energy metabolism and function [109]. Hypertensive disorders of pregnancy represent a unique spectrum of hypertensive disease, only affecting persons becoming pregnant and having developed a placenta. Their long-term effects on maternal cardiovascular structure and function represent another example of a sex-specific pathway to maternal cardiovascular disease for women.

At present, we need more prospective studies to identify more precise mechanisms for the associations, and also to identify better clinical targeting of women at highest risk. We also need to identify if there are specific prevention pathways that are more efficient for all or subgroups of these women, including a focus on microvascular disease and diastolic hypertension. But, even if we lack such knowledge today, this should not stop us from offering women a personalized follow-up, based on their prepregnancy, pregnancy and postpartum risk factors. Programs should encourage women at risk to engage in improving lifestyle habits, such as performing sufficient physical activity, keeping normal weight and diet, as well as restricting alcohol and smoking. A remaining challenge is how to reach such goals and empower women to engage in their own long-term health and to make, if necessary, lifestyle changes that may help avoiding or postponing or reducing the clinical burden of cardiovascular disease.

The time has now come to use pregnancy as an early cardiovascular stress-test that may benefit the woman and her family both in the short and long run. The strive for less female cardiovascular disease and healthier populations should start as early as possible in life, including reducing risk of obesity, hypertension, physical inactivity and diabetes from early ages. A team-based approach is likely optimal in supporting women at risk after hypertensive pregnancy disorders in their optimization of risk factors, including general community health service (e.g. general practitioners, health nurses), specialists (midwives, obstetrician-gynecologists, cardiologists, nephrologists, diabetologists) as well as lifestyle coaches and dietitians.

Key Issues

- Hypertensive disorders of pregnancy and cardiovascular disease share several modifiable risk factors. Many of these risk factors are present at a young age in women prior to, during and following new-onset hypertension in pregnancy.
- Several adverse pregnancy outcomes, including hypertensive disorder of pregnancy, associate with increased maternal cardiovascular mortality and morbidity in a "dose-response" pattern. The mechanisms for these associations are complex and likely include prepregnancy cardiovascular risk factors as well as pregnancy-induced mechanisms, where excessive inflammation may represent a key pathway.
- Known cardiovascular risk factors, such as hypertension and obesity, do not fully explain the elevated risk of future cardiovascular disease after pregnancy hypertension disorders.
- Hypertensive disorders of pregnancy represent an underexploited stress test for female cardiovascular disease world-wide, that could be translated into systematic follow-up programs for affected women at increased risk for cardiovascular disease.
- Educating and empowering women at risk after hypertensive disorders of pregnancy, as well as their health carers, is likely key for successful follow-up programs.
- Suggestions for simple follow-up programs after pregnancy complications associated with increased cardiovascular risk are included in this Chapter, which could be adapted according to personal risk identification and local

health resources. This includes monitoring of blood pressure, blood glucose and lipids, as well as assessing other modifiable risk factors such as body mass index and lifestyle.

- Better biomarkers are needed in young women after hypertensive disorders of pregnancy for risk stratification, in order to offer more precision medicine and follow-up.

Questions and Answers

1. Which modifiable risk factors are shared by hypertensive disorders of pregnancy and cardiovascular disease?
   (A) Several: increased body mass (overweight/obesity), reduced physical activity, dyslipidemia, hypertension, diabetes mellitus. The smoking association differs, but the effect of smoking in "reducing" the risk of preeclampsia is not a straightforward association.
2. What are the mechanisms for the associations between hypertensive disorders of pregnancy and long-term maternal cardiovascular disease?
   (A) They are likely heterogeneous and complex, but hypertension is common after hypertensive disorders of pregnancy and will contribute to further organ damage and cardiovascular disease.
3. Are there any prophylactic pharmacological therapies that could reduce the risk for cardiovascular disease in women after hypertensive disorders of pregnancy?
   (A) Possibly, but none that are clinically documented today. Anti-inflammatory drugs (such as statins and metformin) have been suggested, but not tested in trials.

References

1. Magee LA, Brown MA, Hall DR, Gupte S, Hennessy A, Karumanchi SA, et al. The 2021 International Society for the Study of hypertension in pregnancy classification, diagnosis & management recommendations for international practice. Pregnancy Hypertens. 2022;27:148–69.
2. Roberts JM, Redman CWG. Preeclampsia - more than pregnancy-induced hypertension. Lancet. 1993;341(8858):1447–51.
3. Staff AC. The two-stage placental model of preeclampsia: an update. J Reprod Immunol. 2019;134-135:1–10.
4. Chappell LC, Cluver CA, Kingdom J, Tong S. Pre-eclampsia. Lancet. 2021;398(10297):341–54.
5. Dimitriadis E, Rolnik DL, Zhou W, Estrada-Gutierrez G, Koga K, Francisco RPV, et al. Pre-eclampsia. Nat Rev Dis Primers. 2023;9(1):8.
6. Mol BW, Roberts CT, Thangaratinam S, Magee LA, de Groot CJ, Hofmeyr GJ. Pre-eclampsia. Lancet. 2015;387:999–1011.
7. Poon LC, Shennan A, Hyett JA, Kapur A, Hadar E, Divakar H, et al. The International Federation of Gynecology and Obstetrics (FIGO) initiative on pre-eclampsia: a pragmatic guide for first-trimester screening and prevention. Int J Gynaecol Obstet. 2019;145(Suppl 1):1–33.
8. Staff AC, Redman C. The differences between early- and late-onset preeclampsia. In: Saito S, editor. Preeclampsia. Singapore: Springer; 2018. p. 157–72.
9. Xiong X, Demianczuk NN, Saunders LD, Wang FL, Fraser WD. Impact of preeclampsia and gestational hypertension on birth weight by gestational age. Am J Epidemiol. 2002;155(3):203–9.
10. Redman CW. Current topic: pre-eclampsia and the placenta. Placenta. 1991;12(4):301–8.
11. Redman CW, Sargent IL, Staff AC. IFPA Senior Award Lecture: making sense of pre-eclampsia - two placental causes of preeclampsia? Placenta. 2014;35(Suppl):S20–5.
12. Redman CWG, Staff AC, Roberts JM. Syncytiotrophoblast stress in preeclampsia: the convergence point for multiple pathways. Am J Obstet Gynecol. 2022;226(2s):S907–s27.
13. Redman CW, Staff AC. Preeclampsia, biomarkers, syncytiotrophoblast stress, and placental capacity. Am J Obstet Gynecol. 2015;213(4):9–4.
14. Karumanchi SA. Angiogenic factors in preeclampsia: from diagnosis to therapy. Hypertension. 2016;67(6):1072–9.
15. Awoyemi T, Cerdeira AS, Zhang W, Jiang S, Rahbar M, Logenthiran P, et al. Preeclampsia and syncytiotrophoblast membrane extracellular vesicles (STB-EVs). Clin Sci. 2022;136(24):1793–807.
16. Sole KB, Staff AC, Laine K. The association of maternal country of birth and education with hypertensive disorders of pregnancy: a population-based study of 960 516 deliveries in Norway. Acta Obstet Gynecol Scand. 2018;97(10):1237–47.
17. Hiby SE, Walker JJ, O'Shaughnessy KM, Redman CW, Carrington M, Trowsdale J, et al. Combinations of maternal KIR and fetal HLA-C genes influence the risk of preeclampsia and reproductive success. J Exp Med. 2004;200(8):957–65.
18. Jeyabalan A, Powers RW, Clifton RG, Van DP, Hauth JC, Klebanoff MA, et al. Effect of smoking on circulating angiogenic factors in high risk pregnancies. PLoS ONE. 2010;5(10):e13270.
19. Wikström AK, Stephansson O, Cnattingius S. Tobacco use during pregnancy and preeclamp-

sia risk: effects of cigarette smoking and snuff. Hypertension. 2010;55(5):1254–9.
20. Cudmore M, Ahmad S, Al-Ani B, Fujisawa T, Coxall H, Chudasama K, et al. Negative regulation of soluble Flt-1 and soluble endoglin release by heme oxygenase-1. Circulation. 2007;115(13):1789–97.
21. Jeyabalan A, Powers RW, Durica AR, Harger GF, Roberts JM, Ness RB. Cigarette smoke exposure and angiogenic factors in pregnancy and preeclampsia. Am J Hypertens. 2008;21(8):943–7.
22. Melchiorre K, Giorgione V, Thilaganathan B. The placenta and preeclampsia: villain or victim? Am J Obstet Gynecol. 2022;226(2s):S954–s62.
23. Rolnik DL, Wright D, Poon LC, O'Gorman N, Syngelaki A, de Paco Matallana C, et al. Aspirin versus placebo in pregnancies at high risk for preterm preeclampsia. N Engl J Med. 2017;377(7):613–22.
24. Rolnik DL, Nicolaides KH, Poon LC. Prevention of preeclampsia with aspirin. Am J Obstet Gynecol. 2022;226(2):1108–19.
25. Li X, Milosavljevic A, Elsea SH, Wang CC, Scaglia F, Syngelaki A, et al. Effective aspirin treatment of women at risk for preeclampsia delays the metabolic clock of gestation. Hypertension. 2021;78(5):1398–410.
26. Robson SC, Hunter S, Boys RJ, Dunlop W. Serial study of factors influencing changes in cardiac output during human pregnancy. Am J Phys. 1989;256(4 Pt 2):H1060–5.
27. Shroff SG, Hauspurg A, Hibbard JU, Conrad KP. Cardiovascular alterations in normal and preeclamptic pregnancy. In: Taylor RN, Davidge SD, Staff AC, Roberts JM, editors. Chesley's hypertensive disorders of pregnancy. 5th ed. London: Elsevier; 2022.
28. Staff AC, Fjeldstad HE, Fosheim IK, Moe K, Turowski G, Johnsen GM, et al. Failure of physiological transformation and spiral artery atherosis: their roles in preeclampsia. Am J Obstet Gynecol. 2020. https://doi.org/10.1016/j.ajog.2020.09.026.
29. Melchiorre K, Sutherland GR, Liberati M, Thilaganathan B. Preeclampsia is associated with persistent postpartum cardiovascular impairment. Hypertension. 2011;58(4):709–15.
30. Melchiorre K, Sutherland GR, Watt-Coote I, Liberati M, Thilaganathan B. Severe myocardial impairment and chamber dysfunction in preterm preeclampsia. Hypertens Pregnancy. 2012;31(4):454–71.
31. Sciatti E, Orabona R. A window of opportunity on cardiovascular prevention: pre-eclampsia and fetal growth restriction. Eur J Prev Cardiol. 2022;28(16):e17–e8.
32. Orabona R, Mohseni Z, Sciatti E, Mulder EG, Prefumo F, Lorusso R, et al. Maternal myocardial dysfunction after normotensive fetal growth restriction compared with hypertensive pregnancies: a speckle-tracking study. J Hypertens. 2020;38(10):1955–63.
33. Chesley LC, Annitto JE, Cosgrove RA. The remote prognosis of eclamptic women. Sixth periodic report. Am J Obstet Gynecol. 1976;124(5):446–59.
34. Mann JI, Doll R, Thorogood M, Vessey MP, Waters WE. Risk factors for myocardial infarction in young women. Br J Prev Soc Med. 1976;30(2):94–100.
35. Irgens HU, Reisaeter L, Irgens LM, Lie RT. Long term mortality of mothers and fathers after preeclampsia: population based cohort study. BMJ. 2001;323(7323):1213–7.
36. Smith GC, Pell JP, Walsh D. Pregnancy complications and maternal risk of ischaemic heart disease: a retrospective cohort study of 129,290 births. Lancet. 2001;357(9273):2002–6.
37. Lykke JA, Langhoff-Roos J, Sibai BM, Funai EF, Triche EW, Paidas MJ. Hypertensive pregnancy disorders and subsequent cardiovascular morbidity and type 2 diabetes mellitus in the mother. Hypertension. 2009;53(6):944–51.
38. Wikstrom AK, Haglund B, Olovsson M, Lindeberg SN. The risk of maternal ischaemic heart disease after gestational hypertensive disease. BJOG. 2005;112(11):1486–91.
39. Bellamy L, Casas JP, Hingorani AD, Williams DJ. Pre-eclampsia and risk of cardiovascular disease and cancer in later life: systematic review and meta-analysis. BMJ. 2007;335(7627):974.
40. Sattar N, Greer IA. Pregnancy complications and maternal cardiovascular risk: opportunities for intervention and screening? BMJ. 2002;325(7356):157–60.
41. Rich-Edwards JW. Reproductive health as a sentinel of chronic disease in women. Womens Health. 2009;5(2):101–5.
42. Roberts JM, Hubel CA. Pregnancy: a screening test for later life cardiovascular disease. Womens Health Issues. 2010;20(5):304–7.
43. Staff AC, Redman CW, Williams D, Leeson P, Moe K, Thilaganathan B, et al. Pregnancy and long-term maternal cardiovascular health: progress through harmonization of research cohorts and biobanks. Hypertension. 2016;67(2):251–60.
44. Leon LJ, McCarthy FP, Direk K, Gonzalez-Izquierdo A, Prieto-Merino D, Casas JP, et al. Preeclampsia and cardiovascular disease in a large UK pregnancy cohort of linked electronic health records: a CALIBER study. Circulation. 2019;140(13):1050–60.
45. Scifres CM, Parks WT, Feghali M, Caritis SN, Catov JM. Placental maternal vascular malperfusion and adverse pregnancy outcomes in gestational diabetes mellitus. Placenta. 2017;49:10–5.
46. Riise HK, Sulo G, Tell GS, Igland J, Nygard O, Vollset SE, et al. Incident coronary heart disease after preeclampsia: role of reduced fetal growth, preterm delivery, and parity. J Am Heart Assoc. 2017;6(3):e004158.
47. Auger N, Fraser WD, Schnitzer M, Leduc L, Healy-Profitos J, Paradis G. Recurrent pre-eclampsia and subsequent cardiovascular risk. Heart. 2017;103(3):235–43.
48. Brouwers L, van der Meiden-van Roest AJ, Savelkoul C, Vogelvang TE, Lely AT, Franx A, et al. Recurrence of pre-eclampsia and the risk of future hypertension

and cardiovascular disease: a systematic review and meta-analysis. BJOG. 2018;125(13):1642–54.
49. Wu P, Haththotuwa R, Kwok CS, Babu A, Kotronias RA, Rushton C, et al. Preeclampsia and future cardiovascular health: a systematic review and meta-analysis. Circ Cardiovasc Qual Outcomes. 2017;10(2):e003497.
50. Riise HKR, Sulo G, Tell GS, Igland J, Egeland G, Nygard O, et al. Hypertensive pregnancy disorders increase the risk of maternal cardiovascular disease after adjustment for cardiovascular risk factors. Int J Cardiol. 2019;282:81–7.
51. Ray JG, Vermeulen MJ, Schull MJ, Redelmeier DA. Cardiovascular health after maternal placental syndromes (CHAMPS): population-based retrospective cohort study. Lancet. 2005;366(9499):1797–803.
52. Veerbeek JH, Hermes W, Breimer AY, van Rijn BB, Koenen SV, Mol BW, et al. Cardiovascular disease risk factors after early-onset preeclampsia, late-onset preeclampsia, and pregnancy-induced hypertension. Hypertension. 2015;65(3):600–6.
53. Simon E, Bechraoui-Quantin S, Tapia S, Cottenet J, Mariet AS, Cottin Y, et al. Time to onset of cardiovascular and cerebrovascular outcomes after hypertensive disorders of pregnancy: a nationwide, population-based retrospective cohort study. Am J Obstet Gynecol. 2023;229(3):296.
54. Robbins CL, Hutchings Y, Dietz PM, Kuklina EV, Callaghan WM. History of preterm birth and subsequent cardiovascular disease: a systematic review. Am J Obstet Gynecol. 2014;210(4):285–97.
55. Brown MC, Best KE, Pearce MS, Waugh J, Robson SC, Bell R. Cardiovascular disease risk in women with pre-eclampsia: systematic review and meta-analysis. Eur J Epidemiol. 2013;28(1):1–19.
56. Heida KY, Velthuis BK, Oudijk MA, Reitsma JB, Bots ML, Franx A, et al. Cardiovascular disease risk in women with a history of spontaneous preterm delivery: a systematic review and meta-analysis. Eur J Prev Cardiol. 2016;23(3):253–63.
57. Chappell LC, Brocklehurst P, Green ME, Hunter R, Hardy P, Juszczak E, et al. Planned early delivery or expectant management for late preterm preeclampsia (PHOENIX): a randomised controlled trial. Lancet. 2019;394(10204):1181–90.
58. McCarthy FP, O'Driscoll J, Seed P, Brockbank A, Cox A, Gill C, et al. Efficacy and mechanism evaluation. In: Planned delivery to improve postpartum cardiac function in women with preterm pre-eclampsia: the PHOEBE mechanisms of action study within the PHOENIX RCT. Southampton: NIHR Journals Library; 2021.
59. Moe K, Sugulle M, Dechend R, Staff AC. Risk prediction of maternal cardiovascular disease one year after hypertensive pregnancy complications or gestational diabetes mellitus. Eur J Prev Cardiol. 2020;27(12):1273–83.
60. Behrens I, Basit S, Melbye M, Lykke JA, Wohlfahrt J, Bundgaard H, et al. Risk of post-pregnancy hypertension in women with a history of hypertensive disorders of pregnancy: nationwide cohort study. BMJ. 2017;358:j3078.
61. Egeland GM, Skurtveit S, Staff AC, Eide GE, Daltveit AK, Klungsoyr K, et al. Pregnancy-related risk factors are associated with a significant burden of treated hypertension within 10 years of delivery: findings from a population-based Norwegian cohort. J Am Heart Assoc. 2018;7(10):e008318.
62. Sederholm Lawesson S, Swahn E, Pihlsgård M, Andersson T, Angerås O, Bacsovics Brolin E, et al. Association between history of adverse pregnancy outcomes and coronary artery disease assessed by coronary computed tomography angiography. JAMA. 2023;329(5):393–404.
63. Honigberg MC, Zekavat SM, Raghu VK, Natarajan P. Microvascular outcomes in women with a history of hypertension in pregnancy. Circulation. 2022;145(7):552–4.
64. Barr LC, Pudwell J, Smith GN. Postpartum microvascular functional alterations following severe preeclampsia. Am J Physiol Heart Circ Physiol. 2021;320(4):H1393–h402.
65. Boardman H, Lamata P, Lazdam M, Verburg A, Siepmann T, Upton R, et al. Variations in cardiovascular structure, function, and geometry in midlife associated with a history of hypertensive pregnancy. Hypertension. 2020;75(6):1542–50.
66. Honigberg MC. Understanding heart failure in women with preeclampsia: a call for prevention. J Am Coll Cardiol. 2021;78(23):2291–3.
67. Behrens I, Basit S, Lykke JA, Ranthe MF, Wohlfahrt J, Bundgaard H, et al. Association between hypertensive disorders of pregnancy and later risk of cardiomyopathy. JAMA. 2016;315(10):1026–33.
68. Honigberg MC, Zekavat SM, Aragam K, Klarin D, Bhatt DL, Scott NS, et al. Long-term cardiovascular risk in women with hypertension during pregnancy. J Am Coll Cardiol. 2019;74(22):2743–54.
69. Honigberg MC, Riise HKR, Daltveit AK, Tell GS, Sulo G, Igland J, et al. Heart failure in women with hypertensive disorders of pregnancy: insights from the cardiovascular disease in norway project. Hypertension. 2020;76(5):1506–13.
70. Malek AM, Wilson DA, Turan TN, Mateus J, Lackland DT, Hunt KJ. Incident heart failure within the first and fifth year after delivery among women with hypertensive disorders of pregnancy and prepregnancy hypertension in a diverse population. J Am Heart Assoc. 2021;10(17):e021616.
71. Zakeri R, Cowie MR. Heart failure with preserved ejection fraction: controversies, challenges and future directions. Heart. 2018;104(5):377–84.
72. Taqueti VR, Solomon SD, Shah AM, Desai AS, Groarke JD, Osborne MT, et al. Coronary microvascular dysfunction and future risk of heart failure with preserved ejection fraction. Eur Heart J. 2018;39(10):840–9.
73. Sciatti E, Orabona R. When preclinical data meet epidemiology: preeclampsia and future HFpEF. J Am Coll Cardiol. 2022;79(14):e241.

74. Zoet GA, Koster MP, Velthuis BK, de Groot CJ, Maas AH, Fauser BC, et al. Determinants of future cardiovascular health in women with a history of preeclampsia. Maturitas. 2015;82(2):153–61.
75. Williams D, Stout MJ, Rosenbloom JI, Olsen MA, Joynt Maddox KE, Deych E, et al. Preeclampsia predicts risk of hospitalization for heart failure with preserved ejection fraction. J Am Coll Cardiol. 2021;78(23):2281–90.
76. Kuć A, Kubik D, Kościelecka K, Szymanek W, Męcik-Kronenberg T. The relationship between peripartum cardiomyopathy and preeclampsia – pathogenesis, diagnosis and management. J Multidiscip Healthc. 2022;15:857–67.
77. Gammill HS, Chettier R, Brewer A, Roberts JM, Shree R, Tsigas E, et al. Cardiomyopathy and preeclampsia. Circulation. 2018;138(21):2359–66.
78. Vikse BE, Irgens LM, Leivestad T, Skjaerven R, Iversen BM. Preeclampsia and the risk of end-stage renal disease. N Engl J Med. 2008;359(8):800–9.
79. Barrett PM, McCarthy FP, Kublickiene K, Cormican S, Judge C, Evans M, et al. Adverse pregnancy outcomes and long-term maternal kidney disease: a systematic review and meta-analysis. JAMA Netw Open. 2020;3(2):e1920964.
80. Wu P, Kwok CS, Haththotuwa R, Kotronias RA, Babu A, Fryer AA, et al. Pre-eclampsia is associated with a twofold increase in diabetes: a systematic review and meta-analysis. Diabetologia. 2016;59(12):2518–26.
81. Zhao G, Bhatia D, Jung F, Lipscombe L. Risk of type 2 diabetes mellitus in women with prior hypertensive disorders of pregnancy: a systematic review and meta-analysis. Diabetologia. 2021;64(3):491–503.
82. Lykke JA, Langhoff-Roos J, Lockwood CJ, Triche EW, Paidas MJ. Mortality of mothers from cardiovascular and non-cardiovascular causes following pregnancy complications in first delivery. Paediatr Perinat Epidemiol. 2010;24(4):323–30.
83. Kessous R, Shoham-Vardi I, Pariente G, Sergienko R, Sheiner E. Long-term maternal atherosclerotic morbidity in women with pre-eclampsia. Heart. 2015;101(6):442–6.
84. Bryant AS, Seely EW, Cohen A, Lieberman E. Patterns of pregnancy-related hypertension in black and white women. Hypertens Pregnancy. 2005;24(3):281–90.
85. Fasanya HO, Hsiao CJ, Armstrong-Sylvester KR, Beal SG. A critical review on the use of race in understanding racial disparities in preeclampsia. J Appl Lab Med. 2021;6(1):247–56.
86. Suresh S, Amegashie C, Patel E, Nieman KM, Rana S. Racial disparities in diagnosis, management, and outcomes in preeclampsia. Curr Hypertens Rep. 2022;24(4):87–93.
87. Hinkle SN, Schisterman EF, Liu D, Pollack AZ, Yeung EH, Mumford SL, et al. Pregnancy complications and long-term mortality in a diverse cohort. Circulation. 2023;147(13):1014–25.
88. Malek AM, Wilson DA, Turan TN, Mateus J, Lackland DT, Hunt KJ. Maternal coronary heart disease, stroke, and mortality within 1, 3, and 5 years of delivery among women with hypertensive disorders of pregnancy and pre-pregnancy hypertension. J Am Heart Assoc. 2021;10(5):e018155.
89. Miller EC, Zambrano Espinoza MD, Huang Y, Friedman AM, Boehme AK, Bello NA, et al. Maternal race/ethnicity, hypertension, and risk for stroke during delivery admission. J Am Heart Assoc. 2020;9(3):e014775.
90. Stuart JJ, Tanz LJ, Missmer SA, Rimm EB, Spiegelman D, James-Todd TM, et al. Hypertensive disorders of pregnancy and maternal cardiovascular disease risk factor development: an observational cohort study. Ann Intern Med. 2018;169(4):224–32.
91. Jonsdottir LS, Arngrimsson R, Geirsson RT, Sigvaldason H, Sigfusson N. Death rates from ischemic heart disease in women with a history of hypertension in pregnancy. Acta Obstet Gynecol Scand. 1995;74(10):772–6.
92. Haug EB, Horn J, Markovitz AR, Fraser A, Klykken B, Dalen H, et al. Association of conventional cardiovascular risk factors with cardiovascular disease after hypertensive disorders of pregnancy: analysis of the nord-trondelag health study. JAMA Cardiol. 2019;4(7):628–35.
93. Ahmadi SF, Streja E, Zahmatkesh G, Streja D, Kashyap M, Moradi H, et al. Reverse epidemiology of traditional cardiovascular risk factors in the geriatric population. J Am Med Dir Assoc. 2015;16(11):933–9.
94. Staff AC, Figuero-Filho E, Davidge SD. Long-term effects of preeclampsia on mothers and offsrpings. In: Taylor RN, Davidge SD, Staff AC, Roberts JM, editors. Chesley's hypertensive disorders of pregnancy. 5th ed. London: Elsevier; 2022.
95. Romundstad PR, Magnussen EB, Smith GD, Vatten LJ. Hypertension in pregnancy and later cardiovascular risk: common antecedents? Circulation. 2010;122(6):579–84.
96. Magnussen EB, Vatten LJ, Lund-Nilsen TI, Salvesen KA, Davey SG, Romundstad PR. Prepregnancy cardiovascular risk factors as predictors of preeclampsia: population based cohort study. BMJ. 2007;335(7627):978.
97. Magnussen EB, Vatten LJ, Smith GD, Romundstad PR. Hypertensive disorders in pregnancy and subsequently measured cardiovascular risk factors. Obstet Gynecol. 2009;114(5):961–70.
98. Hubel CA, Wallukat G, Wolf M, Herse F, Rajakumar A, Roberts JM, et al. Agonistic angiotensin II type 1 receptor autoantibodies in postpartum women with a history of preeclampsia. Hypertension. 2007;49(3):612–7.
99. Herse F, Dechend R, Harsem NK, Wallukat G, Janke J, Qadri F, et al. Dysregulation of the circulating and tissue-based renin-angiotensin system in preeclampsia. Hypertension. 2007;49(3):604–11.

100. Staff AC, Dechend R, Redman CW. Review: Preeclampsia, acute atherosis of the spiral arteries and future cardiovascular disease: two new hypotheses. Placenta. 2013;34(Suppl):S73–S8.
101. Alexander BT, South AM, August P, Bertagnolli M, Ferranti EP, Grobe JL, et al. Appraising the preclinical evidence of the role of the renin-angiotensin-aldosterone system in antenatal programming of maternal and offspring cardiovascular health across the life course: moving the field forward: a scientific statement from the American Heart Association. Hypertension. 2023;80(5):e75–89.
102. Cipolla MJ, Liebeskind DS, Chan SL. The importance of comorbidities in ischemic stroke: impact of hypertension on the cerebral circulation. J Cereb Blood Flow Metab. 2018;38(12):2129–49.
103. Rosenbloom JI, Lewkowitz AK, Lindley KJ, Nelson DM, Macones GA, Cahill AG, et al. Expectant management of hypertensive disorders of pregnancy and future cardiovascular morbidity. Obstet Gynecol. 2020;135(1):27–35.
104. Rosenbloom JI, Stwalley D, Lindley KJ, Michael Nelson D, Olsen MA, Stout MJ. Latency of preterm hypertensive disorders of pregnancy and subsequent cardiovascular complications. Pregnancy Hypertens. 2020;21:139–44.
105. Staff AC. Long-term cardiovascular health after stopping pre-eclampsia. Lancet. 2019;394(10204):1120–1.
106. Lindley KJ, Williams D, Davila-Roman VG. Reply: When preclinical data meet epidemiology: pre-eclampsia and future HFpEF. J Am Coll Cardiol. 2022;79(14):e243.
107. Giorgione V, Cauldwell M, Thilaganathan B. Pre-eclampsia and cardiovascular disease: from pregnancy to postpartum. Eur Cardiol. 2023;18:e42.
108. Lew J, Sanghavi M, Ayers CR, McGuire DK, Omland T, Atzler D, et al. Sex-based differences in cardiometabolic biomarkers. Circulation. 2017;135(6):544–55.
109. Gerdts E, Regitz-Zagrosek V. Sex differences in cardiometabolic disorders. Nat Med. 2019;25(11):1657–66.
110. Tromp J, MacDonald MR, Tay WT, Teng TK, Hung CL, Narasimhan C, et al. Heart failure with preserved ejection fraction in the young. Circulation. 2018;138(24):2763–73.
111. Arechvo A, Voicu D, Gil MM, Syngelaki A, Akolekar R, Nicolaides KH. Maternal race and pre-eclampsia: cohort study and systematic review with meta-analysis. BJOG. 2022;129(12):2082–93.
112. Khosla K, Heimberger S, Nieman KM, Tung A, Shahul S, Staff AC, et al. Long-term cardiovascular disease risk in women after hypertensive disorders of pregnancy: recent advances in hypertension. Hypertension. 2021;78(4):927–35.
113. Minhas AS, Ogunwole SM, Vaught AJ, Wu P, Mamas MA, Gulati M, et al. Racial disparities in cardiovascular complications with pregnancy-induced hypertension in the United States. Hypertension. 2021;78(2):480–8.
114. Mosca L, Benjamin EJ, Berra K, Bezanson JL, Dolor RJ, Lloyd-Jones DM, et al. Effectiveness-based guidelines for the prevention of cardiovascular disease in women–2011 update: a guideline from the american heart association. Circulation. 2011;123(11):1243–62.
115. Thakkar A, Hailu T, Blumenthal RS, Martin SS, Harrington CM, Yeh DD, et al. Cardio-obstetrics: the next frontier in cardiovascular disease prevention. Curr Atheroscler Rep. 2022;24(7):493–507.
116. Verghese D, Muller L, Velamakanni S. Addressing cardiovascular risk across the arc of a woman's life: sex-specific prevention and treatment. Curr Cardiol Rep. 2023;25(9):1053–64.
117. Maas A, Rosano G, Cifkova R, Chieffo A, van Dijken D, Hamoda H, et al. Cardiovascular health after menopause transition, pregnancy disorders, and other gynaecologic conditions: a consensus document from European cardiologists, gynaecologists, and endocrinologists. Eur Heart J. 2021;42(10):967–84.
118. Blumer V, Pagidipati NJ. Hypertensive disorders of pregnancy and long-term heart failure risk: a missed opportunity for prevention. Hypertension. 2020;76(5):1420–2.
119. Brown HL, Warner JJ, Gianos E, Gulati M, Hill AJ, Hollier LM, et al. Promoting risk identification and reduction of cardiovascular disease in women through collaboration with obstetricians and gynecologists: a presidential advisory from the American Heart Association and the American College of Obstetricians and Gynecologists. Circulation. 2018;137(24):e843–e52.
120. Khan SS, Brewer LC, Canobbio MM, Cipolla MJ, Grobman WA, Lewey J, et al. Optimizing prepregnancy cardiovascular health to improve outcomes in pregnant and postpartum individuals and offspring: a scientific statement from the American Heart Association. Circulation. 2023;147(7):e76–91.
121. Sharashova E, Gerdts E, Ball J, Espnes H, Jacobsen BK, Kildal S, et al. Sex-specific time trends in incident atrial fibrillation and the contribution of risk factors: the Tromsø Study 1994-2016. Eur J Prev Cardiol. 2023;30(1):72–81.
122. Visseren FLJ, Mach F, Smulders YM, Carballo D, Koskinas KC, Bäck M, et al. 2021 ESC guidelines on cardiovascular disease prevention in clinical practice. Eur Heart J. 2021;42(34):3227–337.
123. Ji H, Kim A, Ebinger JE, Niiranen TJ, Claggett BL, Bairey Merz CN, et al. Sex differences in blood pressure trajectories over the life course. JAMA Cardiol. 2020;5(3):19–26.
124. Ji H, Niiranen TJ, Rader F, Henglin M, Kim A, Ebinger JE, et al. Sex differences in blood pressure associations with cardiovascular outcomes. Circulation. 2021;143(7):761–3.
125. Young B, Hacker MR, Rana S. Physicians' knowledge of future vascular disease in women with pre-eclampsia. Hypertens Pregnancy. 2012;31(1):50–8.
126. Wilkins-Haug L, Celi A, Thomas A, Frolkis J, Seely EW. Recognition by women's health care providers

of long-term cardiovascular disease risk after preeclampsia. Obstet Gynecol. 2015;125(6):1287–92.
127. Seely EW, Rich-Edwards J, Lui J, Nicklas JM, Saxena A, Tsigas E, et al. Risk of future cardiovascular disease in women with prior preeclampsia: a focus group study. BMC Pregnancy Childbirth. 2013;13:240.
128. Skurnik G, Roche AT, Stuart JJ, Rich-Edwards J, Tsigas E, Levkoff SE, et al. Improving the postpartum care of women with a recent history of preeclampsia: a focus group study. Hypertens Pregnancy. 2016;35(3):371–81.
129. Hauspurg A, Seely EW, Rich-Edwards J, Hayduchok C, Bryan S, Roche AT, et al. Postpartum home blood pressure monitoring and lifestyle intervention in overweight and obese individuals the first year after gestational hypertension or pre-eclampsia: a pilot feasibility trial. BJOG. 2023;130(7):715–26.
130. Rich-Edwards JW, Stuart JJ, Skurnik G, Roche AT, Tsigas E, Fitzmaurice GM, et al. Randomized trial to reduce cardiovascular risk in women with recent preeclampsia. J Women's Health. 2019;28(11):1493–504.
131. Horn J, Kolberg M, Rangul V, Magnussen EB, Åsvold BO, Henriksen HB, et al. Feasibility of a postpartum web- and phone-based lifestyle program for women with a history of preeclampsia or gestational diabetes: a pilot intervention study. Women's Health Rep. 2023;4(1):345–57.
132. Rossiter C, Henry A, Roberts L, Brown MA, Gow M, Arnott C, et al. Optimising mothers' health behaviour after hypertensive disorders of pregnancy: a qualitative study of a postnatal intervention. BMC Public Health. 2022;22(1):1259.
133. Celi AC, Seely EW, Wang P, Thomas AM, Wilkins-Haug LE. Caring for women after hypertensive pregnancies and beyond: implementation and integration of a postpartum transition clinic. Matern Child Health J. 2019;23(11):1459–66.
134. Stuart JJ, Tanz LJ, Cook NR, Spiegelman D, Missmer SA, Rimm EB, et al. Hypertensive disorders of pregnancy and 10-year cardiovascular risk prediction. J Am Coll Cardiol. 2018;72(11):1252–63.
135. Timpka S, Fraser A, Schyman T, Stuart JJ, Åsvold BO, Mogren I, et al. The value of pregnancy complication history for 10-year cardiovascular disease risk prediction in middle-aged women. Eur J Epidemiol. 2018;33(10):1003–10.
136. Markovitz AR, Stuart JJ, Horn J, Williams PL, Rimm EB, Missmer SA, et al. Does pregnancy complication history improve cardiovascular disease risk prediction? Findings from the HUNT study in Norway. Eur Heart J. 2019;40(14):1113–20.
137. Fraser A, Nelson SM, Macdonald-Wallis C, Cherry L, Butler E, Sattar N, et al. Associations of pregnancy complications with calculated cardiovascular disease risk and cardiovascular risk factors in middle age: the Avon Longitudinal Study of Parents and Children. Circulation. 2012;125(11):1367–80.
138. Weintraub WS, Daniels SR, Burke LE, Franklin BA, Goff DC Jr, Hayman LL, et al. Value of primordial and primary prevention for cardiovascular disease: a policy statement from the American Heart Association. Circulation. 2011;124(8):967–90.
139. Benschop L, Brouwers L, Zoet GA, Meun C, Boersma E, Budde RPJ, et al. Early onset of coronary artery calcification in women with previous preeclampsia. Circ Cardiovasc Imaging. 2020;13(11):e010340.
140. Giorgione V, Ridder A, Kalafat E, Khalil A, Thilaganathan B. Incidence of postpartum hypertension within 2 years of a pregnancy complicated by pre-eclampsia: a systematic review and meta-analysis. BJOG. 2021;128(3):495–503.
141. Excellence NIfHaC. Hypertension in pregnancy: the management of hypertensive disorders during pregnancy (clinical guideline 107). 2010. www.nice.org.uk/CG107.
142. Staff A, Kvie A, Langesaeter E, Michelsen TM, Moe K, Strand KM, et al. Hypertensive svangerskapskomplikasjoner og eklampsi. 2020. https://www.legeforeningen.no/foreningsledd/fagmed/norsk-gynekologisk-forening/veiledere/veileder-i-fodselshjelp/hypertensive-svangerskapskomplikasjoner-og-eklampsi/.
143. Sheiner E, Kapur A, Retnakaran R, Hadar E, Poon LC, McIntyre HD, et al. FIGO (International Federation of Gynecology and Obstetrics) postpregnancy initiative: long-term maternal implications of pregnancy complications-follow-up considerations. Int J Gynaecol Obstet. 2019;147(Suppl 1):1–31.
144. Arora S, Stouffer GA, Kucharska-Newton AM, Qamar A, Vaduganathan M, Pandey A, et al. Twenty year trends and sex differences in young adults hospitalized with acute myocardial infarction. Circulation. 2019;139(8):1047–56.
145. Jortveit J, Pripp AH, Langorgen J, Halvorsen S. Incidence, risk factors and outcome of young patients with myocardial infarction. Heart. 2020;106(18):1420–6.
146. Benschop L, Schalekamp-Timmermans S, Broere-Brown ZA, Roeters van Lennep JE, Jaddoe VWV, Roos-Hesselink JW, et al. Placental growth factor as an indicator of maternal cardiovascular risk after pregnancy. Circulation. 2019;139(14):1698–709.
147. Lenderink T, Heeschen C, Fichtlscherer S, Dimmeler S, Hamm CW, Zeiher AM, et al. Elevated placental growth factor levels are associated with adverse outcomes at four-year follow-up in patients with acute coronary syndromes. J Am Coll Cardiol. 2006;47(2):307–11.
148. Jacobsen DP, Røysland R, Strand H, Moe K, Sugulle M, Omland T, et al. Circulating cardiovascular biomarkers during and after preeclampsia: Crosstalk with placental function? Pregnancy Hypertens. 2022;30:103–9.
149. Sugulle M, Dechend R, Herse F, Weedon-Fekjaer MS, Johnsen GM, Brosnihan KB, et al. Circulating and placental growth-differentiation factor 15 in pre-

eclampsia and in pregnancy complicated by diabetes mellitus. Hypertension. 2009;54(1):106–12.

150. Staff AC, Dechend R, Pijnenborg R. Learning from the placenta: acute atherosis and vascular remodeling in preeclampsia-novel aspects for atherosclerosis and future cardiovascular health. Hypertension. 2010;56(6):1026–34.
151. Pitz Jacobsen D, Fjeldstad HE, Johnsen GM, Fosheim IK, Moe K, Alnæs-Katjavivi P, et al. Acute atherosis lesions at the fetal-maternal border: current knowledge and implications for maternal cardiovascular health. Front Immunol. 2021;12:791606.
152. Staff AC, Johnsen GM, Dechend R, Redman CW. Preeclampsia and uteroplacental acute atherosis: immune and inflammatory factors. J Reprod Immunol. 2014;101:120–6.
153. Lekva T, Sugulle M, Moe K, Redman C, Dechend R, Staff AC. Multiplex analysis of circulating maternal cardiovascular biomarkers comparing preeclampsia subtypes. Hypertension. 2020;75(6):1513–22.
154. Moe K, Alnaes-Katjavivi P, Storvold GL, Sugulle M, Johnsen GM, Redman CWG, et al. Classical cardiovascular risk markers in pregnancy and associations to uteroplacental acute atherosis. Hypertension. 2018;72(3):695–702.
155. Stevens DU, Al-Nasiry S, Fajta MM, Bulten J, van Dijk AP, van der Vlugt MJ, et al. Cardiovascular and thrombogenic risk of decidual vasculopathy in preeclampsia. Am J Obstet Gynecol. 2014;210(6):545–6.
156. Naseem H, Dreixler J, Mueller A, Tung A, Dhir R, Chibber R, et al. Antepartum aspirin administration reduces activin a and cardiac global longitudinal strain in preeclamptic women. J Am Heart Assoc. 2020;9(12):e015997.
157. Ormesher L, Higson S, Luckie M, Roberts SA, Glossop H, Trafford A, et al. Postnatal enalapril to improve cardiovascular function following preterm Preeclampsia (PICk-UP): a randomised double-blind placebo-controlled feasibility trial. Hypertension. 2020;76(6):1828–37.
158. Benjamin EJ, Virani SS, Callaway CW, Chamberlain AM, Chang AR, Cheng S, et al. Heart disease and stroke statistics-2018 update: a report from the American Heart Association. Circulation. 2018;137(12):67–492.

Menopause and Cardiovascular Changes: A Unique Opportunity for Risk Assessment

Renata Cifkova and Angela H.E.M. Maas

Abstract

Menopause, defined as the permanent cessation of menstrual bleeding for 12 months, is associated with hormonal, cardiovascular and metabolic changes, starting about 2 years before the final menstrual period. Most women experience natural menopause at or around age 50. Natural menopause before age 40 is associated with an increased risk of cardiovascular disease. This is less clear for artificial early menopause, induced by bilateral ovarian surgery or chemotherapy. Weight gain around the menopause is closely related to aging, whereas the development of central obesity seems to be a direct result of the menopause. There is also an increase in endothelial dysfunction, which seems to be age related. The blood pressure increase around the menopause is probably more closely related to age and BMI than to ovarian failure. The changes in lipid profile include an increase in total cholesterol, LDL cholesterol, triglycerides, and a decrease in HDL cholesterol. Insulin resistance and the increase in the prevalence of metabolic syndrome are associated with menopause. Inflammatory co-morbidities often appear in women in their 40s, in association with the decline in estrogen levels. The years around menopause are crucial to initiate preventive measures if needed. The use of the CAC score can be very helpful to discriminate between low- and high-risk women.

Keywords

Obesity · Hypertension · Dyslipidemia · Menopause · Metabolic syndrome

R. Cifkova
First Faculty of Medicine, Center for Cardiovascular Prevention, Thomayer University Hospital, Charles University in Prague, Prague, Czech Republic

Department of Medicine II, First Faculty of Medicine, Charles University in Prague, Prague, Czech Republic
e-mail: renata.cifkova@ftn.cz

A. H.E.M. Maas (✉)
Department of Cardiology, route 616, Radboud University Medical Center, Nijmegen, The Netherlands
e-mail: angela.maas@radboudumc.nl

A. H.E.M. Maas, E. Gerdts (eds.), *Manual of Cardiovascular Disease in Women*,
https://doi.org/10.1007/978-3-031-65952-2_11

Test your learning and check your understanding of this book's contents: use the "Springer Nature Flashcards" app to access questions using ▶ https://sn.pub/51ny7m To use the app, please follow the instructions in chapter 1.

1 Introduction

Menopause is defined as the permanent cessation of menstrual bleeding for 12 months, in most cases resulting from the natural loss of ovarian follicular function. Thus, using this definition, it can be established only retrospectively. Another way of defining menopause is by a consistent elevation in follicular stimulation hormone (FSH) ≥ 30 mIU/mL. However, neither of these definitions is precise, as FSH might be elevated in women with regular menses and, on the other hand, there might be amenorrheic women with normal FSH. Perhaps the most accurate definition of menopause would be the permanent cessation of menstrual bleeding for 12 months accompanied by elevated FSH. Natural menopause is associated with changes in hormonal, inflammatory, cardiovascular, and metabolic factors beginning approximately 2 years before the final menstrual period (FMP). These last 2 years are known as menopausal transition. Menopause can also be artificially induced by bilateral ovarian surgery, such as in BRCA1,2 mutation carriers or caused by chemotherapy treatment. This leads to abrupt cardiometabolic changes and symptoms of estrogen depletion. In many women using oral contraceptives, having an intrauterine levonorgestrel device or after hysterectomy, the exact timing of menopause may be difficult to ascertain.

2 Age at (Natural) Menopause

The median age of natural menopause is 50 years [1]. About 10% of women experience a premature menopause before the age of 45, of which 5% have an early menopause between 40–45 years. Menopause before the age of 40, named as premature ovarian insufficiency (POI) occurs in 1% of women. Women with POI and early menopause were found to have increased risk of non-fatal CVD before 60 years of age [2]. The Korean nationwide cohort study showed that women experiencing menopause under the age of 50 had an increased risk of heart failure and atrial fibrillation compared to women having menopause after 50 [3]. Each year that menopause is delayed, a 2% lower CVD mortality risk is estimated [4]. A recent meta-analysis found that postmenopausal women with early menopause or POI had an increased risk of the development of type 2 diabetes [5]. Current smoking is linked to menopause occurring approximately 1 year earlier than in non-smokers [1, 6].

Natural menopause at a later age (>55 years) has been associated with a longer life expectancy, higher bone mineral density and a lower risk of bone fractures, and a lower total and CVD mortality [7, 8]. These advantages were slightly offset by a greater risk of breast cancer, particularly in obese women, and a greater risk of ovarian cancer [9–12]. Several studies have shown that higher parity was associated with menopause occurring at a later age [6, 7, 13–17]. An important confounding factor is that multiparity is also associated with a lower socio-economic status [18]. In addition, in the Nurses' Health Study it was found that that a bilateral ovariectomy after hysterectomy is associated with a two times higher risk for CVD, especially when performed before 50 years of age [19]. In the Women's Health Initiative (WHI-OS)

Observational Study this disadvantage was found to be importantly associated with a lower socioeconomic status (SES) and a more adverse CVD risk profile in women undergoing a hysterectomy [20]. Large population-based data from Sweden however confirmed a positive association between hysterectomy with/without oophorectomy and CVD in women below 50 years, but not at older age [21]. Age at onset of natural menopause is (partly) heritable with a link to DNA repair and immune mediator pathways [22].

Evidence is currently mounting that early artificial menopause (<45 years), such as caused by a preventive risk reducing salpingo-oophorectomy (RRSO) in women at high risk for breast and ovarian cancer ($BRCA_{1,2}$ mutation carriers) does not lead to an increased CVD risk [19, 23–25]. This is in contrast with early *natural* menopause that seems to be the result of accelerated vascular ageing, explaining its association with an increased CVD risk [26]. There are inconsistent data regarding physical activity and later age at natural menopause [7, 14–16]. A systematic review and meta-analysis found that low and moderate alcohol consumption might be associated with a later onset of menopause [27].

3 Cardiometabolic Changes at Menopause

3.1 Weight Gain

Weight gain around the menopause affects many women. Multiple studies have shown that menopausal transition is not only associated with an increase in BMI, but also with unfavorable changes in body composition, especially with abdominal fat deposition [28]. It has been shown that weight gain in perimenopausal years is closely related to ageing and it does not seem to be affected by the hormonal changes per se. Several studies found a steady weight increase of approximately 0.5 kg per year [29, 30]. Abdominal fat is considered an endocrine organ, secreting adipokines and other substances closely related to insulin resistance and the development of type 2 diabetes and the metabolic syndrome [28, 31]. Increased waist circumference, an indicator of excessive central abdominal fat accumulation, and low serum sex hormone binding globulin (SHBG) are independent predictors of metabolic risk in postmenopausal women. Therefore, central obesity seems to be a direct result of the menopause transition. Dietary weight loss and exercise are the foundation for overweight and obesity treatment in perimenopausal women. Metformin induces a slight weight loss of 1–2 kg over a 1-year period. New anti-diabetic drugs such as glucagon-like peptide-1 receptor agonists (GLP-1RA) are now successfully used for weight reduction also in patients without diabetes [32].

Menopause has been found to be associated with a higher proportion of epicardial and paracardial adipose tissue alike, which are newly emerging risk factors for ischemic heart disease (IHD) [33].

3.2 Blood Pressure

Sex hormonal changes associated with menopause include a decrease in estradiol, an increase in testosterone, and a decrease in the estrogen to testosterone (E/T) ratio. The consequence is the induction of endothelial dysfunction. At the same time, there is also an increase in sympathetic activation, which possibly results in increased renin and angiotensin II release [34–36]. Endothelial dysfunction is associated with a reduction in NO and rise in endothelin, leading to increased oxidative stress. These combined mechanisms induce renal vasoconstriction contributing to the development of hypertension (Fig. 1). The rise in blood pressure around menopause is due to progressive vascular stiffening, but also related to these hormonal changes [36–38]. Higher systolic blood pressure with ageing has a steeper course in women compared to men [39, 40]. Women with normal blood pressure also experience endothelial dysfunction, which seems to be age-related [41]. It is generally assumed that the increase in blood pressure around the menopause is more closely related to ageing and BMI than to ovarian estrogen depletion.

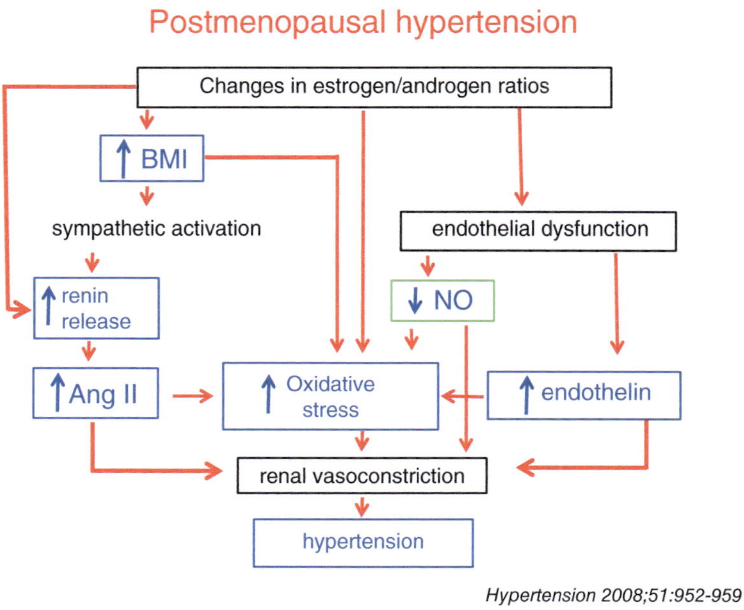

Fig. 1 Postmenopausal hypertension

There are several studies suggesting that women with persistent vasomotor symptoms have higher blood pressures and CVD risk [10, 42–44]. Other frequently reported non-specific symptoms are palpitations, headaches, chest pain, pain between the shoulder blades, tiredness and sleeping disturbances, which are often attributed to menopause [45, 46] (Table 1). Sodium sensitivity increases during menopausal transition, frequently leading to intermittent fluid retention resulting in edema of the legs, hands and/or lower eyelids [47–49]. Many of these symptoms can be, at least partly, managed by treating elevated blood pressure when present. There is currently no evidence to recommend menopausal hormone therapy (MHT) for the prevention or treatment of hypertension. Following the recent ESH guidelines, antihypertensive drug treatment should be initiated in women with insufficient response to lifestyle changes with blood pressure remaining ≥140/90 mmHg. As women have more end-organ damage with comparable blood pressure as men, it is currently discussed whether their thresholds of normal blood pressure should be lower [40].

Table 1 Frequently reported non-specific symptoms in middle-aged women with elevated blood pressure

• Tight, nagging and often continuous chest pain at rest
• Radiating pain to the jaws, left arm, shoulder blades
• Stress-related chest pain, with or without radiation
• Dyspnea at physical exercise (stairs, climbing, hurrying)
• Lack of physical condition, tiredness, lack of energy, exhaustion
• Hot flushes, severe sweating (day and night)
• Headaches, concentration disturbances, dizziness
• Palpitations at rest, paroxysmal supraventricular tachycardia/atrial fibrillation
• Intermittent fluid retention (ankles, hands, eyes)
• Sleeping disorders, inability to lie/sleep on left side
• 'Bra feels too tight'

3.3 Blood Lipids

Important changes in lipid profile occur in menopause transition, including an increase in total cholesterol, LDL cholesterol, triglycerides, and a slight decrease in HDL cholesterol (mostly HDL_2) [5, 50]. A meta-analysis however showed no difference in HDL cholesterol in premenopausal and postmenopausal women [51]. Atherogenic changes in apolipoprotein concentrations and their ratios have been observed after the onset of menopause (increase in apoB and LDL cholesterol/apoB ratio) [50]. There is also an increase in apoA-I and apoA-II, but the ratios of HDL-C/apoA-I and HDL-C/apoA-II decreased indicating a lower cholesterol content in HDL particles. Dyslipidemia in post-menopausal woman is quite common. All women will qualify for lifestyle intervention with specific dietary advice. Drug treatment with statins should be prescribed to women at high or very high CV risk based on SCORE-2 charts. HRT is not recommended for the treatment of dyslipidemia.

3.4 Metabolic Syndrome

Despite the fact that menopause was not shown to be independently associated with increased blood pressure, insulin resistance and hyperglycemia, the prevalence of the metabolic syndrome increases with menopause beyond the effects of chronological aging. An increase in insulin resistance is regularly associated with menopause and is due to changes in adipose tissue such as hypertrophy of adipocytes in subcutaneous and visceral adipose tissue, and increased inflammation and fibrosis [52]. The fat redistribution in postmenopausal women may be due to the upregulation of adipose tissue, lipoprotein, lipase activity, and lower lipolysis, resulting from lower estrogen concentration. Some women may develop impaired glucose tolerance, with the estimated annual incidence of 6% after menopause, independent of BMI, waist to hip ratio, blood pressure, family history of diabetes, age at menopause, and lipid profile [53]. Diabetes in women is associated with a greater risk of CVD mortality in women than in men [54, 55].

3.5 Sleep Disturbances

Poor quality of sleep occurs frequently in the years around the menopause and is found to be associated with an increased risk in the development of metabolic syndrome, carotid plaques, and increased carotid intima-media thickness [56–58]. Self-reported poor-quality sleep has been shown to be linked to a higher risk of aortic calcification in middle-aged women [58]. Shorter sleep duration, poor sleep quality, and greater severity of insomnia were found to be associated with worse AHA Life's Simple 7 scores [59]. Sleep disturbances may also be caused by perimenopausal vasomotor symptoms and the rise in blood pressure [45, 46].

4 Red Flags During the Life-Course of High-Risk Women

As women experience fewer CVD events at any given age, their absolute risks in all age-groups are lower than in men. This does not mean that all perimenopausal women are at low risk. The currently used SCORE2 charts that are used for risk estimation may underestimate true risk in women at middle-age [60]. When considering female-specific risk variables such as hypertensive pregnancies and early menopause as well as gynecologic conditions (PCOS, endometriosis) and inflammatory comorbidities during a woman's life-course, the combined impact of these risk variables is very important. Reproductive and pregnancy-related factors may predispose to earlier signs of endothelial dysfunction, vascular inflammation, and atherosclerosis. Thus far, there is no validated points score available to account for these separate risk variables. When looking at middle-aged women with established ischemic heart disease, a clustering of these risk variables

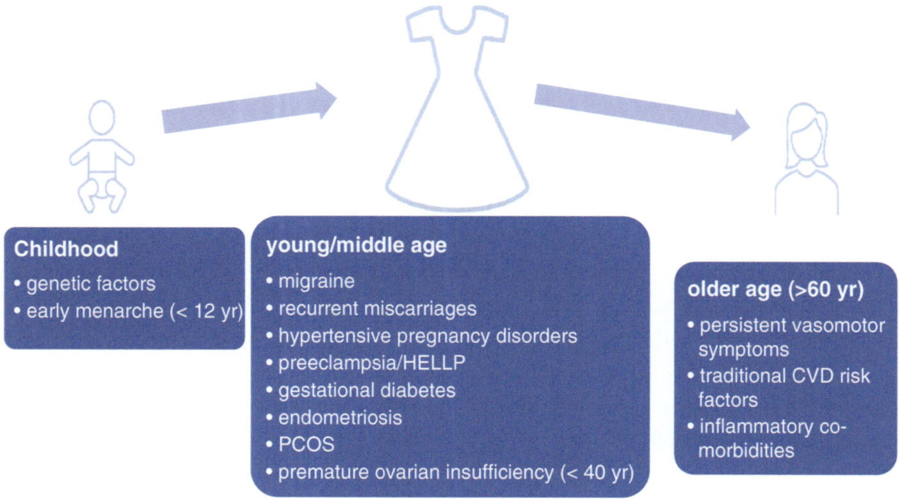

Fig. 2 Risk variables for cardiovascular disease risk in women along the life-course

and co-morbidities is often seen [61] (Fig. 2). These *precursors of individual risk or 'red flags'* become less significant at older age (>65), when the traditional CVD risk factors (lipids, blood pressure, insulin resistance) dominate.

5 Coronary Calcium Score to Tailor Individual Risk

Adding signs of subclinical atherosclerosis by using the coronary artery calcium (CAC) score with CT imaging to routine risk factor assessment significantly improves individual risk prediction and enables to identify high risk women that are overlooked in the commonly used SCORE2 charts [62]. The CAC score has an even higher predictive value in women compared to men [63]. It has been shown that women after preeclampsia have a two-fold elevated risk for a positive CAC score at the age of 50 compared to controls, whereas in women with premature ovarian insufficiency (POI) the presence of CAC was not elevated [64–66]. The additional use of the CAC score is now recommended in individuals at intermediate risk and when there is doubt whether to initiate preventive medication or not [67]. It can equally be done in women requiring menopausal hormone therapy for disabling vasomotor symptoms when there is uncertainty about the individual's safety.

Key Issues

- Menopause is associated with hormonal, cardiovascular, and metabolic changes, starting about 2 years before the final menstrual period.
- The median age of natural menopause is 50 years. Natural menopause, but NOT surgical menopause, before the age of 45 and especially below age 40 is associated with an increased risk of CVD.
- Weight gain around the menopause is closely related to aging, whereas the development of central obesity seems to be a direct result of the menopause.
- The blood pressure increase around the menopause is probably more closely related to ageing, vascular stiffness, and BMI than to ovarian failure per se.
- Hypertension may mimic various perimenopausal symptoms. Advise to measure blood pressure before considering menopausal hormone therapy.
- Adverse changes in lipid profile with atherogenic changes in apolipoprotein concentrations and their ratios occur during menopause transition.
- Ascertain female-specific risk variables and inflammatory co-morbidities in middle-aged women and add a CAC score with CT imaging when there is doubt on individual risk.

Questions and Answers

1. An early *natural* menopause (<40 years) can be considered as a risk variable, whereas a *surgical* menopause at comparable age is not.
   (A) Correct
   (B) Not correct
   A is correct. Growing evidence confirms the theory that a natural menopause is due to an intrinsic higher CVD risk which, importantly, may be mediated by genetic factors.
2. Sophie is 57 years and has many vasomotor symptoms with a blood pressure 150/95 mmHg. What would be the first step in treatment?
   (A) Menopausal hormone therapy (MHT)
   (B) Combination MHT and medication for hypertension
   (C) Reassurance
   (D) Initiate treatment for hypertension
   D is correct. Take elevated blood pressure seriously and start treatment without delay.
3. Which of the following statements is incorrect?
   (A) Coronary calcium score (CAC) significantly improves risk prediction in women
   (B) CAC has a higher predictive value in men
   (C) Women with a history of preeclampsia have a substantially greater chance of having a positive CAC score than their counterparts without a prior preeclampsia
   (D) CAC is recommended in women at intermediate risk to help in the decision to initiate preventive medication
   B is correct. CAC has a higher predictive value in women.
4. SCORE-2 chart may underestimate the true CV risk in women at middle-age.
   (A) Correct
   (B) Not correct
   A is correct. Female-specific risk factors such as hypertensive disorders in pregnancy, early menopause, gynecologic disease (PCOS, endometriosis) and inflammatory diseases further increase the CV risk.

References

1. El Khoudary SR, Aggarwal B, Beckie TM, Hodis HN, Johnson AE, Langer RD, et al. Menopause transition and cardiovascular disease risk: implications for timing of early prevention: a scientific statement from the American Heart Association. Circulation. 2020;142(25):e506–e32.
2. Zhu D, Chung HF, Dobson AJ, Pandeya N, Giles GG, Bruinsma F, et al. Age at natural menopause and risk of incident cardiovascular disease: a pooled analysis of individual patient data. Lancet Public Health. 2019;4(11):e553–64.
3. Shin J, Han K, Jung JH, Park HJ, Kim W, Huh Y, et al. Age at menopause and risk of heart failure and atrial fibrillation: a nationwide cohort study. Eur Heart J. 2022;43(40):4148–57.
4. Atsma F, Bartelink ML, Grobbee DE, van der Schouw YT. Postmenopausal status and early menopause as independent risk factors for cardiovascular disease: a meta-analysis. Menopause. 2006;13(2):265–79.
5. Anagnostis P, Stevenson JC, Crook D, Johnston DG, Godsland IF. Effects of menopause, gender and age on lipids and high-density lipoprotein cholesterol subfractions. Maturitas. 2015;81(1):62–8.
6. Gold EB, Crawford SL, Avis NE, Crandall CJ, Matthews KA, Waetjen LE, et al. Factors related to age at natural menopause: longitudinal analyses from SWAN. Am J Epidemiol. 2013;178(1):70–83.
7. Gold EB. The timing of the age at which natural menopause occurs. Obstet Gynecol Clin North Am. 2011;38(3):425–40.
8. El Khoudari SR. Age at menopause onset and risk of cardiovascular disease around the world. Maturitas. 2020;141:33–8.
9. Ossewaarde ME, Bots ML, Verbeek AL, Peeters PH, van der Graaf Y, Grobbee DE, et al. Age at menopause, cause-specific mortality and total life expectancy. Epidemiology. 2005;16(4):556–62.
10. Muka T, Oliver-Williams C, Kunutsor S, Laven JS, Fauser BC, Chowdhury R, et al. Association of age at onset of menopause and time since onset of menopause with cardiovascular outcomes, intermediate vascular traits, and all-cause mortality: a systematic review and meta-analysis. JAMA Cardiol. 2016;1(7):767–76.
11. Monninkhof EM, van der Schouw YT, Peeters PH. Early age at menopause and breast cancer: are leaner women more protected? A prospective analysis of the Dutch DOM cohort. Breast Cancer Res Treat. 1999;55(3):285–91.
12. Franceschi S, Parazzini F, Negri E, Booth M, La Vecchia C, Beral V, et al. Pooled analysis of 3 European case-control studies of epithelial ovar-

ian cancer: III. Oral contraceptive use. Int J Cancer. 1991;49(1):61–5.
13. Henderson KD, Bernstein L, Henderson B, Kolonel L, Pike MC. Predictors of the timing of natural menopause in the multiethnic cohort study. Am J Epidemiol. 2008;167(11):1287–94.
14. Gold EB, Bromberger J, Crawford S, Samuels S, Greendale GA, Harlow SD, et al. Factors associated with age at natural menopause in a multiethnic sample of midlife women. Am J Epidemiol. 2001;153(9):865–74.
15. Bromberger JT, Matthews KA, Kuller LH, Wing RR, Meilahn EN, Plantinga P. Prospective study of the determinants of age at menopause. Am J Epidemiol. 1997;145(2):124–33.
16. Dorjgochoo T, Kallianpur A, Gao YT, Cai H, Yang G, Li H, et al. Dietary and lifestyle predictors of age at natural menopause and reproductive span in the Shanghai Women's health study. Menopause. 2008;15(5):924–33.
17. Mishra GD, Pandeya N, Dobson AJ, Chung HF, Anderson D, Kuh D, et al. Early menarche, nulliparity and the risk for premature and early natural menopause. Hum Reprod. 2017;32(3):679–86.
18. Huber S, Bookstein FL, Fieder M. Socioeconomic status, education, and reproduction in modern women: an evolutionary perspective. Am J Hum Biol. 2010;22(5):578–87.
19. Parker WH, Broder MS, Chang E, Feskanich D, Farquhar C, Liu Z, et al. Ovarian conservation at the time of hysterectomy and long-term health outcomes in the Nurses' health study. Obstet Gynecol. 2009;113(5):1027–37.
20. Howard BV, Kuller L, Langer R, Manson JE, Allen C, Assaf A, et al. Risk of cardiovascular disease by hysterectomy status, with and without oophorectomy: the Women's Health Initiative observational study. Circulation. 2005;111(12):1462–70.
21. Ingelsson E, Lundholm C, Johansson AL, Altman D. Hysterectomy and risk of cardiovascular disease: a population-based cohort study. Eur Heart J. 2011;32(6):745–50.
22. Stolk L, Perry JR, Chasman DI, He C, Mangino M, Sulem P, et al. Meta-analyses identify 13 loci associated with age at menopause and highlight DNA repair and immune pathways. Nat Genet. 2012;44(3):260–8.
23. Dam V, van der Schouw YT, Onland-Moret NC, Groenwold RHH, Peters SAE, Burgess S, et al. Association of menopausal characteristics and risk of coronary heart disease: a pan-European case-cohort analysis. Int J Epidemiol. 2019;48(4):1275–85.
24. Honigberg MC, Zekavat SM, Aragam K, Finneran P, Klarin D, Bhatt DL, et al. Association of premature natural and surgical menopause with incident cardiovascular disease. JAMA. 2019;322(24):2411–21.
25. Van Bommel MHD, de Jong MA, Steenbeek MP, Bots ML, van Westerop LLM, Hopman MTE, et al. No signs of subclinical atherosclerosis after risk-reducing salpingo-oophorectomy in BRCA1/2 mutation carriers. J Cardiol. 2021;77(6):570–5.
26. Kok HS, van Asselt KM, van der Schouw YT, van der Tweel I, Peeters PH, Wilson PW, et al. Heart disease risk determines menopausal age rather than the reverse. J Am Coll Cardiol. 2006;47(10):1976–83.
27. Taneri PE, Kiefte-de Jong JC, Bramer WM, Daan NM, Franco OH, Muka T. Association of alcohol consumption with the onset of natural menopause: a systematic review and meta-analysis. Hum Reprod Update. 2016;22(4):516–28.
28. Davis SR, Castelo-Branco C, Chedraui P, Lumsden MA, Nappi RE, Shah D, et al. Understanding weight gain at menopause. Climacteric. 2012;15(5):419–29.
29. Guthrie JR, Dennerstein L, Dudley EC. Weight gain and the menopause: a 5-year prospective study. Climacteric. 1999;2(3):205–11.
30. Wing RR, Matthews KA, Kuller LH, Meilahn EN, Plantinga PL. Weight gain at the time of menopause. Arch Intern Med. 1991;151(1):97–102.
31. Wajchenberg BL. Subcutaneous and visceral adipose tissue: their relation to the metabolic syndrome. Endocr Rev. 2000;21(6):697–738.
32. Updike WH, Pane O, Franks R, Saber F, Abdeen F, Balazy DD, et al. Is it time to expand glucagon-like peptide-1 receptor agonist use for weight loss in patients without diabetes? Drugs. 2021;81(8):881–93.
33. Prabakaran S, Schwartz A, Lundberg G. Cardiovascular risk in menopausal women and our evolving understanding of menopausal hormone therapy: risks, benefits, and current guidelines for use. Ther Adv Endocrinol Metab. 2021;12:20420188211013917.
34. Schunkert H, Danser AH, Hense HW, Derkx FH, Kurzinger S, Riegger GA. Effects of estrogen replacement therapy on the renin-angiotensin system in postmenopausal women. Circulation. 1997;95(1):39–45.
35. Yanes LL, Romero DG, Iliescu R, Zhang H, Davis D, Reckelhoff JF. Postmenopausal hypertension: role of the renin-angiotensin system. Hypertension. 2010;56(3):359–63.
36. Vongpatanasin W. Autonomic regulation of blood pressure in menopause. Semin Reprod Med. 2009;27(4):338–45.
37. Staessen JA, van der Heijden-Spek JJ, Safar ME, Den Hond E, Gasowski J, Fagard RH, et al. Menopause and the characteristics of the large arteries in a population study. J Hum Hypertens. 2001;15(8):511–8.
38. Reckelhoff JF, Fortepiani LA. Novel mechanisms responsible for postmenopausal hypertension. Hypertension. 2004;43(5):918–23.
39. Ji H, Kim A, Ebinger JE, Niiranen TJ, Claggett BL, Bairey Merz CN, Cheng S. Sex differences in blood pressure trajectories over the life course. JAMA Cardiol. 2020;5(3):19–26.
40. Gerdts E, Sudano I, Brouwers S, Borghi C, Bruno RM, Ceconi C, Cornelissen V, Diévart F, Ferrini M, Kahan T, Løchen ML, Maas AHEM, Mahfoud F, Mihailidou AS, Moholdt T, Parati G, de Simone G. Sex differences in arterial hypertension. Eur Heart J. 2022;43(46):4777–88.

41. Ghazi L, Bello NA. Hypertension in women across the lifespan. Curr Atheroscler Rep. 2021;23(8):43.
42. Van der Schouw YT, Grobbee DE. Menopausal complaints, oestrogens, and heart disease risk: an explanation for discrepant findings on the benefits of post-menopausal hormone therapy. Eur Heart J. 2005;26(14):1358–61.
43. Gast GC, Grobbee DE, Pop VJ, Keyzer JJ, Wijnands-van Gent CJ, Samsioe GN, Nilsson PM, van der Schouw YT. Menopausal complaints are associated with cardiovascular risk factors. Hypertension. 2008;51(6):1492–8.
44. Gast GC, Pop VJ, Samsioe GN, Grobbee DE, Nilsson PM, Keyzer JJ, Wijnands-van Gent CJ, van der Schouw YT. Vasomotor menopausal symptoms are associated with increased risk of coronary heart disease. Menopause. 2011;18(2):146–51.
45. Maas AHEM. Hormone therapy and cardiovascular disease: benefits and harms. Best Pract Res Clin Endocrinol Metab. 2021;35(6):101576.
46. Maas AHEM, Rosano G, Cifkova R, Chieffo A, van Dijken D, Hamoda H, Kunadian V, Laan E, Lambrinoudaki I, Maclaran K, Panay N, Stevenson JC, van Trotsenburg M, Collins P. Cardiovascular health after menopause transition, pregnancy disorders, and other gynaecologic conditions: a consensus document from European Cardiologists, Gynaecologists, and Endocrinologists. Eur Heart J. 2021;42(10):967–84.
47. Pechere-Bertschi A, Burnier M. Gonadal steroids, salt-sensitivity and renal function. Curr Opin Nephrol Hypertens. 2007;16(1):16–21.
48. Tominaga T, Suzuki H, Ogata Y, Matsukawa S, Saruta T. The role of sex hormones and sodium intake in postmenopausal hypertension. J Hum Hypertens. 1991;5(6):495–500.
49. Pechere-Bertschi A, Burnier M. Female sex hormones, salt, and blood pressure regulation. Am J Hypertens. 2004;17(10):994–1001.
50. Anagnostis P, Stevenson JC, Crook D, Johnston DG, Godsland IF. Effects of gender, age and menopausal status on serum apolipoprotein concentrations. Clin Endocrinol (Oxf). 2016;85(5):733–40.
51. Ambikairajah A, Walsh E, Cherbuin N. Lipid profile differences during menopause: a review with meta-analysis. Menopause. 2019;26(11):1327–33.
52. Anagnostis P, Goulis DG. Menopause and its cardiometabolic consequences: current perspectives. Curr Vasc Pharmacol. 2019;17(6):543–5.
53. Slopien R, Wender-Ozegowska E, Rogowicz-Frontczak A, Meczekalski B, Zozulinska-Ziolkiewicz D, Jaremek JD, et al. Menopause and diabetes: EMAS clinical guide. Maturitas. 2018;117:6–10.
54. Dong X, Cai R, Sun J, Huang R, Wang P, Sun H, et al. Diabetes as a risk factor for acute coronary syndrome in women compared with men: a meta-analysis, including 10 856 279 individuals and 106 703 acute coronary syndrome events. Diabetes Metab Res Rev. 2017;33(5).
55. Berga SL, Bush M, Chandrasekaran S, DeFronzo RA, Einhorn D, Galindo RJ, et al. American Association of Clinical Endocrinology Clinical Practice Guideline: developing a diabetes mellitus comprehensive care Plan—2022 update. Endocr Pract. 2022;28(10):923–1049.
56. Hall MH, Okun ML, Sowers M, Matthews KA, Kravitz HM, Hardin K, et al. Sleep is associated with the metabolic syndrome in a multi-ethnic cohort of midlife women: the SWAN sleep study. Sleep. 2012;35(6):783–90.
57. Thurston RC, Chang Y, von Känel R, Barinas-Mitchell E, Jennings JR, Hall MH, et al. Sleep characteristics and carotid atherosclerosis among midlife women. Sleep. 2017;40(2):zsw052.
58. Matthews KA, Everson-Rose SA, Kravitz HM, Lee L, Janssen I, Sutton-Tyrrell K. Do reports of sleep disturbance relate to coronary and aortic calcification in healthy middle-aged women?: study of women's health across the nation. Sleep Med. 2013;14(3):282–7.
59. Makarem N, St-Onge MP, Liao M, Lloyd-Jones DM, Aggarwal B. Association of sleep characteristics with cardiovascular health among women and differences by race/ethnicity and menopausal status: findings from the American Heart Association go red for women strategically focused research network. Sleep Health. 2019;5(5):501–8.
60. SCORE2 working group and ESC Cardiovascular risk collaboration. SCORE2 risk prediction algorithms: new models to estimate 10-year risk of cardiovascular disease in Europe. Eur Heart J. 2021;42(25):2439–54.
61. Konst RE, Damman P, Pellegrini D, Hartzema-Meijer MJ, van Uden BJC, Jansen TPJ, Brandsma J, Vart P, Gehlmann H, Maas AHEM, van Royen N, Elias-Smale SE. Vasomotor dysfunction in patients with angina and nonobstructive coronary artery disease is dominated by vasospasm. Int J Cardiol. 2021;333:14–20.
62. Cho L, Davis M, Elgendy I, Epps K, Lindley KJ, Mehta PK, Michos ED, Minissian M, Pepine C, Vaccarino V, Volgman AS. ACC CVD Womens committee members. Summary of updated recommendations for primary prevention of cardiovascular disease in women: JACC state-of-the-art review. J Am Coll Cardiol. 2020;75(20):2602–18.
63. Shaw LJ, Min JK, Nasir K, Xie JX, Berman DS, Miedema MD, Whelton SP, Dardari ZA, Rozanski A, Rumberger J, Bairey Merz CN, Al-Mallah MH, Budoff MJ, Blaha MJ. Sex differences in calcified plaque and long-term cardiovascular mortality: observations from the CAC consortium. Eur Heart J. 2018;39(41):3727–35.
64. Zoet GA, Benschop L, Boersma E, Budde RPJ, Fauser B, van der Graaf Y, et al. Prevalence of subclinical coronary artery disease assessed by coronary computed tomography angiography in 45- to 55-year-old women with a history of preeclampsia. Circulation. 2018;137(8):877–9.
65. Benschop L, Brouwers L, Zoet GA, Meun C, Boersma E, Budde RPJ, et al. Early onset of coronary artery calcification in women with previous preeclampsia. Circ Cardiovasc Imaging. 2020;13(11):e010340.

66. Gunning MN, Meun C, van Rijn BB, Maas A, Benschop L, Franx A, et al. Coronary artery calcification in middle-aged women with premature ovarian insufficiency. Clin Endocrinol (Oxf). 2019;91(2):314–22.
67. Dzaye O, Dudum R, Reiter-Brennan C, Kianoush S, Tota-Maharaj R, Cainzos-Achirica M, et al. Coronary artery calcium scoring for individualized cardiovascular risk estimation in important patient subpopulations after the 2019 AHA/ACC primary prevention guidelines. Prog Cardiovasc Dis. 2019;62(5):423–30.

Hormone Replacement Therapy (And Other Options to Treat Menopausal Symptoms)

Irene Lambrinoudaki, Eleni Armeni, and Elina Silionga

Abstract

The transition to menopause is associated with adverse cardiometabolic changes which increase the risk of cardiovascular disease. The decline in estrogen levels is associated with increase in fat mass, predominantly in the abdominal region, with insulin resistance and with dyslipidemia. Furthermore, the prevalence of hypertension increases after menopause. Menopausal symptoms, in particular vasomotor symptoms, are associated with a heightened risk of cardiovascular disease later in life. In this context, cardiovascular risk stratification has a central role in decision-making, concerning the replacement of sex hormones as well as the need for control of traditional cardiovascular risk factors. Women with premature ovarian insufficiency or early menopause should receive hormone replacement therapy until the average age of menopause. Women who transition into menopause after the age of 45 years, are eligible for hormone replacement therapy if they have bothersome menopausal symptoms, symptoms of urogenital atrophy or are at risk for an osteoporotic fracture. If initiated for these indications, hormone replacement therapy has also beneficial effects on cholesterol and glucose levels, insulin resistance and body composition. If hormone therapy is contraindicated or not desired, non-hormonal alternatives can be used to manage menopausal symptoms.

Keywords

Hormone replacement therapy · Menopausal hormone therapy · Estrogen · Cardiovascular Cardiovascular disease · SCORE

Test your learning and check your understanding of this book's contents: use the "Springer Nature Flashcards" app to access questions using ▶ https://sn.pub/51ny7m To use the app, please follow the instructions in chapter 1.

I. Lambrinoudaki (✉) · E. Armeni · E. Silionga
Menopause Unit, 2nd Department of Obstetrics and Gynecology, Medical School, National and Kapodistrian University of Athens, Athens, Greece

A. H.E.M. Maas, E. Gerdts (eds.), *Manual of Cardiovascular Disease in Women*,
https://doi.org/10.1007/978-3-031-65952-2_12

1 Introduction

1.1 Hormone Replacement Therapy

1.1.1 Definitions

Hormone Replacement Therapy (HRT) is the exogenous replacement of the steroid hormones produced by the ovarian follicles [1].

1.1.2 Regimens

HRT regimens consist of two main components, estrogens and progestogens.

- Estrogen is the main component of any regimen, aiming to control symptoms attributed to estrogen deficiency.
- A progestogen should be added to estrogen in women with an intact uterus to prevent endometrial hyperplasia. Bazedoxifene, a selective estrogen receptor modulator, can also be considered in women who are intolerant to progestogens, or who have contraindications to progestogens.
- Tibolone is a synthetic steroid compound, the metabolites of which have estrogenic, progestogenic, and androgenic activity, varying according to the target tissue [2]. The use of tibolone is indicated for the management of menopausal symptoms and postmenopausal bone loss in postmenopausal women independently of hysterectomy status [3].
- Testosterone can be recommended for treating women with hypoactive sexual desire disorder (HSDD) [4]. In postmenopausal women with low libido in the context of hypoactive sexual desire disorder, testosterone treatment can be offered using appropriate approved female preparations or approved male formulations as an off-license use to provide the recommended female replacement dose. In the latter case, the dose should be customized to result in serum testosterone concentrations approximating those in premenopausal women [5, 6].
- Ospemifene, a selective estrogen receptor modulator administered as a daily oral tablet, is indicated for managing symptoms of urogenital atrophy in postmenopausal women who do not wish vaginal hormone therapy [7].
- Bioidentical hormones are molecules structurally modified to resemble the human sex steroids produced by the ovaries [8]. Compounded bioidentical hormones are non-governmentally regulated [9]. Data on the efficacy and safety of the majority of the compounded bioidentical hormones remain insufficient. Hence their use is not recommended [8].

The available hormone regimens are presented in Table 1.

1.1.3 Indications for Treatment

In women experiencing menopause at an age less than 45 years, HRT should be offered at least until the average age at menopause (50–52 years). If left untreated, these women have a higher risk of osteoporotic fractures, cardiovascular disease, depression and cognitive decline [1]. These young women should, in principle, receive higher doses of estrogen than women experiencing menopause later in life in an attempt to restore estrogen levels to the premenopausal state (mid-follicular phase, 120 pg/mL) [10].

In women experiencing menopause at an age older than 45 years, HRT is indicated for the management of bothersome menopausal symptoms, for the management of symptoms of urogenital atrophy and for women transitioning to menopause at risk for osteoporosis [1]. An effective HRT regimen employs the lowest dose of hormones required to control symptoms and to manage the menopause-associated bone loss [1, 11–13].

This chapter describes the effect of HRT on the cardiovascular system and the customization of therapy according to the individual patient's risk profile.

Table 1 Menopause hormone therapy regimens (adapted from [1, 13])

Regimen	Dose	Route of administration
Estrogens		
17-beta-estradiol	*Standard dose*: 2–4 mg (oral) or 50–100 μg (transdermal) *Low dose*: 1 mg (oral) or 25 μg (transdermal) *Ultra-low dose*: 0.25–0.5 mg (oral) or 14 μg transdermal) Vaginal dose: 5–10 μg	Tablet, patch, gel, vaginal cream or gel
Conjugated estrogen	*Standard oral dose*: 0.625–1.25 mg *Low oral dose*: 0.300–0.400 mg Vaginal dose: 0.300–1.25 mg	Oral tablet or vaginal cream or gel
Estriol	50 μg	Vaginal gel or disk
Progestogens		
Chlormadinone acetate	15–20 mg	Oral tablet
Dienogest	Sequential: 3–4 mg	Oral tablet
Drospirenone	1–2 mg	Oral tablet
Dydrogesterone	2.5–20 mg	Oral tablet
Micronized progesterone	50–200 mg orally or vaginally	Oral or vaginal tablet
Nomegestrol acetate	2.5–5 mg	Oral tablet
Norethisterone acetate	0.5–1.0 mg (orally) or 125–250 μg (transdermally)	Oral tablet or patch
Norgestrel	0.25–0.5 mg	Oral tablet
Norgestimate	0.5 mg	Oral tablet
Levonorgestrel	30–40 μg (orally) 150 μg (transdermally) 14–20 mg (intrauterine device)	Oral tablet or transdermal patch or intrauterine system device
Medroxyprogesterone acetate	2.5–10 mg	Oral tablet
Promegestone	Sequential: 5–10 mg or continuous: 2.5 mg	Oral tablet
Trimegestone	0.25 mg	Oral tablet
Other		
Selective estrogen receptor modulators – Bazedoxifene	20 mg	Oral tablet combined with CEE 0.45 mg
Ospemifene	60 mg	Oral tablet
Tibolone	1.25–2.5 mg	Oral tablet
Dehydroepiandrosterone sulfate (prasterone)	6.5 mg	Vaginal tablet

2 Theory

2.1 Cardiovascular Effects of HRT

2.1.1 Effect of HRT on Vascular Cells

The beneficial effect of estrogen on the vascular vessel wall has been demonstrated by a vast amount of data retrieved from in vitro studies, which showed that the effect of estradiol on the vessels is multidimensional [14]. *First*, endogenous estradiol has been described to promote angiogenesis as well as vasodilation. *Second*, estrogen has been linked with a decrease in migration and proliferation of fibroblasts as well as reduced collagen deposition. *Third*, estrogen has been shown to promote mitochondrial survival and exert anti-apoptotic effects by decreasing the production of reactive oxygen species and promoting the oxidation of fatty acid, which ultimately leads to a decrease in the size of the infarct. *Fourth*, estrogen has also been shown to regulate the degree of oxidative stress by exerting anti-oxidant properties and consequently improving cell survival.

Many studies have investigated the effect of progestins on vascular cells. In vivo, data have demonstrated that administration of different progestogens has a different effect on the expression of vascular inflammation markers since progestins such as medroxyprogesterone acetate (MPA), norethindrone acetate, levonorgestrel increase the expression of vascular inflammation markers, which is not the case for micronized progesterone and dienogest [15]. In particular, the expression of vascular cell adhesion molecule-1 in human vascular endothelial cells was induced by progesterone but not following the administration of MPA [16]. Similarly, progestogens exert a differing effect on nitric oxide production in aortas from ovariectomized rats and isolated human endothelial cells. The production was increased following treatment with progesterone and drospirenone, while it remained unaffected or was even downregulated by MPA [17, 18]. Platelet aggregation and the interaction with endothelial cells are inhibited by progesterone and stimulated by MPA [18].

2.1.2 Effect of HRT on Blood Lipids

The effect of HRT on blood lipids is summarized in Table 2. The choice of hormone treatment depends on the severity of dyslipidemia, whereas the type and route of administration should be established according to the individual cardiovascular risk [19, 20]. Oral estrogens increase levels of high-density lipoprotein cholesterol (HDL-C) and triglycerides while they decrease levels of low-density lipoprotein cholesterol (LDL-C) [21, 22]. In comparison to oral agents, transdermal estradiol has comparable but less potent effect on LDL-C and HDL-C [21, 22]. In addition, transdermal estradiol does not increase plasma levels of triglycerides and is likely to even reduce their levels [21, 22]. The latter effect has been attributed to an increase in the clearance of the VLDL-TG (very-low density lipoprotein and triglycerides) [23]. Conjugated equine estrogens (CEE) increase HDL-C levels (12-week change, 16–18%) and triglyceride levels (12-week change, by 24–38%), while they decrease LDL-C levels (12-week change, by approximately 15–19%) [22]. Progestogens may mitigate the beneficial effects of estrogens on lipids in a degree dependent on the potency of the progestogen [19]. Among the available choices, micronized progesterone and dydrogesterone have the mildest effect on blood lipids [24]. Second in line, norethisterone acetate appears to have a rather favorable effect on LDL-C and triglyceride levels, but may decrease HDL-C [19, 25–27]. Levonorgestrel administered through an intravaginal device has only a mild effect on triglycerides and LDL-C levels, while a mild fluctuation in total cholesterol and HDL-C can be noted within the first 6 months after the insertion of the device, with a return to normal at 12 months [19, 25, 27, 28]. Oral levonorgestrel or medroxyprogesterone acetate can compromise the beneficial effect of estrogen on the lipid profile [29, 30].

Table 2 Effect of menopause hormone therapy on cardiovascular risk factors (adapted from [2, 28, 39, 113–119])

	Oral E2	Tts-E2	CEE	17-bE2	Tibolone
Blood lipids					
TC	↓↓	↓	Mild ↓	↓	↓
TG	↑	N	↑	Oral: ↑ Tts: ↓	↓
HDL-C	↑↑	↑	↑	↑	↓
LDL-C	↓↓	↓	↓	↓	↓
LpA	↓↓	↓	↓	↓	↓
Insulin resistance	↓↓	↓	↓	Oral: ↓ Tts: N	N

CEE conjugated estrogen, *E2* estradiol, *Tts* transdermal, *N* neutral, *TC* total cholesterol, *TG* triglycerides, *HDL-C* high density lipoprotein cholesterol, *LDL-C* low density lipoprotein cholesterol, *LpA* lipoprotein alpha
N neutral, ↓ lower, ↑ increased

2.1.3 Effect of HRT on Blood Pressure

HRT appears to have a neutral effect on blood pressure and it is not contraindicated in women with controlled arterial hypertension. However, the effect of HRT on blood pressure blood pressure with regard to regimen, route of administration and timing of initiation remains controversial [31]. Interestingly, initiation of CEE treatment within the 10 years, so within the known "window of opportunity" after the discontinuation of menses, is associated with lower risk for hypertension compared to those starting HRT within the 10 years after the final menstrual period (WHI observational study, WHI-OS and Postmenopausal Estrogen/Progestin Interventions Trial, PEPI) [32, 33].

More recently, the role of the treatment route has been investigated in updated analyses of the E3N and the Women's Health Initiative trial, WHI [32, 34]. Accordingly, users of oral estrogen have a 7–9% higher risk for developing new onset hypertension when compared to never-users of HRT [32, 34]. The use of transdermal estrogen has a neutral effect on blood pressure, as users have only 3% higher readings which are comparable to women who have never used HRT [34]. The risk of incident new onset hypertension does not vary according to the dose of estrogen [32]. The type of estrogen is associated with a differing effect on blood pressure regulation; women treated with transdermal estradiol or estrone sulphate preparations had 15% and 17% lower risk in comparison to those treated with CEE with or without progestin [32]. The risk for new onset hypertension appears to be altered by the addition of pregnane or norpregnane derives as opposed to estrogen monotherapy [32, 34]. Micronized progesterone, on the other hand, has a neutral effect on blood pressure and the risk for new onset hypertension (Kronos Early Estrogen Prevention study, KEEPS) [35].

2.1.4 Effect of HRT on Glucose Metabolism and Body Composition

Overall, HRT is associated with lower risk for new onset diabetes in later life in comparison with the risk of women who have never used HRT [36]. An earlier large meta-analysis has shown that HRT-use decreased the incidence of type 2 diabetes mellitus by 30%, and the rates of insulin resistance by 13% [37]. More specifically, women on treatment with CEE or transdermal estradiol in combination with progestogen exhibit an average decrease in fasting blood glucose levels of 11.5% and an average decrease in homeostasis model assessment of insulin resistance levels by 35.8% [37]. The use of oral estradiol has been associated with a greater reduction in the risk of diabetes mellitus (DM) compared to the use of transdermal estrogen, with or without added progestogens (E3N study) [38]. In trials reporting the metabolic effect of CEE monotherapy, patients experienced a decrease in glucose and insulin levels (PEPI trial [39], WHI at year 1 of observation [40], KEEPS at year 4 of observation [41]). The use of progestogens is likely to mitigate the estrogen-induced metabolic effect; women on CEE or 17β-estradiol plus medroxyprogesterone were less protected against incident DM compared to women on treatment with estrogen-monotherapy only [42, 43].

Body composition changes during the transition to menopause. In the perimenopausal period, the rate of adipose tissue proliferation increases up to twofold and the lean mass decreases compared to the premenopausal state [44]. The changes continue to take place up until 2 years after the last final menstrual period [44, 45]. Simultaneously, energy expenditure decreases secondary to lower lipid oxidation [46]. In an estrogen deficient environment, lower activation of estrogen receptor alpha downregulates the signals transmitted by the sympathetic nervous system targeting brown adipose tissue thermogenesis and result in weight dysregulation [47]. HRT has been shown to exert a favorable effect on body composition [20]. Moreover, menopause has also been associated with lower energy expenditure in the context of lower physical activity, which can result to sarcopenia [48]. In this context, the available data is still inconclusive and cannot supporting a beneficial or detrimental link between HRT-use and maintenance of muscle mass in middle-aged women [49].

2.1.5 Effect of HRT on Coagulation

The risk of venous thromboembolism (VTE) is 1.5–2 times higher in women treated with HRT in comparison to women who were never treated with HRT [50, 51]. For women aged 50–59 years, treatment with CEE alone is associated with 5 additional events of deep vein thrombosis (DVT), 3 additional events of pulmonary embolism (PE) and 1 less events of stroke per 10,000 women annually compared to controls (WHI trial) [52].

On the other hand, combined treatment with CEE and medroxyprogesterone is associated with 10 additional cases of DVT, 6 cases of PE and 5 cases of stroke per 10,000 women annually (WHI trial) [52]. These rates correspond to a rare complication, as per the classification of drug reactions by the World Health Organization Council for International Organizations of Medical Sciences [53]. In particular, oral estrogen only preparations can increase the risk of VTE 1.48 times on average compared to non-treated patients [54]. Women receiving transdermal estrogen have similar VTE risk with women who remain untreated [54]. Recurrent VTE is up to 6.4 times more common in users of oral estrogens, while there is no risk associated with the use of transdermal estrogens [50]. The type of progestogen can also affect VTE risk. Micronized progesteterone and dydrogesterone are associated with lower risk compared to more potent progestins like levonorgestrel or medroxyprogesterone acetate [54, 55].

2.2 Landmark Studies on the Effect of HRT on Cardiovascular Disease Outcomes

Towards the end of the 1990s, many observational studies emphasized the favorable effect of HRT on cardiovascular disease [56]. Following these observations, the first large-scale randomized controlled trial was designed in the United States of America to investigate the effect of HRT on death from coronary heart disease or non-fatal myocardial infarction. The Women's Health Initiative evaluated 27,347 postmenopausal women aged 50–79 years, with a mean age of 63 years at the time of entering the study. The participants randomized to either 0.625 mg conjugated equine estrogens (CEE-only arm) or 0.625 mg CEE and 2.5 mg medroxyprogesterone acetate (CEE + P arm) were not free of cardiovascular disease or related risk factors at baseline [57]. The estrogen-progestogen (E + P) arm of the study was terminated early, namely after an average of 5.6 years, due to the observed higher incidence of breast cancer [58]. The estrogen-only arm (E) was terminated after 7.2 years due to the observed higher incidence of stroke [59]. The results of the study received significant attention until the understanding that the number of coronary heart disease (CHD) events were only marginally higher for those started on E + P treatment at an age <70 years vs. older women (absolute number of events vs. placebo, age 50–59 years +5 events; age 60–69 years, +1 event; age 70–79 years, +23 events). Interestingly, E-only treatment was protective in younger but not in older postmenopausal women (absolute number of events, age 50–59 years, −10 events; age 60–69 years, −4 events; age 70–79 years, +10 events). The postintervention analysis showed similar results, highlighting the protective effect of estrogen-only treatment regarding future CHD events [52], but also the modifying effect of the menopausal age at the time of treatment initiation concerning cardiovascular outcomes. This data also highlighted that cardiovascular outcomes of MHT treatment are significantly associated with the type and the dose of the administered progestin [60, 61].

The theory of the "window of opportunity" is supported by a large body of evidence. A meta-regression analysis [62] reported 28% lower rates of all-cause mortality, 39% lower rates of cardiac mortality, and 36% lower rates of all coronary events in postmenopausal women who started HRT early after menopause as compared to late postmenopausal women. Early and, in particular, late initiators had higher thromboembolic risk (late HR = 1.54, 95%CI: 1.39–1.79; early HR = 1.40, 95%CI: 1.10–1.78) [62]. The ELITE trial (Effects of Early versus Late Postmenopausal Treatment with Estradiol) showed that estradiol + progesterone treatment reduced the age-accelerated increase in carotid intima-media thickness (CIMT) in women who initiated treatment within the first 6 years after menopause. On the contrary, treatment had no effect in women who started treatment more than 10 years after their last menstrual period [63, 64]. In addition, a re-analysis of the WHI cohort showed that treatment with CEE initiated at the age of 50–59 years was associated with a reduction of all-cause mortality, which remained significant at 18 years of cumulative follow-up (HR 0.79, 95% CI 0.64–0.96) [52, 65]. The cardioprotective effect was even more obvious in women with a history of bilateral oophorectomy who started CEE-treatment at age 50–59 years compared to women on placebo (HR = 0.68, 95% CI: 0.48–0.96); a finding that could not be replicated in the group of older women (aged >70 years) [66].

2.3 Effect of HRT on the Risk of Breast Cancer

The HRT-associated risk of breast cancer should be addressed in the context of patient's age at the time of ovarian senescence or oophorectomy and the individual risk stratification [67]. Overall, the evidence is reassuring for women with premature ovarian insufficiency or early menopause who initiate HRT, as the risk of breast cancer is similar to their age-matched premenopausal women [13, 68, 69]. For older women, the effect of HRT on the risk of breast cancer depends mainly on the presence and type of the progestogen [67]. The risk appears to be higher for women receiving combined estrogen-progestogen preparations. Vaginal estrogens are not associated with an increase in the risk of breast cancer, irrespective of the duration of use [13]. Newer progestogens, like micronized progesterone and dydrogesterone, are associated with lower breast cancer risk than older progestogens like medroxyprogesterone acetate [67].

From a practical perspective, breast cancer risk can be assessed using internet-based calculators. Women with a low 5-year risk for breast cancer can safely be treated with HRT. However, caution is advised in women with an intermediate risk for breast cancer, while women with a higher risk should not be offered HRT [67]. Simultaneously, the presence of other risk factors like obesity or alcohol intake and inactivity should also be assessed, as these factors are likely to contribute to the risk for breast cancer to a more significant proportion than the risk conferred by HRT [70–73].

3 Clinical Praxis

Accurate estimation of cardiovascular risk is crucial in guiding the management and treatment options for individuals. Electronic algorithms have been developed to stratify the risk for of future cardiovascular events based on various factors. In the United States of America, the US Framingham score is a commonly used algorithm, available online at (http://cvdrisk.nhlbi.nih.gov) [74, 75]. Similarly, the European Society of Cardiology (ESC) provides an equivalent algorithm known as SCORE (Systematic Coronary Risk Evaluation) to quantify cardiovascular risk in the general population, and is available online at (http://www.heartscore.org/) [76].

Recently, the ESC published the updated SCORE2 risk prediction algorithm, which has been calibrated and validated to predict the 10-year risk of a first-onset cardiovascular event specifically for European populations. The algorithm takes into account gender-specific risk factors, providing a more individualized risk estimation [77]. Additionally, the SCORE2-OP toolkit estimates the 5- and 10-year risk of cardiovascular events in individuals aged over 70 years, with validated results for different geographical regions representing varying levels of cardiovascular risk [78]. It is important to note that when considering cardiovascular risk, specific factors unique to women, such as a history of hypertensive disease during pregnancy or radiation therapy for breast cancer, should also be considered [79].

Cardiovascular risk stratification plays a vital role in the discussion of treatment options, particularly in the context of hormone replacement therapy (HRT) [80]. Based on the level of cardiovascular risk, different approaches to HRT can be recommended (Fig. 1):

- *Women with low cardiovascular risk* (<1%) can be offered any type of HRT.
- *Women with moderate cardiovascular risk* (≥1% up to <5%) can be offered any type of systemic HRT, with or without primary prevention strategies for the management of CRFs.

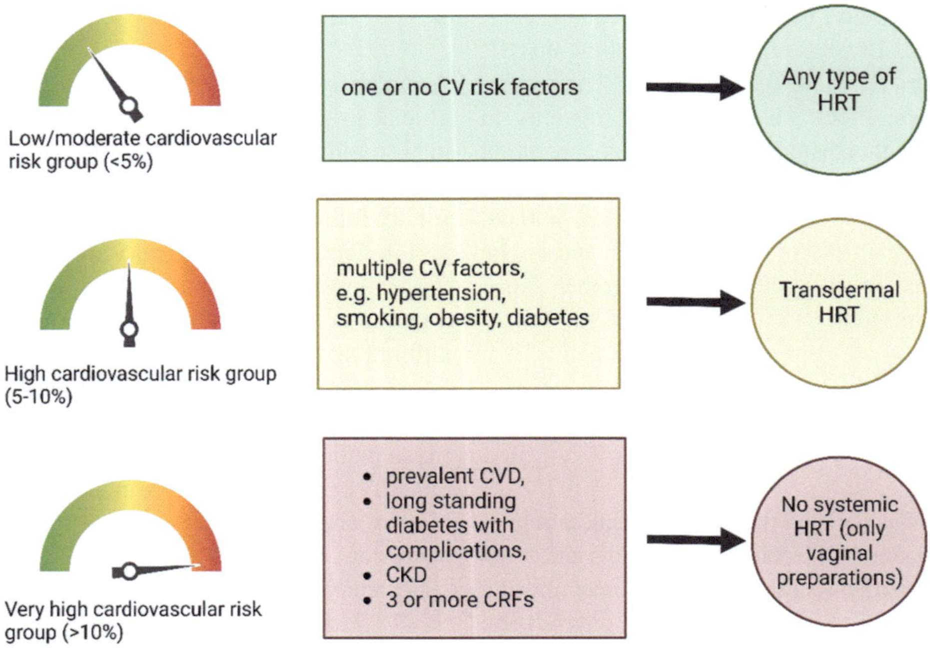

Fig. 1 HRT customization according to cardiovascular risk. Note: *CRFs* cardiovascular risk factors, *TOD* terminal organ damage, *DM* diabetes mellitus, *CVD* cardiovascular disease, *HRT* hormone replacement therapy, *CKD* chronic kidney disease. (The figure was created using Biorender.com)

- *Women with high cardiovascular risk* (SCORE 5% to <10%) can receive topical HRT (vaginal) in combination with primary or secondary prevention strategies for CRFs. If systemic HRT is required, transdermal regimens can be offered on an individual basis.
- *Women with very high cardiovascular risk* (SCORE ≥ 10%) should only receive topical HRT (vaginal) in combination with secondary prevention strategies for managing cardiovascular risk factors (CRFs).

4 Non-Hormonal Therapies

4.1 Pharmacological Alternatives for Vasomotor Symptoms

This group includes alternatives that can be used as valid options for second-line treatment in women for whom estrogen treatment is contraindicated, as well as a summary of the available evidence on the effect of these agents on the cardiovascular system (Table 3).

A large body of evidence has indicated that the use of selective Serotonin Reuptake Inhibitors (SSRIs, e.g., paroxetine, citalopram, sertraline, paroxetine, fluoxetine or escitalopram) and Serotonin Norepinephrine Reuptake Inhibitors (SNRIs, e.g., venlafaxine or desvenlafaxine) are the preferred first-line option for the management of hot flashes [9, 81–84]. Interestingly, paroxetine mesylate is the only agent approved by the FDA for the control of the severity of moderate to severe vasomotor hot flashes [85]. Side effects are dose-dependent and include fatigue, dizziness, and nausea [85]. Citalopram has no significant effect on levels of blood lipids, while fluoxetine may decrease concentrations of TC, triglyceride, and LDL-C [86, 87]. Sertraline and paroxetine exert a pro-atherogenic or neutral effect on TC and LDL-C but increased levels of triglycerides [86, 87].The use of SSRIs should be adjusted in patients treated with aspirin to minimize the risk of bleeding [88]. Caution is advised in prescribing paroxetine/fluoxetine for women with breast cancer treated with tamoxifen, as these types of SSRIs are known to inhibit P450

Table 3 Non-hormonal treatment options for vasomotor symptoms and effects on the cardiovascular system (adapted from [9, 81–84, 88, 89, 92, 95–98]

Treatment agents	Recommended daily dose	Cardiovascular adverse effects	Contraindications
SSRI	• Paroxetine 7.5 mg • Citalopram 10–20 mg • Escitalopram 10–20 mg	• Increased risk of bleeding in patients treated with aspirin • Risk of hypertension or palpitations • Risk for QT interval prolongation specific for citalopram	• Caution in women with known CVD
SNRI	• Venlafaxin 37.5–150 mg • Desvenlafaxine 100–150 mg	• Small risk for hypertension or orthostatic hypotension in older patients, no effect on ECG	• Caution in women with known CVD
Gabapentinoids	• Gabapentin, starting dose 100–300 mg at night, titrated to a maximum of 2400 mg	• May exacerbate peripheral edema	• No adverse effects on CVD
Central alpha-2 adrenergic agonist	• Clonidine 50 μg two—three times	• Orthostatic hypotension Hypotension	• Only if BP regulation is mandatory
Anticholinergic modulators	• Oxybutinin 5–15 mg	• Moderate risk for arrhythmia with or without palpitations • Risk for worsening congestive heart failure	• Caution in women with known CVD
Neurokinin B antagonists	• Fezolinetant 45 mg/day	• Under investigation	• Under investigation

SSRI selective serotonin reuptake inhibitor, *SNRI* Serotonin norepinephrine reuptake inhibitors, *ECG* electrocardiogram, *CVD* cardiovascular disease, *BP* blood pressure

cytochrome activity, interfering with tamoxifen metabolism [83]. The use of venlafaxine has been associated with a modest risk of hypertension, evident only in older adults, but no significant changes in the parameters of an electrocardiogram [89]. Venlafaxine may increase levels of blood lipids, while duloxetine has no apparent effect, whereas gabapentin may moderately increase LDL-C levels only [86, 90, 91].

Alternatively, commonly used antiepileptic agents like gabapentin may be a better option for women experiencing disruptive sleep due to hot flashes occurring primarily at night [83]. Gabapentin has it has been reported to reduce the frequency of vasomotor symptoms by 31–89.5% [84]. Side effects include unsteadiness, dizziness, and drowsiness, which tend to improve after 4 weeks of treatment [84]. Both pregabalin and gabapentin have a relatively neutral effect on the cardiovascular system [92]. As reported by an earlier trial, venlafaxine appears to be the preferable option as opposed to gabapentin regarding the control of menopausal hot flashes, as it was found to improve the score of hot flash severity by 41% [93]. Concerns about gabapentin and pregabalin misuse and dependence need to be taken into consideration before their recommendation for vasomotor symptoms [94].

Another valid option for the control of menopausal hot flashes is the use of centrally active alpha-2 adrenergic agonists, like clonidine [95]. This agent, approved by the FDA for the control of hypertension, is used less frequently for the control of vasomotor symptoms, with moderate effectiveness of 20–35% [83, 95, 96]. The use of clonidine is limited by side effects like orthostatic hypotension and hypotension [95].

Oxybutinin is an emerging agent for the control of menopausal symptoms, acting as an anticholinergic modulator. This option has also been shown to decrease the severity of vasomotor symptoms, as well as the frequency of hot flushes, by 50–77% [97]. The use of oxybutynin has been associated with side effects such as palpitations (1–10%) as well as constipation, dry mouth, urinary issues, higher risk of dementia, and anticholinergic effects, which are better tolerated when using lower doses [85, 96, 97].

Selective neurokinin-3 receptor antagonists are a novel group of agents for the management of vasomotor symptoms which act on the temperature regulating zone in hypothalamus. The main representatives of these medicines are fezolinetant and elinzanetant [98]. Fezolinetant has been recently approved by the FDA (Food and Drug Association) [99] and is undergoing regulatory review by the European Medicines Agency (EMA) [100]. The second agent, elinzanetant, is still in development. A growing amount of data is highlighting the efficacy of fezolinetant for the control of moderate-to-severe hot flahses [101–104]. The 52 week randomized, double-blind trial SKYLIGHT 4 (Study to Find out how safe long-term treatment with fezolinetant is in women with hot flashes going through menopause) evaluated the efficacy of fezolinetant 30 mg compared to the 45 mg dose or placebo [103]. From cardiovascular perspective, the study assessed 1830 participants with an electrocardiogram and did not report any meaningful alterations [103]. As participants with clinical evidence of cardiovascular disease were excluded from the large randomized controlled trials evaluating fezolinetant [102], the long-term cardiovascular implications remain to be investigated.

4.2 Alternative and Complementary Therapies

Clinical hypnosis, weight loss, stellate ganglion block and possibly homeopathic medicine have been used for the management of menopausal symptoms [98, 105–108]. These therapies have modest effects on menopausal symptoms, yet the evidence is limited by the quality and heterogeneity of studies [109, 110]. Healthcare providers should take into consideration possible interactions with standard medicines such as anticancer therapies, anticoagulants, and antiepileptics [95]. Finally, cognitive behavioral therapy (CBT), initially developed for patients suffering from depression and anxiety, has recently been considered an effective treatment for the control of health problems like chronic pain, insomnia as well as vasomotor symptoms [12, 111]. Two small randomized controlled trials described the possible role of a dedicated cognitive-behavioral therapy protocol for menopause (CBT-Meno) and the experience of climacteric symptoms. The CBT-Meno protocol was found to be effective in improving the rates of self-reported hot flashes, night sweats as well as sleep disorders, sexual concerns, as well as problematic beliefs about menopause, and attitudes related to depression [112].

5 Conclusions

The transition into menopause is associated with adverse cardiometabolic changes which increase the risk of CVD. HRT is indicated for all women with early menopause and POI and for women older than 45 years with bothersome menopausal symptoms or for women at risk of fracture. HRT has a beneficial effect on the lipid profile, on glucose metabolism and on body composition. HRT should be customized according to cardiovascular risk. Women with low/moderate CV risk are eligible for any HRT regimen, whereas women with high CV risk can receive transdermal treatment after carefully assessing CV risk factors. Women with very high CV risk should not receive systemic HRT and are eligible for non-hormonal options for the management of menopausal symptoms.

Key Issues

- All women with premature ovarian insufficiency or early menopause should be offered HRT, at least until the age of natural menopause.
- Perimenopausal and postmenopausal women experiencing bothersome menopausal symptoms or at risk of an osteoporotic fracture can be offered HRT.
- If offered perimenopausally or shortly after menopause, so within the “window of opportunity”, HRT can be cardioprotective.
- Cardiovascular risk assessment can guide the individualization of HRT.

- Women who are not eligible for HRT or are not wishing to receive HRT can use non-hormonal alternatives.

Questions and Answers

1. A 54 years old woman with last menstrual period before 6 months presents to the Menopause clinic with severe hot flashes and night sweats. She is a non-smoker, has a blood pressure of 120/70 mmHg and her BMI is 24 kg/m^2. LDL-C 100 mg/dL. How would you treat the vasomotor symptoms?
   (A) Oral estradiol
   (B) Oral estradiol and micronized progesterone
   (C) Tibolone
   (D) Venlafaxine
   Answer: B—Given the fact that the patient is perimenopausal and has a low cardiovascular risk, the best choice is combined HRT with oral estradiol and micronized progesterone.
2. A 33 years old woman underwent bilateral oophorectomy and hysterectomy. She has a BMI of 35 kg/m^2 and type 2 diabetes mellitus on treatment with metformin 500 mg twice a day. HbA1c is 6.4%. She is a non-smoker. The lady presents to the clinic seeking advise for hormone replacement options, and describes brain fog and low libido. What is the next step?
   (A) Offer transdermal 17beta-estradiol because the patient is obese and has diabetes.
   (B) Offer oral 17beta-estradiol, as the oral route is more beneficial for the management of diabetes.
   (C) Offer transdermal 17beta-estradiol combined with micronized progesterone
   (D) Offer raloxifene, a selective estrogen receptor modulator
   Answer: A—Offer estrogen-only therapy as the patient is hysterectomized and a progestogen is not needed. The patient is stratified in the high CV risk category, so therapy should be administered through the transdermal route.
3. A 72 years old woman comes to the Menopause clinic asking for HRT, as she has vaginal dryness and pain during intercourse. Her menstruation stopped at the age of 56 years. She is a current smoker, despite having suffered a myocardial infarction 4 years ago. Current treatment includes simvastatin 40 mg daily, amlodipine 10 mg per day for hypertension. What would you advise her?
   (A) Oral HRT
   (B) Offer transdermal estradiol and micronized progesterone
   (C) Offer vaginal estrogen
   (D) Gabapentin
   Answer: C–Given the fact that the complaints are mainly genitourinary and she belongs to a very high CV risk category, local estrogen can be a safe option which will not affect the cardiovascular risk.

Acknowledgments Figure 1 was created using Biorender.com

References

1. Armeni E, et al. Hormone therapy regimens for managing the menopause and premature ovarian insufficiency. Best Pract Res Clin Endocrinol Metab. 2021;35(6):101561.
2. Formoso G, et al. Short-term and long-term effects of tibolone in postmenopausal women. Cochrane Database Syst Rev. 2016;10(10):Cd008536.
3. Cummings SR, et al. The effects of tibolone in older postmenopausal women. N Engl J Med. 2008;359(7):697–708.
4. Hamoda H, et al. The British Menopause Society & Women's health concern 2020 recommendations on hormone replacement therapy in menopausal women. Post Reprod Health. 2020;26(4):181–209.
5. Davis SR. Testosterone for women: certainties and uncertainties. Climacteric. 2022;26:1–4.
6. Marko KI, Simon JA. Androgen therapy for women after menopause. Best Pract Res Clin Endocrinol Metab. 2021;35(6):101592.
7. Archer DF, et al. Ospemifene for the treatment of menopausal vaginal dryness, a symptom of the genitourinary syndrome of menopause. Expert Rev Endocrinol Metab. 2019;14(5):301–14.
8. Stanczyk FZ, Matharu H, Winer SA. Bioidentical hormones. Climacteric. 2021;24(1):38–45.

9. Stuenkel CA. Compounded bioidentical hormone therapy: new recommendations from the 2020 National Academies of sciences, engineering, and medicine. Menopause. 2021;28(5):576–8.
10. Goldfarb NM. Mosby's diagnostic & laboratory test reference. Maryland Heights, MO: Mosby; 2009.
11. de Villiers TJ, et al. Revised global consensus statement on menopausal hormone therapy. Maturitas. 2016;91:153–5.
12. The North American Menopause Society. Statement on continuing use of systemic hormone therapy after age 65. Menopause. 2015;22(7):693.
13. Lambrinoudaki I, et al. Menopause, wellbeing and health: a care pathway from the European Menopause and Andropause Society. Maturitas. 2022;163:1–14.
14. Iorga A, et al. The protective role of estrogen and estrogen receptors in cardiovascular disease and the controversial use of estrogen therapy. Biol Sex Differ. 2017;8(1):33.
15. Tatsumi H, et al. Lack of stimulatory effect of dienogest on the expression of intercellular adhesion molecule-1 and vascular cell adhesion molecule-1 by endothelial cell as compared with other synthetic progestins. Maturitas. 2002;42(4):287–94.
16. Otsuki M, et al. Progesterone, but not medroxyprogesterone, inhibits vascular cell adhesion molecule-1 expression in human vascular endothelial cells. Arterioscler Thromb Vasc Biol. 2001;21(2):243–8.
17. Simoncini T, et al. Differential signal transduction of progesterone and medroxyprogesterone acetate in human endothelial cells. Endocrinology. 2004;145(12):5745–56.
18. Cutini PH, Campelo AE, Massheimer VL. Differential regulation of endothelium behavior by progesterone and medroxyprogesterone acetate. J Endocrinol. 2014;220(3):179–93.
19. Anagnostis P, et al. Menopause symptom management in women with dyslipidemias: an EMAS clinical guide. Maturitas. 2020;135:82–8.
20. Shufelt CL, Manson JE. Menopausal hormone therapy and cardiovascular disease: the role of formulation, dose, and route of delivery. J Clin Endocrinol Metab. 2021;106(5):1245–54.
21. Palmisano BT, Zhu L, Stafford JM. Role of estrogens in the regulation of liver lipid metabolism. Adv Exp Med Biol. 2017;1043:227–56.
22. Walsh BW, et al. Effects of postmenopausal estrogen replacement on the concentrations and metabolism of plasma lipoproteins. N Engl J Med. 1991;325(17):1196–204.
23. Smith GI, et al. Systemic delivery of estradiol, but not testosterone or progesterone, alters very low density lipoprotein-triglyceride kinetics in postmenopausal women. J Clin Endocrinol Metab. 2014;99(7):E1306–10.
24. Prior JC, et al. Progesterone therapy, endothelial function and cardiovascular risk factors: a 3-month randomized, placebo-controlled trial in healthy early postmenopausal women. PLoS One. 2014;9(1):e84698.
25. Polyzos SA, Lambrinoudaki I, Goulis DG. Menopausal hormone therapy in women with dyslipidemia and nonalcoholic fatty liver disease. Hormones. 2022;21(3):375–81.
26. Zhao X, et al. Exploration of the relationship between gut microbiota and polycystic ovary syndrome (PCOS): a review. Geburtshilfe Frauenheilkd. 2020;80(2):161–71.
27. Stanczyk FZ, et al. Progestogens used in postmenopausal hormone therapy: differences in their pharmacological properties, intracellular actions, and clinical effects. Endocr Rev. 2013;34(2):171–208.
28. Jiang Y, Tian W. The effects of progesterones on blood lipids in hormone replacement therapy. Lipids Health Dis. 2017;16(1):219.
29. Ågren UM, et al. Effects of a monophasic combined oral contraceptive containing nomegestrol acetate and 17β-oestradiol compared with one containing levonorgestrel and ethinylestradiol on haemostasis, lipids and carbohydrate metabolism. Eur J Contracept Reprod Health Care. 2011;16(6):444–57.
30. Terauchi M, et al. Effects of oral estradiol and levonorgestrel on cardiovascular risk markers in postmenopausal women. Arch Gynecol Obstet. 2012;285(6):1647–56.
31. Srivaratharajah K, Abramson BL. Hypertension in menopausal women: the effect and role of estrogen. Menopause. 2019;26(4):428–30.
32. Wild RA, et al. Hormone therapy formulation, dose, route of delivery, and risk of hypertension: findings from the Women's Health Initiative observational study (WHI-OS). Menopause. 2021;28(10):1108–16.
33. The Writing Group for the PEPI Trial. Effects of estrogen or estrogen/progestin regimens on heart disease risk factors in postmenopausal women. The Postmenopausal Estrogen/Progestin Interventions (PEPI) Trial. JAMA. 1995;273(3):199–208.
34. Madika AL, et al. Menopausal hormone therapy and risk of incident hypertension: role of the route of estrogen administration and progestogens in the E3N cohort. Menopause. 2021;28(11):1204–8.
35. Miller VM, et al. The Kronos early estrogen prevention study (KEEPS): what have we learned? Menopause. 2019;26(9):1071–84.
36. Lambrinoudaki I, et al. The interplay between diabetes mellitus and menopause: clinical implications. Nat Rev Endocrinol. 2022;18(10):608–22.
37. Salpeter SR, et al. Meta-analysis: effect of hormone-replacement therapy on components of the metabolic syndrome in postmenopausal women. Diabetes Obes Metab. 2006;8(5):538–54.
38. de Lauzon-Guillain B, et al. Menopausal hormone therapy and new-onset diabetes in the French etude Epidemiologique de femmes de la Mutuelle Générale de l'Education Nationale (E3N) cohort. Diabetologia. 2009;52(10):2092–100.

39. Fineberg SE. Glycaemic control and hormone replacement therapy: implications of the postmenopausal estrogen/progestogen intervention (PEPI) study. Drugs Aging. 2000;17(6):453–61.
40. Rossouw JE, et al. Inflammatory, lipid, thrombotic, and genetic markers of coronary heart disease risk in the women's health initiative trials of hormone therapy. Arch Intern Med. 2008;168(20):2245–53.
41. Harman SM, et al. Arterial imaging outcomes and cardiovascular risk factors in recently menopausal women: a randomized trial. Ann Intern Med. 2014;161(4):249–60.
42. Gartlehner G, et al. Hormone therapy for the primary prevention of chronic conditions in postmenopausal women: evidence report and systematic review for the US preventive services task force. JAMA. 2017;318(22):2234–49.
43. Prentice RL, et al. Dual-outcome intention-to-treat analyses in the Women's Health Initiative randomized controlled hormone therapy trials. Am J Epidemiol. 2020;189(9):972–81.
44. Greendale GA, et al. Changes in body composition and weight during the menopause transitionI. JCI Insight. 2019;4(5):e124865.
45. Greendale GA, et al. Changes in regional fat distribution and anthropometric measures across the menopause transition. J Clin Endocrinol Metab. 2021;106(9):2520–34.
46. Rogers NH, et al. Reduced energy expenditure and increased inflammation are early events in the development of ovariectomy-induced obesity. Endocrinology. 2009;150(5):2161–8.
47. Heine PA, et al. Increased adipose tissue in male and female estrogen receptor-alpha knockout mice. Proc Natl Acad Sci U S A. 2000;97(23):12729–34.
48. Geraci A, et al. Sarcopenia and menopause: the role of estradiol. Front Endocrinol (Lausanne). 2021;12:682012.
49. Javed AA, et al. Association between hormone therapy and muscle mass in postmenopausal women: a systematic review and meta-analysis. JAMA Netw Open. 2019;2(8):e1910154.
50. Olié V, et al. Hormone therapy and recurrence of venous thromboembolism among postmenopausal women. Menopause. 2011;18(5):488–93.
51. Tremollieres F, et al. EMAS position statement: managing menopausal women with a personal or family history of VTE. Maturitas. 2011;69(2):195–8.
52. Manson JE, et al. Menopausal hormone therapy and health outcomes during the intervention and extended poststopping phases of the Women's Health Initiative randomized trials. JAMA. 2013;310(13):1353–68.
53. (CIOMS), C.f.I.O.o.M.S. Report of CIOMS Working Group IV. Benefit-risk balance for marketed drugs: evaluating safety signals. https://cioms.ch/working-groups/working-group-xii/. Accessed 20 May 2023.
54. Scarabin PY. Progestogens and venous thromboembolism in menopausal women: an updated oral versus transdermal estrogen meta-analysis. Climacteric. 2018;21(4):341–5.
55. Vinogradova Y, Coupland C, Hippisley-Cox J. Use of hormone replacement therapy and risk of venous thromboembolism: nested case-control studies using the QResearch and CPRD databases. BMJ. 2019;364:k4810.
56. Falkeborn M, et al. The risk of acute myocardial infarction after oestrogen and oestrogen-progestogen replacement. Br J Obstet Gynaecol. 1992;99(10):821–8.
57. The Women's Health Initiative Study Group. Design of the Women's health initiative clinical trial and observational study. Control Clin Trials. 1998;19(1):61–109.
58. Rossouw JE, et al. Risks and benefits of estrogen plus progestin in healthy postmenopausal women: principal results from the Women's Health Initiative randomized controlled trial. JAMA. 2002;288(3):321–33.
59. Anderson GL, et al. Effects of conjugated equine estrogen in postmenopausal women with hysterectomy: the Women's Health Initiative randomized controlled trial. JAMA. 2004;291(14):1701–12.
60. Odmark IS, et al. Long-term effects of two different continuous combined regimens of hormone replacement therapy on well-being. Gynecol Endocrinol. 2004;18(6):305–17.
61. Liu L, et al. Clinically relevant progestins regulate neurogenic and neuroprotective responses in vitro and in vivo. Endocrinology. 2010;151(12):5782–94.
62. Nudy M, Chinchilli VM, Foy AJ. A systematic review and meta-regression analysis to examine the 'timing hypothesis' of hormone replacement therapy on mortality, coronary heart disease, and stroke. Int J Cardiol Heart Vasc. 2019;22:123–31.
63. Hodis HN, et al. Vascular effects of early versus late postmenopausal treatment with estradiol. N Engl J Med. 2016;374(13):1221–31.
64. Karim R, et al. Effect of menopausal hormone therapy on arterial wall echomorphology: results from the early versus late intervention trial with estradiol (ELITE). Maturitas. 2022;162:15–22.
65. Manson JE, et al. Menopausal hormone therapy and long-term all-cause and cause-specific mortality: the Women's Health Initiative randomized trials. JAMA. 2017;318(10):927–38.
66. Manson JE, et al. Menopausal estrogen-alone therapy and health outcomes in women with and without bilateral oophorectomy: a randomized trial. Ann Intern Med. 2019;171(6):406–14.
67. Rozenberg S, et al. Menopausal hormone therapy and breast cancer risk. Best Pract Res Clin Endocrinol Metab. 2021;35(6):101577.
68. Webber L, et al. ESHRE guideline: management of women with premature ovarian insufficiency. Hum Reprod. 2016;31(5):926–37.
69. Panay N, et al. Premature ovarian insufficiency: an international menopause society white paper. Climacteric. 2020;23(5):426–46.
70. Eheman C, et al. Annual report to the nation on the status of cancer, 1975-2008, featuring cancers

associated with excess weight and lack of sufficient physical activity. Cancer. 2012;118(9):2338–66.
71. Lee IM, et al. Effect of physical inactivity on major non-communicable diseases worldwide: an analysis of burden of disease and life expectancy. Lancet. 2012;380(9838):219–29.
72. Hamajima N, et al. Alcohol, tobacco and breast cancer—collaborative reanalysis of individual data from 53 epidemiological studies, including 58,515 women with breast cancer and 95,067 women without the disease. Br J Cancer. 2002;87(11):1234–45.
73. Chan DSM, et al. World Cancer Research Fund international: continuous update project—systematic literature review and meta-analysis of observational cohort studies on physical activity, sedentary behavior, adiposity, and weight change and breast cancer risk. Cancer Causes Control. 2019;30(11):1183–200.
74. Jahangiry L, Farhangi MA, Rezaei F. Framingham risk score for estimation of 10-years of cardiovascular diseases risk in patients with metabolic syndrome. J Health Popul Nutr. 2017;36(1):36.
75. Andersson C, et al. Framingham heart study: JACC focus seminar, 1/8. J Am Coll Cardiol. 2021;77(21):2680–92.
76. Conroy RM, et al. Estimation of ten-year risk of fatal cardiovascular disease in Europe: the SCORE project. Eur Heart J. 2003;24(11):987–1003.
77. group, S.w. and E.C.r. collaboration. SCORE2 risk prediction algorithms: new models to estimate 10-year risk of cardiovascular disease in Europe. Eur Heart J. 2021;42(25):2439–54.
78. ESC. SCORE2-OP risk prediction algorithms: estimating incident cardiovascular event risk in older persons in four geographical risk regions. Eur Heart J. 2021;42(25):2455–67.
79. Maas A, et al. Cardiovascular health after menopause transition, pregnancy disorders, and other gynaecologic conditions: a consensus document from European Cardiologists, Gynaecologists, and Endocrinologists. Eur Heart J. 2021;42(10):967–84.
80. Maas A. Hormone therapy and cardiovascular disease: benefits and harms. Best Pract Res Clin Endocrinol Metab. 2021;35(6):101576.
81. Riemma G, et al. Efficacy of low-dose paroxetine for the treatment of hot flushes in surgical and physiological postmenopausal women: systematic review and meta-analysis of randomized trials. Medicina (Kaunas). 2019;55(9):554.
82. Orleans RJ, et al. FDA approval of paroxetine for menopausal hot flushes. N Engl J Med. 2014;370(19):1777–9.
83. Woyka J. Consensus statement for non-hormonal based treatments for menopausal symptoms. Post Reprod Health. 2020;26(3):137–41.
84. Nonhormonal management of menopause-associated vasomotor symptoms: 2015 position statement of the North American Menopause Society. Menopause. 2015;22(11):1155–72; quiz 1173–4, 1174.
85. David PS, et al. A clinical review on paroxetine and emerging therapies for the treatment of vasomotor symptoms. Int J Womens Health. 2022;14:353–61.
86. McIntyre RS, et al. The effect of antidepressants on lipid homeostasis: a cardiac safety concern? Expert Opin Drug Saf. 2006;5(4):523–37.
87. Colotto M, et al. Effect of treatment with selective serotonin reuptake inhibitors on lipid profile: state of the art. Clin Ter. 2012;163(1):e41–5.
88. Buda V, et al. An up-to-date article regarding particularities of drug treatment in patients with chronic heart failure. J Clin Med. 2022;11(7).
89. Behlke LM, Lenze EJ, Carney RM. The cardiovascular effects of newer antidepressants in older adults and those with or at high risk for cardiovascular diseases. CNS Drugs. 2020;34(11):1133–47.
90. Hummel J, et al. Serum lipoproteins improve after successful pharmacologic antidepressant treatment: a randomized open-label prospective trial. J Clin Psychiatry. 2011;72(7):885–91.
91. Agarwal N, et al. Safety and efficacy of gabapentin in management of psychosomatic and sexual symptoms in postmenopausal women: a pilot study. J Midlife Health. 2015;6(1):10–5.
92. Mareti E, et al. Non-hormonal replacement therapy regimens: do they have an effect on cardiovascular risk? Curr Vasc Pharmacol. 2019;17(6):573–8.
93. Bordeleau L, et al. Multicenter, randomized, cross-over clinical trial of venlafaxine versus gabapentin for the management of hot flashes in breast cancer survivors. J Clin Oncol. 2010;28(35):5147–52.
94. Evoy KE, Morrison MD, Saklad SR. Abuse and misuse of pregabalin and gabapentin. Drugs. 2017;77(4):403–26.
95. Pinkerton JV, Santen RJ. Managing vasomotor symptoms in women after cancer. Climacteric. 2019;22(6):544–52.
96. Hirsch H, Manson JE. Menopausal symptom management in women with cardiovascular disease or vascular risk factors. Maturitas. 2022;161:1–6.
97. Leon-Ferre RA, et al. Oxybutynin vs placebo for hot flashes in women with or without breast cancer: a randomized, double-blind clinical trial (ACCRU SC-1603). JNCI Cancer Spectr. 2020;4(1):pkz088.
98. The 2023 nonhormone therapy position statement of the North American Menopause Society. Menopause. 2023;30(6):573–90.
99. FDA. FDA approves novel drug to treat moderate to severe hot flashes caused by menopause. 2023. https://www.fda.gov/news-events/press-announcements/fda-approves-novel-drug-treat-moderate-severe-hot-flashes-caused-menopause#:~:text=The%20FDA%20approved%20Veozah%20%28fezolinetant%29%2C%20an%20oral%20medication,treat%20moderate%20to%20severe%20hot%20flashes%20from%20menopause. Accessed 18 Jun 2023.
100. EMA. Applications for new human medicines under evaluation by the CHMP: June 2023.

2023. https://www.ema.europa.eu/en/medicines/medicines-human-use-under-evaluation.
101. Lederman S, et al. Fezolinetant for treatment of moderate-to-severe vasomotor symptoms associated with menopause (SKYLIGHT 1): a phase 3 randomised controlled study. Lancet. 2023;401(10382):1091–102.
102. Johnson KA, et al. Efficacy and safety of Fezolinetant in moderate-to-severe vasomotor symptoms associated with menopause: a phase 3 RCT. J Clin Endocrinol Metab. 2023;108:1981–97.
103. Neal-Perry G, et al. Safety of Fezolinetant for vasomotor symptoms associated with menopause: a randomized controlled trial. Obstet Gynecol. 2023;141(4):737–47.
104. LaCroix A, Ensrud K. The flash dance of midlife: the Skylight 1 trial. Nat Med. 2023;29:1324–5.
105. Rees M, et al. European menopause and Andropause society (EMAS) and international gynecologic cancer society (IGCS) position statement on managing the menopause after gynecological cancer: focus on menopausal symptoms and osteoporosis. Maturitas. 2020;134:56–61.
106. Hunter MS. EMAS position statement: non-hormonal management of menopausal vasomotor symptoms. Maturitas. 2015;82(4):443.
107. Mintziori G, et al. Non-hormonal management of menopausal vasomotor symptoms: psychosocial interventions. Maturitas. 2015;82(4):444–5.
108. Baber RJ, Panay N, Fenton A. 2016 IMS recommendations on women's midlife health and menopause hormone therapy. Climacteric. 2016;19(2):109–50.
109. Panay N, Kalu E. Management of premature ovarian failure. Best Pract Res Clin Obstet Gynaecol. 2009;23(1):129–40.
110. Tran S, et al. Nonpharmacological therapies for the management of menopausal vasomotor symptoms in breast cancer survivors. Support Care Cancer. 2021;29(3):1183–93.
111. Hunter MS. Cognitive behavioral therapy for menopausal symptoms. Climacteric. 2021;24(1):51–6.
112. Donegan E, et al. Impact of the CBT-meno protocol on menopause-specific beliefs, dysfunctional attitudes, and coping behaviors. Menopause. 2022;29(8):963–72.
113. Kotani K, et al. Tibolone decreases lipoprotein(a) levels in postmenopausal women: a systematic review and meta-analysis of 12 studies with 1009 patients. Atherosclerosis. 2015;242(1):87–96.
114. Godsland IF. Effects of postmenopausal hormone replacement therapy on lipid, lipoprotein, and apolipoprotein (a) concentrations: analysis of studies published from 1974–2000. Fertil Steril. 2001;75(5):898–915.
115. Tang Z, et al. The effect of 17β-estradiol plus norethisterone acetate treatment on lipoprotein (a), atherogenic and anti-atherogenic apolipoproteins levels in postmenopausal women: a meta-analysis of randomized controlled trials. Exp Gerontol. 2023;172:112055.
116. Lobo RA, et al. Effects of lower doses of conjugated equine estrogens and medroxyprogesterone acetate on plasma lipids and lipoproteins, coagulation factors, and carbohydrate metabolism. Fertil Steril. 2001;76(1):13–24.
117. Slopien R, et al. Menopause and diabetes: EMAS clinical guide. Maturitas. 2018;117:6–10.
118. Spencer CP, et al. Effects of oral and transdermal 17β-estradiol with cyclical oral norethindrone acetate on insulin sensitivity, secretion, and elimination in postmenopausal women. Metabolism. 2000;49(6):742–7.
119. Godsland IF, et al. Insulin resistance, secretion, and elimination in postmenopausal women receiving oral or transdermal hormone replacement therapy. Metabolism. 1993;42(7):846–53.

Migraine and Cardiovascular Risk in Women

Linda Al-Hassany
and Antoinette MaassenVanDenBrink

Abstract

Migraine is a neurovascular headache disorder that affects women disproportionately. Apart from its direct burden, it is a cardiovascular risk factor associated with major cardiovascular events, including stroke, myocardial infarction, arterial dissection, atrial fibrillation, and even cardiovascular mortality. While migraine does not show an obvious association with traditional cardiovascular risk factors or mechanisms, such as obesity, diabetes mellitus, hypertension, and atherosclerosis, exact pathophysiological mechanisms remain elusive. Paradoxically, clinical and epidemiological data show that active migraine is rather associated with favorable risk scores, while pointing towards microvascular dysfunction and an altered neuropeptide activity as a putative biological mechanism. Clear-cut medical therapies and recommendations to mitigate the risk associated with migraine are currently lacking. However, healthy lifestyle modifications are generally recommended, while smoking and the use of combined contraceptives should be discouraged, especially in young females suffering from migraine with aura. In this chapter, we dive into the pathophysiology of the cardiovascular risk associated with migraine and provide clinical directions and implications on the increased cardiovascular risk associated with migraine.

Keywords

Migraine · Cardiovascular risk · Cardiovascular disease · Females · Microvasculature

Test your learning and check your understanding of this book's contents: use the "Springer Nature Flashcards" app to access questions using ▶ https://sn.pub/51ny7m
To use the app, please follow the instructions in chapter 1.

L. Al-Hassany · A. MaassenVanDenBrink (✉)
Division of Vascular Medicine and Pharmacology, Department of Internal Medicine, Erasmus MC University Medical Center,
Rotterdam, The Netherlands
e-mail: l.alhassany@erasmusmc.nl; a.vanharen-maassenvandenbrink@erasmusmc.nl

A. H.E.M. Maas, E. Gerdts (eds.), *Manual of Cardiovascular Disease in Women*,
https://doi.org/10.1007/978-3-031-65952-2_13

1 Introduction

Migraine is a chronic neurovascular disorder characterized by attacks of moderate to severe pulsating one-sided headache, often accompanied by nausea and photophobia, that may last up to 72 h [1]. One-third of migraine patients experience migraine auras, most commonly transient visual or sensory neurological disturbances [2, 3]. With a global prevalence of 14–15%, the prevalence of migraine is two to three times higher in women compared with men [4]. Importantly, it is the most disabling disease in women under the age of 50 due to the high number of years lived with disability, resulting in a substantially high global socioeconomic burden in young women [5, 6]. After the age of 50, the prevalence declines but remains high in comparison to men. Besides differences in prevalence, women have been described to report longer attack durations, higher recurrence rates, greater disability, and symptoms that accompany migraine attacks (including nausea, vomiting, phonophobia, and photophobia) compared to men with migraine [7–10].

Migraine pathophysiology involves incompletely understood yet complex neurobiological mechanisms originating from trigeminal activation and the subsequent release of neuropeptides, including calcitonin gene-related peptide (CGRP) and pituitary adenylate cyclase-activating polypeptide (PACAP), associated with vasodilation, inflammation, and pain [11]. Cortical spreading depression, a wave of sustained depolarization slowly spreading across the cerebral cortex, has also been shown to be an activator of the trigeminal neurons and is an important mechanism underlying migraine auras [12]. These processes are thought to be influenced by sex hormone fluctuations [13].

Apart from its direct burden, it has now clearly been demonstrated that migraine, especially migraine with aura, is linked to long-term cardiovascular complications, as apparent from increased risk of cardiovascular disease, including ischemic stroke (odds ratio (OR)/relative risk (RR) 1.70 [95% confidence interval (CI) 1.47–1.98] [14]), hemorrhagic stroke (OR/RR 1.35 [95% CI 1.11–1.63] [14]), cervical artery dissection (OR 1.74 [95% CI 1.38–2.19] [15]), myocardial infarction (hazard ratio (HR) 1.36 [95% CI 1.23–1.51] [16]), atrial fibrillation or atrial flutter (OR 1.25 [95% CI 1.16–1.36] [17]), and even cardiovascular mortality (HR 1.27 [95% CI 1.14–1.42] [16]). In this chapter, we discuss potential pathophysiological mechanisms, microvascular dysfunction in particular, that could be involved in the relationship between cardiovascular disease and migraine. Further, we elaborate on the clinical relevance and implications of this association, while providing directions for future research.

2 Theory

As mentioned above, migraine has consistently been associated with cardiovascular disease in epidemiological studies. Interestingly, this relationship is not confined to cerebrovascular disease, which might be expected to be related to migraine in view that the cranial circulation seems to be involved in this disorder, but also includes cardiac disease. This suggests that not only local cranial processes are pivotal in the relationship between migraine and cardiovascular disease, but also systemic factors. While the mechanism involved in the increased cardiovascular risk of migraine remains elusive, epidemiological studies have shed some light on this relation, providing circumstantial evidence for a relationship between migraine and microvascular disease.

2.1 Microvascular Dysfunction Underlying Migraine as a Cardiovascular Risk Factor

Migraine, which is more common in women, has a notable association with cardiovascular disease, which is often linked to nonobstructive coronary artery disease or microvascular arterial dysfunction, a condition more frequently observed in women than in men [18, 19]. The strongest link between migraine with aura and major cardiovascular diseases was further observed in individuals with the lowest Framingham risk scores [20]—a sex-specific risk score including traditional cardiovascular risk factors (e.g. cholesterol levels, systolic blood pressure, age, current smoking) that predicts the 10-year risk of coronary artery disease [21]. These results imply that the relationship between migraine and cardiovascular risk probably does not exclusively involve traditional cardiovascular risk factors. This is also exemplified by studies indicating that migraine is not linked to atherosclerosis in large vessels and coronary artery calcification [22–26]. Moreover, the relationship between migraine with aura and ischemic stroke is more commonly observed in women with lower cardiovascular risk, including those who are younger. In contrast, the association between migraine with aura and myocardial infarction predominantly occurs in women with higher cardiovascular risk, often seen in older individuals [20].

Interestingly, data from the Women's Health Study indicated that elevated Framingham Risk Scores categories are exclusively observed in women who had a prior history of migraine, while such associations were not observed in those with active migraine or in individuals with incident migraine (i.e. individuals who developed migraine later during follow-up)—independent from potential age differences between the groups [27]. Thus, changes in migraine activity status during the life course seem to be associated with divergent cardiovascular risk scores in migraine patients, and should, therefore, be taken into account. Whether this could be explained by the hypothesis that the increased cardiovascular risk associated with migraine is rather expressed by measures of microvascular dysfunction than conventional risk scores (including the Framingham Risk Score) representing traditional, atherogenic cardiovascular risk factors, remains to be demonstrated [27]. Also, it cannot be excluded that pharmacologic treatment with antihypertensive drugs, also serving as prophylactic treatment for migraine, could have affected the cardiovascular risk score. Additionally, migraine patients—especially women—treated with triptans and ergotamines show a reduced risk of ischemic cerebrovascular and cardiovascular diseases compared to migraine patients who do not use these drugs [28]. Yet, it cannot be excluded that a certain form of selection bias might be present, considering that having a pre-existing high cardiovascular risk or a positive cardiovascular history serves as a contraindication for the use of triptans and ergot alkaloids [29, 30].

Another indirect indication for the role of microvascular dysfunction has been provided by the fact that the aforementioned vasodilating neuropeptide CGRP is more potent and efficacious in small arteries than in large arteries [31]. Also, specifically diastolic blood pressure as a measure of microvascular resistance, rather than systolic blood pressure as a measure of macrovascular pressure, has recently been proposed to play a critical role in migraine susceptibility [32, 33]. Interestingly, such microvascular dysfunction may be attributed to both endothelial dysfunction, as well as to impaired vascular smooth muscle cell relaxation [34]. We recently set out a translational study to assess potential microvascular dysfunction in women with migraine, aiming to distinguish between endothelial (presumably nitric oxide-related) and smooth muscle (presumably related to peptidergic innervation) components. The study was performed in middle-aged women with polycystic ovary syndrome (PCOS), as this condition has previously been suggested to be related to an increased cardiovascular risk [35, 36], although this was not confirmed by others [37]. The results of our study indicated that, in women with migraine, the peptidergic innervation of the microvasculature is impaired, showing an altered neuropeptide activity [38]. While larger studies are obviously warranted, our findings provide a potential mechanism supporting previous findings that cardiovascular risk associated with migraine may be independent of traditional risk factors.

2.2 Alternative Mechanisms Underlying Migraine as a Cardiovascular Risk Factor

As mentioned previously, migraine (with aura in particular) has also been associated with incident atrial fibrillation, which has been proposed as a mechanism underlying the association between migraine and other cardio- and cerebrovascular diseases [39, 40]. A state of autonomic dysfunction has been implied to play a pathophysiological role herein [41, 42]. Further, there is a tendency for migraine symptoms to reduce following ablation therapy of atrial fibrillation [43], while migraine-like headache has been reported as a possible complication of transseptal puncture for catheter ablation [44].

Several genome-wide association studies have also explored mechanisms that might explain the connection between migraine and the increased risk of cardiovascular disease, suggesting shared genetic factors could underlie this association, especially in migraine without aura [45, 46], and for coronary artery disease [47, 48] and ischemic stroke [46], while no significant association was detected for atrial fibrillation [48]. Interestingly, two large-scale genome-wide association studies showed a significant overlap of genetic risk loci between migraine and coronary artery disease, but this overlap was only observed in migraine without aura, and it even appears to be protective—indicating that migraine patients have a lower genetic risk of coronary artery disease compared to controls [47]. In addition, Daghlas et al. identified novel genetic loci associated with migraine, stroke, and cervical arterial dissection with a profound role of LRP1, which is part of the low-density lipoprotein receptor gene family, suggesting that migraine may have a causal influence on cervical artery dissection but a protective effect against large artery stroke [49].

Together with environmental factors, small-effect genetic variants also contribute to the susceptibility of migraine [50]. Microvascular dysfunction has been demonstrated in specific disorders that also present an increased migraine prevalence, such as cerebral autosomal dominant arteriopathy with subcortical infarcts and leukoencephalopathy (CADASIL), and Retinal Vasculopathy With Cerebral Leukoencephalopathy and Systemic Manifestations (RVCL-S) [34, 51]. Further, disrupted cardiac metabolism and signaling have been shown in mice with a mutation associated with familial hemiplegic migraine—a genetically heterogeneous and rare subtype of migraine with aura [52, 53]. More specifically, it concerned a mutation in the ATP1A2 gene encoding Na,K-ATPase, which might therefore be a cardiovascular risk gene [53].

Further, migraine auras have been described to cause ischemic stroke immediately, i.e. migrainous infarction due to insufficient or reduced cerebral blood flow, metabolism, and oxygen supply [54]. It has been argued that the treatment of cortical spreading depression might, therefore, also prevent ischemic infarction in vulnerable brains [55, 56]. Other mechanisms that might form the biological link between migraine and cardiovascular disease is a hypercoagulable state, including shortages of coagulation proteins, polycythemia, increased platelet activation, and higher levels of fibrinogen and Von Willebrand Factor—possibly due to a rise in estrogen levels. Yet, no evidence exists on the efficacy of antithrombotic drugs in the treatment of migraine [57, 58]. Moreover, inconclusive evidence was found for patent foramen ovale, which was hypothesized to serve as a shared risk factor between migraine, with aura in particular, and cardiovascular disease [59–61], However, foramen ovale closure is not recommended as a treatment to reduce migraine headache frequency or to accomplish migraine cessation based on three trials [62–64]. Finally, several studies suggest a proinflammatory state in migraine with a key role for neurogenic neuroinflammation in the progression from episodic to chronic migraine, while providing weak biological evidence for changes in tumor necrosis factor and other interleukines and cytokines in migraine patients [2, 65–67]. Possibly, a proinflammatory state may also co-occur with comorbidities of migraine that are associated with an increased cardiovascular risk, e.g. depression [68, 69] and obesity [70, 71].

3 Clinical Practice

As discussed, robust cohort data demonstrating the association between migraine and cardiovascular and cerebrovascular disease, ischaemic stroke in particular, have mainly emerged in the last 15 years. The development and validation of the cardiovascular risk score QRISK3, which estimates the 10-year risk of cardiovascular disease in both sexes, has led to including and acknowledging migraine as a cardiovascular risk factor [72]. Further, the 2021 guidelines on cardiovascular disease prevention released by the European Society of Cardiology recommended including migraine with aura in assessing cardiovascular risk [73]. It should be acknowledged that the absolute increased risk of migraine is small on an individual level but high at a population level, given its high overall prevalence [74, 75]. A recent study by Kurth et al. placed the contribution of migraine as a cardiovascular risk factor into perspective, demonstrating that the incidence rate of major cardiovascular disease (i.e., first myocardial infarction, stroke, or cardiovascular death) among women with migraine with aura is significantly higher than the adjusted incidence rate among those with obesity, high triglycerides, and low high-density lipoprotein cholesterol [76]. The increased cardiovascular risk is more profound in younger populations with migraine and has not been demonstrated in elderly [77, 78] unless the migraine onset is late in life [79]. Whether this can be explained by the hypothesis that cardiovascular aging and the high prevalence of atherosclerosis in the elderly [80] mask the increased cardiovascular risk of migraine, remains to be demonstrated.

This risk of ischemic stroke has been demonstrated to be amplified in females with aura, aged 45 years or younger, who use high-dose estrogen contraceptives and smoke—leading up to a more than tenfold increased risk [81–83]. Several studies suggest that the association between migraine and stroke mainly exists among individuals without traditional cardiovascular risk factors for stroke, such as hypertension, myocardial infarction, and diabetes [84, 85]. Moreover, the association between migraine and conventional cardiovascular risk factors, including hypertension [86], metabolic syndrome [87], diabetes mellitus, and obesity [88, 89] remains controversial [90]. Nevertheless, several of these risk factors do contribute to an increase in episodic migraine attack frequency, leading to the chronification of migraine [91, 92].

The question automatically arises of how to mitigate and even prevent the elevated cardiovascular risk in migraine patients. Yet, while evidence on the association between migraine and cardiovascular disease is robust, there are no clear-cut recommendations on adequate therapies. The association between migraine and cardiovascular disease has been demonstrated to vary by migraine frequency, mainly among women with migraine with aura [93, 94]. A higher frequency of white matter hyperintensities has been demonstrated in chronic migraine patients, rather than in episodic migraine patients. Longer disease duration and frequent attacks, in contrast to the severity or duration of migraine attacks, have also been demonstrated to be risk factors for an increased frequency of white matter hyperintensities in migraine patients [95]. Such associations are yet debated, considering that results from the Cerebral Abnormalities in Migraine, an Epidemiological Risk Analysis (CAMERA) study showed no differences in white matter hyperintensities between migraine patients compared to controls [96].

Treating the increased cardiovascular risk associated with migraine is further complicated by the cardiovascular concerns of several acute and prophylactic treatments of migraine (e.g. antihypertensives, frequent use of non-steroid anti-inflammatory drugs (NSAIDs), but also the recently approved monoclonal antibodies and small molecules targeting CGRP or its receptor, i.e. CGRP(-receptor) antibodies or gepants [97, 98]. Further, a placebo-controlled trial on 100 mg aspirin every other day, conducted as part of the Women's Health Study, showed no significant decrease in migraine severity, duration, and migraine-related disability [99]. Yet, aspirin has been shown to offer comparable protection against ischemic stroke in women, regardless of their migraine status, as demonstrated by post-hoc subgroup analyses of the Women's Health Study. These analyses also revealed that women with migraine with aura who take aspirin may have a heightened risk of myocardial infarction—especially in women with a smoking history or a history of hypertension [100]. Another randomized double-blind trial compared aspirin and metoprolol as prophylactics in migraine, and showed that metoprolol was superior but had more side effects and lower tolerability [101].

Most general healthy lifestyle modifications for migraine management are usually recommendable and effective in lowering the cardiovascular risk of migraine patients, e.g. a healthy lifestyle including sufficient physical exercise, adequate sleep, and avoidance of alcohol, smoking, or drug abuse [102]. Further, additional attention is required in young females with migraine with comorbidities or diseases that are well-known to be associated with an increased cardiovascular risk as well, including gestational hypertension, pre-eclampsia, and pulmonary embolism [103, 104] or those with circulating antiphospholipid antibodies, which are an independent predictor of risk of recurrent vascular events [105]. Interestingly, a few studies have also suggested a link between migraine, stroke, and livedo reticularis (dermatopathy due to blood status of the superficial venous systems) as well as Sneddon's syndrome (a non-inflammatory thrombotic vasculopathy) [106–108]. Current recommendations include the advice to avoid the use of combined oral contraceptives in female migraine patients, as the risk seems to correlate with the estrogen dose [109], while the desogestrel 75 μg/day pill might be the safest option [83, 110]. There is, however, a lack of high-quality research on the risk of stroke associated with the use of low-dose estrogen in women with migraine [111]. While recommendations on the use of hormone replacement therapy are insufficiently supported by data, estrogen-containing menopausal hormone therapy should be avoided for patients at high risk, such as those with migraine with aura or a history of stroke. However, its use is acceptable for patients with migraine without aura and for those who are at low risk of cardiovascular disease. In cases where progestogen is necessary, a continuous delivery method (levonorgestrel intrauterine system (Mirena®)) is the recommended approach as it is better tolerated than cyclical progestogens [112, 113]. In light of evidence from a previous study showing that migraine sufferers have a higher risk of ischemic stroke during the perioperative period, it is advisable to take a migraine history into account when evaluating the risk for perioperative ischemic stroke [114].

Lastly, being an underreported and stigmatized disorder among men [115], this patient category should not be forgotten in the treatment of the additional cardiovascular burden associated with migraine. Indeed, previous studies also showed an elevated cardiovascular risk of major cardiovascular disease, especially myocardial infarction, in males [116, 117]. While direct estimate comparisons between males and females are lacking, and data on migraine in men are either scarce or incomplete, it is currently impossible to directly compare the estimates between both sexes [74]. Nevertheless, a meta-analysis of 16 cohort studies, including 1,152,407 subjects revealed no sex differences in the adjusted hazard ratio of stroke, myocardial infarction, and all-cause mortality [118].

4 Conclusions

Migraine is a clearly demonstrated, yet still underrecognized cardiovascular risk factor, and mechanisms mediating the increased cardiovascular risk in migraine have not yet been identified. More basic research is needed to elucidate the underlying biological mechanisms. Further, clinical and epidemiological studies are warranted to disentangle the temporality of these associations while paying special attention to underlying assumptions of analyses performed in observational studies when working within the causal framework. As an example, migraine could be considered a cause of hypertension, but also a consequence of it, leading to different analysis strategies [119]. This knowledge will facilitate the development of strategies that may mitigate the increased cardiovascular risk in migraine, and the possibility to screen and identify subgroups of migraine patients who are at particular high cardiovascular risk. To perform such future research as effectively as possible, it should also be kept in mind that, in the abovementioned studies, migraine was often defined as lifetime migraine (i.e., current migraine or history of migraine). Thus, it is crucial to take lifetime changes in migraine patterns into account while performing future studies, while incorporating differences between migraine with and without aura. Lastly, as the increased cardiovascular risk seems to be mainly present among females with a possible role for sex steroids, it is important that future studies take biology-related sex differences into account [8], while distinguishing these aspects adequately from gender aspects (i.e.culturally determined characteristics related to behaviors and role patterns) [120].

Key Issues

For a graphical summary of the key issues with regards to putative pathophysiological mechanisms below, please refer to Fig. 1.

- Migraine, with aura in particular, is a neurovascular headache disorder with a substantial individual and societal burden, especially among females under the age of 50 years.
- Besides its direct burden due to its incapacitating headache attacks, migraine is a cardiovascular risk factor with a higher incidence rate of major cardiovascular disease than other well-known cardiovascular risk factors, including obesity and an unfavorable lipid profile.
- This increased cardiovascular risk is especially amplified in young female migraine patients with aura, who smoke and use combined oral contraceptives.
- While exact underlying mechanisms are not elucidated yet, microvascular dysfunction is a possible link between migraine and cardiovascular disease.
- Other suggested pathophysiological mechanisms include atrial fibrillation, a shared genetic basis, and a hypercoagulable or pro-inflammatory state.
- No evidence-based pharmacological therapies exist yet to effectively treat the elevated cardiovascular risk in migraine patients.
- Future studies are warranted to disentangle the underlying biology while paying attention to the migraine activity status and diversity aspects—including sex and gender—in order to, ultimately, mitigate the cardiovascular risk in migraine patients.

Questions and Answers

1. Mention two aspects that distinguish migraine from other cardiovascular risk factors, like diabetes mellitus and hypertension.

   Answer: (i) Migraine is mainly associated with an increased risk of cardiovascular diseases, stroke in particular, in young females. Other cardiovascular risk factors usually have a higher prevalence in elderly and male patients. (ii) Migraine is not linked with tradi-

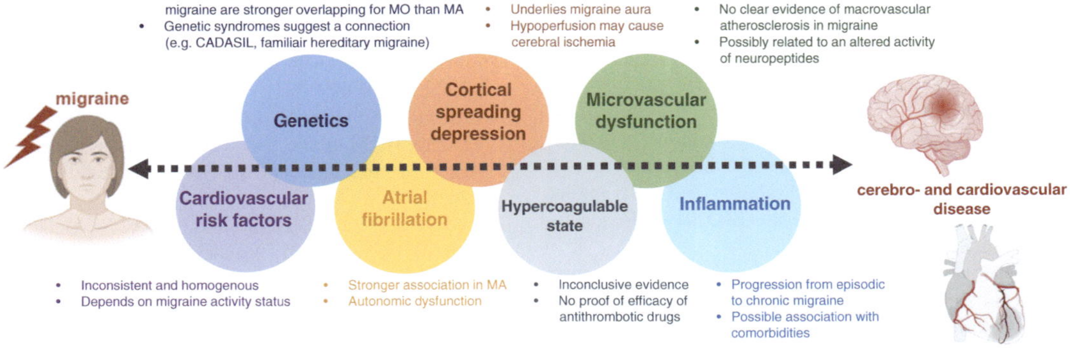

Fig. 1 Illustration of putative mechanisms, including a short summary, of the association between migraine and cerebrovascular and cardiovascular disease. *MA* migraine with aura, *MO* migraine without aura, *SNP* single nucleotide polymorphism. (Created with BioRender.com)

tional cardiovascular risk factors and an increased prevalence of atherosclerosis, in contrast to most other cardiovascular risk factors.

2. Mention three possible pathophysiological mechanisms that might underlie migraine as a cardiovascular risk factor.

   Answer: (i) Microvascular dysfunction; (ii) Genetics; (iii) Inflammation

3. Mention two clinical pieces of advice that you would give a female migraine patient aged 32 years who suffers from migraine with aura.

   Answer: (i) Stop and avoid smoking, as the cardiovascular risk of migraine with aura is considerably augmented in women who smoke. (ii) When discussing contraception, take the increased cardiovascular risk in women with migraine with aura who use combined oral contraception into account.

4. What Is the Name of the Cardiovascular Risk Score Calculator that Includes Migraine as a Risk Factor?

   Answer: The QRISK3

References

1. Headache Classification Committee of the International Headache Society (IHS). The International Classification of headache disorders, 3rd edition. Cephalalgia. 2018;38(1):1–211.
2. Goadsby PJ, Holland PR, Martins-Oliveira M, Hoffmann J, Schankin C, Akerman S. Pathophysiology of migraine: a disorder of sensory processing. Physiol Rev. 2017;97(2):553–622.
3. Dodick DW. A phase-by-phase review of migraine pathophysiology. Headache. 2018;58(Suppl 1):4–16.
4. Steiner TJ, Stovner LJ. Global epidemiology of migraine and its implications for public health and health policy. Nat Rev Neurol. 2023;19(2):109–17.
5. Steiner TJ, Stovner LJ, Jensen R, Uluduz D, Katsarava Z. Lifting the burden: the global campaign against headache. Migraine remains second among the world's causes of disability, and first among young women: findings from GBD2019. J Headache Pain. 2020;21(1):137.
6. GBD 2019 Diseases and Injuries Collaborators. Global burden of 369 diseases and injuries in 204 countries and territories, 1990-2019: a systematic analysis for the Global Burden of Disease Study 2019. Lancet. 2020;396(10258):1204–22.
7. Allais G, Chiarle G, Sinigaglia S, Airola G, Schiapparelli P, Benedetto C. Gender-related differences in migraine. Neurol Sci. 2020;41(Suppl 2):429–36.
8. Al-Hassany L, Haas J, Piccininni M, Kurth T, Maassen Van Den Brink A, Rohmann JL. Giving researchers a headache - sex and gender differences in migraine. Front Neurol. 2020;11:549038.
9. Vetvik KG, MacGregor EA. Sex differences in the epidemiology, clinical features, and pathophysiology of migraine. Lancet Neurol. 2017;16(1):1234.
10. Verhagen IE, van der Arend BWH, van Casteren DS, le Cessie S, MaassenVanDenBrink A, Terwindt GM. Sex differences in migraine attack characteristics: a longitudinal E-diary study. Headache. 2023;63(3):333–41.
11. Puledda F, Silva EM, Suwanlaong K, Goadsby PJ. Migraine: from pathophysiology to treatment. J Neurol. 2023;270(7):3654–66.
12. Charles AC, Baca SM. Cortical spreading depression and migraine. Nat Rev Neurol. 2013;9(11):637–44.
13. Labastida-Ramírez A, Rubio-Beltrán E, Villalón CM, MaassenVanDenBrink A. Gender aspects of CGRP in migraine. Cephalalgia. 2019;39(3):435–44.
14. Zhang S, Liu H, Shi T. Association between migraine and risk of stroke: a systematic review and meta-analysis. Neurol Sci. 2022;43(8):4875–89.
15. Sun Z, Kleine-Borgmann J, Suh J, McDermott GC, Vishnevetsky A, Rist PM. Migraine and the risk of cervical artery dissection: a systematic review and meta-analysis. Eur Stroke J. 2023;8(4):904–14.
16. Ng CYH, Tan BYQ, Teo YN, Teo YH, Syn NLX, Leow AST, et al. Myocardial infarction, stroke and cardiovascular mortality among migraine patients: a systematic review and meta-analysis. J Neurol. 2022;269(5):2346–58.
17. Adelborg K, Szépligeti SK, Holland-Bill L, Ehrenstein V, Horváth-Puhó E, Henderson VW, et al. Migraine and risk of cardiovascular diseases: Danish population based matched cohort study. BMJ. 2018;360:k96.
18. Reynolds HR, Bairey Merz CN, Berry C, Samuel R, Saw J, Smilowitz NR, et al. Coronary arterial function and disease in women with no obstructive coronary arteries. Circ Res. 2022;130(4):529–51.
19. Waheed N, Elias-Smale S, Malas W, Maas AH, Sedlak TL, Tremmel J, et al. Sex differences in non-obstructive coronary artery disease. Cardiovasc Res. 2020;116(4):829–40.
20. Kurth T, Schürks M, Logroscino G, Gaziano JM, Buring JE. Migraine, vascular risk, and cardiovascular events in women: prospective cohort study. BMJ. 2008;337:a636.
21. Wilson PW, D'Agostino RB, Levy D, Belanger AM, Silbershatz H, Kannel WB. Prediction of coronary heart disease using risk factor categories. Circulation. 1998;97(18):1837–47.
22. Ahmed B, Bairey Merz CN, McClure C, Johnson BD, Reis SE, Bittner V, et al. Migraines, angiographic coronary artery disease and cardiovascular outcomes in women. Am J Med. 2006;119(8):670–5.

23. Filippopulos FM, Schoeberl F, Becker HC, Becker-Bense S, Eren O, Straube A, et al. Coronary artery calcification score in migraine patients. Sci Rep. 2019;9(1):14069.
24. Stam AH, Weller CM, Janssens ACJ, Aulchenko YS, Oostra BA, Frants RR, et al. Migraine is not associated with enhanced atherosclerosis. Cephalalgia. 2013;33(4):228–35.
25. Gollion C, Guidolin B, Lerebours F, Rousseau V, Barbieux-Guillot M, Larrue V. Migraine and large artery atherosclerosis in young adults with ischemic stroke. Headache. 2022;62(2):191–7.
26. Wen KX, Ikram MA, Franco OH, Vernooij M, MaassenVanDenBrink A, Bos D, et al. Association of migraine with calcification in major vessel beds: the Rotterdam study. Cephalalgia. 2019;39(8):1041–8.
27. Ibrahimi K, Rist PM, Carpenet C, Lee Rohmann J, Buring JE, Maassen van den Brink A, et al. Vascular risk score and associations with past, current, or future migraine in women: cohort study. Neurology. 2022;99(16):e1694–701.
28. Kim Y, Shin SJ, Lee JW, Kim YS, You HS, Kim J, et al. Association between migraine and ischemic cardio-cerebrovascular disease (CCVD) and effects of Triptans and ergotamine on the risk of ischemic CCVD in patients with migraine in the Korean NHIS-HEALS cohort. Clin Drug Investig. 2023;43(7):541–50.
29. Diener HC. The risks or lack thereof of migraine treatments in vascular disease. Headache. 2020;60(3):649–53.
30. Roberto G, Raschi E, Piccinni C, Conti V, Vignatelli L, D'Alessandro R, et al. Adverse cardiovascular events associated with triptans and ergotamines for treatment of migraine: systematic review of observational studies. Cephalalgia. 2015;35(2):118–31.
31. MaassenVanDenBrink A, Meijer J, Villalón CM, Ferrari MD. Wiping out CGRP: potential cardiovascular risks. Trends Pharmacol Sci. 2016;37(9):779–88.
32. Guo Y, Rist PM, Daghlas I, Giulianini F, International Headache Genetics Consortium, 23andMe Research Team, et al. A genome-wide cross-phenotype meta-analysis of the association of blood pressure with migraine. Nat Commun. 2020;11(1):3368.
33. Barral JP, Croibier A. 2. Circulatory physiology. In: Barral JP, Croibier A, editors. Visceral vascular manipulations. Oxford: Churchill Livingstone; 2011. p. 27–45.
34. de Boer I, Stam AH, Buntinx L, Zielman R, van der Steen I, van den Maagdenberg AMJM, et al. RVCL-S and CADASIL display distinct impaired vascular function. Neurology. 2018;91(10):e956–63.
35. Zhao L, Zhu Z, Lou H, Zhu G, Huang W, Zhang S, et al. Polycystic ovary syndrome (PCOS) and the risk of coronary heart disease (CHD): a meta-analysis. Oncotarget. 2016;7(23):33715–21.
36. Zhang J, Xu JH, Qu QQ, Zhong GQ. Risk of cardiovascular and cerebrovascular events in polycystic ovarian syndrome women: a meta-analysis of cohort studies. Front Cardiovasc Med. 2020;7:552421.
37. Meun C, Gunning MN, Louwers YV, Peters H, Roos-Hesselink J, Roeters van Lennep J, et al. The cardiovascular risk profile of middle-aged women with polycystic ovary syndrome. Clin Endocrinol (Oxf). 2020;92(2):150–8.
38. Al-Hassany L, Linstra KM, Meun C, van den Berg J, Boersma E, Danser AHJ, et al. Decreased role of neuropeptides in the microvascular function in migraine patients with polycystic ovary syndrome. Atherosclerosis. 2023;384:117172.
39. Sen S, Androulakis M, Duda V, Alonso A, Chen LY, Soliman EZ, et al. Migraine with visual aura is a risk factor for incident atrial fibrillation: a cohort study. Neurology. 2018;91(24):E2202–10.
40. Scutelnic A, Mattle HP, Branca M, Jung S, Reichlin T, Fischer U, et al. Migraine and atrial fibrillation: a systematic review. Eur J Neurol. 2022;29(3):910–20.
41. Chen J, Wasmund SL, Hamdan MH. Back to the future: the role of the autonomic nervous system in atrial fibrillation. Pacing Clin Electrophysiol. 2006;29(4):413–21.
42. Melek IM, Seyfeli E, Duru M, Duman T, Akgul F, Yalcin F. Autonomic dysfunction and cardiac repolarization abnormalities in patients with migraine attacks. Med Sci Monit. 2007;13(3):RA47–9.
43. Mohanty S, Mohanty P, Rutledge JN, Di Biase L, Yan RX, Trivedi C, et al. Effect of catheter ablation and periprocedural anticoagulation regimen on the clinical course of migraine in atrial fibrillation patients with or without pre-existent migraine. Circ Arrhythm Electrophysiol. 2015;8(2):279–87.
44. Kato Y, Hayashi T, Kato R, Takao M. Migraine-like headache after transseptal puncture for catheter ablation: a case report and review of the literature. Intern Med. 2019;58(16):2393–5.
45. Schürks M, Buring JE, Ridker PM, Chasman DI, Kurth T. Genetic determinants of cardiovascular events among women with migraine: a genome-wide association study. PLoS One. 2011;6(7):e22106.
46. Malik R, Freilinger T, Winsvold BS, Anttila V, Vander Heiden J, Traylor M, et al. Shared genetic basis for migraine and ischemic stroke: a genome-wide analysis of common variants. Neurology. 2015;84(21):2132–45.
47. Winsvold BS, Nelson CP, Malik R, Gormley P, Anttila V, Vander Heiden J, et al. Genetic analysis for a shared biological basis between migraine and coronary artery disease. Neurol Genet. 2015;1(1):e10.
48. Daghlas I, Guo Y, Chasman DI. Effect of genetic liability to migraine on coronary artery disease and atrial fibrillation: a Mendelian randomization study. Eur J Neurol. 2020;27(3):550–6.
49. Daghals I, Sargurupremraj M, Danning R, Gormley P, Malik R, Amouyel P, et al. Migraine, stroke, and cervical arterial dissection: shared genetics for a triad of brain disorders with vascular involvement. Neurol Genet. 2022;8(1):e653.

50. de Boer I, van den Maagdenberg AMJM, Terwindt GM. Advance in genetics of migraine. Curr Opin Neurol. 2019;32(3):413–21.
51. Mulder IA, Rubio-Beltran E, Ibrahimi K, Dzyubachyk O, Khmelinskii A, Hoehn M, et al. Increased mortality and vascular phenotype in a Knock-in mouse model of retinal vasculopathy with cerebral leukoencephalopathy and systemic manifestations. Stroke. 2020;51(1):300–7.
52. Pelzer N, Stam AH, Haan J, Ferrari MD, Terwindt GM. Familial and sporadic hemiplegic migraine: diagnosis and treatment. Curr Treat Options Neurol. 2013;15(1):13–27.
53. Staehr C, Rohde PD, Krarup NT, Ringgaard S, Laustsen C, Johnsen J, et al. Migraine-associated mutation in the Na, K-ATPase leads to disturbances in cardiac metabolism and reduced cardiac function. J Am Heart Assoc. 2022;11(7):e021814.
54. Friberg L, Olesen J, Lassen NA, Olsen TS, Karle A. Cerebral oxygen extraction, oxygen consumption, and regional cerebral blood flow during the aura phase of migraine. Stroke. 1994;25(5):974–9.
55. Bousser MG, Welch KMA. Relation between migraine and stroke. Lancet Neurol. 2005;4(9):533–42.
56. Yemisci M, Eikermann-Haerter K. Aura and Stroke: relationship and what we have learnt from preclinical models. J Headache Pain. 2019;20(1):63.
57. Tietjen GE, Collins SA. Hypercoagulability and migraine. Headache. 2018;58(1):173–83.
58. Fahmy EM, Hamdy MSE, Mahmoud RM, Elshebawy H. Association between blood coagulability and migraine. Egypt J Neurol Psychiatry Neurosurg. 2022;58(1):1–7.
59. Rundek T, Elkind MSV, Di Tullio MR, Carrera E, Jin Z, Sacco RL, et al. Patent foramen ovale and migraine: a cross-sectional study from the northern Manhattan study (NOMAS). Circulation. 2008;118(14):1419–24.
60. Takagi H, Umemoto T. ALICE (all-literature investigation of cardiovascular evidence) group. A meta-analysis of case-control studies of the association of migraine and patent foramen ovale. J Cardiol. 2016;67(6):493–503.
61. Pezzini A, Grassi M, Lodigiani C, Patella R, Gandolfo C, Casoni F, et al. Predictors of migraine subtypes in young adults with ischemic stroke: the Italian Project on Stroke in young adults. Stroke. 2011;42(1):17–21.
62. Mattle HP, Evers S, Hildick-Smith D, Becker WJ, Baumgartner H, Chataway J, et al. Percutaneous closure of patent foramen ovale in migraine with aura, a randomized controlled trial. Eur Heart J. 2016;37(26):2029–36.
63. Dowson A, Mullen MJ, Peatfield R, Muir K, Khan AA, Wells C, et al. Migraine intervention with STARFlex technology (MIST) trial. Circulation. 2008;117(11):1397–404.
64. Tobis JM, Charles A, Silberstein SD, Sorensen S, Maini B, Horwitz PA, et al. Percutaneous closure of patent foramen ovale in patients with migraine: the PREMIUM trial. J Am Coll Cardiol. 2017;70(22):2766–74.
65. Edvinsson L, Haanes KA, Warfvinge K. Does inflammation have a role in migraine? Nat Rev Neurol. 2019;15(8):483–90.
66. Kurth T, Ridker PM, Buring JE. Migraine and biomarkers of cardiovascular disease in women. Cephalalgia. 2008;28(1):49–56.
67. Acarsoy C, Ruiter R, Bos D, Ikram MK. No association between blood-based markers of immune system and migraine status: a population-based cohort study. BMC Neurol. 2023;23(1):445.
68. Shao M, Lin X, Jiang D, Tian H, Xu Y, Wang L, et al. Depression and cardiovascular disease: shared molecular mechanisms and clinical implications. Psychiatry Res. 2020;285:112802.
69. de Vries LS, Louter MA, van Oosterhout W, van Zwet EW, van Noorden MS, Terwindt GM. Depressive symptoms during the different phases of a migraine attack: a prospective diary study. J Affect Disord. 2022;297:502–7.
70. Khafagy R, Dash S. Obesity and cardiovascular disease: the emerging role of inflammation. Front Cardiovasc Med. 2021;8:768119.
71. Peres MFP, Lerário DDG, Garrido AB, Zukerman E. Primary headaches in obese patients. Arq Neuropsiquiatr. 2005;63(4):931–3.
72. Hippisley-Cox J, Coupland C, Brindle P. Development and validation of QRISK3 risk prediction algorithms to estimate future risk of cardiovascular disease: prospective cohort study. BMJ. 2017;357:j2099.
73. Visseren FLJ, Mach F, Smulders YM, Carballo D, Koskinas KC, Bäck M, et al. 2021 ESC guidelines on cardiovascular disease prevention in clinical practice. Eur Heart J. 2021;42(34):3227–337.
74. Sacco S, Kurth T. Migraine and the risk for stroke and cardiovascular disease. Curr Cardiol Rep. 2014;16(9):524.
75. Kurth T, Diener HC. Migraine and stroke: perspectives for stroke physicians. Stroke. 2012;43(12):3421–6.
76. Kurth T, Rist PM, Ridker PM, Kotler G, Bubes V, Buring JE. Association of migraine with aura and other risk factors with incident cardiovascular disease in women. JAMA. 2020;323(22):2281–9.
77. Mosek A, Marom R, Korczyn AD, Bornstein N. A history of migraine is not a risk factor to develop an ischemic stroke in the elderly. Headache. 2001;41(4):399–401.
78. Acarsoy C, Fani L, Al-Hassany L, Berghout B, Koudstaal PJ, Maassen Van Den Brink A, et al. Migraine and the risk of stroke in a middle-aged and elderly population: a prospective cohort study. Cephalalgia. 2023;43(1):3331024221132008.
79. Androulakis XM, Sen S, Kodumuri N, Zhang T, Grego J, Rosamond W, et al. Migraine age of onset and association with ischemic stroke in

late life: 20 years follow-up in ARIC. Headache. 2019;59(4):556–66.
80. Wang JC, Bennett M. Aging and atherosclerosis: mechanisms, functional consequences, and potential therapeutics for cellular senescence. Circ Res. 2012;111(2):245–59.
81. Tzourio C, Tehindrazanarivelo A, Iglésias S, Alpérovitch A, Chedru F, d'Anglejan-Chatillon J, et al. Case-control study of migraine and risk of ischaemic stroke in young women. BMJ. 1995;310(6983):830–3.
82. Chang CL, Donaghy M, Poulter N. Migraine and stroke in young women: case-control study. The World Health Organisation collaborative study of cardiovascular disease and steroid hormone contraception. BMJ. 1999;318(7175):13–8.
83. Sacco S, Merki-Feld GS, Ægidius KL, Bitzer J, Canonico M, Kurth T, et al. Hormonal contraceptives and risk of ischemic stroke in women with migraine: a consensus statement from the European headache federation (EHF) and the European Society of Contraception and Reproductive Health (ESC). J Headache Pain. 2017;18(1):108.
84. Henrich JB, Horwitz RI. A controlled study of ischemic stroke risk in migraine patients. J Clin Epidemiol. 1989;42(8):773–80.
85. MacClellan LR, Giles W, Cole J, Wozniak M, Stern B, Mitchell BD, et al. Probable migraine with visual aura and risk of ischemic stroke: the stroke prevention in young women study. Stroke. 2007;38(9):2438–45.
86. Wang YF, Wang SJ. Hypertension and migraine: time to revisit the evidence. Curr Pain Headache Rep. 2021;25(9):58.
87. Salmasi M, Amini L, Javanmard SH, Saadatnia M. Metabolic syndrome in migraine headache: a case-control study. J Res Med Sci. 2014;19(1):13–7.
88. Rivera-Mancilla E, Al-Hassany L, Villalón CM, Maassen Van Den Brink A. Metabolic aspects of migraine: association with obesity and diabetes mellitus. Front Neurol. 2021;12:686398.
89. López-De-Andrés A, Del Barrio JL, Hernández-Barrera V, De Miguel-Díez J, Jimenez-Trujillo I, Martinez-Huedo MA, et al. Migraine in adults with diabetes; is there an association? Results of a population-based study. Diabetes Metab Syndr Obes. 2018;11:367–74.
90. Kurth T, Winter AC, Eliassen AH, Dushkes R, Mukamal KJ, Rimm EB, et al. Migraine and risk of cardiovascular disease in women: prospective cohort study. BMJ. 2016;353:i2610.
91. Fava A, Pirritano D, Consoli D, Plastino M, Casalinuovo F, Cristofaro S, et al. Chronic migraine in women is associated with insulin resistance: a cross-sectional study. Eur J Neurol. 2014;21(2):267–72.
92. Ojha P, Malhotra V. Implication of high body fat percentage on migraine Chronification in premenopausal females. Neurol Res Int. 2022;2022:8219254.
93. Kurth T, Schürks M, Logroscino G, Buring JE. Migraine frequency and risk of cardiovascular disease in women. Neurology. 2009;73(8):581–8.
94. Donaghy M, Chang CL, Poulter N. European collaborators of the World Health Organisation collaborative study of cardiovascular disease and steroid hormone contraception. Duration, frequency, recency, and type of migraine and the risk of ischaemic stroke in women of childbearing age. J Neurol Neurosurg Psychiatry. 2002;73(6):747–50.
95. Al-Hashel JY, Alroughani R, Gad K, Al-Sarraf L, Ahmed SF. Risk factors of white matter hyperintensities in migraine patients. BMC Neurol. 2022;22(1):159.
96. Arkink EB, Palm-Meinders IH, Koppen H, Milles J, van Lew B, Launer LJ, et al. Microstructural white matter changes preceding white matter hyperintensities in migraine. Neurology. 2019;93(7):e688–94.
97. Kalkman DN, Couturier EGM, El Bouziani A, Dahdal J, Neefs J, Woudstra J, et al. Migraine and cardiovascular disease: what cardiologists should know. Eur Heart J. 2023;44(30):2815–28.
98. Favoni V, Giani L, Al-Hassany L, Asioli GM, Butera C, de Boer I, et al. CGRP and migraine from a cardiovascular point of view: what do we expect from blocking CGRP? J Headache Pain. 2019;20(1):27.
99. Benseñor IM, Cook NR, Lee IM, Chown MJ, Hennekens CH, Buring JE. Low-dose aspirin for migraine prophylaxis in women. Cephalalgia. 2001;21(3):175–83.
100. Kurth T, Diener HC, Buring JE. Migraine and cardiovascular disease in women and the role of aspirin: subgroup analyses in the Women's Health Study. Cephalalgia. 2011;31(10):1106–15.
101. Diener HC, Hartung E, Chrubasik J, Evers S, Schoenen J, Eikermann A, et al. A comparative study of oral acetylsalicyclic acid and metoprolol for the prophylactic treatment of migraine. A randomized, controlled, double-blind, parallel group phase III study. Cephalalgia. 2001;21(2):120–8.
102. Agbetou M, Adoukonou T. Lifestyle modifications for migraine management. Front Neurol. 2022;13:719467.
103. Facchinetti F, Allais G, Nappi RE, D'Amico R, Marozio L, Bertozzi L, et al. Migraine is a risk factor for hypertensive disorders in pregnancy: a prospective cohort study. Cephalalgia. 2009;29(3):286–92.
104. Sacco S, Carolei A. Burden of atherosclerosis and risk of venous thromboembolism in patients with migraine. Neurology. 2009;72(23):2056–7; author reply 2057.
105. Pezzini A, Grassi M, Lodigiani C, Patella R, Gandolfo C, Zini A, et al. Predictors of long-term recurrent vascular events after ischemic stroke at young age: the Italian project on stroke in young adults. Circulation. 2014;129(16):1668–76.
106. Tietjen GE, Al-Qasmi MM, Shukairy MS. Livedo reticularis and migraine: a marker for stroke risk? Headache. 2002;42(5):352–5.
107. Tietjen GE, Al-Qasmi MM, Gunda P, Herial NA. Sneddon's syndrome: another migraine-stroke association? Cephalalgia. 2006;26(3):225–32.

108. Tietjen GE. Migraine as a systemic vasculopathy. Cephalalgia. 2009;29(9):987–96.
109. Lidegaard Ø, Løkkegaard E, Jensen A, Skovlund CW, Keiding N. Thrombotic stroke and myocardial infarction with hormonal contraception. N Engl J Med. 2012;366(24):2257–66.
110. Sacco S, Merki-Feld GS, Ægidius KL, Bitzer J, Canonico M, Gantenbein AR, et al. Effect of exogenous estrogens and progestogens on the course of migraine during reproductive age: a consensus statement by the European headache federation (EHF) and the European Society of Contraception and Reproductive Health (ESCRH). J Headache Pain. 2018;19(1):76. http://www.embase.com/search/results?subaction=viewrecord&from=export&id=L623688022.
111. Sheikh HU, Pavlovic J, Loder E, Burch R. Risk of stroke associated with use of estrogen containing contraceptives in women with migraine: a systematic review. Headache. 2018;58(1):5–21.
112. MacGregor EA. Migraine, menopause and hormone replacement therapy. Post Reprod Health. 2018;24(1):11–8.
113. Facchinetti F, Nappi RE, Tirelli A, Polatti F, Nappi G, Sances G. Hormone supplementation differently affects migraine in postmenopausal women. Headache. 2002;42(9):924–9.
114. Timm FP, Houle TT, Grabitz SD, Lihn AL, Stokholm JB, Eikermann-Haerter K, et al. Migraine and risk of perioperative ischemic stroke and hospital readmission: hospital based registry study. BMJ. 2017;356:i6635. http://www.embase.com/search/results?subaction=viewrecord&from=export&id=L614047569.
115. Scher AI, Wang SJ, Katsarava Z, Buse DC, Fanning KM, Adams AM, et al. Epidemiology of migraine in men: results from the chronic migraine epidemiology and outcomes (CaMEO) study. Cephalalgia. 2019;39(2):296–305.
116. Kurth T, Gaziano JM, Cook NR, Bubes V, Logroscino G, Diener HC, et al. Migraine and risk of cardiovascular disease in men. Arch Intern Med. 2007;167(8):795–801.
117. Schürks M, Rist PM, Bigal ME, Buring JE, Lipton RB, Kurth T. Migraine and cardiovascular disease: systematic review and meta-analysis. BMJ. 2009;339:b3914.
118. Mahmoud AN, Mentias A, Elgendy AY, Qazi A, Barakat AF, Saad M, et al. Migraine and the risk of cardiovascular and cerebrovascular events: a meta-analysis of 16 cohort studies including 1 152 407 subjects. BMJ Open. 2018;8(3):e020498.
119. Kurth T, Rohmann JL. Studying migraine as a risk factor for stroke: the importance of working with an explicit causal framework. Cephalalgia. 2023;43(1):3331024221132007.
120. Al-Hassany L, Verdonk P, VanDenBrink AM. Studying sex and gender in neurological disease. Lancet Neurol. 2023;22(1):32–3.

Rheumatic and Autoimmune Disorders and CVD Risk in Women

Helga Midtbø and Marie Wahren-Herlenius

Abstract

Rheumatic diseases are musculoskeletal diseases, of which most, but not all are also autoimmune. Rheumatic and autoimmune diseases are more common in women than in men. The general risk of cardiovascular (CV) disease (CVD) is increased in patients with rheumatic disorders with a factor of 1.5 in both women and men, but the CVD risk varies across the different diseases. The increased CVD risk is related to a combination of high prevalence of traditional CV risk factors, adverse effects of medication, and presence of chronic systemic inflammation. Reduction of inflammation is beneficial in this patient group and antirheumatic therapy has been associated with reduced CVD risk. Corticosteroids and non-steroid anti-inflammatory drugs should be used with caution. Awareness of CVD risk is vital in this patient group as CV risk scores developed for the general population do not fully capture the CV risk. Management of traditional CV risk factors should be done in accordance with national guidelines and is important for improved CV prognosis.

Keywords

Autoimmunity · Rheumatic diseases
Cardiovascular risk · Anti-rheumatic therapy

Test your learning and check your understanding of this book's contents: use the "Springer Nature Flashcards" app to access questions using ▶ https://sn.pub/51ny7m
To use the app, please follow the instructions in chapter 1.

H. Midtbø (✉)
Department of Clinical Science, Center for Research on Cardiac Disease in Women, University of Bergen, Bergen, Norway

Department of Heart Disease, Haukeland University Hospital, Bergen, Norway
e-mail: helga.midtbo@uib.no

M. Wahren-Herlenius
Division of Rheumatology, Department of Medicine, Karolinska Institutet, Stockholm, Sweden

Broegelmann Research Laboratory, Department of Clinical Science, University of Bergen, Bergen, Norway
e-mail: marie.wahren@ki.se

A. H.E.M. Maas, E. Gerdts (eds.), *Manual of Cardiovascular Disease in Women*,
https://doi.org/10.1007/978-3-031-65952-2_14

1 Introduction

Rheumatic and autoimmune diseases are more common in women than in men and associated with increased risk of cardiovascular (CV) disease (CVD) [1–3]. Rheumatic diseases are an umbrella term covering over 100 diseases of the joints, tendons, ligaments, and muscle, but systemic variants may also affect inner organs [4]. Most, but not all, rheumatic diseases are also autoimmune diseases [5]. Autoimmune diseases are characterized by loss of immunological tolerance to self and the presence of autoantibodies and autoreactive T cells. These auto-reactive lymphocytes cause tissue damage leading to diseases such as arthritis [5]. Autoimmune diseases include a wide range of over 70 diseases, but chronic inflammation may also occur without an autoimmune component [6]. Thus, the term chronic inflammatory diseases are used as a broader term for diseases where inflammation and dysregulation of the immune system is central in the pathogenesis and covers both autoimmune and rheumatic diseases. Although many individual rheumatic and autoimmune diseases are rare, their combined prevalence is high, affecting up to 5–9% of the adult population [6, 7].

Rheumatic autoimmune diseases have systemic manifestations beyond the primary affected organs [8]. Although cardiac and arterial manifestations have been recognized for decades, it was not until the late 1990ties that the increased risk of CVD was fully recognized [9]. Although all rheumatic inflammatory diseases have increased risk of CVD, this has been most extensively studied for rheumatoid arthritis (RA). In a meta-analysis of observational studies including 41,490 patients with RA, the risk of CVD was increased with 48% [2]. The risk of myocardial infarction was increased by 70% compared to the general population with no differences between men and women. In a Danish nationwide study, the risk of atrial fibrillation was increased with 40% in RA [10]. Thus, in 2016, RA was included as a risk factor for CVD in the European Society of Cardiology guidelines for CVD prevention in clinical practice [11]. The same year the European Alliance of Associations for Rheumatology (EULAR) published their guidelines on CVD prevention in patients with RA and other inflammatory joint diseases [12]. During the last 10 years, new observational studies have indicated that the excess risk of CVD in patients with RA is declining [13–15], which has been attributed to improvements in arthritis treatment, especially the use of biological disease modifying antirheumatic drugs (bDMARDs).

2 Theory

2.1 Why Are There Sex Differences in Rheumatic Autoimmune Diseases?

There is a well-known female predominance in the prevalence of autoimmune and rheumatic diseases. This is most noted in primary Sjögren's syndrome, systemic lupus erythematous, autoimmune thyroid disease, and scleroderma where over 80% of patients are women [3]. It is also recognized that women and men have differences in risk factors, disease presentation, comorbidities, and outcome in rheumatic and autoimmune diseases. The mechanisms behind these sex-differences are complex and multifactorial, although incomplete understood. Differences in immune function are thought to be central [5]. Females usually have stronger immune response than men, observed in e.g., higher vaccine-specific antibody titers following vaccination, which could increase the susceptibility to autoimmune diseases [16]. On the other hand, the female immune system is capable to adapt during pregnancy to a less reactive state, to allow the fetus to coexist with the mother [3]. This could also explain why some autoimmune diseases such as RA and multiple sclerosis tend to improve during pregnancy. Differences in sex-hormones have also been proposed [17]. Oestrogen has been shown to promote inflammation through an enhanced immune response, while testosterone could have immunosuppressive effects [18]. Also, genetic factors, and in particular the sex chromosomes, have been implicated in the development of autoimmune diseases. Several genes encoding proteins with immune functions are located on the X chromosome. Notably, around 20% of genes on the X chromosome escape X inactivation, leading to a higher gene dosage in females which again could increase susceptibility to autoimmunity [18]. Environmental factors, like smoking and infections are also implied in the pathogenesis of rheumatic and autoimmune disease and could contribute to the observed sex-differences [17]. Taken together, sex-differences in autoimmune and rheumatic diseases are complex and the underlying mechanism may vary between different diseases.

2.2 What Are the Mechanisms Behind the Increased Risk for CVD?

The increased risk of CVD in rheumatic and autoimmune diseases is multifactorial. There is substantial overlap in genetic susceptibility between autoimmune diseases, but an overlap with genetic risk factors for CVD is less obvious [19]. Rather, the chronic and systemic inflammation associated with immune dysregulation is believed to be the main cause of the observed excess CVD risk in rheumatic autoimmune diseases, in combination with traditional CV risk factors and adverse effects of medication [1, 20].

2.3 Prevalence of CV Risk Factors in Autoimmune and Rheumatic Diseases

The prevalence of traditional CV risk factors including smoking, dyslipidemia, hypertension, diabetes mellitus and obesity are increased in many rheumatic autoimmune diseases. Among 502, 649 participants in UK Biobank, the risk of hypertension was 19% higher and diabetes 18% higher in patients with RA compared to the general population [21]. In an American database study of 33,117 patients with RA, psoriasis arthritis or ankylosing spondylitis, the risk of type 2 diabetes, hyperlipidaemia and hypertension was increased by 20–50% compared to the matched control group [22]. There is, however, heterogeneity between studies especially regarding the prevalence of hypertension [23]. The excess systemic inflammation in rheumatic autoimmune diseases could modify CV risk factors such as blood pressure. In addition, rheumatic diseases could lead to inactivity and predispose for overweight, but also rheumatic cachexia which again affects traditional CV risk factors [20]. Inflammation also lowers the lipid levels in inflammatory diseases, thus patients with low lipid levels could have high CVD risk, referred to as the lipid paradox [24]. Smoking is a shared risk factor for development of both rheumatic autoimmune diseases, but the prevalence of smoking is declining both among patients with rheumatic autoimmune diseases and in the general population [8].

2.4 Chronic Inflammation

In patients with autoimmune diseases, it well documented that the excess risk of CVD is not only due to CV risk factors. In a recent population-based study of 19 autoimmune diseases in 22 million individuals in the UK, having any autoimmune disease was associated with a 56% increased risk of CVD [1]. The risk of CVD was highest in patients with systemic sclerosis, systemic lupus erythematosus and in Sjögren's syndrome where there was a two to threefold increased risk of CVD. The excess CVD risk was higher in younger individuals, and the risk was the same in women and men. Further, autoimmune diseases were associated with an increased prevalence of all types of CVD examined including aortic aneurysm, atrial fibrillation, heart failure, myocarditis, pericarditis, and venous thromboembolism. Of note, in adjusted sensitivity analyses, traditional CV risk factors only slightly attenuated the excess CVD risk observed. Several studies in patients with RA have demonstrated that the CVD risk is associated with the degree of RA disease activity and inflammation. In 24,989 patients with RA followed for 2.7 years by the Consortium of Rheumatology Researchers of North America, reduction in RA disease activity was found to be associated with fewer CVD events, after adjusting for CVD risk factors and medication [25]. Similarly, in a population-based cohort of 525 patients with RA, the CVD risk of RA patients in remission was similar to the control subjects without RA, while patients with RA flares had significantly higher CVD risk [26].

Also in the general population, chronic inflammation is well known to be associated with increased risk of CVD. In the Women's Health Study performed in 28 thousand apparently healthy, postmenopausal women, having CRP in the highest quartile was associated with a 50% increased risk of CVD compared to those with CPR in the lowest quartile [27]. In a substudy of the Women's Health Study, women on hormone replacement therapy, Black women and women with increased body mass index had the highest levels of CRP [28]. Other biomarkers of inflammation, such as serum amyloid A, interleukins and fibrinogen has also been associated with increased CVD risk, although CRP is by far the most studied and most robust biomarker of inflammation in CVD risk assessment [29].

3 Clinical Practice

3.1 Management of CV Risk Factors

Optimal management of traditional CVD risk factors in patients with rheumatic autoimmune diseases is important. Lifestyle advice including physical activity, healthy diet and smoking cessation is advised in all patients [12]. Antihypertensive and lipid-lowering treatment should be initiated according to national guidelines, as there is no conclusive evidence that this patient group benefits from a different primary prevention strategy. It is important to be aware that traditional risk scores underestimate the CVD risk in patients with rheumatic autoimmune diseases. Considerable work has been done to establish CVD risk scores specific for RA, but the results have been somewhat disappointing [12, 20]. Several of the established CV risk scores include RA as a risk modifier, but if this is not the case, EULAR recommends using a 1.5 multiplication factor to calculate CVD risk in RA patients [12].

Lipid-lowering treatment has been found to be underused as primary prevention in RA patients. In a multinational survey of 14,503 RA patients, 52% of patients had indication for lipid-lowering treatment, but only 44% were on therapy [30]. The use of statins as primary prevention in all patients with RA was investigated in the randomized controlled TRACE-RA trial [31]. Comparing atorvastatin with placebo, the trial was stopped early due to low cardiovascular event rates. However, the use of statins was associated with a 34% reduction in CVD events. Although not significant, these results are in line with estimated risk reduction of statin therapy in the general population.

Management of hypertension is often suboptimal in patients with rheumatic autoimmune diseases. In the multinational survey of CVD risk factors in RA, only 50% of the hypertensive patients were treated to their BP target [30]. Use of ambulatory BP is little studied in this patient group, but one study of 214 RA patients suggests that the awareness and control of hypertension is poor, and that ambulatory BP measurements is associated with an increased detection rate of hypertension [32]. If there is doubt as to whether antihypertensive treatment should be initiated, referral to echocardiography for detection of hypertension-mediated cardiac organ damage could be indicated [33]. The prevalence of cardiac organ damage is higher in patients with rheumatic organ damage, independent of traditional CVD risk factors including hypertension [34, 35]. Presence of cardiac organ damage is associated with high CVD risk, and antihypertensive treatment is indicated in this group [33].

3.2 Management of Clinical CVD

In patients with rheumatic and autoimmune diseases, clinical CVD should be managed as in the general population. A study of 1135 RA patients showed that the short-term mortality in acute coronary syndromes was 40% higher in RA patients compared to controls [36]. Change or pause in anti-rheumatic medication might be indicated during CVD admissions, and it is recommended that management of anti-rheumatic medication is done in close cooperation with the treating rheumatologist. Specific considerations regarding the different anti-rheumatic medications are detailed below.

3.3 Management of Anti-Rheumatic Medication in Regard to CVD Risk

Anti-rheumatic drug therapy could influence the CVD risk. There is agreement that lowering the inflammatory load and disease activity is beneficial for CVD risk, in particular the risk of atherosclerotic CVD. Observational data indicated that DMARD treatment is beneficial, but therapies with glucocorticoids or non-steroidal anti-inflammatory drugs (NSAIDs) could be harmful [37, 38].

3.3.1 Glucocorticoids

Glucocorticoids remain central to manage acute flares and exacerbations in inflammatory diseases. However, they have side effects that are harmful to the CV system including weight gain, increased blood pressure and blood glucose levels. A recent population-based registry study of 87,794 patients with immune-mediated inflammatory diseases and no prior CVD, showed that even doses as low as <5 mg daily prednisolone equivalent dose, was associated with a doubled absolute risk of CVD, including atrial fibrillation, heart failure and myocardial infarction [39]. For patients using 25 mg or higher doses, the risk of CVD was 6 times higher. Thus, it is recommended to use the minimal effective dose of glucocorticoids for the shortest possible duration.

3.3.2 NSAIDs

NSAIDs are associated with increased CVD risk in the general population as well as in patients with rheumatic and autoimmune diseases. In a nation-wide Danish registry study, the excess risk of CVD was lower in RA patients compared to the general population, possible because of a reduction in inflammation in RA patients [40]. NSAIDs could increase bleeding risk and interact negatively with antiplatelet therapy. It is recommended to use NSAIDs with caution, especially in persons with increased CVD risk or established CVD.

3.3.3 DMARDs

Several non-randomized studies in patients with RA have demonstrated a favorable association between anti-rheumatic treatment and CVD events. In a meta-analysis from 2015 of eight observational studies, methotrexate use was associated with a 21% reduced risk of CVD [38]. Another meta-analysis using observational data, demonstrated that the use of tumor necrosis factor-α (TNF) inhibitors was associated with a 54% reduction of CVD events [37]. Safety studies comparing the effect of the interleukin-6 inhibitor tocilizumab with TNF inhibitor treatment showed similar CVD event rate in the two groups, although blood lipids were higher with tocilizumab treatment [41]. The janus kinase inhibitor tofacitinib, failed to reach noninferiority criteria when compared to treatment with a TNF inhibitor, and tofacitinib was associated with 33% higher risk of major CV events compared to TNF inhibitor treatment [42]. To date there are no randomized clinical trials demonstrating the effectiveness of anti-rheumatic therapy on CVD outcomes in patients with autoimmune rheumatic diseases.

3.4 Anti-Inflammatory Medication and CVD in the General Population

In the general population, several randomized clinical trials have studied whether reduction of inflammation can result in reduction of CVD. The Canakinumab Anti-inflammatory Thrombosis Outcome Study tested if canakinumab, an interleukin-1β inhibitor, could prevent recurrent CVD events in 10, 061 patients with previous myocardial infarction and a persistent proinflammatory response [43].

After a median follow-up of 3.7 years, treatment with canakinumab was associated with a 15% percent reduction in the prevalence of myocardial infarction, ischemic stroke, and CV death. Treatment with canakinumab did not reduce all-cause mortality and was associated with increased risk of severe infections. Colchicine is an old drug with a broad cellular anti-inflammatory effect. In the Colchicine Cardiovascular outcome trials (COLCOT) almost 5000 patients were randomized to colchicine or placebo as secondary prevention after myocardial infarction [44]. Treatment with colchicine was associated with a 23% reduction of the primary endpoint of CVD death, cardiac arrest, myocardial infarction, stroke, or revascularization of unstable angina. Similar favorable results with colchicine treatment for patients with chronic coronary disease was demonstrated in the low-dose colchicine trial [45]. Cardiovascular Inflammation Reduction Trial (CIRT) tested if treatment with low-dose methotrexate was associated with lower prevalence of CVD in almost 5000 patients with established coronary artery disease and concomitant type 2 diabetes or metabolic syndrome [46]. Treatment with methotrexate was not associated with a reduction in CVD but resulted in increased prevalence of adverse events such as non-basal-cells skin cancers compared to placebo. Treatment with anti-inflammatory medication has also been attempted for heart failure. In heart failure, levels of TNF are increased in proportion to the severity of the disease. In the Anti-TNF Therapy Against Congestive Heart failure (ATTACH) Trial, 150 patients with stable heart failure and ejection fraction ≤35% were randomized to treatment with the TNF inhibitor infliximab or placebo [47]. After 28 weeks of treatment, the risk of heart failure hospitalization or all-cause mortality was increased with infliximab treatment. Summarized, these trials demonstrate that anti-inflammatory treatment is associated with a reduction in atherosclerotic CVD. The Food and Drug Administration (FDA) recently approved the use of colchicine as CVD prevention in patients with established atherosclerotic disease or multiple CV risk factors. However, the clinical benefit of other types of anti-inflammatory treatment for CVD prevention in patients without other indications for anti-inflammatory treatment is hampered by side effects and drug cost.

4 Conclusions

Autoimmune and rheumatic diseases affect women more than men. In both genders, the risk of CVD is increased with a factor of 1.5 and the highest CVD risk is found in patients with systemic sclerosis and systemic lupus erythematosus. The increased CVD risk is multifactorial and associated with inflammatory load and disease activity, traditional CV risk factors and medication. Awareness of CVD risk, management of CV risk factors and reduction of inflammation is central for improving the CVD risk and outcome in patients with autoimmune rheumatic diseases (Fig. 1).

Key Issues

- Autoimmune and rheumatic diseases are more prevalent in women than in men.
- The risk of atherosclerotic CVD is increased in autoimmune and rheumatic diseases with a factor of about 1.5, but the risk varies according to disease type.
- The prevalence of traditional CV risk factors is high.

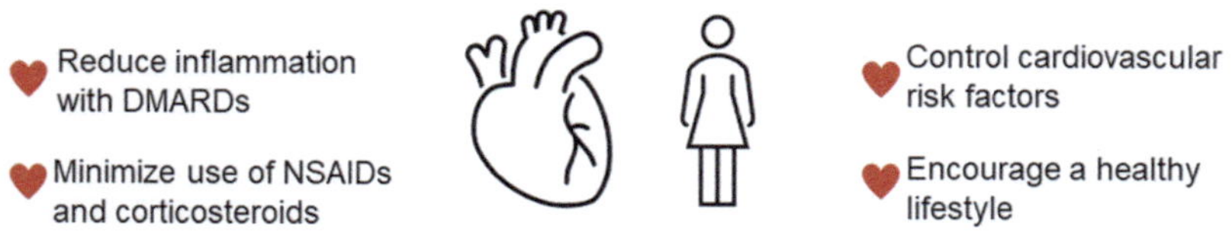

Fig. 1 Management of CVD risk in rheumatic autoimmune diseases. *CVD* cardiovascular disease, *DMARDs* disease modifying antirheumatic drugs, *NSAIDs* nonsteroidal anti-inflammatory drugs

- Management of CV risk factors is vital for improvement of CV risk and should follow national guidelines.
- Reduction of inflammation is positive for CVD risk, and antirheumatic medication is considered beneficial for CVD risk in observational studies.
- Treatment with glucocorticoids and NSAIDs could be harmful.

Questions and Answers

1. Sex-differences in rheumatic autoimmune diseases are related to
   (A) Differences in the musculoskeletal system
   (B) Genetic factors linked to gene expression of joints, tendons, ligaments and bones
   (C) Multifactorial and incompletely understood involving the immune system, sex hormones and genetic factors
   Correct answer: C
2. The excess CVD risk in rheumatic autoimmune diseases is mostly related to
   (A) High prevalence of traditional CV risk factors in combination with excess systemic inflammation
   (B) Mostly related to side effects of antirheumatic medication
   (C) Mostly related to a high prevalence of smoking and poor diet
   Correct answer: A
3. What is correct regarding anti-inflammatory treatment and CVD
   (A) Randomized clinical trials have shown reduction in CVD risk with DMARD treatment in patients with rheumatic autoimmune diseases
   (B) NSAID treatment is more harmful for CVD risk in patients with RA than in the general population
   (C) Colchicine has been approved for CV prevention in patients with established CVD or multiple CV risk factors
   Correct answer: C

References

1. Conrad N, Verbeke G, Molenberghs G, Goetschalckx L, Callender T, Cambridge G, et al. Autoimmune diseases and cardiovascular risk: a population-based study on 19 autoimmune diseases and 12 cardiovascular diseases in 22 million individuals in the UK. Lancet. 2022;400(10354):733–43.
2. Avina-Zubieta JA, Thomas J, Sadatsafavi M, Lehman AJ, Lacaille D. Risk of incident cardiovascular events in patients with rheumatoid arthritis: a meta-analysis of observational studies. Ann Rheum Dis. 2012;71(9):1524–9.
3. Whitacre CC. Sex differences in autoimmune disease. Nat Immunol. 2001;2(9):777–80.
4. WHO. Musculoskeletal health 2022. https://www.who.int/news-room/fact-sheets/detail/musculoskeletal-conditions.
5. Szekanecz Z, McInnes IB, Schett G, Szamosi S, Benkő S, Szűcs G. Autoinflammation and autoimmunity across rheumatic and musculoskeletal diseases. Nat Rev Rheumatol. 2021;17(10):585–95.
6. Davidson A, Diamond B. Autoimmune diseases. N Engl J Med. 2001;345(5):340–50.
7. Cooper GS, Bynum ML, Somers EC. Recent insights in the epidemiology of autoimmune diseases: improved prevalence estimates and understanding of clustering of diseases. J Autoimmun. 2009;33(3–4):197–207.
8. Scott DL, Wolfe F, Huizinga TW. Rheumatoid arthritis. Lancet. 2010;376(9746):1094–108.
9. Peters MJ, van Halm VP, Voskuyl AE, Smulders YM, Boers M, Lems WF, et al. Does rheumatoid arthritis equal diabetes mellitus as an independent risk factor for cardiovascular disease? A prospective study. Arthritis Rheum. 2009;61(11):1571–9.
10. Lindhardsen J, Ahlehoff O, Gislason GH, Madsen OR, Olesen JB, Svendsen JH, et al. Risk of atrial fibrillation and stroke in rheumatoid arthritis: Danish nationwide cohort study. BMJ. 2012;344:e1257.
11. Piepoli MF, Hoes AW, Agewall S, Albus C, Brotons C, Catapano AL, et al. 2016 European Guidelines on cardiovascular disease prevention in clinical practice. Eur Heart J. 2016;37(29):2315–81.
12. Agca R, Heslinga SC, Rollefstad S, Heslinga M, McInnes IB, Peters MJ, et al. EULAR recommendations for cardiovascular disease risk management in patients with rheumatoid arthritis and other forms of inflammatory joint disorders: 2015/2016 update. Ann Rheum Dis. 2016;76:17–28.
13. Myasoedova E, Gabriel SE, Matteson EL, Davis JM 3rd, Therneau TM, Crowson CS. Decreased cardiovascular mortality in patients with incident rheumatoid arthritis (RA) in recent years: Dawn of a new era in cardiovascular disease in RA? J Rheumatol. 2017;44:732–9.

14. Kerola AM, Nieminen TV, Virta LJ, Kautiainen H, Kerola T, Pohjolainen T, et al. No increased cardiovascular mortality among early rheumatoid arthritis patients: a nationwide register study in 2000-2008. Clin Exp Rheumatol. 2015;33(3):391–8.
15. Alsing CL, Nystad TW, Igland J, Gjesdal CG, Midtbø H, Tell GS, et al. Trends in the occurrence of ischaemic heart disease over time in rheumatoid arthritis: 1821 patients from 1972 to 2017. Scand J Rheumatol. 2023;52(3):233–42.
16. Fischinger S, Boudreau CM, Butler AL, Streeck H, Alter G. Sex differences in vaccine-induced humoral immunity. Semin Immunopathol. 2019;41(2):239–49.
17. Björk A, Mofors J, Wahren-Herlenius M. Environmental factors in the pathogenesis of primary Sjögren's syndrome. J Intern Med. 2020;287(5):475–92.
18. Taneja V. Sex hormones determine immune response. Front Immunol. 2018;9:1931.
19. Perrotti PP, Aterido A, Fernández-Nebro A, Cañete JD, Ferrándiz C, Tornero J, et al. Genetic variation associated with cardiovascular risk in autoimmune diseases. PLoS One. 2017;12(10):e0185889.
20. Kerola AM, Rollefstad S, Semb AG. Atherosclerotic cardiovascular disease in rheumatoid arthritis: impact of inflammation and antirheumatic treatment. Eur Cardiol. 2021;16:e18.
21. Siebert S, Lyall DM, Mackay DF, Porter D, McInnes IB, Sattar N, et al. Characteristics of rheumatoid arthritis and its association with major comorbid conditions: cross-sectional study of 502 649 UK biobank participants. RMD Open. 2016;2(1):e000267.
22. Han C, Robinson DW, Hackett MV, Paramore LC, Fraeman KH, Bala MV. Cardiovascular disease and risk factors in patients with rheumatoid arthritis, psoriatic arthritis, and ankylosing spondylitis. J Rheumatol. 2006;33(11):2167–72.
23. Kerola AM, Kerola T, Kauppi MJ, Kautiainen H, Virta LJ, Puolakka K, et al. Cardiovascular comorbidities antedating the diagnosis of rheumatoid arthritis. Ann Rheum Dis. 2013;72(11):1826–9.
24. Rollefstad S, Ikdahl E, Hisdal J, Olsen IC, Holme I, Hammer HB, et al. Rosuvastatin-induced carotid plaque regression in patients with inflammatory joint diseases: the Rosuvastatin in rheumatoid arthritis, ankylosing spondylitis and other inflammatory joint diseases study. Arthritis Rheumatol. 2015;67(7):1718–28.
25. Solomon DH, Reed GW, Kremer JM, Curtis JR, Farkouh ME, Harrold LR, et al. Disease activity in rheumatoid arthritis and the risk of cardiovascular events. Arthritis Rheumatol. 2015;67(6):1449–55.
26. Myasoedova E, Chandran A, Ilhan B, Major BT, Michet CJ, Matteson EL, et al. The role of rheumatoid arthritis (RA) flare and cumulative burden of RA severity in the risk of cardiovascular disease. Ann Rheum Dis. 2015;74:245.4–246.
27. Ridker PM, Hennekens CH, Buring JE, Rifai N. C-reactive protein and other markers of inflammation in the prediction of cardiovascular disease in women. N Engl J Med. 2000;342(12):836–43.
28. Albert MA, Glynn RJ, Buring J, Ridker PM. C-reactive protein levels among women of various ethnic groups living in the United States (from the Women's health study). Am J Cardiol. 2004;93(10):1238–42.
29. Libby P, Ridker PM. Inflammation and atherosclerosis: role of C-reactive protein in risk assessment. Am J Med. 2004;116(Suppl 6A):9s–16s.
30. Semb AG, Rollefstad S, Ikdahl E, Wibetoe G, Sexton J, Crowson C, et al. Diabetes mellitus and cardiovascular risk management in patients with rheumatoid arthritis: an international audit. RMD Open. 2021;7(2):e001724.
31. Kitas GD, Nightingale P, Armitage J, Sattar N, Belch JJF, Symmons DPM. A multicenter, randomized, placebo-controlled trial of atorvastatin for the primary prevention of cardiovascular events in patients with rheumatoid arthritis. Arthritis Rheumatol. 2019;71(9):1437–49.
32. Protogerou AD, Panagiotakos DB, Zampeli E, Argyris AA, Arida K, Konstantonis GD, et al. Arterial hypertension assessed "out-of-office" in a contemporary cohort of rheumatoid arthritis patients free of cardiovascular disease is characterized by high prevalence, low awareness, poor control and increased vascular damage-associated "white coat" phenomenon. Arthritis Res Ther. 2013;15(5):R142.
33. Williams B, Mancia G, Spiering W, Agabiti Rosei E, Azizi M, Burnier M, et al. 2018 ESC/ESH guidelines for the management of arterial hypertension. Eur Heart J. 2018;39(33):3021–104.
34. Midtbø H, Gerdts E, Kvien TK, Olsen IC, Hirth A, Davidsen ES, et al. Disease activity and left ventricular structure in patients with rheumatoid arthritis. Rheumatology. 2015;54(3):511–9.
35. Midtbø H, Gerdts E, Berg IJ, Rollefstad S, Jonsson R, Semb AG. Ankylosing spondylitis is associated with increased prevalence of left ventricular hypertrophy. J Rheumatol. 2018;45(9):1249–55.
36. Mantel Ä, Holmqvist M, Jernberg T, Wållberg-Jonsson S, Askling J. Rheumatoid arthritis is associated with a more severe presentation of acute coronary syndrome and worse short-term outcome. Eur Heart J. 2015;36(48):3413–22.
37. Barnabe C, Martin BJ, Ghali WA. Systematic review and meta-analysis: anti-tumor necrosis factor alpha therapy and cardiovascular events in rheumatoid arthritis. Arthritis Care Res. 2011;63(4):522–9.
38. Micha R, Imamura F, Wyler von Ballmoos M, Solomon DH, Hernán MA, Ridker PM, et al. Systematic review and meta-analysis of methotrexate use and risk of cardiovascular disease. Am J Cardiol. 2011;108(9):1362–70.
39. Pujades-Rodriguez M, Morgan AW, Cubbon RM, Wu J. Dose-dependent oral glucocorticoid cardiovascular risks in people with immune-mediated inflammatory diseases: a population-based cohort study. PLoS Med. 2020;17(12):e1003432.

40. Lindhardsen J, Gislason GH, Jacobsen S, Ahlehoff O, Olsen AM, Madsen OR, et al. Non-steroidal anti-inflammatory drugs and risk of cardiovascular disease in patients with rheumatoid arthritis: a nationwide cohort study. Ann Rheum Dis. 2014;73:1515–21.
41. Giles JT, Sattar N, Gabriel S, Ridker PM, Gay S, Warne C, et al. Cardiovascular safety of tocilizumab versus Etanercept in rheumatoid arthritis: a randomized controlled trial. Arthritis Rheumatol. 2020;72(1):31–40.
42. Ytterberg SR, Bhatt DL, Mikuls TR, Koch GG, Fleischmann R, Rivas JL, et al. Cardiovascular and cancer risk with Tofacitinib in rheumatoid arthritis. N Engl J Med. 2022;386(4):316–26.
43. Ridker PM, Everett BM, Thuren T, MacFadyen JG, Chang WH, Ballantyne C, et al. Antiinflammatory therapy with Canakinumab for atherosclerotic disease. N Engl J Med. 2017;377(12):1119–31.
44. Tardif JC, Kouz S, Waters DD, Bertrand OF, Diaz R, Maggioni AP, et al. Efficacy and safety of low-dose colchicine after myocardial infarction. N Engl J Med. 2019;381(26):2497–505.
45. Nidorf SM, Fiolet ATL, Mosterd A, Eikelboom JW, Schut A, Opstal TSJ, et al. Colchicine in patients with chronic coronary disease. N Engl J Med. 2020;383(19):1838–47.
46. Ridker PM, Everett BM, Pradhan A, MacFadyen JG, Solomon DH, Zaharris E, et al. Low-dose methotrexate for the prevention of atherosclerotic events. N Engl J Med. 2019;380(8):752–62.
47. Chung ES, Packer M, Lo KH, Fasanmade AA, Willerson JT. Randomized, double-blind, placebo-controlled, pilot trial of infliximab, a chimeric monoclonal antibody to tumor necrosis factor-alpha, in patients with moderate-to-severe heart failure: results of the anti-TNF therapy against congestive heart failure (ATTACH) trial. Circulation. 2003;107(25):3133–40.

Psychosocial Risk in Women with Heart Disease

Dinah van Schalkwijk, Paula M. C. Mommersteeg, and Nina Kupper

Abstract

Psychosocial risk factors such as chronic stress, depression, anxiety, post-traumatic stress, anger, hostility, and distressed personality increase the risk of acute and chronic ischemic heart diseases (obstructive and non-obstructive), heart failure (HF), and atrial fibrillation (AF). In general, women (with or without heart disease) are particularly vulnerable to the sequelae of stress and show higher prevalence of psychological risk factors compared to men. Important sex differences exist in the physiological stress response and its socio-cultural moderation. These notable differences have enticed the hypothesis that psychological stress may influence cardiovascular health differently in women versus men and therefore also lead to dissimilar cardiovascular risk and illness profiles. It is therefore crucial to take these differences into account in cardiologic clinical practice. The implementation of a comprehensive psychosocial screening instrument and the development of a more women-focused cardiac rehabilitation program, sensitive to women-specific stress-inducing barriers and treatment preferences, are important first steps to address the higher risk and prevalence of psychosocial risk factors in women.

Keywords

Psychosocial risk factors · Sex

Test your learning and check your understanding of this book's contents: use the "Springer Nature Flashcards" app to access questions using ▶ https://sn.pub/51ny7m To use the app, please follow the instructions in chapter 1.

D. van Schalkwijk · P. M. C. Mommersteeg · N. Kupper (✉)
CoRPS—Department of Medical and Clinical Psychology, Tilburg University, Tilburg, The Netherlands
e-mail: h.m.kupper@tilburguniversity.edu

A. H.E.M. Maas, E. Gerdts (eds.), *Manual of Cardiovascular Disease in Women*,
https://doi.org/10.1007/978-3-031-65952-2_15

1 Introduction

When Helen Flanders-Dunbar, an accomplished physician, founded the American Psychosomatic Society, and was the first editor of its journal *Psychosomatic Medicine* in mid-twentieth century, she did so because she believed that psyche and soma were closely connected, and should be clinically addressed in an integrated manner [1]. The same decade, the World Health Organization published a new definition of health, stating that *health is a state of complete physical, mental, and social well-being*. To date, the multidisciplinary biopsychosocial approach to health and disease is still gaining ground and remains essential to understand the dynamic nature of cardiovascular health and disease, to practice patient-centred care, and to develop effective interventions.

Psychological stress is fundamental to life. As Hans Selye, the founder of modern stress theory, explained; stress is a non-specific bodily response to any kind of demand, which can be either negative (distress), or positive (eustress), and includes any disruption of homeostasis (biological or psychological; [2]). Selye provided evidence that stress, through the workings of stress hormones, might cause physical disease, including heart disease [3]. Later theories, such as the seminal theory of Bruce McEwen on allostatic load, provided a more in-depth notion of the health cost of adaptation, in terms of the allostatic process by which chronic stress leads to illness [4].

Since several decades, the importance of studying sex differences in the relationship between stress and cardiovascular disease is acknowledged [5, 6]. Women appear to have greater susceptibility to psychological stress [7, 8], and altered patterns of cardiovascular risk and illness [9, 10]. Biologically, sex differences are present at all stages of stress processing, with differences being evident in perception, appraisal, central and peripheral physiological, and emotional response patterns, as well as in its effects on longer-term cardiovascular pathophysiology and clinical outcomes [11]. These notable differences have enticed the hypothesis that psychological stress may influence cardiovascular health differently in women compared to men and therefore also lead to altered cardiovascular risk and illness profiles.

The current chapter embraces the role of psychological stress in the development and progression of heart disease and highlights the latest state-of-the-art literature on sex differences in this link. We also provide a concise overview of purported psychobiological and sociocultural mechanisms that may explain some of the reported sex differences. Finally, we will make recommendations for clinical practice.

2 Sex Differences in Psychosocial Risk Factors

Psychosocial risk factors generally comprise two categories: emotional factors and chronic stress. In general, we speak about experiencing psychological stress when demands tax or exceed available psychological resources or adaptive capacity, endangering well-being [12]. Patients with emotional problems will show symptoms of depression, anxiety, anger/hostility, or post-traumatic stress [12]. Psychosocial risk factors are extended by a variety of life circumstances responsible for increased levels of chronic stress, such as low social support, marital stress, financial hardship, job insecurity, and poor housing conditions (i.e., low SES), but also work strain and caregiving strain, or having stress-prone personality characteristics [13].

Sex differences exist in the prevalence of psychosocial risk factors of emotional origin; most are more prevalent in women than in men. Depression may either include going through a period of major depressive disorder (MDD) or having an elevated score on a questionnaire measuring depressive symptoms. Multi-nation, meta-analytic evidence on sex differences has shown that the likelihood of being diagnosed with MDD was about double in women [14]. Similar sex differences were reported for sub-clinical depressive symptoms, though with smaller effects [14]. Anxiety is also more prevalent in women, with a lifetime risk ratio of about 1.7:1 for women versus men [15]. Post-traumatic stress disorder (PTSD) is twice as likely to be diagnosed in women as well [16]. In contrast, a consistently higher prevalence in men has been observed for hostility and aggression. Whereas experiencing anger is not different between the (adult) sexes, physical and verbal aggression are more often used by men. Even though indirect aggression showed no sex differences, displaced aggression (aimed at someone or something other than the provoker) could be a way for women to express their anger [17].

With respect to chronic stressors, results are more inconsistent, in terms of type of stressor, and reported presence of sex differences. Women seem to suffer more extensively from work stress. A large Canadian study showed that while men typically show increased risk of being absent from work in high demand-low control job strain situations, women *also* show increased risk of absenteeism in case of high demand-high control job strain [18]. In patients with chronic coronary syndrome, female patients reported heightened experienced stress over the past year and more social stress (relational, loneliness), while no sex differences were shown for early negative life events and work stress [19], nor in Type D personality traits [20]. Sex differences in work stress and how it affects health are shaped by social mechanisms [21]. In adolescents, it was shown that although there were no sex differences in early negative life events, negative life events predicted anxiety more strongly in female youth [22]. Overall, this suggest that differences in stress processing rather than exposure may be at the roots of stress-related cardiovascular problems in women.

3 Psychosocial Risk of Cardiovascular Disease Incidence and Prognosis

Psychosocial risk factors contribute to the development and progression of a variety of cardiovascular diseases which are relevant to women. Below we summarize the elevated risk associated with psychosocial risk factors for obstructive and non-obstructive ischemic heart diseases (IHD), stress-related acute coronary syndromes, heart failure (HF), and atrial fibrillation (AF). Furthermore, sex differences will be described for each of these cardiac disease groups.

3.1 Obstructive Ischemic Heart Disease

Large-scale studies like the INTERHEART and the PURE study, along with several meta-analyses, have underscored the importance of chronic stress in increasing IHD risk [23–25]. Overall, chronic stress experienced throughout the lifespan (due to early-life stressors, and/or adult stressors) has been related to a higher risk of IHD, with the risk ranging between 40–60% [26]. This risk increases with age, in already at-risk groups, and with repeated exposure to early-life stressors [27]. Additionally, research has shown an impact of acute stressors (e.g., intense anger, fear, panic, heightened excitement, natural disasters) on the incidence of cardiac events [28]. Combined data indicated a 2.5-fold increased risk of an acute cardiac event among patients who had experienced an acute stressor right before [28]. Moreover, a meta-analysis of 62 studies showed that presenting with elevated scores on a broad range of psychological factors was associated with the development of IHD [29]. Besides increasing the risk of IHD onset, psychological stressors have also been linked to disease progression, adverse events, and cardiovascular mortality [24, 28, 30].

3.1.1 Sex Differences

Although depression is twice as prevalent among female patients with IHD [31], sex differences in the cardiovascular risk associated with depression have been inconsistent. Doyle and coworkers showed in an individual patient data meta-analysis that depression was associated with a larger risk of all-cause mortality in men, while no sex differences were present in the depression-associated risk of cardiac events [32]. Two meta-analyses by Smaardijk and colleagues examined sex differences in the impact of the broad range of psychosocial risk factors on the onset and progression of obstructive IHD [29, 30]. Results showed an about equal psychosocial risk factors-associated increased risk of IHD incidence in men and women [29]. A more recent study showed that when psychological distress variables (depression, anxiety, PTSD, anger, hostility, and perceived stress) were combined in one index score, this score was associated with an increased risk of adverse cardiovascular events and death in women, but not men [33]. In terms of disease progression, a large meta-analysis for all psychosocial risk factors combined showed a stronger effect on the risk of adverse cardiac events in men with IHD compared to women [30]. However, some literature also suggests that women with IHD, especially younger women, are more susceptible to the impact of depression and stress on adverse cardiac events [31, 34, 35]. Future studies are needed to examine the role of risk factor profiles on IHD incidence and progression, and sex differences therein.

3.2 Non-Obstructive Ischemic Heart Diseases

Cardiac ischemia without obstructed coronary arteries (INOCA) is more common in women and presumably caused by microvascular dysfunctions or vasospasms [36]. While several earlier studies have shown that patients with INOCA experience more anxiety and depression than the general population [37], and than patients with obstructive IHD [38], other studies have not reported such differences [39–42]. INOCA is related to a reduced quality of life [43], and a decreased functional capacity [44].

3.2.1 Sex Differences

The decline in physical, mental, and social functioning experienced after the onset of INOCA symptoms was found to be comparable in women and men, while the observed days lost were more abundant in men [44]. With respect to hard medical outcomes, no sex differences were observed in event rates and all-cause mortality [45, 46]. Though studies on sex-specific effects of psychosocial risk factors on outcomes after INOCA diagnosis are lacking, there are suggestions that psychological factors play a role in INOCA subtypes. A population-based study found that anxiety and depression contributed to a higher risk of developing coronary vasospasm compared to incident obstructive CAD and a healthy control group, and this effect was similar in both sexes [47]. The role of acute *mental* stress in INOCA etiology is based on research into mental stress-induced myocardial ischemia (MSIMI), which is explained next.

3.3 Stress-Related Acute Coronary Syndromes

Stress-related acute coronary syndromes are conditions in which emotional stress triggers a cardiac event, often due to a sudden surge of stress hormones causing changes in coronary arteries and heart muscle function. These conditions have a high female predominance (75%–95%) and include mental stress-induced myocardial ischemia (MSIMI), spontaneous coronary artery dissection (SCAD), takotsubo cardiomyopathy, and coronary artery vasospasm (see INOCA) [48, 49].

MSIMI refers to a condition where acute mental or emotional stress provokes ischemia in patients with and without preexisting obstructive IHD [34, 49, 50]. Based on previous studies it is estimated that MSIMI occurs in 30–60% of the patients with obstructive IHD and is two-three times more prevalent in women younger than 50 years. During (induced) mental stress, women showed higher microvascular vasoconstriction compared to men [49]. Furthermore, among women, patients with MSIMI exhibited more *peripheral* vasoconstriction in contrast to those without MSIMI, whereas there was no such distinction within men [49]. Finally, angina symptoms appear to be related to psychological triggers in women, but not men, which is supported by a positive relation between angina frequency and more severe MSIMI [34, 49].

SCAD is defined as a spontaneous, non-traumatic and non-iatrogenic separation of the coronary artery wall, creating a false lumen [51, 52]. SCAD is increasingly recognized as a cause of acute coronary syndrome, particularly in younger women. The term SCAD in contemporary medicine is predominantly used to refer to SCAD from non-atherosclerotic origins, while coronary artery dissections also may have atherosclerotic origins [52]. Interestingly, research has shown that emotional triggers precipitated SCAD in over 55% of patients, while only 24% of patients experienced a physical trigger [53], [54]. Other evidence shows that while physical and combined stress was more often reported in men, emotional stress was more often reported as a trigger in women [55]. Furthermore, experiencing SCAD is associated with higher levels of stress [53], and has greater psychosocial impact on patients when compared to a 'traditional' obstructive myocardial infarction [56].

Takotsubo cardiomyopathy or broken-heart syndrome is a severe acute physical or mental stress induced cardiomyopathy, which 'stuns' the muscles of the heart. An estimated 30% of takotsubo cases have a physical etiological stressor, such as infection, surgery, or exercise, which is associated with a worse prognosis [57]. Triggering events indicating emotional stress (also an estimated 30%) have a relatively better prognosis [58]. Excessive high levels of the stress hormones adrenaline and noradrenaline are hypothesized to start the takotsubo process [59]. Given that physical triggers were more often observed in men, and emotional triggers or an absence of a clear trigger in women [60], this could explain the observed higher mortality in men with takotsubo [61, 62]. Having experienced SCAD or takotsubo can have a profound psychological impact, with people experiencing post-traumatic stress disorder, depression, and anxiety [51]. However, estimates are not necessarily higher compared with people who experienced a myocardial infarction, in part due to uncertainty on causes and recommendations [63].

3.4 Heart Failure

Regarding heart failure (HF), more controversy exists and less studies have been performed. We need to distinguish between HF with a *reduced* ejection fraction (HFrEF = systolic heart failure, LVEF ≤40%), which is more prevalent in men, and HF with a *preserved* ejection fraction (HFpEF = diastolic heart failure, preserved LVEF), more prevalent in women, while most studies examine a combination of both [64–66]. Whereas HFrEF often has an obstructive ischemic etiology, recent literature suggests the etiology for HFpEF to be related to coronary microvascular dysfunction [36].

Depression has been linked to both onset and progression of HF. For anxiety, this relationship is less clear. The Nord-Trondelag Health Study (HUNT 2) included 62,567 healthy individuals and found that symptoms of depression, but not anxiety, were associated with a 41% higher risk of incident HF after an 11-year follow-up [67]. In another mega-cohort study of people with depression, a twofold higher risk of a newly diagnosed HFrEF, and 1.6 times higher risk for HFpEF was found [68]. The Multiethnic Study of Atherosclerosis (MESA) found no significant association between psychosocial risk factors (anger, anxiety, chronic stress, depressive symptoms) and HF incidence [69]. In patients with HF, the prevalence of depression (20%–45%) and anxiety (20%–50%) are higher than in the general population [70–72]. A meta-analysis by Rutledge et al. (2006) found a twofold higher increased risk of HF outcomes (death or cardiac events) in patients with depressive symptoms/disorder [73].

3.4.1 Sex Differences

It is unclear whether the relation between psychological risk factors and HF incidence differ between men and women. The sex-specific analysis of the MESA cohort indicated that women but not men exhibited a heightened risk of HF when they reported high hostility. Another study [74] reported a relation between depression and HF incidence in older women. In contrast, a cohort study of cardiovascular healthy 1.9 million people without cardiovascular diseases in the UK found that depression is related to a higher risk of HF occurrence, without sex differences [75]. In patients with existing HF, higher incidences of anxiety and depression and a lower quality of life are observed in women [76, 77]. However, no significant sex-differences in survival were observed, which may be limited by the number of women included in studies with HF.

3.5 Atrial Fibrillation

There are clear differences between the sexes in epidemiology, pathophysiology, presentation, and prognosis of atrial fibrillation (AF). AF is less common in women, showing a 1.5 to 2 times lower incidence in women. The age-adjusted prevalence of AF is also lower in women, with a difference of about 3% [78]. In terms of pathophysiology, there appear to be sex differences in both risk factors and disease processes, symptom presentation (more atypical symptoms, more symptoms in general), as well as in disease outcomes. For example, women with AF more often develop cardiovascular sequelae such as stroke and myocardial infarction and might die sooner [78]. Health-related quality of life tends to be worse in women compared to men with AF [79]. Psychological risk factors, such as depression, anxiety, anger, work strain, and chronic stress may increase the incidence of AF in both men and women. A recent meta-analysis concluded that psychosocial risk factors such as depression, anxiety, work stress, and anger were associated with a 25%, 10%, 18%, and 15% increased risk of atrial fibrillation (AF) respectively [80]. In men, anger and hostility have shown to be associated with early development of AF [80]. Differences have also been found in the impact that AF has in women versus men, with women reporting more symptoms, increased symptoms severity, and elevated levels of anxiety and depression, which in turn contributes to increased reports of symptom severity, poorer quality of life, and AF recurrence [81].

4 How Do Psychosocial Risk Factors Impact Cardiovascular Disease in Women and Men?

Psychosocial risk factors, in this section reffered to as stress, can lead to the development and worsening of cardiovascular diseases through a complex interplay of multiple mechanisms. In this section, we will provide a brief description of the primary mechanisms involved, as well as discuss the sex-dependent stress response and its contribution to cardiovascular diseases differently in women and men.

4.1 Biological Mechanisms Underlying Psychosocial Risk Factors and Cardiac Diseases

While chronic stress gradually promotes progression of cardiac diseases, acute stressors can cause acute cardiac events. Chronic stress affects cardiac diseases through multiple pathways, which can be distinguished into behavioral, autonomic, and neuroendocrine [82]. The behavioral pathway involves lifestyle behaviors, such as unhealthy eating habits, smoking, decreased physical activity, and poor medication adherence, but also (not) seeking social support [26, 28, 82]. The autonomic pathway is immediate and involves activating sympathetic and restorative parasympathetic actions. The neuroendocrine response to stress involves a cascade of physiological changes mediated by the hypothalamic-pituitary-adrenal (HPA) axis and the sympathetic-adrenal-medullary (SAM) system [26, 28, 82]. Neuroendocrine activation can affect cardiac diseases through increased cathecholamines (noradrenaline, adrenaline, and dopamine) and cortisol levels, as well as via autonomic nervous system dysregulation, and subsequent promotion of inflammatory responses. Chronic sympathetic nervous system activation and parasympathetic withdrawal has been related to higher blood pressure and a lower heart rate variability [82]. Also, chronically elevated cortisol affects vascular function negatively [11]. Furthermore, prolonged stress is related to higher circulating pro-inflammatory markers and endothelial dysfunction [83]. All of these factors play a critical role in the development of atherosclerosis [28, 84]. In the case of acute stress, the autonomic nervous system, neurohormonal and immune system also contribute to acute cardiac events. Following the onset of the stress response (activation of the SAM- and HPA-axis), an increase in inflammatory biomarkers and elevated sympathetic activity has been found to trigger plaque rupture by disrupting the fibrous cap [27]. Moreover, it was found that patients with ischemic heart disease more often show vasoconstriction in reaction to acute mental stress, particularly in the stenosed segments [28, 49, 84].

It must be acknowledged that this is an oversimplification of a much more complex mechanism, which serves as an introduction to importantly sex differences in the biological stress response.

4.2 Sex Differences in the Biological Stress Response and Interplay with Sociocultural Mechanisms

How stress exerts its effects on heart disease is distinct for women and men. This is due to differences in stress response, involving a complex interplay between socio-cultural (gender) factors and biological (sex) mechanisms. Helman and colleagues summarized how sex could affect the cardiac disease [11]. In short, the stress response differs at the level of stress perception, behavioral reactions (what people do), cognitions (how people think), and biological mechanisms. Women and men perceive different situations as stressful. While men are more sensitive to achievement and competitive situations, women are more sensitive to situations impacting their social position (e.g. group exclusion) [8, 85]. These norms about gender expectations, how women and men are 'supposed' to behave based on their gender, influences the experience of stressors. Women more often experience ongoing stress related to disparities in household and caregiving tasks, whereas men are more often not showing vulnerability and minimizing their emotional distress [86]. These initial stress perceptions combined with different stressors also influence how women and men react to stress. Women may exhibit a 'tend and befriend' reaction, seeking emotional and social support interactions, while men tend to employ a 'fight or flight' response, more often engaging in physical activities, risky behavior, or drug abuse [8].

Biological sex differences include different physiological responses within the HPA-axis, sympathetic nervous system, and neuro-inflammatory pathways. Neurological variations, including neuroplasticity, are also notable. Structural differences in brain areas that release noradrenaline, as well as the observation that estrogens affect noradrenaline release and prevent noradrenaline breakdown all point toward increased arousal in females [87]. Furthermore, genetic makeup and epigenetic modifications, stemming from early life experiences, as well as later-life environmental experiences play a role in shaping the divergent stress responses observed in women and men [88].

A comprehension of distinct socio-cultural and biological factors is relevant to understand how stress affects cardiac diseases differently in women and men. The physical, hormonal, and emotional responses to stress are sex-dependent and therefore contribute to differential effects on cardiac health. The behavioral and biological stress-mechanisms contributing to CAD vary by sex and gender [11]. For example, variations in coping strategies contribute to sex-specific stress-related risk behaviors (e.g., decreased physical activity, changed sleep and dietary habits). Studies show that stress has a greater impact on disturbed sleeping and eating behavior among women compared men [89–91]. Premenopausal women have higher levels of advantageous HDL cholesterol than men, though stress may cancel out its protective effects [92, 93].

Stress hormones contribute to endothelial dysfunction via impaired vasodilation and augmented vasoconstriction, and studies show that women with CAD have a higher microvascular dysfunction in response to stress compared to men [34, 94]. Accordingly, microvascular dysfunction has been linked to stress-susceptible cardiac diseases such as INOCA, MSIMI, takotsubo cardiomyopathy, and HFpEF [36, 49, 95, 96]. These conditions are heavily influenced by sex and more prevalent in women. This aligns with the salient sex differences in stress physiology, and how this translates into effects on the cardiovascular system. Therefore, the interaction between sex-dependent stress response and baseline physiology is a good candidate to contribute to the sex-dependent development of CAD, and particularly cardiac diseases linked to vascular dysfunction.

Although it is widely recognized that biological stress mechanisms differ between women and men, it is less commonly understood that the stress reactivity is also concurrently influenced by external socio-cultural and gender-related factors [97, 98]. This has implications for cardiovascular prevention whereby biological and sociocultural factors should be taken into account.

5 Clinical Practice

Psychosocial risk factors confer a greater likelihood of developing a cardiovascular condition, and heightened risk of poor prognosis and quality of life once cardiovascular disease has been diagnosed. Sex-specific differences in stress processes and myocardial and coronary physiology interact in the development of sex-dependent cardiovascular disorders. In addition to the underlying biology, differences in sociocultural gender roles remain a strong explanatory factor in the report of heightened stress in women. It is therefore eminent to take these differences into account in cardiological and medical-psychology practice.

5.1 Implications for Cardiac Rehabilitation

Cardiac rehabilitation (CR) holds a class 1A recommendation from the American Heart Association for risk reduction, and women tend to benefit more than men [99]. Yet, in women, referral to CR is significantly lower [100]. Moreover, physician communication is an important determinant of participation, as health care providers may aid (by recommending and endorsing) or hinder (by informing patients they are either too well, too old, or too sick) CR [101]. Women experience distinct stress-inducing barriers to CR participation, including (lack of) transportation options, care-giving responsibilities, and perceptions towards exercise, that should be addressed beforehand [102]. Women in CR also report exercise to be more tiring and painful [103, 104]. As described extensively above, women experience a larger psychosocial burden than men, so women-focused CR programs should take inventory of psychosocial risk during intake and should offer psychological treatment. We recommend that cardiologists and cardiac nurses be mindful about communication aspects and stress-inducing barriers to cardiac rehabilitation participation, focus on participation of minority women, and address fatigue and pain adequately when referring women to cardiac rehabilitation. Automated referral and assisted enrollment may facilitate participation in women [105].

5.2 Implications for Psychosocial Screening Practices

In addition to poorer referral and attendance to CR, women with heart disease have adverse psychological profiles, and suboptimal social support. These latter factors may be recognized by screening for psychosocial risk. From available guidelines, the European Society of Cardiology (ESC) guideline on Cardiovascular Prevention has robustly recommended a comprehensive assessment of psychosocial risk to prevent heart disease or progression thereof, including screening for depression, anxiety, chronic stress, Distressed personality (Type D), hostility, anger, low socioeconomic status, lack of social support, post-traumatic stress disorder, and a history of psychiatric disorders over the past decade [106–108]. For chronic coronary syndromes, psychological treatment is given a Class IA recommendation as part of lifestyle management recommendation, and Class IB for improvement in depression and anxiety [108]. The 2020 ESC guideline on AF summarized the effects of anxiety, depression, and poorer health-related quality of life, especially when having a Type D personality [109], and recommends integrated patient-centred management, including psychosocial assessment and treatment. Other guidelines are more hesitant, with the 2021 ESC guideline on diagnosis and treatment of acute and chronic HF and the 2020 guideline on the management of acute coronary syndromes recommending assessment and treatment for depression only [65], while the American Heart Association guideline for chronic coronary artery disease indicates the same longlist of risk factors to be important [110], and recommend their assessment (although in particular depression is used as example).

We thus may conclude that screening for psychosocial risk factors is widely supported. It serves as an indication of whether psychological/psychiatric evaluation is advisable, but also can identify a patient's unique needs and lay bare the barriers that need to be overcome to successfully change health behaviors [111]. It seems necessary to progress from current practice (screening for depression and anxiety) and broaden the screening scope to include all psychological risk factors, while taking sex and gender differences into account. A recently developed screener comprehensively assesses all nine psychosocial risk factors identified in the ESC Cardiovascular Prevention guidelines [106, 112]. A within-person analysis examining psychological risk profiles using the comprehensive screener revealed that women showed an increased likelihood for a profile characterized by high levels of anxiety and depression, and negative affectivity, but not anger and hostility [20].

While screening for psychological risk factors after an acute cardiac event is undisputedly useful, it is more diffuse whether routine screening may benefit stable IHD patients. A recent depression-oriented trial (CODIACS-QoL) showed no differences between a screen-notify-treat group versus a screen-notify group and a usual care (no screening) group in terms of quality-adjusted life years [113]. It is important to add a critical note though. The patients in the screen-notify-treat and screen-notify groups predominantly (~93%) screened negative, which may have been too scant to show benefit. A secondary analysis of the trial showed that the stepped care treatment (in the screen-notify-treat group) was more effective in reducing depressive symptoms than just screening and notifying [114]. Cardiologists may take into account the general disposition towards experiencing negative emotions and the greater risk of emotional instability following a cardiac event. This could be done by using a standardized comprehensive screener as part of a stepped care process, in which patients who screen positive are invited for an interview with a medical psychologist, and then are directed towards appropriate treatment (individual, group therapy), as just notifying and leaving it up to the patient does not seem to work.

5.3 Implications for Psychological Treatment

There are several indications for sex differences in the effectiveness of psychological treatment. The ENRICHD study was one of the largest efforts to treat depression and low social support existing in the first month after acute MI, randomizing patients to cognitive behavior therapy (CBT) vs. usual medical care. Secondary analyses showed that treatment efficacy for mortality or recurrent MI was only significant in white men, not in women, though depressed affect improved in all participants who received CBT treatment [115]. The authors suggested that more aggressive medical treatment in white men, originating from underlying perceived differences in risk factors and disease severity may have been one of the causes. Other offered explanations included treatment design and delivery, such as demographic matching of therapists, group vs. individual therapy, and offering single-sex group sessions. Emerging research is now showing what was still anecdotal in the ENRICHD era. Effectiveness of psychotherapy is reported to be dependent upon group composition, as women tend to profit more from same-sex group sessions [105]. This was shown to improve openness and willingness to share. Importantly, there are also sex differences in how effective pharmaceutical therapies are for psychiatric problems like anxiety and depression. For example, SSRIs may be more effective in younger than older (postmenopausal) women, and in men [116]. We recommend psychological treatment to be tailored to the patients' needs such that effectiveness for female and male patients is maximized. Psychosocial modules in the context of cardiac rehabilitation could be offered in single-sex format, with flexible (gym)-hours and online options to tackle planning and transportation issues.

6 Conclusion

Psychosocial risk factors are more abundantly present in female than in male patients with heart disease. The literature is still inconclusive as to whether women and men differ in the risk psychosocial factors convey towards increased incidence, progression, and impact of IHD. However, stress-related acute coronary syndromes, such as MSIM, SCAD, and takotsubo, in which emotional stress triggers a cardiac event are highly female-dominated. In patients with heart failure, women have a higher incidence of anxiety and depressive symptoms, but mixed evidence exists about risk differences between women and men. Finally, in patients with AF, psychosocial risk factors increase the risk of incident AF, with psychological characteristics specifically being associated with a heightened risk in men vs. women. A complex interplay between socio-cultural (gender) factors and biological (sex) mechanisms explains sex differences in both the prevalence of psychosocial risk factors and mechanistic pathways that increase the risk of heart disease. Based on this body of evidence, several recommendations for research and clinical practice have been made that are summarized in Table 1.

Table 1 Recommendations

Recommendations for research and practice
• Health care professionals should be mindful about communication aspects and stress-inducing barriers to CR participation. Automated referral and assisted enrollment may facilitate female participation
• Tailored interventions and educational programs should be developed to meet the specific needs of women, with attention for the intervention design and delivery
• Physicians training programs should include the recognition of psychosocial risk factors together with a biopsychosocial perspective to optimize clinical care
• A broader inclusion of ischemic conditions in research may facilitate insight in the complex mechanisms through which sex and gender affect cardiovascular etiology and prognosis

Key Issues

- Psychosocial risk factors are more prevalent in women, both in the general population as well as in women with heart disease.
- Psychosocial risk factors play a significant role in the development and progression of cardiac diseases in women and men.
- Differences in stress response pathways are essential to understand how psychosocial risk factors impact the cardiovascular system differently between women and men.
- Women are less often referred to CR and less inclined to participate due to stress-inducing barriers; including options for transportation, care-giving responsibilities, perceptions towards exercise, and due to intervention characteristics (therapist, single-sex groups).
- Effectiveness of psychological treatment in heart disease may be different as a function of therapy fit (see above), differences in medical treatment, and due to hormonal interactions with pharmaceutical medications.

Questions and Answers

1. Which psychosocial risk factors are more prevalent in women compared to men?
   (A) Chronic work stress, negative early life events, and Type D personality traits
   (B) Major depressive disorder, anxiety, and experiencing anger
   (C) **Posttraumatic stress disorder, depressive symptoms, and anxiety**
   (D) Experiencing anger, anxiety, and Type D personality traits

   Feedback Q1: C. Women consistently more often experience major depression disorder, depressive symptoms, anxiety, and posttraumatic stress disorder. For chronic stressors, findings are less consistent. Though women may experience more work stress, findings for negative early life events and Type D personality traits are not clearly different between the sexes.
2. Depressive symptoms have consistently been observed to be associated with worse cardiovascular outcomes in patients with obstructive heart disease. Which sentence below best describes the potential sex differences in the risk for adverse outcomes related to depression in these patients?
   (A) Depressive symptoms are much more prevalent in women with obstructive heart disease, and the risk for adverse outcomes related to depression is consistently higher for women than for men.
   (B) Findings on sex differences in depressive symptoms in patients with obstructive heart disease are mixed, though depressive symptoms in especially younger women confer a risk for adverse outcomes.
   (C) In contrast to expectations, depressive symptoms are more prevalent in for men with obstructive heart disease compared to women, though no consistent significant sex differences with adverse outcomes are observed.
   (D) **Though depressive symptoms are much more prevalent in women with obstructive heart disease, the risk for adverse outcomes related to depression is higher for men.**

   Feedback Q2: D. Depressive symptoms are much more prevalent in women compared to men, also in patients with obstructive heart disease. For obstructive IHD, depressive symptoms are associated with a higher risk in men. Though more recent studies find a higher risk for depressive symptoms in younger women for adverse outcomes compared to men.
3. Examples of stress-related acute coronary syndromes with a high female predominance include:
   (A) Atrial fibrillation, SCAD, coronary vasospasm
   (B) **Coronary vasospasm, SCAD, MSIMI**
   (C) HFpEF, atrial fibrillation, takotsubo cardiomyopathy
   (D) MSIMI, HFpEF, takotsubo cardiomyopathy

   Feedback Q3: B. Atrial fibrillation (AF) is more prevalent in men. Still psychosocial factors are associated with a higher prevalence of AF. SCAD, MSIMI, takotsubo cardiomyopathy, and coronary vasospasm (INOCA) are more prevalent in women and potentially associated with stress triggering evens. Though HFpEF is more prevalent in women, an immediate association of acute stress with HFpEF is not confirmed.
4. Which of the following is a biological mechanism underlying the association between psychosocial risk factors and cardiac diseases?
   (A) Lifestyle behaviors, like exercise
   (B) Impaired vasodilation
   (C) **Increased levels of cortisol and catecholamines (stress hormones)**
   (D) Social support, hormones of social affiliation (oxytocin)

   Feedback Q4: C. Lifestyle behaviors and social support are not biological mechanisms, but potential moderators in the association between psychological risk factors and cardiac disease. Though impaired vasodilation is part of a biological mechanism, all stress responses start at least with an increase in levels of HPA-axis hormone cortisol, and SAM-system catecholamines (dopamine, noradrenaline, adrenaline).

5. Which of the following stress-inducing barriers for cardiac rehabilitation are more often experienced by women?
   (A) Addressing pain and fatigue experiences in women
   (B) **Challenges related to transportation options, care-giving responsibilities, and perceptions towards exercise**
   (C) Provide CR group sessions for women and men separately
   (D) Using a comprehensive screener to assess psychosocial risk factors, and follow-up on the outcomes of the screener

   Feedback Q5: B. Women are less often referred to CR and less inclined to participate due to stress-inducing barriers; including options for transportation, care-giving responsibilities, perceptions towards exercise, and due to intervention characteristics (therapist, single-sex groups).

References

1. Kaplan RM. Helen Flanders Dunbar: the mother of psychosomatic medicine—psychiatry in history. Br J Psychiatry. 2023;222(2):81.
2. Selye H. The stress of life; 1956.
3. Selye H. The evolution of the stress concept: stress and cardiovascular disease. Am J Cardiol. 1970;26(3):289–99.
4. McEwen BS. Stress, adaptation, and disease. Allostasis and allostatic load. Ann N Y Acad Sci. 1998;840:33–44.
5. Stoney CM, Davis MC, Matthews KA. Sex differences in physiological responses to stress and in coronary heart disease: a causal link? Psychophysiology. 1987;24(2):127–31.
6. Orth-Gomer K, Chesney MA, Wenger NK, editors. Women, stress, and heart disease. 1st ed. London: Psychology Press; 1998.
7. Folkman S. The Oxford handbook of stress, health, and coping. Oxford: Oxford University Press; 2011.
8. Taylor SE, Klein LC, Lewis BP, Gruenewald TL, Gurung RA, Updegraff JA. Biobehavioral responses to stress in females: tend-and-befriend, not fight-or-flight. Psychol Rev. 2000;107(3):411–29.
9. Gao Z, Chen Z, Sun A, Deng X. Gender differences in cardiovascular disease. Med Novel Technol Devices. 2019;4:100025.
10. Maas AHEM, Appelman YEA. Gender differences in coronary heart disease. Neth Heart J. 2010;18(12):598–603.
11. Helman TJ, Headrick JP, Stapelberg NJC, Braidy N. The sex-dependent response to psychosocial stress and ischaemic heart disease. Front Cardiovasc Med. 2023;10:1072042.
12. Ben-Zur H. Transactional model of stress and coping. In: Zeigler-Hill V, Shackelford TK, editors. Encyclopedia of personality and individual differences. Cham: Springer International; 2019. p. 1–4.
13. Rozanski A, Blumenthal JA, Davidson KW, Saab PG, Kubzansky L. The epidemiology, pathophysiology, and management of psychosocial risk factors in cardiac practice: the emerging field of behavioral cardiology. J Am Coll Cardiol. 2005;45(5):637–51.
14. Salk RH, Hyde JS, Abramson LY. Gender differences in depression in representative national samples: meta-analyses of diagnoses and symptoms. Psychol Bull. 2017;143(8):783–822.
15. McLean CP, Asnaani A, Litz BT, Hofmann SG. Gender differences in anxiety disorders: prevalence, course of illness, comorbidity and burden of illness. J Psychiatr Res. 2011;45(8):1027–35.
16. Ravi M, Stevens JS, Michopoulos V. Neuroendocrine pathways underlying risk and resilience to PTSD in women. Front Neuroendocrinol. 2019;55:100790.
17. Archer J. Sex differences in aggression in real-world settings: a meta-analytic review. Rev Gen Psychol. 2004;8(4):291–322.
18. Gilbert-Ouimet M, Trudel X, Aubé K, Ndjaboue R, Duchaine C, Blanchette C, et al. Differences between women and men in the relationship between psychosocial stressors at work and work absence due to mental health problem. Occup Environ Med. 2020;77(9):603–10.
19. Doedee F, van den Houdt S, Widdershoven J, Kupper N. Chronic stress exposure in men and women, and implications for the course of fatigue after percutaneous coronary intervention; the THORESCI study. Gen Hosp Psychiatry. 2021;72:45–52.
20. van den Houdt SCM, Mommersteeg PMC, Widdershoven J, Kupper N. Sex and gender differences in psychosocial risk profiles among patients with coronary heart disease—the THORESCI-Gender Study. Int J Behav Med. 2023;31:130–44.
21. Padkapayeva K, Gilbert-Ouimet M, Bielecky A, Ibrahim S, Mustard C, Brisson C, et al. Gender/sex differences in the relationship between psychosocial work exposures and work and life stress. Ann Work Expo Health. 2018;62(4):416–25.
22. Madhavan S, Stewart LC, Birk SL, Nielsen JD, Olino TM. Positive and negative life events in association with psychopathology: an examination of sex differences in early adolescence. Child Psychiatry Hum Dev. 2023.
23. Vahedian-Azimi A, Moayed MS. Updating the meta-analysis of perceived stress and its association with the incidence of coronary heart disease. Int J Med Rev. 2019;6(4):146–53.
24. Santosa A, Rosengren A, Ramasundarahettige C, Rangarajan S, Gulec S, Chifamba J, et al.

Psychosocial risk factors and cardiovascular disease and death in a population-based cohort from 21 low-, middle-, and high-income countries. JAMA Netw Open. 2021;4(12):e2138920.
25. Anand SS, Islam S, Rosengren A, Franzosi MG, Steyn K, Yusufali AH, et al. Risk factors for myocardial infarction in women and men: insights from the INTERHEART study. Eur Heart J. 2008;29(7):932–40.
26. Steptoe A, Kivimäki M. Stress and cardiovascular disease: an update on current knowledge. Annu Rev Public Health. 2013;34:337–54.
27. Kivimäki M, Steptoe A. Effects of stress on the development and progression of cardiovascular disease. Nat Rev Cardiol. 2018;15(4):215–29.
28. Levine GN. Psychological stress and heart disease: fact or folklore? Am J Med. 2022;135(6):688–96.
29. Smaardijk VR, Lodder P, Kop WJ, van Gennep B, Maas A, Mommersteeg PMC. Sex- and gender-stratified risks of psychological factors for incident ischemic heart disease: systematic review and meta-analysis. J Am Heart Assoc. 2019;8(9):e010859.
30. Smaardijk VR, Maas AHEM, Lodder P, Kop WJ, Mommersteeg PMC. Sex and gender-stratified risks of psychological factors for adverse clinical outcomes in patients with ischemic heart disease: a systematic review and meta-analysis. Int J Cardiol. 2020;302:21–9.
31. Vaccarino V, Badimon L, Bremner JD, Cenko E, Cubedo J, Dorobantu M, et al. Depression and coronary heart disease: 2018 position paper of the ESC working group on coronary pathophysiology and microcirculation. Eur Heart J. 2019;41(17):1687–96.
32. Doyle F, McGee H, Conroy R, Conradi HJ, Meijer A, Steeds R, et al. Systematic review and individual patient data meta-analysis of sex differences in depression and prognosis in persons with myocardial infarction: a MINDMAPS study. Psychosom Med. 2015;77(4):419–28.
33. Pimple P, Lima BB, Hammadah M, Wilmot K, Ramadan R, Levantsevych O, et al. Psychological distress and subsequent cardiovascular events in individuals with coronary artery disease. J Am Heart Assoc. 2019;8(9):e011866.
34. Vaccarino V, Sullivan S, Hammadah M, Wilmot K, Al Mheid I, Ramadan R, et al. Mental stress-induced-myocardial ischemia in Young patients with recent myocardial infarction: sex differences and mechanisms. Circulation. 2018;137(8):794–805.
35. Shah AJ, Ghasemzadeh N, Zaragoza-Macias E, Patel R, Eapen DJ, Neeland IJ, et al. Sex and age differences in the association of depression with obstructive coronary artery disease and adverse cardiovascular events. J Am Heart Assoc. 2014;3(3):e000741.
36. Mehta PK, Huang J, Levit RD, Malas W, Waheed N, Bairey Merz CN. Ischemia and no obstructive coronary arteries (INOCA): a narrative review. Atherosclerosis. 2022;363:8–21.
37. Mommersteeg PMC, Arts L, Zijlstra W, Widdershoven JW, Aarnoudse W, Denollet J. Impaired health status, psychological distress, and personality in women and men with nonobstructive coronary artery disease: sex and gender differences: the TWIST (Tweesteden Mild Stenosis) Study. Circ Cardiovasc Qual Outcomes. 2017;10(2):e003387.
38. Asbury EA, Creed F, Collins P. Distinct psychosocial differences between women with coronary heart disease and cardiac syndrome X. Eur Heart J. 2004;25(19):1695–701.
39. van Schalkwijk DL, Widdershoven J, Magro M, Smaardijk V, Bekendam M, Vermeltfoort I, et al. Clinical and psychological characteristics of patients with ischemia and non-obstructive coronary arteries (INOCA) and obstructive coronary artery disease. Am Heart J Plus. 2023;27:100282.
40. Konst RE, Elias-Smale SE, Lier A, Bode C, Maas AH. Different cardiovascular risk factors and psychosocial burden in symptomatic women with and without obstructive coronary artery disease. Eur J Prev Cardiol. 2020;26(6):657–9.
41. Bekendam MT, Vermeltfoort IAC, Kop WJ, Widdershoven JW, Mommersteeg PMC. Psychological factors of suspect coronary microvascular dysfunction in patients undergoing SPECT imaging. J Nucl Cardiol. 2022;29(2):768–78.
42. Daniel M, Agewall S, Berglund F, Caidahl K, Collste O, Ekenbäck C, et al. Prevalence of anxiety and depression symptoms in patients with myocardial infarction with non-obstructive coronary arteries. Am J Med. 2018;131(9):1118–24.
43. Ford TJ, Yii E, Sidik N, Good R, Rocchiccioli P, McEntegart M, et al. Ischemia and no obstructive coronary artery disease: prevalence and correlates of coronary vasomotion disorders. Circ Cardiovasc Interv. 2019;12(12):e008126.
44. Ranasinghe S, Merz CNB, Khan N, Wei J, George M, Berry C, et al. Sex differences in quality of life in patients with ischemia with no obstructive coronary artery disease (INOCA): a patient self-report retrospective survey from INOCA international. J Clin Med. 2023;12(17):5646.
45. Ouellette ML, Löffler AI, Beller GA, Workman VK, Holland E, Bourque JM. Clinical characteristics, sex differences, and outcomes in patients with Normal or near-Normal coronary arteries, non-obstructive or obstructive coronary artery disease. J Am Heart Assoc. 2018;7(10).
46. Huang Z, Cao B, Zhu J, Du X, Yang Y, Li M, et al. Non-obstructive CAD and risk of all-cause mortality in middle-aged and older patients: a nine-year follow-up and multicentre study Curr Med Imaging. 2023;20.
47. Hung MY, Mao CT, Hung MJ, Wang JK, Lee HC, Yeh CT, et al. Coronary artery spasm as related to anxiety and depression: a nationwide population-based study. Psychosom Med. 2019;81(3):237–45.
48. Mehilli J, Presbitero P. Coronary artery disease and acute coronary syndrome in women. Heart. 2020;106(7):487–92.

49. Mehta PK, Sharma A, Bremner JD, Vaccarino V. Mental stress-induced myocardial ischemia. Curr Cardiol Rep. 2022;24(12):2109–20.
50. Arri SS, Ryan M, Redwood SR, Marber MS. Mental stress-induced myocardial ischaemia. Heart. 2016;102(6):472–80.
51. Hayes SN, Tweet MS, Adlam D, Kim ESH, Gulati R, Price JE, et al. Spontaneous coronary artery dissection: JACC state-of-the-art review. J Am Coll Cardiol. 2020;76(8):961–84.
52. Saw J. Spontaneous coronary artery dissection. Interv Cardiol. 2015;10(3):142–3.
53. Smaardijk VR, Mommersteeg PMC, Kop WJ, Adlam D, Maas A. Psychological and clinical characteristics of female patients with spontaneous coronary artery dissection. Neth Heart J. 2020;28(9):485–91.
54. Saw J, Aymong E, Sedlak T, Buller CE, Starovoytov A, Ricci D, et al. Spontaneous coronary artery dissection: association with predisposing arteriopathies and precipitating stressors and cardiovascular outcomes. Circ Cardiovasc Interv. 2014;7(5):645–55.
55. Daoulah A, Al-Faifi SM, Hersi AS, Dinas PC, Youssef AA, Alshehri M, et al. Spontaneous coronary artery dissection in relation to physical and emotional stress: a retrospective study in 4 Arab gulf countries. Curr Probl Cardiol. 2021;46(3):100484.
56. Murphy BM, Rogerson MC, Hesselson S, Iismaa SE, Hoover V, Le Grande M, et al. Prevalence of anxiety, depression, and distress in SCAD and non-SCAD AMI patients: a comparative study. J Cardiopulm Rehabil Prev. 2023;43(5):338–45.
57. Uribarri A, Nunez-Gil IJ, Conty DA, Vedia O, Almendro-Delia M, Duran Cambra A, et al. Short- and long-term prognosis of patients with Takotsubo syndrome based on different triggers: importance of the physical nature. J Am Heart Assoc. 2019;8(24):e013701.
58. Ghadri JR, Kato K, Cammann VL, Gili S, Jurisic S, Di Vece D, et al. Long-term prognosis of patients with Takotsubo syndrome. J Am Coll Cardiol. 2018;72(8):874–82.
59. Al Houri HN, Jomaa S, Jabra M, Alhouri AN, Latifeh Y. Pathophysiology of stress cardiomyopathy: a comprehensive literature review. Ann Med Surg (Lond). 2022;82:104671.
60. Agdamag AC, Patel H, Chandra S, Rao A, Suboc TM, Marinescu K, et al. Sex differences in Takotsubo syndrome: a narrative review. J Womens Health (Larchmt). 2020;29(8):1122–30.
61. Vincent LT, Grant J, Ebner B, Maning J, Montana P, Olorunfemi O, et al. Effect of gender on prognosis in patients with Takotsubo syndrome (from a Nationwide perspective). Am J Cardiol. 2022;162:6–12.
62. Abuelazm M, Saleh O, Hassan AR, Ahmad S, Albarakat MM, Abdalshafy H, et al. Sex difference in clinical and management outcomes in patients with Takotsubo syndrome: a systematic review and meta-analysis. Curr Probl Cardiol. 2023;48(4):101545.
63. Olliges E, Burgdorf C, Ladwig KH, Moeller C, Deftu-Kloes D, Pohl S, et al. Psychosocial and physical long-term outcome in patients with a history of takotsubo cardiomyopathy or myocardial infarction—a multi-centered case control study. Psychol Health Med. 2020;25(8):989–1003.
64. McDonagh TA, Metra M, Adamo M, Gardner RS, Baumbach A, Böhm M, et al. 2023 focused update of the 2021 ESC guidelines for the diagnosis and treatment of acute and chronic heart failure: developed by the task force for the diagnosis and treatment of acute and chronic heart failure of the European Society of Cardiology (ESC) with the special contribution of the heart failure association (HFA) of the ESC. Eur Heart J Fail. 2024;26:5–17.
65. McDonagh TA, Metra M, Adamo M, Gardner RS, Baumbach A, Böhm M, et al. 2021 ESC guidelines for the diagnosis and treatment of acute and chronic heart failure: developed by the task force for the diagnosis and treatment of acute and chronic heart failure of the European Society of Cardiology (ESC) with the special contribution of the heart failure association (HFA) of the ESC. Eur Heart J. 2021;42(36):3599–726.
66. Tadic M, Cuspidi C, Plein S, Belyavskiy E, Heinzel F, Galderisi M. Sex and heart failure with preserved ejection fraction: from pathophysiology to clinical studies. J Clin Med. 2019;8(6):792.
67. Gustad LT, Laugsand LE, Janszky I, Dalen H, Bjerkeset O. Symptoms of anxiety and depression and risk of heart failure: the HUNT study. Eur J Heart Fail. 2014;16(8):861–70.
68. Bobo WV, Ryu E, Petterson TM, Lackore K, Cheng Y, Liu H, et al. Bi-directional association between depression and HF: an electronic health records-based cohort study. J Comorb. 2020;10:2235042x20984059.
69. Ogilvie RP, Everson-Rose SA, Longstreth WT Jr, Rodriguez CJ, Diez-Roux AV, Lutsey PL. Psychosocial factors and risk of incident heart failure: the multi-ethnic study of atherosclerosis. Circ Heart Fail. 2016;9(1):e002243.
70. Celano CM, Villegas AC, Albanese AM, Gaggin HK, Huffman JC. Depression and anxiety in heart failure: a review. Harv Rev Psychiatry. 2018;26(4):175–84.
71. Tsabedze N, Kinsey JH, Mpanya D, Mogashoa V, Klug E, Manga P. The prevalence of depression, stress and anxiety symptoms in patients with chronic heart failure. Int J Ment Health Syst. 2021;15(1):44.
72. Rashid S, Gulfam A, Noor TA, Yaseen K, Sheikh MAA, Malik M, et al. Anxiety and depression in heart failure: an updated review. Curr Probl Cardiol. 2023;48(11):101987.
73. Rutledge T, Reis VA, Linke SE, Greenberg BH, Mills PJ. Depression in heart failure a meta-analytic review of prevalence, intervention effects, and associations with clinical outcomes. J Am Coll Cardiol. 2006;48(8):1527–37.
74. Williams SA, Kasl SV, Heiat A, Abramson JL, Krumholz HM, Vaccarino V. Depression and risk

of heart failure among the elderly: a prospective community-based study. Psychosom Med. 2002;64(1):6–12.
75. Daskalopoulou M, George J, Walters K, Osborn DP, Batty GD, Stogiannis D, et al. Depression as a risk factor for the initial presentation of twelve cardiac, cerebrovascular, and peripheral arterial diseases: data linkage study of 1.9 million women and men. PLoS One. 2016;11(4):e0153838.
76. Dewan P, Rørth R, Jhund PS, Shen L, Raparelli V, Petrie MC, et al. Differential impact of heart failure with reduced ejection fraction on men and women. J Am Coll Cardiol. 2019;73(1):29–40.
77. Lewis EF, Lamas GA, O'Meara E, Granger CB, Dunlap ME, McKelvie RS, et al. Characterization of health-related quality of life in heart failure patients with preserved versus low ejection fraction in CHARM. Eur J Heart Fail. 2007;9(1):83–91.
78. Ko D, Rahman F, Schnabel RB, Yin X, Benjamin EJ, Christophersen IE. Atrial fibrillation in women: epidemiology, pathophysiology, presentation, and prognosis. Nat Rev Cardiol. 2016;13(6):321–32.
79. Bazemore TC, Bolger LE, Sears SF, Sadaf MI, Gehi AK. Gender differences in symptoms and functional status in patients with atrial fibrillation undergoing catheter ablation. Pacing Clin Electrophysiol. 2019;42(2):224–9.
80. Wu H, Li C, Li B, Zheng T, Feng K, Wu Y. Psychological factors and risk of atrial fibrillation: a meta-analysis and systematic review. Int J Cardiol. 2022;362:85–92.
81. McCabe PJ. Psychological distress in patients diagnosed with atrial fibrillation: the state of the science. J Cardiovasc Nurs. 2010;25(1):40–51.
82. Mommersteeg PMC, Whittaker AC, Rohleder N. Stress and biological pathways of health and disease. In: Pedersen SS, Roessler KK, Anderse TE, Johnsen AT, Pouwer F, editors. Textbook of applied medical psychology a multidisciplinary approach. Odense: University Press of Southern Denmark; 2022. p. 35–60.
83. Sher LD, Geddie H, Olivier L, Cairns M, Truter N, Beselaar L, et al. Chronic stress and endothelial dysfunction: mechanisms, experimental challenges, and the way ahead. Am J Physiol Heart Circ Physiol. 2020;319(2):H488–506.
84. Vaccarino V, Shah AJ, Mehta PK, Pearce B, Raggi P, Bremner JD, et al. Brain-heart connections in stress and cardiovascular disease: implications for the cardiac patient. Atherosclerosis. 2021;328:74–82.
85. Stroud LR, Salovey P, Epel ES. Sex differences in stress responses: social rejection versus achievement stress. Biol Psychiatry. 2002;52(4):318–27.
86. Ervin J, Taouk Y, Alfonzo LF, Hewitt B, King T. Gender differences in the association between unpaid labour and mental health in employed adults: a systematic review. Lancet Public Health. 2022;7(9):e775–e86.
87. Bangasser DA, Wiersielis KR, Khantsis S. Sex differences in the locus coeruleus-norepinephrine system and its regulation by stress. Brain Res. 2016;1641(Pt B):177–88.
88. Iannuzzi V, Bacalini MG, Franceschi C, Giuliani C. The role of genetics and epigenetics in sex differences in human survival. Genus. 2023;79(1):1.
89. Kuo WC, Bratzke LC, Oakley LD, Kuo F, Wang H, Brown RL. The association between psychological stress and metabolic syndrome: a systematic review and meta-analysis. Obes Rev. 2019;20(11):1651–64.
90. Cotter EW, Kelly NR. Stress-related eating, mindfulness, and obesity. Health Psychol. 2018;37(6):516–25.
91. Gargiulo AT, Jasodanand V, Luz S, O'Mara L, Kubin L, Ross RJ, et al. Sex differences in stress-induced sleep deficits. Stress. 2021;24(5):541–50.
92. Djekic K, Ipp E. Loss of sex difference in high-density lipoprotein cholesterol in diabetic women during acute stress. J Clin Endocrinol Metab. 2014;99(11):E2357–61.
93. Ancelin ML, Carrière I, Boulenger JP, Malafosse A, Stewart R, Cristol JP, et al. Gender and genotype modulation of the association between lipid levels and depressive symptomatology in community-dwelling elderly (the ESPRIT study). Biol Psychiatry. 2010;68(2):125–32.
94. Sullivan S, Young A, Garcia M, Almuwaqqat Z, Moazzami K, Hammadah M, et al. Sex differences in vascular response to mental stress and adverse cardiovascular events among patients with ischemic heart disease. Arterioscler Thromb Vasc Biol. 2023;43(4):e112–e20.
95. Lyon AR, Citro R, Schneider B, Morel O, Ghadri JR, Templin C, et al. Pathophysiology of Takotsubo syndrome: JACC state-of-the-art review. J Am Coll Cardiol. 2021;77(7):902–21.
96. Shah SJ, Lam CSP, Svedlund S, Saraste A, Hage C, Tan RS, et al. Prevalence and correlates of coronary microvascular dysfunction in heart failure with preserved ejection fraction: PROMIS-HFpEF. Eur Heart J. 2018;39(37):3439–50.
97. Cohen S, Murphy MLM, Prather AA. Ten surprising facts about stressful life events and disease risk. Annu Rev Psychol. 2019;70:577–97.
98. Pruessner JC. The interplay of sex and gender on the reactivity of the endocrine stress axis in humans. Curr Opin Behav Sci. 2018;23:191–5.
99. Colbert JD, Martin BJ, Haykowsky MJ, Hauer TL, Austford LD, Arena RA, et al. Cardiac rehabilitation referral, attendance and mortality in women. Eur J Prev Cardiol. 2015;22(8):979–86.
100. Colella TJ, Gravely S, Marzolini S, Grace SL, Francis JA, Oh P, et al. Sex bias in referral of women to outpatient cardiac rehabilitation? A meta-analysis. Eur J Prev Cardiol. 2015;22(4):423–41.
101. Ghisi GLM, Kin SMR, Price J, Beckie TM, Mamataz T, Naheed A, et al. Women-focused cardiovascular rehabilitation: an International Council of Cardiovascular Prevention and Rehabilitation Clinical Practice Guideline. Can J Cardiol. 2022;38(12):1786–98.

102. Moore SM. Women's views of cardiac rehabilitation programs. J Cardiopulm Rehabil. 1996;16(2):123–9.
103. Firoozabadi MG, Mirzaei M, Grace SL, Vafaeinasab M, Dehghani-Tafti M, Sadeghi A, et al. Sex differences in cardiac rehabilitation barriers among nonenrollees in the context of lower gender equality: a cross-sectional study. BMC Cardiovasc Disord. 2023;23(1):329.
104. Grace SL, Gravely-Witte S, Kayaniyil S, Brual J, Suskin N, Stewart DE. A multisite examination of sex differences in cardiac rehabilitation barriers by participation status. J Womens Health (Larchmt). 2009;18(2):209–16.
105. Supervía M, Medina-Inojosa JR, Yeung C, Lopez-Jimenez F, Squires RW, Pérez-Terzic CM, et al. Cardiac rehabilitation for women: a systematic review of barriers and solutions. Mayo Clin Proc. 2017;92:565–77.
106. Piepoli MF, Hoes AW, Agewall S, Albus C, Brotons C, Catapano AL, et al. 2016 European guidelines on cardiovascular disease prevention in clinical practice: the sixth joint task force of the European Society of Cardiology and Other Societies on cardiovascular disease prevention in clinical practice (constituted by representatives of 10 societies and by invited experts)developed with the special contribution of the European Association for Cardiovascular Prevention & rehabilitation (EACPR). Eur Heart J. 2016;37(29):2315–81.
107. Perk J, De Backer G, Gohlke H, Graham I, Reiner Z, Verschuren M, et al. European guidelines on cardiovascular disease prevention in clinical practice (version 2012). The fifth joint task force of the European Society of Cardiology and Other Societies on cardiovascular disease prevention in clinical practice (constituted by representatives of nine societies and by invited experts). Eur Heart J. 2012;33(13):1635–701.
108. Knuuti J, Wijns W, Saraste A, Capodanno D, Barbato E, Funck-Brentano C, et al. 2019 ESC guidelines for the diagnosis and management of chronic coronary syndromes. Eur Heart J. 2019;41(3):407–77.
109. Hindricks G, Potpara T, Dagres N, Arbelo E, Bax JJ, Blomström-Lundqvist C, et al. 2020 ESC guidelines for the diagnosis and management of atrial fibrillation developed in collaboration with the European Association for Cardio-Thoracic Surgery (EACTS): the task force for the diagnosis and management of atrial fibrillation of the European Society of Cardiology (ESC) developed with the special contribution of the European heart rhythm association (EHRA) of the ESC. Eur Heart J. 2021;42(5):373–498.
110. Virani SS, Newby LK, Arnold SV, Bittner V, Brewer LC, Demeter SH, et al. 2023 AHA/ACC/ACCP/ASPC/NLA/PCNA guideline for the Management of Patients with Chronic Coronary Disease: a report of the American Heart Association/American College of Cardiology Joint Committee on clinical practice guidelines. Circulation. 2023;148(9):e9–e119.
111. Brouwers RWM, van Exel HJ, van Hal JMC, Jorstad HT, de Kluiver EP, Kraaijenhagen RA, et al. Cardiac telerehabilitation as an alternative to centre-based cardiac rehabilitation. Neth Heart J. 2020;28(9):443–51.
112. van den Houdt S, Albus C, Herrmann-Lingen C, Widdershoven J, Kupper N. Validity of a multidimensional comprehensive psychosocial screening instrument based on the ESC cardiovascular prevention guidelines—evidence from the general and cardiovascular patient population. J Psychosom Res. 2022;157:110791.
113. Kronish IM, Moise N, Cheung YK, Clarke GN, Dolor RJ, Duer-Hefele J, et al. Effect of depression screening after acute coronary syndromes on quality of life: the CODIACS-QoL randomized clinical trial. JAMA Intern Med. 2020;180(1):45–53.
114. Riehm KE, Davidson KW, Moise N, Margolis KL, Clarke GN, Dolor RJ, et al. Effectiveness of stepped depression care among patients with screen-identified depression after acute coronary syndromes: a secondary analysis of the CODIACS-QoL randomized clinical trial. Gen Hosp Psychiatry. 2022;78:126–7.
115. Schneiderman N, Saab PG, Catellier DJ, Powell LH, DeBusk RF, Williams RB, et al. Psychosocial treatment within sex by ethnicity subgroups in the enhancing recovery in coronary heart disease clinical trial. Psychosom Med. 2004;66(4):475–83.
116. Sramek JJ, Murphy MF, Cutler NR. Sex differences in the psychopharmacological treatment of depression. Dialogues Clin Neurosci. 2016;18(4):447–57.

Domestic Violence, Psychosocial Stress, Socio-Economic Status and CVD Risk in Women

Nicole van Gelder and Sabine Oertelt-Prigione

Abstract

Many women experience at least one type (psychological, physical, sexual, and economic) of intimate partner violence (IPV) during their lifetime. Women who experience(d) IPV are at increased risk of developing CVD, therefore knowledge about IPV and how to address it during clinical consultation is important for healthcare professionals. In this chapter, we discuss the link between IPV and CVD via various pathways (e.g. risk behavior, stress, mental health issues, coping mechanisms, and injuries). Furthermore, we describe options for detecting, screening, and disclosure of IPV in the clinical context.

Keywords

Intimate partner violence · Domestic violence Cardiovascular disease · Mental health · Socioeconomic status

Test your learning and check your understanding of this book's contents: use the "Springer Nature Flashcards" app to access questions using ▶ https://sn.pub/51ny7m To use the app, please follow the instructions in chapter 1.

1 Introduction: Types and Incidence of Intimate Partner Violence (IPV)

Domestic violence (DV) is an umbrella term for a diverse range of interpersonal violence and abuse dynamics, for example: intimate partner violence (IPV), child abuse, elder abuse, and honor-based violence. This chapter will focus on IPV defined as "any behavior by a current or former intimate partner within the context of marriage, cohabitation or any other formal or informal union, that causes physical, sexual or psychological harm." (p. 4; [1]).

N. van Gelder
Gender Unit, Department of Primary and Community Care, Radboudumc, Nijmegen, The Netherlands

S. Oertelt-Prigione (✉)
Gender Unit, Department of Primary and Community Care, Radboudumc, Nijmegen, The Netherlands

AG10 Sex- and Gender-Sensitive Medicine, Medical Faculty OWL, University of Bielefeld, Bielefeld, Germany
e-mail: sabine.oertelt-prigione@radboudumc.nl

A. H.E.M. Maas, E. Gerdts (eds.), *Manual of Cardiovascular Disease in Women*,
https://doi.org/10.1007/978-3-031-65952-2_16

IPV consists of various forms of violence and abuse: psychological (e.g. controlling behaviors, manipulating, humiliating, stalking, making threats), physical (e.g. hitting, strangulation, using weapons), sexual (e.g. assault, rape, stealthing, image-based sexual abuse), and economic (e.g. preventing from access to money and resources, preventing from study or paid employment, committing fraud or making debts in the survivor's name) [1–3]. IPV can be perpetrated in person but also with the use of technology, for example hacking, online stalking, or spreading intimate photos of the survivor online (or threatening to do so (i.e. sextortion)) [4, 5]. It occurs in all layers of society, in heterosexual and non-heterosexual relationships. While both men and women can be survivors of IPV, yet women experience this type of violence more often, especially when it comes to structural IPV. Also, women sustain more severe physical injuries from IPV and they are more often killed by their male (ex-) partner [1, 6, 7]. People belonging to the LGBTQ+ community are also at higher risk for experiencing IPV, possibly due to a combination of factors, among them discrimination, stigma, and homo-, bi- and transphobia [8].

Globally, approximately one in four women aged 15 years and older experiences physical and/ or sexual violence by an intimate partner at least once during their lifetime [1]. With regards to psychological IPV, data from European countries show that 44% of women experiences this type of abuse [2]. Approximately 15%–20% of women in the United States and Europe reported having experienced economic abuse by an intimate (ex-)partner [9–12]. Vulnerable groups experience a higher risk of IPV, for example: women with a refugee or migration background [13, 14], women with physical and / or mental disabilities [15], and women who do not identify as heterosexual [8, 16].

IPV has detrimental consequences on multiple levels such as physical health, mental health, social life, and economic situation. The impact on physical health can entail injuries, disabilities, (chronic) illness, fatigue, psychosomatic complaints, sleeping problems, joint conditions, gastrointestinal problems, traumatic brain injury, sexual and reproductive problems, and sexually transmitted diseases [17–21]. The survivor's mental health can be affected by depression, anxiety, high levels of stress, posttraumatic stress disorder, self-harm, suicidality, low self-esteem, and problems with executive functioning [19, 20, 22, 23]. Survivors of IPV can to be isolated and alienated from family, friends, colleagues, neighbors etc. This could be directly due to actions of the abusive (ex-) partner, for example not allowing the survivor to leave the house or threatening to hurt the survivor's loved ones. A survivor could also withdraw from their social network because they are ashamed of their partnership situation, or afraid of someone finding out and the possible consequences [24, 25]. IPV can also affect the survivor's economic situation, for example through loss of paid employment, loss of money and resources, debt, and discontined studies [3, 26]. Last, a form of IPV that is of particular importance for the healthcare sector is chemical restraint. In this situation, the abusive partner controls or denies the survivor access to medications and treatment, or coerces the survivor into using unnecessary medications or illegal drugs [27]. Women experiencing IPV who seek medical care for CVD could be exposed to this particular type of violence as well and it might impact their ability to adhere to their necessary medication regimen.

2 Theoretical Background

IPV can occur in diverse partnership dynamics (for example intimate terrorism or situational couple violence) and can include various forms of abuse. Therefore, the presentation of IPV can differ significantly depending on the survivor's unique experience. For example, one could encounter a survivor whose abusive partner asserts coercive control and abuses them psychologically and economically, but has never perpetrated physical or sexual violence. This survivor would not match the stereotypical picture of a "victim of IPV" and potentially not obtain the support they might need. One could also encounter IPV in the form of a couple in which both partners are verbally and physically violent towards each other, complicating the identification of support needs. Regardless of the specific nature of the IPV experience, all forms of IPV represent a constant stressor in a survivor's life. The constant stress is caused by the recurrence of abusive events. Some survivors experience a form of IPV every day, while others only experience IPV sporadically and unpredictably. However, in both situations the survivor will experience constant stress, either because they are constantly being abused (for example in the case of coercive control) or because they are stressed and worried about when the next escalation will occur, as they are feeling tension building up knowing that it will eventually lead to acts of abuse and violence [28].

2.1 IPV and Psychosocial Stress

Experiencing IPV is linked to mental health complaints, in particular depression, anxiety, and posttraumatic stress disorder (PTSD) [20, 23, 29]. Experiencing IPV is strongly linked to a higher risk of experiencing symptoms of depression, with the severity of the depression being influenced by the duration and severity of the IPV situation and the amount of IPV types the survivor was exposed to. Similar trends are observed for PTSD and anxiety, and a high comorbidity with symptoms of depression is found as well for both PTSD and anxiety [20, 23]. Survivors of IPV consistently report lower levels of mental and social wellbeing, and higher levels of psychological distress [20, 23, 30]. Mental health complaints related to IPV victimization can be long lasting, persisting for years after having left the abusive partner [20, 30–32]. Furthermore, ending the relationship with an abusive partner does not mean that the IPV will (immediately) end as well.

2.2 IPV and Socio-Economic Status

Both IPV and economic hardship have a negative influence on women's mental health [20, 23, 33, 34]. Women with a lower socio-economic status (SES) tend to experience IPV more often than women with a higher SES, and a lower SES hinders the process of leaving an abusive partner due to e.g. economic dependency and possibly limited resources to navigate the help-seeking process [35–38]. However, women with a higher education and income level than their male partner can also experience a high risk of experiencing IPV if the male partner embraces traditional gender role beliefs that could be triggered by a potentially equal partner [39–41]. IPV can influence a survivor's SES directly, through economic abuse, and indirectly, for example by not being able to sustain paid employment due to physical and / or mental health issues caused by IPV [3, 42].

Women survivors of IPV experience between 19% and 42% higher healthcare costs than non-abused women [43]. This difference in healthcare costs persists for 3 years after the violence has ended [44] but, as an Australian study found, the impact on healthcare costs could also last a lifetime: *"Women who experience IPV have AUD 48,413 higher lifetime health costs per person"* [45]. A study from the United States estimates the lifetime costs of IPV at $103,767 per women survivor and $23,414 per men survivor. Most costs would come from medical care (59%), followed by productivity loss at work for both survivors and perpetrators (37%; [46]).

2.3 IPV and CVD

IPV has been linked to an increased risk of CVD, for example heart attack and thrombosis [20, 21, 47, 48]. Adolescents and young adults who experienced IPV have an increased risk of CVD years after having been exposed to IPV [49]. Chandan and colleagues [47] recently described how women who experienced IPV were at a 31% higher risk for future CVD in comparison to non-victimized women. The largest disparity between the victimized and non-victimized group appeared for ischemic heart disease, with a 50% higher risk [47]. Importantly, the IPV group displayed an overall higher prevalence of comorbidities, such as type 2 diabetes mellitus, hypertension, hyperlipidemia, as well as a history of excessive drinking. This highlights the complexity of in investigating the nexus between IPV and CVD. Available research data often do not allow to disentangle whether specific risk factors are present in the population of IPV and CVD *a priori*, or if coping mechanisms and associated risk factors for IPV translate into an increased risk for CVD. For example, were women survivors of IPV with CVD more likely to smoke (before having experienced IPV) or do they start smoking as a coping mechanism due to IPV experiences, increasing their CVD risk? Overall, the potential risk pathways for CVD include both biological and psychological factors. Biological aspects can be inflammatory pathways leading to co-morbidities or antecedents such as atherosclerosis, hypertension, diabetes or hyperlipidemia. Psychological factors include different forms of stress, anxiety, depression, and other mental health issues.

Regardless of whether the mechanism is common to IPV and CVD or a causal pathway leading from IPV to CVD, biological mechanisms appear plausible, but have been seldom documented in the literature. For example, although a potential correlation between IPV and the development of hypertension seems likely, studies have failed to identify clear ties between the two this far [21]. Several studies have reported a potential correlation between IPV and hyperlipidemia and obesity [50, 51]. However, large (ideally prospective) study populations will be needed to confirm these findings. A potential link with endocrinological disruption and emergence of diabetes could also not be confirmed. These findings can be influenced by several factors. First, the available studies into the biological consequences of IPV are often limited in participant size. Second, many studies are cross-sectional rather than long-term cohort investigations that could identify potential causal links. Third, underreporting of IPV is a well-known limitation to its systematic investigation. Specifically, some forms of IPV, such as psychological and economic abuse, are under- or unreported potentially skewing correlations identified in the available data.

The association of different forms of stress and mental health issues with IPV has been documented more extensively. However, also in this case, most studies describe associations rather than causal pathways linking IPV experiences with the development of these conditions. The most commonly hypothesized connections between IPV and CVD in the field of mental health, are psychological distress, depression, PTSD, and maladaptive coping strategies. Especially maladaptive coping strategies are themselves risk factors for CVD, such as alcohol abuse and smoking. Both are more prevalent amongst survivors of IPV and can directly increase their CVD risk [21, 48, 52–55]. Furthermore, survivors can experience diverse other stressors that can be linked to IPV and can affect their health, for example: worries about the impact of witnessing IPV on their children, co-occurring child abuse, fear of losing their children, fear of the consequences if anyone finds out about the abuse, fear of loved ones being hurt by the abusive partner, negative reactions when disclosing IPV, feeling guilty about the situation (self-blaming), worries about their pet's wellbeing (when the abusive partner harms their pet or threatens to do so), economic dependency, financial issues, dependency for a residence permit, and (gender, sexual, cultural etc.) minority stress and discrimination [56–60]. All these factors can lead to the lower levels of mental and social wellbeing, and higher levels of psychological distress [20, 23, 30] described above. Subsequently, the heightened levels of stress might increase the risk for cardiovascular disease, as described in the literature [61–63]. Importantly, the role of stress as a cardiovascular risk factor might be more pronounced in women, especially of young age [64], the group mostly affected by IPV. Hence, overall, IPV should be considered a substantial risk factor for CVD in female patients.

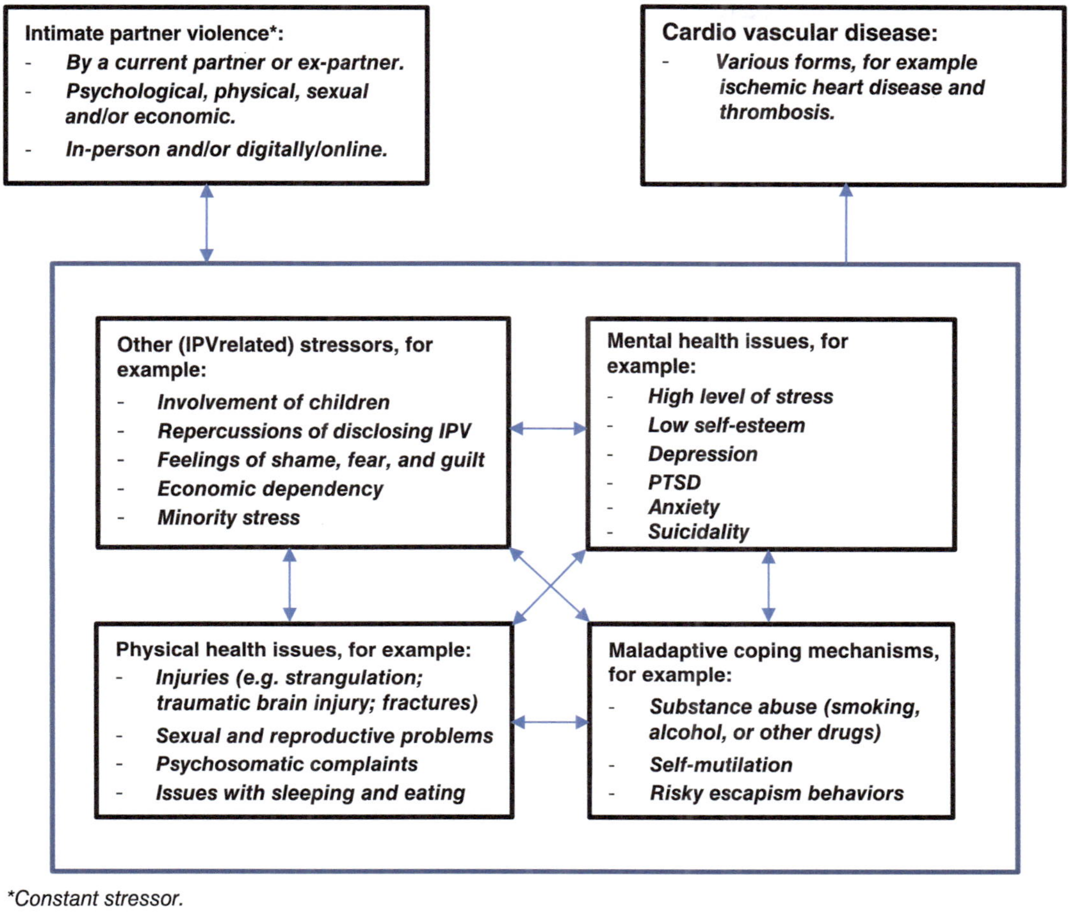

3 Recommendations for Detection of IPV in Clinical Practice

Healthcare professionals frequently are the first professional a survivor decides to disclose the IPV experience to [65]. Disclosure is a complex process, often the consequence of a number of previous unsuccessful attempts due to being afraid and/or ashamed. Sometimes survivors are also unaware that the abuse they have experienced is indeed IPV and seek validation of their trauma. In any case, the moment of disclosure is a vulnerable and confidential situation, which requires specific attention from the healthcare provider [66–68].

To detect IPV in a clinical setting several signs should be considered:

- The presence of physical signs of aggression, for example different types of bruises or injuries (*always look for petechial hemorrhaging as a sign of strangulation and, hence, potentially life-threatening situation*), sexually transmitted diseases, and psychosomatic complaints (e.g. unexplained headaches or stomach aches, hyperventilation, heart palpitations, muscle tension, sleeping issues).
- The patient provides an explanation of the injury that does not comply with how such an injury is likely to be sustained.
- The patient often cancels appointments with the healthcare professional or their partner will not leave them alone with the healthcare professional. Their partner might also be dominant in the conversation with the healthcare

professional and for example speak for the patient.
- The patient often looks to their partner for approval or, if their partner is not present, says things like "I have to ask my partner first" or "my partner does not allow me to …".
- The patient might constantly receive phone calls or messages from their partner during the consultation.
- The patient may seem nervous or very quiet, avoid eye contact, or pull away / react startled during physical examination.
- The patient might avoid talking about their personal situation with regard to their partner, relationship, or family.
- The patient shows signs of (extreme) fatigue, malnourishment, poor hygiene, and neglect taking care of themselves.
- The patient shows symptoms of mental health problems, for example symptoms of a high level of stress, low self-esteem, burnout, depression, anxiety, PTSD, suicidality, maladaptive coping mechanisms (e.g. substance abuse, self-mutilation).
- The patient shows problems with executive functioning.
- Social isolation.
- Not being allowed to study or work, or to have access to money and resources.

These signs do not provide a definitive diagnosis of IPV and can potentially correlate with other diseases or life situations, however, especially the presence of multiple of them at the same time should be considered as a red flag for IPV in need of further investigation.

When it comes to screening for IPV and disclosure, women express certain needs and wishes. For example, they value the healthcare professional creating a safe space and promoting connection, acknowledging their complex situation, addressing their personal context, and being non-judgmental, non-minimizing, and non-directive [66–69]. If a healthcare professional suspects that a patient might be experiencing IPV and wants to discuss this, they could for example use the following statements or questions [70, 71]:

- "I have seen women with problems like yours who have been experiencing trouble at home."
- "Do you sometimes feel unsafe or not free in your relationship?"
- "Is there anyone who is hurting, threatening, or controlling you in any way?"
- "Are you afraid of your partner?"

If IPV is disclosed, the healthcare professional might be obliged to report it. Handling of IPV and disclosure obligations differ between countries and might represent a complex situation and/or choice for the healthcare provider. In fact, a report from the World Health Organization (WHO) states that in 44 out of 174 countries healthcare professionals are obliged to report signs of IPV. However, the WHO advises against mandatory reporting for violence against women (VAW; this includes IPV against women) *"on grounds that it can violate women's autonomy and confidentiality and act as a deterrent for survivors to disclose their experiences to healthcare providers and thus can prevent them from accessing timely health services. Instead, WHO recommends that healthcare providers provide information on the legal process so that women can make an informed decision about reporting, and then offer to report violence on their behalf or assist those women who wish to report for themselves* [20]." (p. 18; [72]).

4 Conclusions

While it is clear that IPV and CVD are correlated, possibly through factors such as stress, mental health issues, and maladaptive coping, the link between them remains complex. Longitudinal studies and a proper assessment of IPV in all its complexity are needed to clarify direct, indirect, and bidirectional relations. However, the disentanglement of common risk factors and causality pathways is difficult. Systematic screening could help to enlighten certain patterns and increase insight on the combined prevalence of IPV and CVD.

With the current knowledge, stress appears as a causal pathway and this could be used as a trigger to investigate IPV (if appropriate). Especially when other signs that could be IPV-related are present as well. For example, physical signs of injury and a patient's explanation that does not match how such an injury is likely to be sustained; or a patient that avoids talking about their personal situation. Currently, IPV is still a topic that many physicians avoid due to a lack of preparedness, a lack of awareness, and fear of re-traumatization. Therefore, it is essential to educate healthcare professionals on how to appropriately address IPV and handle disclosure [65].

Key Issues

- IPV occurs frequently, in all layers of society, and consists of physical, psychological, sexual, and economic abuse.
- IPV is related to increased risk for CVD via various pathways, such as stress and maladaptive coping mechanisms (e.g. smoking, alcohol abuse).
- CVD in combination with stress could be a sign to investigate if IPV is present. Especially when this is accompanied by other signs that are listed in the paragraph on clinical practice.
- Healthcare professionals need to be educated on IPV to promote adequate detecting, screening, discussing, reporting, referring, and advising; and to reduce lack of preparedness and awareness, and fear or re-traumatization and harming the physician-patient relationship.

Questions and Answers

1. How many women in the general population are likely to experience IPV in their lifetime?
   (A) 1 every 2
   (B) 1 every 4
   (C) 1 every 10
   (D) 1 every 20
   Correct answer: B

   Globally, approximately one in four women aged 15 years and older experiences physical and/or sexual violence by an intimate partner at least once during their lifetime [1].

2. Which forms of IPV exist and can affect patients with CVD?
   (A) Physical violence
   (B) Sexual violence
   (C) Psychological violence
   (D) A and B
   (E) All of the above
   Correct answer: E

   IPV consists of various forms of violence and abuse: psychological (e.g. controlling behaviors, manipulating, humiliating, stalking, making threats), physical (e.g. hitting, strangulation, using weapons), sexual (e.g. assault, rape, stealthing, image-based sexual abuse), and economic (e.g. preventing from access to money and resources, preventing from study or paid employment, committing fraud or making debts in the survivor's name) [1–3].

3. Which risk pathways have been described for the connection between IPV and CVD?
   (A) Patients that experience IPV are more likely to develop diabetes, which increases their risk of CVD.
   (B) Patients that experience IPV are more likely to experience chronic stress, which increases their risk of CVD.
   (C) Patients that experience IPV are more likely to develop unhealthy coping mechanisms, like smoking and consuming drugs and alcohol, which increases their risk of CVD.
   (D) All of the above
   (E) B and C
   Correct answer: E

   Overall, the potential risk pathways for CVD include both biological and psychological factors. Biological aspects can be inflammatory pathways leading to co-morbidities or antecedents such as atherosclerosis, hypertension or hyperlipidemia. Psychological factors include different forms of stress, anxiety, depression, and other mental health issues.

4. What attitudes are important for a healthcare provider when asking about IPV?
   (A) Always actively asking all female patients about potential experiences of IPV
   (B) Creating a safe space and maintaining a non-judgmental attitude throughout the consultation
   (C) Always questioning both partners about the situation to maintain an impartial attitude
   (D) Reminding the patient that as soon as all information has been gathered the healthcare provider will notify the authorities on behalf of the survivor

   Correct answer: B

   Survivors of IPV value the healthcare professional creating a safe space and promoting connection, acknowledging their complex situation, addressing their personal context, and being non-judgmental, non-minimizing, and non-directive [66–69].

References

1. WHO. Global, regional and national prevalence estimates for intimate partner violence against women and global and regional prevalence estimates for non-partner sexual violence against women, vol. Violence against women prevalence estimates, 2018. Geneva: WHO; 2021.
2. European Institute for Gender Equality. Combating coercive control and psychological violence against women in the EU Member States; 2022.
3. Postmus JL, Hoge GL, Breckenridge J, Sharp-Jeffs N, Chung D. Economic abuse as an invisible form of domestic violence: a multicountry review. Trauma Violence Abuse. 2020;21(2):261–83.
4. Kim C, Ferraresso R. Examining technology-facilitated intimate partner violence: a systematic review of journal articles. Trauma Violence Abuse. 2023;24(3):1325–43.
5. Fernet M, Lapierre A, Hébert M, Cousineau M-M. A systematic review of literature on cyber intimate partner victimization in adolescent girls and women. Comput Hum Behav. 2019;100:11–25.
6. Stockl H, Devries K, Rotstein A, Abrahams N, Campbell J, Watts C, et al. The global prevalence of intimate partner homicide: a systematic review. Lancet. 2013;382(9895):859–65.
7. Hardesty JL, Ogolsky BG. A socioecological perspective on intimate partner violence research: a decade in review. J Marriage Fam. 2020;82(1):454–77.
8. Decker M, Littleton HL, Edwards KM. An updated review of the literature on LGBTQ+ intimate partner violence. Curr Sex Health Rep. 2018;10(4):265–72.
9. FRA E. Violence against women: an EU-wide survey. Report for European Union Agency for Fundamental Rights; 2014.
10. Kutin J, Russell R, Reid M. Economic abuse between intimate partners in Australia: prevalence, health status, disability and financial stress. Aust N Z J Public Health. 2017;41(3):269–74.
11. Sharp-Jeffs N. Money matters : research into the extent and nature of financial abuse within intimate relationships in the UK. London: London Metropolitan University; 2015.
12. Voth Schrag RJ. Economic abuse and later material hardship:is depression a mediator? Affilia. 2015;30(3):341–51.
13. Freedman J. Sexual and gender-based violence against refugee women: a hidden aspect of the refugee "crisis". Reprod Health Matters. 2016;24(47):18–26.
14. Wachter K, Cook Heffron L, Dalpe J, Spitz A. "Where is the Women's center here?": the role of information in refugee Women's help seeking for intimate partner violence in a resettlement context. Violence Against Women. 2021;27(12–13):2355–76.
15. García-Cuéllar MM, Pastor-Moreno G, Ruiz-Pérez I, Henares-Montiel J. The prevalence of intimate partner violence against women with disabilities: a systematic review of the literature. Disabil Rehabil. 2023;45(1):1–8.
16. Russell B. Intimate partner violence and the LGBT+ community. Understanding power dynamics. Cham: Springer Nature Switzerland AG; 2020.
17. Murray CE, Lundgren K, Olson LN, Hunnicutt G. Practice update: what professionals who are not brain injury specialists need to know about intimate partner violence-related traumatic brain injury. Trauma Violence Abuse. 2016;17(3):298–305.
18. Haag HL, Jones D, Joseph T, Colantonio A. Battered and brain injured: traumatic brain injury among women survivors of intimate partner violence-a scoping review. Trauma Violence Abuse. 2022;23(4):1270–87.
19. Ellsberg M, Jansen HA, Heise L, Watts CH, Garcia-Moreno C. Intimate partner violence and women's physical and mental health in the WHO multi-country study on women's health and domestic violence: an observational study. Lancet. 2008;371(9619):1165–72.
20. Dillon G, Hussain R, Loxton D, Rahman S. Mental and physical health and intimate partner violence against women: a review of the literature. Int J Family Med. 2013;2013:313909.
21. Stubbs A, Szoeke C. The effect of intimate partner violence on the physical health and health-related behaviors of women: a systematic review of the literature. Trauma Violence Abuse. 2022;23(4):1157–72.
22. Twamley EW, Allard CB, Thorp SR, Norman SB, Hami Cissell S, Hughes Berardi K, et al. Cognitive impairment and functioning in PTSD related to

intimate partner violence. J Int Neuropsychol Soc. 2009;15(6):879–87.
23. Lagdon S, Armour C, Stringer M. Adult experience of mental health outcomes as a result of intimate partner violence victimisation: a systematic review. Eur J Psychotraumatol. 2014;5(1):24794.
24. Peterman A, Potts A, O'Donnell M, Thompson K, Shah N, Oertelt-Prigione S, et al. Pandemics and violence against women and children. Washington, DC: Center for Global Development; 2020.
25. O'Doherty LJ, Taft A, McNair R, Hegarty K. Fractured identity in the context of intimate partner violence: barriers to and opportunities for seeking help in health settings. Violence Against Women. 2016;22(2):225–48.
26. Johnson L, Chen Y, Stylianou A, Arnold A. Examining the impact of economic abuse on survivors of intimate partner violence: a scoping review. BMC Public Health. 2022;22(1):1014.
27. Walker S-J, Hester M, McCarthy L. The use of 'chemical restraints' in the context of domestic abuse: widening our understanding of coercive control. In: European conference on domestic violence, Ljubljana; 2021.
28. Boxall H, Lawler S. How does domestic violence escalate over time? In: Trends & issues in crime and criminal justice. Canberra: Australian Institute of Criminology; 2021. p. 626.
29. Chandan JS, Thomas T, Bradbury-Jones C, Russell R, Bandyopadhyay S, Nirantharakumar K, et al. Female survivors of intimate partner violence and risk of depression, anxiety and serious mental illness. Br J Psychiatry. 2020;217(4):562–7.
30. Loxton D, Dolja-Gore X, Anderson AE, Townsend N. Intimate partner violence adversely impacts health over 16 years and across generations: a longitudinal cohort study. PLoS One. 2017;12(6):e0178138.
31. Ford-Gilboe M, Wuest J, Varcoe C, Davies L, Merritt-Gray M, Campbell J, et al. Modelling the effects of intimate partner violence and access to resources on women's health in the early years after leaving an abusive partner. Soc Sci Med. 2009;68(6):1021–9.
32. Blasco-Ros C, Sánchez-Lorente S, Martinez M. Recovery from depressive symptoms, state anxiety and post-traumatic stress disorder in women exposed to physical and psychological, but not to psychological intimate partner violence alone: a longitudinal study. BMC Psychiatry. 2010;10(1):98.
33. Voth Schrag RJ, Robinson SR, Ravi K. Understanding pathways within intimate partner violence: economic abuse, economic hardship, and mental health. J Aggress Maltreat Trauma. 2019;28(2):222–42.
34. Frankham C, Richardson T, Maguire N. Psychological factors associated with financial hardship and mental health: a systematic review. Clin Psychol Rev. 2020;77:101832.
35. Yakubovich AR, Stöckl H, Murray J, Melendez-Torres GJ, Steinert JI, Glavin CEY, et al. Risk and protective factors for intimate partner violence against women: systematic review and meta-analyses of prospective-longitudinal studies. Am J Public Health. 2018;108(7):e1–e11.
36. Capaldi DM, Knoble NB, Shortt JW, Kim HK. A systematic review of risk factors for intimate partner violence. Partn Abus. 2012;2:231–80.
37. Davies L, Ford-Gilboe M, Willson A, Varcoe C, Wuest J, Campbell J, et al. Patterns of cumulative abuse among female survivors of intimate partner violence: links to women's health and socioeconomic status. Violence Against Women. 2015;21(1):30–48.
38. Reichel D. Determinants of intimate partner violence in Europe: the role of socioeconomic status, inequality, and partner behavior. J Interpers Violence. 2017;32(12):1853–73.
39. Anderson KL. Conflict, power, and violence in families. J Marriage Fam. 2010;72(3):726–42.
40. Sanders CK. Economic abuse in the lives of women abused by an intimate partner: a qualitative study. Violence Against Women. 2015;21(1):3–29.
41. Eggers Del Campo I, Steinert JI. The effect of female economic empowerment interventions on the risk of intimate partner violence: a systematic review and meta-analysis. Trauma Violence Abuse. 2022;23(3):810–26.
42. Stylianou AM. Economic abuse within intimate partner violence: a review of the literature. Violence Vict. 2018;1:3–22.
43. Bonomi AE, Anderson ML, Rivara FP, Thompson RS. Health care utilization and costs associated with physical and nonphysical-only intimate partner violence. Health Serv Res. 2009;44(3):1052–67.
44. Fishman PA, Bonomi AE, Anderson ML, Reid RJ, Rivara FP. Changes in health care costs over time following the cessation of intimate partner violence. J Gen Intern Med. 2010;25(9):920–5.
45. William J, Loong B, Hanna D, Parkinson B, Loxton D. Lifetime health costs of intimate partner violence: a prospective longitudinal cohort study with linked data for out-of-hospital and pharmaceutical costs. Econ Model. 2022;116:106013.
46. Peterson C, Kearns MC, McIntosh WL, Estefan LF, Nicolaidis C, McCollister KE, et al. Lifetime economic burden of intimate partner violence among U.S. adults. Am J Prev Med. 2018;55(4):433–44.
47. Chandan JS, Thomas T, Bradbury-Jones C, Taylor J, Bandyopadhyay S, Nirantharakumar K. Risk of cardiometabolic disease and all-cause mortality in female survivors of domestic abuse. J Am Heart Assoc. 2020;9(4):e014580.
48. El-Serag R, Thurston RC. Matters of the heart and mind: interpersonal violence and cardiovascular disease in women. J Am Heart Assoc. 2020;9(4):e015479.
49. Clark CJ, Alonso A, Everson-Rose SA, Spencer RA, Brady SS, Resnick MD, et al. Intimate partner violence in late adolescence and young adulthood and subsequent cardiovascular risk in adulthood. Prev Med. 2016;87:132–7.
50. Bosch J, Weaver TL, Arnold LD, Clark EM. The impact of intimate partner violence on Women's physical health: findings from the Missouri behavioral

risk factor surveillance system. J Interpers Violence. 2017;32(22):3402–19.
51. Stene LE, Jacobsen GW, Dyb G, Tverdal A, Schei B. Intimate partner violence and cardiovascular risk in women: a population-based cohort study. J Womens Health. 2013;22(3):250–8.
52. O'Neil A, Fisher AJ, Kibbey KJ, Jacka FN, Kotowicz MA, Williams LJ, et al. Depression is a risk factor for incident coronary heart disease in women: an 18-year longitudinal study. J Affect Disord. 2016;196:117–24.
53. Wright EN, Hanlon A, Lozano A, Teitelman AM. The impact of intimate partner violence, depressive symptoms, alcohol dependence, and perceived stress on 30-year cardiovascular disease risk among young adult women: a multiple mediation analysis. Prev Med. 2019;121:47–54.
54. Liu X, Logan J, Alhusen J. Cardiovascular risk and outcomes in women who have experienced intimate partner violence: an integrative review. J Cardiovasc Nurs. 2020;35(4):400–14.
55. Frank P, Batty GD, Pentti J, Jokela M, Poole L, Ervasti J, et al. Association between depression and physical conditions requiring hospitalization. JAMA Psychiatry. 2023;80(7):690–9.
56. O'Doherty L, Taket A, Valpied J, Hegarty K. Receiving care for intimate partner violence in primary care: barriers and enablers for women participating in the weave randomised controlled trial. Soc Sci Med. 2016;160:35–42.
57. Rose D, Trevillion K, Woodall A, Morgan C, Feder G, Howard L. Barriers and facilitators of disclosures of domestic violence by mental health service users: qualitative study. Br J Psychiatry. 2011;198(3):189–94.
58. Cleary M, Thapa DK, West S, Westman M, Kornhaber R. Animal abuse in the context of adult intimate partner violence: a systematic review. Aggress Violent Behav. 2021;61:101676.
59. Briddick C. Combatting or enabling domestic violence? Evaluating the residence rights of migrant victims of domestic violence in Europe. Int Compar Law Q. 2020;69(4):1013–34.
60. Caceres BA, Streed CG, Corliss HL, Lloyd-Jones DM, Matthews PA, Mukherjee M, et al. Assessing and addressing cardiovascular health in LGBTQ adults: a scientific statement from the American Heart Association. Circulation. 2020;142(19):e321–e32.
61. Steptoe A, Kivimäki M. Stress and cardiovascular disease. Nat Rev Cardiol. 2012;9(6):360–70.
62. Dimsdale JE. Psychological stress and cardiovascular disease. J Am Coll Cardiol. 2008;51(13):1237–46.
63. Osborne MT, Shin LM, Mehta NN, Pitman RK, Fayad ZA, Tawakol A. Disentangling the links between psychosocial stress and cardiovascular disease. Circ Cardiovasc Imaging. 2020;13(8):e010931.
64. Vaccarino V, Wilmot K, Mheid IA, Ramadan R, Pimple P, Shah AJ, et al. Sex differences in mental stress-induced myocardial ischemia in patients with coronary heart disease. J Am Heart Assoc. 2016;5(9):e003630.
65. Jenner SC, Etzold SS, Oesterhelweg L, Stickel A, Kurmeyer C, Reinemann D, et al. Barriers to active inquiry about intimate partner violence among German physicians participating in a mandatory training. J Fam Violence. 2016;31(1):109–17.
66. Feder GS, Hutson M, Ramsay J, Taket AR. Women exposed to intimate partner violence: expectations and experiences when they encounter health care professionals: a meta-analysis of qualitative studies. Arch Intern Med. 2006;166(1):22–37.
67. Heron RL, Eisma MC. Barriers and facilitators of disclosing domestic violence to the healthcare service: a systematic review of qualitative research. Health Soc Care Community. 2021;29(3):612–30.
68. Tarzia L, Bohren MA, Cameron J, Garcia-Moreno C, O'Doherty L, Fiolet R, et al. Women's experiences and expectations after disclosure of intimate partner abuse to a healthcare provider: a qualitative metasynthesis. BMJ Open. 2020;10(11):e041339.
69. Melendez-Torres GJ, Dowdell EB, Kelley SJ, Lewis-O'Connor A. Strategies for identification of intimate partner violence in healthcare settings: overview of reviews and realist synthesis. J Fam Violence. 2022;38:1457–68.
70. World Health Organization. Health care for women subjected to intimate partner violence or sexual violence: a clinical handbook. Luxembourg: World Health Organization; 2014.
71. Basile KC, Hertz MF, Back SE. Intimate partner violence and sexual violence victimization assessment instruments for use in healthcare settings: version 1. Atlanta, GA: Centers for Disease Control and Prevention, National Center for Injury Prevention and Control; 2007.
72. World Health Organization. Addressing violence against women in health and multisectoral policies: a global status report. Geneva: World Health Organization; 2021.

Cardiovascular Health Issues in Transgender Persons

C. C. van Bunderen
and H. L. Claahsen- van der Grinten

Abstract

In the last 10 years increasing numbers of trans- and gender diverse individuals (TGDs) seek treatment to align their body to their gender identity. Treatment may consist, among others, of mental health support, hormonal treatment and surgical intervention. Gender-affirming hormone treatment (GAHT) aims to develop characteristics of the identified gender and thereby diminishing feelings of gender dysphoria. GAHT with testosterone/estrogens should be provided only after careful counseling about the advantages and disadvantages. GAHT in TGDs is generally considered to be safe and well tolerated. However, there is evidence that sex hormones influence several cardiovascular (CV) risk factors such as BMI, lipide profile, and blood pressure. Also, the risk for venous thromboembolic events is influenced. Therefore, GAHT for TGDs requires a multidisciplinary approach in which CV risk assessment is part of the counseling prior to treatment initiation (besides the evaluation of fertility). The contribution of (life style) factors (comorbidities, estrogen types, smoking, alcohol abuse) is addressed to balance the advantages against the disadvantages of treatment together. During GAHT, TGDs have to be carefully monitored lifelong for adverse effects in this area.

In this chapter we describe the CV risk factors and CV disease in TGDs who are treated with feminizing and in TGDs treated with masculinizing GAHT.

Keywords

Gender-affirming hormone therapy (GAHT) · Transgender · Gender diverse · Cardiovascular risk · Thromboembolic events

C. C. van Bunderen · H. L. C.- van der Grinten (✉)
Radboudumc Center Sex and Gender,
Radboudumc Amalia Children's Hospital,
Nijmegen, The Netherlands
e-mail: christa.vanbunderen@radboudumc.nl;
Hedi.Claahsen@radboudumc.nl

A. H.E.M. Maas, E. Gerdts (eds.), *Manual of Cardiovascular Disease in Women*,
https://doi.org/10.1007/978-3-031-65952-2_17

Test your learning and check your understanding of this book's contents: use the "Springer Nature Flashcards" app to access questions using ▶ https://sn.pub/51ny7m
To use the app, please follow the instructions in chapter 1.

1 Introduction

1.1 Genderdysphoria

The number of transgender and gender diverse identifying persons (TGDs) is growing, with a current estimated proportion of 0.1% to 2.7% [1]. TGDs are individuals whose sex assigned at birth does not align with their experienced gender identity, named gender incongruence (see Table 1). While transgender persons typically feel they identify more with the opposite sex than their sex assigned at birth, gender diverse individuals such as non-binary, genderfluid or gender non-conforming persons can fall anywhere on the gender spectrum [2]. TGDs can experience gender dysphoria (GD) when they feel discomfort or distress due to the gender incongruence often leading to significant mental health problems [3]. Health care is available for this population to help diminish the GD, and consequently, make TGDs feel more aligned with their gender identity after careful evaluation by experienced (mental) health care providers. The current care that can be offered consists among others mainly of mental health support, hormonal treatment and surgical intervention based on the needs of the individual. A medical treatment that is often initiated is gender-affirming hormone treatment (GAHT) [4]. Feminizing GAHT is available for individuals >15 years after careful evaluation, and who fulfill criteria for medical treatment. These criteria include careful mental assessment, fertility counseling and a medical screening including evaluation of the cardiovascular (CV) risk profile. Gender reassignment surgery is optional to further align physical appearances. GAHT, usually testosterone or a combination of estrogen and anti-androgens, provides the desired masculinizing or feminizing effects on certain body characteristics (see Table 2) [2]. In adolescents in whom pubertal development is not yet completed GAHT is most often preceded by a period of GnRH analogues to postpone endogenous puberty and thereby expanding the diagnostic phase before making final decisions about hor-

Table 1 Terms and definitions [20]

Cisgender, non-transgender	Adjectives for individuals whose gender identity is aligned with sex assigned at birth
Gender-affirming or gender-confirming hormone treatment (GAHT) and surgery	Medical/surgical interventions performed to align appearances with gender identity
Gender dysphoria	Mental health term for the discomfort felt by some transgender individuals due to lack of alignment between gender identity and sex assigned at birth
Gender expression	How an individual communicates gender identity internally and to others
Gender identity	An individual's internal sense of one's own sex
Transgender, transsexual, trans, trans- and gender diverse (TGD), gender-nonbinary, gender incongruent/incongruence, gender-nonconfirming, genderqueer	Adjectives for individuals whose gender identity is not aligned with sex assigned at birth
Transgender women, transwomen	Individuals who self-identify as female, but whose sex was assigned male at birth
Transgender men, transmen	Individuals who self-identify as male, but whose sex was assigned female at birth

Adopting language specific to transgender health care that includes definitions with consensus is essential for communicating with patients and within the medical field

Table 2 Gender-affirming hormone regimens in transgender and gender diverse persons

Feminization	Effect	Route of administration	Drug and dose
Estrogens	Breast growth, reduction in facial and body hair, softening of skin, change in body composition	Oral	Estradiol valerate 2–6 mg/day
		Transdermal	Estradiol patch 0.025–0.2 mg/day
			Estradiol gel 0.06% 0.75–1.5 mg/day
			Estradiol spray 1.53–4.59 mg/day
		Parenteral	Estradiol valerate or cypionate 5–30 mg/2-weekly or 2–10 mg/week (IM)
Antiandrogens	Additional suppressing of testosterone into the female range	Oral	Cyproterone acetate 10–50 mg/day
			Spironolactone 100–300 mg/day
		Parenteral	GnRH analogue 3.75 mg (SC/IM) monthly/11.25 mg 3-monthly (IM)
Progesterone	Alleged enhancement of breast development	Oral	Progesterone 200 mg/day
Masculinization			
Testosterone	Male pattern hair growth, muscle development, cessation of uterine bleeding	Transdermal	Testosterone gel 20–100 mg/day
		Parenteral	Testosterone esters 250 mg (IM) every 2–3 weeks
			Testosterone undecanoate 1000 mg (IM) every 10–12 weeks
Progesterone	Additional suppression of menstrual bleeds	Oral	Lynestrenol 5–10 mg/day
			Medroxyprogesterone 5–10 mg/day
			Norethisterone 5–10 mg/day
		Parenteral	Medroxyprogesterone 150 mg/mL (IM) every 12 weeks
			GnRH analogue 3.75 mg (SC/IM) monthly/11.25 mg 3-monthly (IM)

IM intramuscular, *SC* subcutaneously

monal treatment with irreversible changes. Furthermore, it has to be realized that GAHT affects fertility in both sexes. However, GAHT is considered beneficial for the quality of life and reduction of depression in TGDs, but high-quality data are limited [5]. Although GAHT has been prescribed by gender clinics for approximately 50 years, long-term data on efficacy, safety, and clinically relevant outcomes remain scarce. In this chapter we review the CV effects of sex hormones used for GAHT in TGDs after a short introduction into the current treatment guidelines.

1.2 Feminizing Hormonal Treatment

Mostly, the feminization implies suppression of the endogenous sex hormone production (androgen lowering) and replacement with sex hormone levels of the desired gender (estrogens) (see Table 2). The synthetic estrogen ethinyl estradiol was widely used in Europe prior to 2003. However, given safety concerns regarding thromboembolic and CV disease risk, most gender clinics have switched to oral or transdermal or intramuscular conjugated estradiol [6]. Studies comparing efficacy between different routes of estradiol application in feminization are sparse [7]. Depending on the outcome measure, no significant difference in effect is observed so far [8]. Next to estrogens, TGDs seeking feminization often require the addition of medication to lower testosterone levels into the female range [2]. Until recently, in most European countries oral cyproterone acetate (CPA), an androgen receptor blocker with some progesterone-like activity, was predominantly prescribed. However, since reports of increased risk of meningiomas [9], association with depression, and increased risk of hyperprolactinemia [10], GnRH agonists to suppress the pituitary gonadal axis with consequently decreasing testosterone concentrations are now predominantly prescribed in European countries. In the US, where GnRH agonists are not available, spironolactone is often used due to its antiandrogen effect in high dosage. Some transgender women request additional progesterone suppletion besides estrogens to enhance breast development, yet no clinical studies to date have demonstrated this effect. Furthermore, there are concerns that high doses of progesterone increase thromboembolic risk based on studies in cisgender postmenopausal women [11]. Therefore, its use is not incorporated in clinical guidelines and routine clinical practice at time. GAHT will need to be continued lifelong to maintain the achieved feminization and to avoid symptoms of hypogonadism, especially when gonadectomy has been performed. After optional gonadectomy, androgen-lowering therapy can be stopped.

1.3 Masculinizing Hormonal Treatment

Masculinization can be achieved by different testosterone formulations (see Table 2). Most prescribed preparations are parenteral testosterone esters and long-acting testosterone undecanoate, or daily administered topical testosterone gel. Aim of the treatment is to achieve testosterone levels within the normal male range. This will lead to increased muscle mass and facial and body hair but also growth of the clitoris and affect sexual desire. If menstrual bleeding does not stop after initiation of testosterone within 6 to 9 months, a progesterone such as oral lynestrenol or medroxyprogesterone, or a GnRH analogue, might be added.

1.4 GAHT in Adolescents

In adolescents in which endogenous puberty leads to an increase in sex hormone production and the development of sexual characteristics, a progression of GD and mental problems such as depression and decrease of quality of life can be observed. At this stage, pubertal suppression can be offered to prevent further development of pubertal signs leading to improvement of GD and mental health of the adolescent [12, 13]. Pubertal suppression using long acting GnRH analogues is considered to be fully reversible although there are concerns about a prolonged state of hypogonadism. Little is known about the CV effects of pubertal suppression at this age [14, 15]. Arterial hypertension has been reported in single cases. Therefore, blood pressure monitoring is recommended before and during treatment.

GAHT is usually available from the age of 16 years although current guidelines recommend to start earlier in patients with consistent gender incongruence who fulfill the treatment criteria but only after careful counseling about the irreversible body changes and informed consent [4, 16]. A multidisciplinary team of medical and mental health providers should be involved in the process of indication and follow up. In contrast to adults, adolescents usually start with lower dosages of sex hormones that gradually increase every 3–6 months similar to the recommendations for patients with absence of puberty. Especially in adolescents who did not reach final height, biometric parameters should be carefully monitored.

1.5 GAHT in Gender Diverse Individuals

For gender diverse individuals (e.g. non-binary), medical interventions may vary depending on the person's dysphoria and often a personalized treatment plan will be made taking into consideration both efficacy and safety issues.

1.6 General Concerns

GAHT in TGDs is generally considered to be safe [17]. Nevertheless, since sex hormones are well known to be able to influence several CV risk factors, TGDs are carefully screened before and monitored during medical treatment for adverse effects in this area (BMI, blood pressure, lipid profile), to prevent increased CV morbidity and mortality. However, long-term data on this topic are scarce. A recent retrospective cohort study on five decades of 4568 adult transgender people receiving GAHT showed an increased mortality risk regardless of treatment type (Standardized Mortality Ratio (SMR) 1.8 (95% CI 1.6–2.0) for transgender women compared to cismen and SMR 2.8 (95% 2.5–3.1) compared to ciswomen; and SMR 1.8 (95% CI 1.3–2.4) for transgender men compared to ciswomen and SMR 1.2 (95% CI 0.9–1.6) compared to cismen). The cause-specific mortality risk showed no specific effect of GAHT. Also, social stressors have been suggested to be important contributors [18]. Subsequently, next to fertility preservation counseling, prior to initiation, medical professionals should evaluate all transgender individuals for conditions that can be exacerbated by GAHT. Next to thromboembolic and CV risk factors, for estradiol this includes hormone-sensitive cancers (including mamma), hyperprolactinemia, and cholelithiasis. Medical conditions that are influenced by testosterone therapy include mostly risk factors that increase CV risk, e.g. dyslipidemia, hypertension, sleep apnea, and polycythemia [19]. Since gonadectomy is not always performed, cancers of ovary and uterus can still occur and thorough counseling on pertaining in relevant screening programs is important.

2 Theory

2.1 The Effect of Feminizing GAHT on CV Risk Factors

Despite the limited amount of research performed on this subject, evidence suggests that TGDs in general have an increased mortality risk. The before mentioned Dutch study by de Blok et al. (2021) found an increased mortality risk in TGDs using GAHT, especially in transgender women, together with a high cause-specific mortality for CV disease [18]. Glintborg et al. (2022) found that the risk of CV disease was also increased in Danish transgender men and women, which increased even further after initiation of GAHT mainly in transgender men [21]. More studies have conducted research on the short and longer term effect of GAHT on classic CV risk factors, mostly by examining body mass index, blood pressure, and lipid profile (see Table 3). Cocchetti et al. (2021) performed a study on the 30-year CV risk of transgender individuals who received GAHT in Ghent, Belgium. They found that in transgender women blood pressure decreased and lipid profile improved during GAHT [22]. In 2017, a systematic review including studies from 1980 onwards reported that transfeminine hormone therapy was associated with increased serum triglyceride levels in transgender women treated for >24 months with no changes in serum low-density lipoprotein or high-density lipoprotein [23]. The increase in triglycerides was not found in more recent studies with data from ENIGI (European Network for the Investigation of Gender Incongruence) on feminizing GAHT [24]. In a meta-analysis of studies published prior to 2015, transfeminine hormone therapy was associated with increased body fat and a decrease in lean body mass [25]. More recent studies from Europe have documented that BMI increases in transgender women after transfeminine hormone therapy [26, 27]. Klaver et al. [28] also demonstrated increases in body weight in 179 transgender women, and transfeminine hormone therapy was associated with an increase in body fat, specifically in the android, leg, and gynoid regions.

2.2 The Effect of Masculinizing GAHT on CV Risk Factors

In general, the use of testosterone in different applications is relatively safe with only a small number of studies reporting severe adverse effects. An increase in BMI is reported but

Table 3 An minimalistic overview of the reported effects of gender-affirming hormone regimens on cardiovascular risk factors in transgender and gender diverse persons

Parameter	Masculinizing GAHT	Feminizing GAHT
BMI	↑↑	↑
Blood pressure	↑	↓
Total cholesterol	↑	↓
LDL cholesterol	↑↑	↓↓
HDL cholesterol	↓↓	↓↑
Triglycerides	↑	↑↓
Hematocrit	↑↑	↓

↑/↓ increasing/decreasing effect demonstrated in some studies

↑/↓↓ increasing/decreasing effect demonstrated in all studies

↓/↑ decreasing and increasing effect demonstrated in some studies

mostly due to increased lean body mass [29]. The encountered alterations in the lipid profile should be taken into account. Most studies report an increase in triglyceride levels combined with a decrease in HDL cholesterol levels and an increase in LDL cholesterol levels after the introduction of testosterone [30, 31] (see Table 3). This alteration in lipid profile might contribute to an increased CV risk and patients should be counseled about the additional risk to develop atherosclerosis and/or coronary heart disease especially in the presence of other risk factors such as overweight, hypertension or smoking. Therefore, although hypertension is not a common feature in testosterone treatment, blood pressure should be monitored regularly.

Erythrocytosis defined as an hematocrit >50% is a known complication in the treatment with testosterone [32], and more common with parenteral administration compared to transdermal [33]. Erythrocytosis increases the risk of thromboembolic disease by an increase in blood viscosity. Therefore, current guidelines recommend to measure hematocrit regularly [4]. When a hematocrit levels exceeds levels >54% testosterone dose has to be lowered or reconsidered to reduce the risk to develop CV events [32].

2.3 The Effect of GAHT on CV Disease

Whether the above described findings result in clinically relevant adverse health outcomes is unclear. For instance, feminizing hormone therapy presents an interesting paradox: while it improves blood pressure and lipid profile, transgender women still experience a higher incidence of CV events [18]. To date, a definite explanation for this contradiction remains elusive. Next to the classic CV risk factors, limited number of studies have demonstrated an altering effect of GAHT on inflammation and hemostasis [34, 35], suggesting a possible role in the underlying mechanism explaining the increased CV risk in this population which merits further research. Also, it is apparent that socioeconomic and lifestyle factors may have substantial impact on CV risk. Evidence shows that TGDs are more likely to smoke, drink alcohol, use drugs, have unhealthy diet, or have poor exercise behaviors compared to the general population [36, 37]. Next to this, they might also experience excess stress due to a stigmatized social position, so called minority stress [38]. Karalexi et al. (2022), for instance, demonstrated an increased incidence of CV disease in Swedish TGDs, but this incidence did not seem to differ between TGDs who had started GAHT and those who had not [39]. This result indicates that other factors, such as lifestyle or minority stress, could also contribute to the increased risk for developing CV disease described in mainly transgender women.

In addition, most patients described in these long term observational studies were prescribed older treatment regimes, e.g. including the chronical use of CPA, which may increase the risk for CV disease more than the currently used treatment to lower testosterone levels, such as GnRH analogues [40, 41]. Consequently, the effect of GAHT on the CV risk might currently be less severe, necessitating long-term follow up studies to be repeated or continued and different treatment regimens should compared or, at least, be taken into account.

2.4 The Effect of GAHT on Venous Thromboembolic Events (VTE)

Although data of VTE risk in transgender women is much less comprehensive than in cisgender women, the smaller cohort and retrospective studies available seem to confirm the increased VTE risk associated with oral GAHT. For example, the largest cohort study published to date investigated over 2800 U.S. adult transgender women and more than 2100 U.S. adult transgender men for a period of 4 years, and matched them to cisgender women in a 1:10 ratio [42]. In transgender women, the 2- and 8-year VTE risk differences were 4.1 and 16.7 per 1000 person-years, respectively, relative to cisgender men, and 3.4 and 13.7 per 1000 person-years relative to cisgender women. The adjusted hazard ratio for VTE with oral estrogen use for transwomen was 3.2 (1.5–6.2) and 2.5 (1.2–5.0), compared to matched cisgender men and cisgender women respectively. A recent meta-analysis on VTE risk in transgender women included 18 studies, collectively providing information on 11.542 individuals [43]. The (absolute) overall pooled VTE incidence was 2 per 1000 person-years (95%CI 1–3%), which is similar to the incidence rates for VTE in transgender women found in an earlier meta-analysis of 2.3 (95%CI 0.8–6.9) per 1000 person-years [44]. Both meta-analyses are however affected by large and significant heterogeneity. Interestingly, in these studies the VTE risk increased with longer duration of GAHT use, which differs from hormone replacement therapy (HRT) in cisgender women in whom VTE risk is highest in the first year of use and decreases over time. In addition, it is suggested that different types of estrogen preparations may have different procoagulant profiles. Transdermal estrogen therapy seems not to be associated with a procoagulant phenotype. There is some evidence that conjugated equin estrogen and 17β-estradiol may be more safe than ethinyl estradiol, although this is based on smaller observational studies with no head-to-head comparisons and some conflicting results [45–47]. VTE risk during masculinizing GAHT appears to be similar to the published rates in cisgender men on hormone replacement therapy, and should therefore also be taken into account during counseling and monitoring of TGDs on GAHT [48].

3 Clinical Practice

3.1 CV Risk Screening and Suggested Adjustments

The improvement of quality of life and decrease in GD upon initiation of GAHT should always be weighed against the potential risk of CV disease among transgender people relative to cisgender people of the same birth sex. The underlying causes for this increased risk profile are not yet fully understood. However, given the potential implications for the long-term health outcome of this population, aiming to minimize CV risk by implementing lifestyle interventions and CV risk management in transgender healthcare is imperative. TGDs must be informed about the possibilities, consequences, limitations, and risks of GAHT by a medical professional. Nowadays, due to longer waiting lists to access professional gender health care more and more TGDs have reach out to self-prescribed hormone therapy without medical or psychological supervision. The long-term effects on health outcomes within this group is unknown. On the other hand, available evidence from the U.S. and Europe suggests that hormone therapy initiated and monitored under the supervision of a medical professional is associated with very low rates of adverse events [49, 50].

Transgender persons should maintain hormone levels within the expected physiologic female or male reference range. The Endocrine Society guidelines recommend hormone measurements every 3 months in the first year after initiating treatment until hormone concentrations reach the desired level [4]. Consequently, measurements can be repeated once yearly. Screening for conditions that can be exacerbated by GAHT needs to be continued. However, recommendations for actions when relative contraindications arise are lacking. With feminizing GAHT in high-risk patients, or above the age of 40 years, transdermal estrogens are advised to bypass the first-pass effect and to reduce the presumed risks. Over the age of 50 years, together with the patient, one might consider halving the dose of estrogen to reduce CV risk with maintaining feminization. With masculinizing GAHT, the effects of the different testosterone formulations were not found to be different regarding short-term safety, compliance, body composition, metabolic parameters, and general life satisfaction [51]. Testosterone therapy will have to be continued lifelong to maintain the achieved virilization and to avoid symptoms of hypogonadism such as vasomotor symptoms or osteoporosis. When erythrocytosis occurs, transdermal testosterone can be chosen above intramuscular due to the lower risk on polycythemia, next to weight reduction and smoking cessation.

3.2 VTE Risk Screening and Suggested Adjustments

Although absolute VTE risk is low, the two to fourfold increased VTE risk associated with oral feminizing GAHT becomes clinically relevant when other VTE risk factors are present such as obesity, thrombophilia, or smoking (e.g. odds ratios for VTE in obese cisgender women taking HRT increased from 2.6 (95%CI 2.1–3.3) to 5.4 (2.9–10.0), and in cisgender women with inherited thrombophilia like factor V Leiden taking HRT from 3.3 (2.6–4.2) to 8.0 (5.4–11.9) [52, 53]. Current guidelines do not address questions regarding transgender women with additional VTE risk factors who will start with GAHT, and individual risk factors should be weighed against optimal GAHT treatment. Whereas discontinuation of HRT can relatively easily be advised in cisgender women with a history of VTE or known inherited thrombophilia, this is not the case for TGDs as the benefit of GAHT is much more pronounced. Therefore, it seems reasonable to advise GAHT associated with the lowest possible VTE risk (e.g. transdermal estrogen) in patients with risk factors that moderately increase VTE risk. In line, the recent Thrombophilia guidelines suggest to consider thrombophilia testing in cisgender women who want to start HRT when they have first- or second-degree relatives with known high-risk thrombophilia such as antithrombin, protein C or protein S deficiency and recommends to not start HRT in those patients who are diagnosed with one of these defects (ASH Draft Recommendations for Thrombophilia Testing). This is extrapolated from studies on the overall risk for VTE [54], impact of inherited thrombophilia [55, 56], and estimated effect of HRT on VTE risk [52], and based on an estimated reduction of more than 10 VTE events per 1000 patient years in high-risk thrombophilia, prevented by this screening strategy and subsequent avoidance of HRT in women with high-risk thrombophilia. In all other individuals starting with HRT, thrombophilia testing is not recommended. It is unclear whether this advice also counts for TGDs, but with lack of data, this could be extrapolated. In individuals with a very high VTE risk (e.g. history of VTE, the presence of several VTE risk factors or high-risk thrombophilia) the benefits of GAHT should therefore be carefully weighed against the high VTE risk and treatment should be individualized after thorough counseling. As an alternative to discontinuation of GAHT, risks and benefits of concomitant administration of pharmacological thromboprophylaxis by means of anticoagulation could be considered, particularly for women who have a history of VTE.

The increased risk of thromboembolism in TGDs may be partially attributed to surgeries involved in the transition process for many individuals, as it is known that major surgery and immobilization are risk factors for VTE. The annual number of gender-affirming surgeries increases worldwide. There remains, however, a lack of evidence-based guidelines related to perioperative VTE prophylaxis for TGDs. While symptomatic VTE incidence is estimated at less than 1–2% for cisgender surgical patients, little is known about the incidence of VTE in transgender persons undergoing surgery [57]. Next to optimizing adjustable risk factors (e.g. BMI), discontinuing GAHT in the perioperative period has historically been recommended to reduce VTE risk after gender-affirming surgery [58]. Most surgeons withheld hormone therapy from 2 to 6 weeks before surgery, and resumed GAHT once patients were reliably ambulating (generally 2 to 3 weeks after surgery). However, prolonged GAHT cessation may lead to adverse emotional and physiologic effects, including an exacerbation of GD [59]. There is little evidence to support the discontinuation of masculinizing hormones, however, data on the risk of feminizing hormones in the perioperative setting are conflicting and often based on outdated studies not addressing the types of estrogens and anti-androgens most often used at present [60]. Current evidence does not support routine discontinuation of all GAHT prior to surgery, particularly given the lack of information on risks associated with resuming these medications after they have been stopped. Nowadays, shared-decision making is advised, taking into consideration general risk factors (e.g. pelvic surgery, immobility, age, morbidities) of perioperative VTE, together with detailed information on GAHT (e.g. administration route and dosing), to balance and outweigh the risks together.

4 Conclusions

GAHT helps to ameliorate gender dysphoria and promote well-being in TGD individuals. GAHT potentially increases the risk to develop CV disease. Therefore, medical treatment requires a multidisciplinary approach in which endocrinologists play a crucial role as cardiovascular and venous thromboembolic risk assessment is part of the counseling prior to treatment initiation. The short-term effects of GAHT on basic CV risk factors seem to be detrimental in masculinizing and favorable in feminizing GAHT. However, these effects are difficult to evaluate due to the limited number of extensive longitudinal studies focusing on CV disease and VTE outcomes in this population. More recently, in several cohort studies, in all TGDs the risk for developing CV disease and VTE seems to increase during GAHT, mainly in transgender women. However, these studies are mainly observational and difficult to interpret due to a variety of hormone regimens and observation periods, together with possible bias by confounding factors (comorbidities, estrogen types, smoking, alcohol abuse). The long-term risks of GAHT remain to be further elucidated and other risk-inducing factors (e.g. lifestyle, minority stress) need to be addressed simultaneously.

In conclusion, future research should join forces to obtain data from prospective controlled studies, including larger samples. Also, studies should consider including younger patients initiating GAHT, as well as the gender diverse (non-binary) population yearning a more personalized treatment regime, in order to improve knowledge of the CV effects of GAHT in all TGDs.

Key Issues

- The number of trans- and gender diverse persons (TGDs) seeking medical treatment increases worldwide.
- Gender-affirming hormonal treatment (GAHT) consists of feminizing or masculinizing hormones.
- In TGDs seeking for feminization, GAHT is often a combination of estrogens with anti-androgens to suppress endogenous androgen levels.
- In TGDs seeking for masculinization, GAHT consists of testosterone, sometimes in combination with progesterone preparations to suppression menstrual cycle.
- In adolescents with gender dysphoria in which endogenous puberty started, pubertal suppression with GnRH analogues can be used to prevent further development of puberty signs and to prolong diagnostic evaluation.
- GAHT is generally considered to be safe, however the use of sex hormones can influence the CV and VTE risk profile.
- Feminizing GAHT with estrogens is associated with an increased CV risk profile with higher BMI, increased body fat and increased triglyceride levels.
- Masculinizing GAHT with androgens is associated with an alterations of lipid profile and the development of erythrocytosis.
- Oral estrogens used in transgender women increase VTE risk.

Questions and Answers

1. What are the treatment regimes for feminizing and for masculinizing GAHT?
   (A1) Feminization: estrogens (oral, transdermal) + anti-androgen (GnRH analogue, CPA, spironolactone). Masculinization: testosterone (parenteral, transdermal)
2. What are the main effects of estrogens in feminizing GAHT considering CV and VTE risk?
   (A2) Estrogens increase body fat, possibly increase triglyceride level, and induce procoagulant effects (especially oral administration). CV mortality risk and VTE risk seem to be increased.
3. What are the main effects of androgens in masculinizing GAHT considering CV and VTE risk?
   (A3) Testosterone deteriorates lipid profile, and increases blood pressure and hematocrit. Mortality rate is increased compared to ciswomen, but comparable to cismen. The risk for VTE is comparable to cismen on hormone replacement therapy.
4. What are important caveats when studying the effect of GAHT on long-term health outcomes in TGDs?
   (A4) Long-term studies on relevant health outcomes remain scarce and might describe a different composition of the TGD population, including different treatment regimens administered, and therefore might not fully represent current clinical practice. Other risk-inducing factors, such as lifestyle and minority stress, are not included.

References

1. Goodman M, Adams N, Corneil T, Kreukels B, Motmans J, Coleman E. Size and distribution of transgender and gender nonconforming populations: a narrative review. Endocrinol Metab Clin North Am. 2019;48(2):303–21.
2. T'Sjoen G, Arcelus J, Gooren L, Klink DT, Tangpricha V. Endocrinology of transgender medicine. Endocr Rev. 2019;40(1):97–117.
3. D'Hoore L, T'Sjoen G. Gender-affirming hormone therapy: an updated literature review with an eye on the future. J Intern Med. 2022;291(5):574–92.
4. Hembree WC, Cohen-Kettenis PT, Gooren L, Hannema SE, Meyer WJ, Murad MH, et al. Endocrine treatment of gender-dysphoric/gender-incongruent persons: an Endocrine Society clinical practice guideline. J Clin Endocrinol Metab. 2017;102(11):3869–903.
5. Baker K, Wilson L, Sharma R, Dukhanin V, McArthur K, Robinson K. Hormone therapy, mental health, and quality of life among transgender people: a systematic review. J Endocr Soc. 2021;5:5.
6. Asscheman H, T'Sjoen G, Lemaire A, Mas M, Meriggiola MC, Mueller A, et al. Venous thrombo-embolism as a complication of cross-sex hormone treatment of male-to-female transsexual subjects: a review. Andrologia. 2014;46(7):791–5.
7. Haupt C, Henke M, Kutschmar A, Hauser B, Baldinger S, Saenz S, et al. Antiandrogen or estradiol treatment or both during hormone therapy in transitioning transgender women. Cochrane Database Syst Rev. 2020;11:CD013138.
8. Glintborg D, T'Sjoen G, Ravn P, Andersen MS. Management of endocrine disease: optimal feminizing hormone treatment in transgender people. Eur J Endocrinol. 2021;185(2):R49–63.
9. Mancini I, Rotilio A, Coati I, Seracchioli R, Martelli V, Meriggiola MC. Presentation of a meningioma in a transwoman after nine years of cyproterone acetate and estradiol intake: case report and literature review. Gynecol Endocrinol. 2018;34(6):456–9.
10. Defreyne J, Nota N, Pereira C, Schreiner T, Fisher AD, den Heijer M, et al. Transient elevated serum prolactin in trans women is caused by Cyproterone acetate treatment. LGBT Health. 2017;4(5):328–36.
11. Manson JE, Hsia J, Johnson KC, Rossouw JE, Assaf AR, Lasser NL, et al. Estrogen plus progestin and the risk of coronary heart disease. N Engl J Med. 2003;349(6):523–34.
12. de Vries AL, Steensma TD, Doreleijers TA, Cohen-Kettenis PT. Puberty suppression in adolescents with gender identity disorder: a prospective follow-up study. J Sex Med. 2011;8(8):2276–83.
13. de Vries AL, McGuire JK, Steensma TD, Wagenaar EC, Doreleijers TA, Cohen-Kettenis PT. Young adult psychological outcome after puberty suppression and gender reassignment. Pediatrics. 2014;134(4):696–704.
14. Schagen SE, Cohen-Kettenis PT, Delemarre-van de Waal HA, Hannema SE. Efficacy and safety of gonadotropin-releasing hormone agonist treatment to suppress puberty in gender dysphoric adolescents. J Sex Med. 2016;13(7):1125–32.
15. Klaver M, de Mutsert R, van der Loos M, Wiepjes CM, Twisk JWR, den Heijer M, et al. Hormonal treatment and cardiovascular risk profile in transgender adolescents. Pediatrics. 2020;145(3):e20190741.
16. Coleman E, Radix AE, Bouman WP, Brown GR, de Vries ALC, Deutsch MB, et al. Standards of Care for the Health of transgender and gender diverse people,

version 8. Int J Transgend Health. 2022;23(Suppl 1):S1–s259.
17. Braun H, Nash R, Tangpricha V, Brockman J, Ward K, Goodman M. Cancer in transgender people: evidence and methodological considerations. Epidemiol Rev. 2017;39(1):93–107.
18. de Blok CJ, Wiepjes CM, van Velzen DM, Staphorsius AS, Nota NM, Gooren LJ, et al. Mortality trends over five decades in adult transgender people receiving hormone treatment: a report from the Amsterdam cohort of gender dysphoria. Lancet Diabetes Endocrinol. 2021;9(10):663–70.
19. Irwig MS. Cardiovascular health in transgender people. Rev Endocr Metab Disord. 2018;19(3):243–51.
20. Safer JD, Tangpricha V. Care of the transgender patient. Ann Intern Med. 2019;171(1):ITC1–ITC16.
21. Glintborg D, Rubin KH, Petersen TG, Lidegaard Ø, T'Sjoen G, Hilden M, et al. Cardiovascular risk in Danish transgender persons: a matched historical cohort study. Eur J Endocrinol. 2022;187(3):463–77.
22. Cocchetti C, Castellini G, Iacuaniello D, Romani A, Maggi M, Vignozzi L, et al. Does gender-affirming hormonal treatment affect 30-year cardiovascular risk in transgender persons? A two-year prospective European study (ENIGI). J Sex Med. 2021;18(4):821–9.
23. Maraka S, Singh Ospina N, Rodriguez-Gutierrez R, Davidge-Pitts CJ, Nippoldt TB, Prokop LJ, et al. Sex steroids and cardiovascular outcomes in transgender individuals: a systematic review and meta-analysis. J Clin Endocrinol Metab. 2017;102(11):3914–23.
24. Klaver M, van Velzen D, de Blok C, Nota N, Wiepjes C, Defreyne J, et al. Change in visceral fat and total body fat and the effect on cardiometabolic risk factors during transgender hormone therapy. J Clin Endocrinol Metab. 2022;107(1):e153–e64.
25. Klaver M, Dekker M, de Mutsert R, Twisk JWR, den Heijer M. Cross-sex hormone therapy in transgender persons affects total body weight, body fat and lean body mass: a meta-analysis. Andrologia. 2017;49(5).
26. Fisher AD, Castellini G, Ristori J, Casale H, Cassioli E, Sensi C, et al. Cross-sex hormone treatment and psychobiological changes in transsexual persons: two-year follow-up data. J Clin Endocrinol Metab. 2016;101(11):4260–9.
27. Quirós C, Patrascioiu I, Mora M, Aranda GB, Hanzu FA, Gómez-Gil E, et al. Effect of cross-sex hormone treatment on cardiovascular risk factors in transsexual individuals. Experience in a specialized unit in Catalonia. Endocrinol Nutr. 2015;62(5):210–6.
28. Klaver M, de Blok CJM, Wiepjes CM, Nota NM, Dekker M, de Mutsert R, et al. Changes in regional body fat, lean body mass and body shape in trans persons using cross-sex hormonal therapy: results from a multicenter prospective study. Eur J Endocrinol. 2018;178(2):163–71.
29. Jarin J, Pine-Twaddell E, Trotman G, Stevens J, Conard LA, Tefera E, et al. Cross-sex hormones and metabolic parameters in adolescents with gender dysphoria. Pediatrics. 2017;139(5):e20163173.
30. van Velzen DM, Paldino A, Klaver M, Nota NM, Defreyne J, Hovingh GK, et al. Cardiometabolic effects of testosterone in transmen and estrogen plus Cyproterone acetate in transwomen. J Clin Endocrinol Metab. 2019;104(6):1937–47.
31. Tack LJ, Craen M, Dhondt K, Vanden Bossche H, Laridaen J, Cools M. Consecutive lynestrenol and cross-sex hormone treatment in biological female adolescents with gender dysphoria: a retrospective analysis. Biol Sex Differ. 2016;7:14.
32. Bhasin S, Cunningham GR, Hayes FJ, Matsumoto AM, Snyder PJ, Swerdloff RS, et al. Testosterone therapy in adult men with androgen deficiency syndromes: an endocrine society clinical practice guideline. J Clin Endocrinol Metab. 2006;91(6):1995–2010.
33. Madsen MC, van Dijk D, Wiepjes CM, Conemans EB, Thijs A, den Heijer M. Erythrocytosis in a large cohort of trans men using testosterone: a long-term follow-up study on prevalence, determinants, and exposure years. J Clin Endocrinol Metab. 2021;106(6): 1710–7.
34. Schutte MH, Kleemann R, Nota NM, Wiepjes CM, Snabel JM, T'Sjoen G, et al. The effect of transdermal gender-affirming hormone therapy on markers of inflammation and hemostasis. PLoS One. 2022;17(3):e0261312.
35. Tsatsanis C, Elenkov A, Leijonhufvud I, Vaporidi K, Tivesten Å, Giwercman A. Sex hormone-dependent and -independent regulation of serum BAFF and TNF in cohorts of transgender and cisgender men and women. Endocr Connect. 2023;12(3):e220456.
36. Newcomb ME, Hill R, Buehler K, Ryan DT, Whitton SW, Mustanski B. High burden of mental health problems, substance use, violence, and related psychosocial factors in transgender, non-binary, and gender diverse youth and young adults. Arch Sex Behav. 2020;49(2):645–59.
37. Bishop A, Overcash F, McGuire J, Reicks M. Diet and physical activity behaviors among adolescent transgender students: school survey results. J Adolesc Health. 2020;66(4):484–90.
38. Tan KKH, Treharne GJ, Ellis SJ, Schmidt JM, Veale JF. Gender minority stress: a critical review. J Homosex. 2020;67(10):1471–89.
39. Karalexi MA, Frisell T, Cnattingius S, Holmberg D, Holmberg M, Kollia N, et al. Cardiovascular outcomes in transgender individuals in Sweden after initiation of gender-affirming hormone therapy. Eur J Prev Cardiol. 2022;29(15):2017–26.
40. Gava G, Mancini I, Alvisi S, Seracchioli R, Meriggiola MC. A comparison of 5-year administration of cyproterone acetate or leuprolide acetate in combination with estradiol in transwomen. Eur J Endocrinol. 2020;183(6):561–9.
41. Fung R, Hellstern-Layefsky M, Tastenhoye C, Lega I, Steele L. Differential effects of Cyproterone acetate vs spironolactone on serum high-density lipoprotein and prolactin concentrations in the hormonal treatment of transgender women. J Sex Med. 2016;13(11):1765–72.

42. Getahun D, Nash R, Flanders WD, Baird TC, Becerra-Culqui TA, Cromwell L, et al. Cross-sex hormones and acute cardiovascular events in transgender persons: a cohort study. Ann Intern Med. 2018;169(4):205–13.
43. Totaro M, Palazzi S, Castellini C, Parisi A, D'Amato F, Tienforti D, et al. Risk of venous thromboembolism in transgender people undergoing hormone feminizing therapy: a prevalence meta-analysis and meta-regression study. Front Endocrinol (Lausanne). 2021;12:741866.
44. Khan J, Schmidt RL, Spittal MJ, Goldstein Z, Smock KJ, Greene DN. Venous thrombotic risk in transgender women undergoing estrogen therapy: a systematic review and metaanalysis. Clin Chem. 2019;65(1):57–66.
45. Wierckx K, Mueller S, Weyers S, Van Caenegem E, Roef G, Heylens G, et al. Long-term evaluation of cross-sex hormone treatment in transsexual persons. J Sex Med. 2012;9(10):2641–51.
46. Seal LJ, Franklin S, Richards C, Shishkareva A, Sinclaire C, Barrett J. Predictive markers for mammoplasty and a comparison of side effect profiles in transwomen taking various hormonal regimens. J Clin Endocrinol Metab. 2012;97(12):4422–8.
47. van Kesteren PJ, Asscheman H, Megens JA, Gooren LJ. Mortality and morbidity in transsexual subjects treated with cross-sex hormones. Clin Endocrinol (Oxf). 1997;47(3):337–42.
48. Kotamarti VS, Greige N, Heiman AJ, Patel A, Ricci JA. Risk for venous thromboembolism in transgender patients undergoing cross-sex hormone treatment: a systematic review. J Sex Med. 2021;18(7):1280–91.
49. Weinand JD, Safer JD. Hormone therapy in transgender adults is safe with provider supervision; a review of hormone therapy sequelae for transgender individuals. J Clin Transl Endocrinol. 2015;2(2):55–60.
50. Wierckx K, Van Caenegem E, Schreiner T, Haraldsen I, Fisher AD, Toye K, et al. Cross-sex hormone therapy in trans persons is safe and effective at short-time follow-up: results from the European network for the investigation of gender incongruence. J Sex Med. 2014;11(8):1999–2011.
51. Pelusi C, Costantino A, Martelli V, Lambertini M, Bazzocchi A, Ponti F, et al. Effects of three different testosterone formulations in female-to-male transsexual persons. J Sex Med. 2014;11(12):3002–11.
52. Marjoribanks J, Farquhar C, Roberts H, Lethaby A, Lee J. Long-term hormone therapy for perimenopausal and postmenopausal women. Cochrane Database Syst Rev. 2017;1:CD004143.
53. Canonico M, Plu-Bureau G, Lowe GD, Scarabin PY. Hormone replacement therapy and risk of venous thromboembolism in postmenopausal women: systematic review and meta-analysis. BMJ. 2008;336(7655):1227–31.
54. Couturaud F, Leroyer C, Julian JA, Kahn SR, Ginsberg JS, Wells PS, et al. Factors that predict risk of thrombosis in relatives of patients with unprovoked venous thromboembolism. Chest. 2009;136(6):1537–45.
55. Couturaud F, Leroyer C, Tromeur C, Julian JA, Kahn SR, Ginsberg JS, et al. Factors that predict thrombosis in relatives of patients with venous thromboembolism. Blood. 2014;124(13):2124–30.
56. Cushman M. Thrombophilia testing in women with venous thrombosis: the 4 P's approach. Clin Chem. 2014;60(1):134–7.
57. Kozato A, Fox GWC, Yong PC, Shin SJ, Avanessian BK, Ting J, et al. No venous thromboembolism increase among transgender female patients remaining on estrogen for gender-affirming surgery. J Clin Endocrinol Metab. 2021;106(4):e1586–e90.
58. Hontscharuk R, Alba B, Manno C, Pine E, Deutsch MB, Coon D, et al. Perioperative transgender hormone management: avoiding venous thromboembolism and other complications. Plast Reconstr Surg. 2021;147(4):1008–17.
59. Lawrence AA. Patient-reported complications and functional outcomes of male-to-female sex reassignment surgery. Arch Sex Behav. 2006;35(6):717–27.
60. Boskey ER, Taghinia AH, Ganor O. Association of surgical risk with exogenous hormone use in transgender patients: a systematic review. JAMA Surg. 2019;154(2):159–69.

Part III

Heart Disease in Women

Valvular Heart Disease in Women

Shauna L. Newton and Catherine M. Otto

Abstract

Valvular heart disease (VHD) is a major cause of cardiovascular mortality and morbidity worldwide in both women and men, despite medical and interventional management improvements over the past two decades. The pathophysiology of VHD is similar in women compared to men, but there are some important differences in clinical presentation and management as summarized in this chapter. In women with VHD who become pregnant, the hemodynamic changes of pregnancy may precipitate symptoms or lead to hemodynamic decompensation. Management during pregnancy of women with known VHD or a prosthetic valve can be challenging. Outcomes after surgical or transcatheter intervention are not always the same in women compared to men. Although women historically have been underrepresented in cardiovascular clinical trials, recent clinical trials of new interventions for VHD have an appropriate sex balance.

Keywords

Valvular heart disease · Aortic stenosis · Mitral regurgitation · Valvular heart disease in pregnancy

Test your learning and check your understanding of this book's contents: use the "Springer Nature Flashcards" app to access questions using ▶ https://sn.pub/51ny7m
To use the app, please follow the instructions in chapter 1.

S. L. Newton · C. M. Otto (✉)
Division of Cardiology, Department of Medicine, University of Washington School of Medicine, Seattle, WA, USA
e-mail: snewton6@uw.edu; cmotto@uw.edu

A. H.E.M. Maas, E. Gerdts (eds.), *Manual of Cardiovascular Disease in Women*,
https://doi.org/10.1007/978-3-031-65952-2_18

1 Introduction

Valvular heart disease (VHD) is a major cause of cardiovascular mortality and morbidity worldwide in both women and men, despite medical and interventional management improvements over the past two decades.

2 Theory

2.1 Aortic Stenosis

Aortic stenosis (AS) is the most common type of valvular heart disease that eventually requires intervention [1–5]. The predominant etiologies of AS are calcific stenosis of a trileaflet valve, superimposed fibro-calcific changes of a congenital bicuspid aortic valve, and rheumatic valve disease, which invariably is associated with mitral valve involvement. Calcific stenosis of a trileaflet or congenital bicuspid valve predominates in high-income counties [5]. Rheumatic valve disease typically involves the mitral valve but a subset of patients also have aortic valve involvement with stenosis, regurgitation, or mixed aortic valve disease [6].

Etiology Calcific AS has similar risk factors as atherosclerosis [2], including male gender, but also hypertension, shorter height, serum cholesterol levels, smoking, and diabetes. Genetic variants in Lp(a) and serum Lp(a) also are associated with AS risk. The prevalence of calcific AS of a trileaflet aortic valve appears to be similar in women and men. However, for hemodynamically similar degrees of stenosis, women tend to have greater leaflet fibrosis and less calcification when compared to men, as measured by multidetector computed tomography (MDCT) imaging [7–9]. Given these differences, current guidelines recommend sex-specific thresholds for the calcium score on MDCT that defines severe AS [10, 11]. It has been postulated that sex-specific differences in leaflet fibrosis/calcification are due, in part, to differences in hormone levels and gene expression [8].

Bicuspid aortic valve disease is three times more prevalent in men than women [2, 10, 12], resulting in more men than women with calcific AS and underlying bicuspid valve anatomy. Bicuspid valve leaflet morphology does not differ between the sexes but women are less likely to have associated aortopathy when compared to men (6.7% vs. 14.7% for isolated aortic sinus dilation, 7.3% vs. 16.7% for diffuse dilation of the aorta $P < 0.001$) [12]. In patients presenting with significant dysfunction of a bicuspid aortic valve, women less often present with aortic regurgitation compared to men (22.2% vs. 33.8%, $P = 0.033$) [12]. The X-chromosome is considered somewhat protective against significant aortopathy, as patients with Turner's syndrome (a single X chromosome) frequently have aortopathy and dissection [12].

Clinical Presentation Women typically are diagnosed with calcific AS at an older age than men (Table 1) [13, 14]. This could be partly due to decreased awareness of aortic valve disease in women but underdiagnosis and underestimation of stenosis severity also are likely. Women have lower rates of diagnostic testing and referral to subspecialists for treating AS [1]. Generally, women are likelier to have small left ventricular (LV) outflow tracts and smaller valve areas even when these parameters are indexed to body surface area [3, 12]. As aortic valve disease progresses, there are significant differences in LV remodeling in response to pressure overload between women and men. Men more often develop LV dilation and systolic dysfunction. In contrast, women have increased LV wall thickness with small LV chambers resulting in a low stroke volume despite a normal ejection fraction. Women have greater ventricular fibrosis at similar valve gradients compared to men [3, 15, 16], which is associated with higher filling pressures and more severe diastolic dysfunction [3, 16]. Despite earlier symptom onset in women [3], given lower levels of valvular calcification and smaller chamber sizes, symptoms are more likely to be attributed to normal aging or ignored, leading to underdiagnosis of severe AS. Low-flow states can make the diagnosis of severe AS challenging, requiring a multimodality approach (Fig. 1).

Table 1 Special considerations in women with valvular heart disease

	Causes and clinical presentation	Diagnostic features to consider in women	Potential treatment issues
Aortic stenosis (AS)	• Bicuspid aortic valve (BAV) disease less common overall but high incidence of BAV in women with Turner's syndrome • Older age in women with AS at symptom onset • Symptoms more often due to LV diastolic dysfunction	• Smaller LVOT and smaller aortic valve areas on echocardiogram • Low flow states are more common in women. Evaluate for evidence of low stroke volume index (<35 mL/m^2) • Sex specific CT valve calcium scores for diagnosis of severe AS [>1300 (AHA/ACC) or >1200 (ESC)] • Consider low dose dobutamine stress echocardiogram to diagnose low-flow low-gradient AS in patients with reduced LV ejection fraction	• Surgical referral in women with asymptomatic or symptomatic severe aortic stenosis • TAVI may offer a survival benefit over SAVR in women
Aortic regurgitation (AR)	• BAV less common in women • No sex differences in prevalence of inherited aortopathies	• LV size is smaller at symptom onset compared to men • Aortic size measurements may be smaller in women • Report indexed measurements of aorta size, sinus of Valsalva size, and LV dimensions	• Avoid delays in surgical referral for women with severe AR and: – Symptoms or – Reduced LV ejection fraction (≤55%) or – LV dilation (LVESD >50 mm or LVESDi >25 mm/m^2)
Mitral stenosis (MS)	• Rheumatic MS mainly occurs in women (80% of cases) • Calcific MS is a disease of older women with AF	• Evaluate for evidence of rheumatic valve disease when heart failure symptoms occur in pregnancy • Circumferential mitral annular calcification is more common in women	• Early commissurotomy for rheumatic MS with favorable anatomy and valve area ≤1.5 cm^2 • Surgical mitral valve repair when a transcatheter approach is not possible • Treatment of calcific MS is medical; unclear whether intervention provides any benefit
Mitral regurgitation (MR)	• Mitral valve prolapse is common but less often results in severe MR in women	• Quantitative measurement of regurgitant severity is recommended • Intervention recommended earlier in disease course when surgical valve repair is feasible	• Higher rates of mitral valve replacement instead of repair and worse surgical outcomes; refer women to valve centers of excellence • Mitral transcatheter edge-to-edge repair reserved for patients with intractable symptoms and prohibitive surgical risk
Tricuspid regurgitation (TR)	• Mild TR is common • Significant TR typically occurs with AF • Pacer lead related TR is increasingly seen	• Women are less likely to have ascites or hospitalizations for right sided heart failure	• Treatment of severe TR is in evolution; current recommendation is medical treatment in most patients

ACC American College of Cardiology, *AHA* American Heart Association, *AS* aortic stenosis, *AR* aortic regurgitation, *AF* atrial fibrillation, *BAV* bicuspid aortic valve, *ESC* European Society of Cardiology, *LV* left ventricular, *LVOT* left ventricular outflow tract diameter, *MR* mitral regurgitation, *MS* mitral stenosis, *TR* tricuspid regurgitation

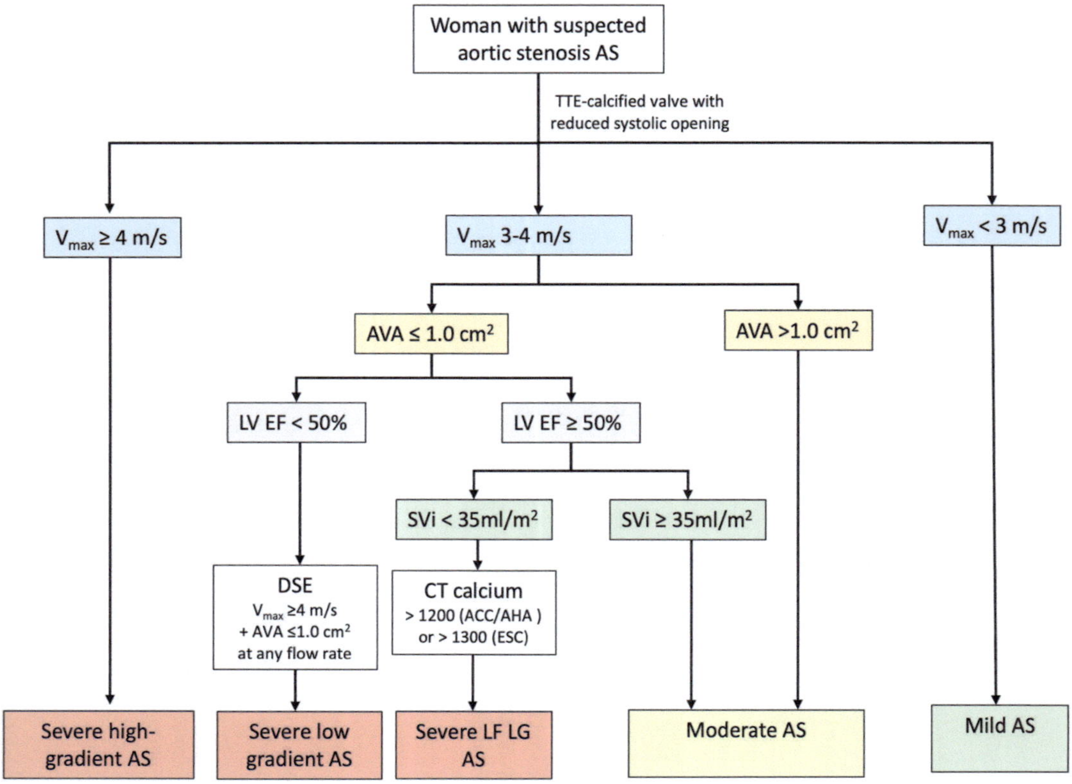

Fig. 1 Flowchart for evaluation of aortic stenosis in women. Women are more likely to have an intermediate velocity (and mean gradient) so that evaluation of valve area, LV ejection fraction and stroke volume index is important to ensure detection of severe AS with a low gradient, either in the context of a low ejection fraction or with a low stroke volume index. If the dobutamine stress echocardiogram (DSE) does not show a velocity over 4 m/s, AS likely is moderate with primary myocardial dysfunction. With a low stroke volume index and small valve area but a calcium score on computed tomographic (CT) imaging that is not severe, again AS is likely only moderate in severity. *Vmax* maximum aortic velocity, *AVA* aortic valve area, *TTE* transthoracic echocardiography, *LF* low flow, *LG* low gradient, *LV* left ventricular

Management Current indications for timing of intervention for severe AS are the same in women and men, given the absence of data to support sex-specific recommendations. The primary indication for intervention in adults with severe AS is the onset of even mild symptoms, most often decreased exercise capacity or dyspnea on exertion. The presence of LV systolic dysfunction (ejection fraction <50%) also is an indication for intervention when severe AS is present. Intervention also is reasonable in patients at low surgical risk with very severe AS (maximum velocity > 5 m/s), an abnormal exercise test, serum B-natriuretic peptide level > 3X normal, or rapid disease progression. Improved recognition of symptom onset in women likely will reduce any apparent disparities in treatment.

Currently, there is no medical therapy to prevent or slow AS disease progression, although treatment of standard cardiovascular risk factors, including hypertension, is recommended. The only effective therapy for women with symptoms due to severe AS is surgical aortic valve replacement (SAVR) or transcatheter aortic valve implantation (TAVI). Some studies have suggested that TAVI may have superior 1-year outcomes in women compared to men [17, 18], regardless of women often having smaller and more tortuous blood vessels, resulting in an increased risk of vascular complications and periprocedural bleeding [14, 17, 18]. TAVI also is associated with lower rates of patient-prosthesis mismatch, valve embolization, and paravalvular leak in women [4, 14, 17].

Despite similar prevalence [5] and hemodynamic profiles of AS [4] in both sexes, the majority of patients who undergo SAVR for treatment of AS are men (63% vs. 37%) [19]. A retrospective analysis of almost 4000 patients with AS suggests that the differences in surgical referral may be driven by management differences in women with low-flow low-gradient severe AS [4]. For example, women with high-gradient severe AS had similar referral rates for aortic valve intervention and long-term mortality during a mean follow-up of 4.33 ± 2.53 years [4]. In contrast, women with low-flow, low-gradient severe AS were referred for intervention less often than men (37% vs. 43%; $P = 0.03$) and experienced higher mortality than men (IPW-HR: 2.17 [1.19–3.95]; $P = 0.01$) [4]. In patients referred for SAVR, women are more likely to be older with unfavorable preoperative baseline characteristics due to higher rates of non-cardiac comorbidities [4, 17, 19], which likely drives the associated longer hospital stays and higher in-hospital mortality in women (5.6% vs. 4%, $P < 0.001$) [19], and higher long-term mortality (16.7% vs. 8.2%) [20]. Similar to TAVI, there are higher rates of bleeding and vascular complications in women who undergo SAVR.

Given the apparent outcomes differences in women undergoing SAVR vs. TAVI to treat severe AS, the RHEIA trial (Randomized researcH in womEn All comers With AS) is a prospective, randomized, controlled trial seeking to evaluate efficacy differences between the two interventions in women with severe, symptomatic AS [21] NCT04160130 clinicaltrials.gov.

2.2 Aortic Regurgitation

Etiology Mild aortic regurgitation (AR) is common with aging and does not usually require monitoring or intervention. Significant AR is classified as primary, when due to disease of the valve leaflets, and secondary, when due to aortic dilation. Primary AR is most often due to a congenital bicuspid valve or rheumatic disease and is less common in women [2, 22], perhaps due to higher rates of bicuspid valve disease in men. In patients with significant secondary AR, causes include aortic dilation due to inherited connective tissue disorders such as Marfan or Loeys-Dietz syndrome. In patients with hypertensive or atherosclerotic aortic dilation, AR is typically mild to moderate in severity although aortic dissection of any cause can present with acute severe AR.

Clinical Presentation Despite similar AR severity, women are more likely to be older with lower diastolic blood pressure, advanced New York Heart Association (NYHA) functional class, higher estimated pulmonary artery systolic pressures, and higher estimated LV filling pressures at the time of diagnosis [22, 23]. Women with moderate-severe or severe AR have lower 10-year survival rates than men (64% ± 5% vs. 76% ± 2%; $P = 0.004$) [22], possibly due to the underestimation of AR severity from the use of non-indexed echocardiographic parameters. When not indexed for body size, women with AR have smaller aortic sinus diameters, ascending aorta size, and LV end-systolic dimensions (LVESD) [22]. However, the opposite is true when indexed values are used during diagnosis [22]. Current ACC/AHA guidelines do include correction for body size in patients with LV dilation due to AR, recommending consideration of surgical referral when the LV is severely enlarged (defined by LVESD of greater than 50 mm or indexed LVESD of greater than 25 mm/m^2) [10].

Management Similar to AS, women have lower SAVR referral rates for treatment of AR. When referred, women are more likely to be symptomatic with a higher NYHA functional class than men [22, 23]. Older studies demonstrated increased postoperative mortality in women undergoing SAVR for treatment of aortic regurgitation, with female sex identified as a risk factor for operative mortality (OR 1.6 [1.14–2.25]; $P = 0.01$) [23]. However, when adjusting for age, symptoms, comorbidities, and indexed LVESD, female sex no longer predicted mortality [22], emphasizing the importance of timely referral for surgical intervention. Newer analyses demonstrate no differences in post-SAVR survival between men and women for AR [22]. Approaches to avoiding placement of a prosthetic valve in patients with severe AR include aortic valve repair procedures, use of a pulmonic autograft (e.g., Ross procedure), or valve reimplantation in patients undergoing replacement of a dilated aorta (e.g., David procedure).

2.3 Rheumatic Mitral Stenosis

Etiology Mitral stenosis (MS) is 3–4× more prevalent in women [24] and primarily due to rheumatic heart disease. Rheumatic heart disease is estimated to affect 40.5 (95% CI 32.1–50.1) million people worldwide and is significantly more prevalent in low-income countries [5]. While the exact pathophysiology is poorly understood, rheumatic heart disease develops in some patients with untreated Streptococcal pharyngitis. Rheumatic fever predominately impacts young adults and children, in which there is an abnormal autoimmune reaction to group A streptococcal infection. Carditis from rheumatic fever has a predilection for the mitral and aortic valves, often initially presenting with valve regurgitation followed later by valve stenosis [5]. Valve inflammation results in leaflet and chordal fibrosis and subsequent commissural fusion, leading to mitral valve stenosis.

Clinical Presentation The age at clinical presentation in women with rheumatic MS shows significant geographic variation, presenting in young adults or teenagers in low- and middle-income countries with a high prevalence of rheumatic fever versus later in life in high income countries with a low prevalence of rheumatic fever. Some women present with the insidious onset of reduced exercise capacity and exertional shortness of breath as valve obstruction becomes severe. More often, the clinical presentation is acute with heart failure precipitated by the superimposed hemodynamic load of infection or pregnancy in a woman with previously unrecognized rheumatic MS. Screening programs for detection of rheumatic valve disease in countries with a high prevalence of disease may reduce the likelihood of an acute presentation.

Management Medical management includes secondary prevention of recurrent rheumatic fever and treatment of complications, such as atrial fibrillation. Interventional management is reserved for patients with moderate to severe MS, defined as a mitral valve area less than 1.5 cm^2. Transcatheter balloon mitral commissurotomy is recommended when valve morphology is favorable [10, 11]. If surgical intervention is needed due to unfavorable valve morphology or coexisting regurgitation, a surgical repair may be possible. If a prosthetic valve is required, a mechanical valve is preferred over a bioprosthetic valve, except in young women planning a future pregnancy, patients with a contraindication to anticoagulation, or patients over age 65 years [10].

2.4 Calcific Mitral Stenosis

Etiology Severe mitral annular calcification (MAC) causing functional MS is a disease of the elderly found predominately in high income countries. Although both rheumatic and calcific MS obstruct flow from the left atrium into the LV, the clinical presentation and management are quite different for these two diseases [10]. Women are more likely than men to have circumferential calcification around the entire mitral annulus, rather than the more typical U-shaped posterior pattern of calcification. While MAC is a common echocardiography finding and is a marker of increased atherosclerotic risk, MAC rarely leads to significant MS [5, 25]. Loss of oestrogen at menopause and abnormal calcium metabolism are thought to play a role in the development of MAC. Women with MAC have a significantly higher prevalence of severe osteoporosis compared to women without MAC (65.2% vs. 17.1%; $P < 0.001$) [26]. MAC is strongly associated with an increased likelihood of atrial fibrillation, mitral regurgitation and left atrial enlargement [25, 27].

Clinical Presentation Calcific MS primarily presents in older women with multiple cardiac and noncardiac comorbidities. In addition to calcific MS, these patients often are in atrial fibrillation, have concurrent mitral regurgitation, LV diastolic and/or systolic dysfunction and elevated pulmonary pressures. Often, pulmonary disease, renal insufficiency and other noncardiac comorbid conditions also are present. Thus, these patients present with chronic heart failure symptoms, with calcific MS being one contributing factor.

Management Management of calcific MS relies on control of atrial fibrillation rate, anticoagulation to prevent embolic events and medical therapy to optimize LV filling pressures. Intervention might be considered in severely symptomatic patients with severe calcific MS who are not responsive to medical therapy, but surgical and transcatheter options are associated with high mortality and uncertain benefit. Surgical intraoperative mortality rates range from 6% to 14% [27]. Transcatheter mitral valve replacement (valve in MAC) procedures have estimated 30-day mortality rates of 21.8%–34.5% [27]. No differences in outcomes with women compared to men have been reported.

2.5 Mitral Regurgitation

Etiology Mitral regurgitation (MR) is a frequent diagnosis, with trace to mild MR being present in 80% of patients with an otherwise normal echocardiogram. Mild mitral regurgitation with normal valve anatomy rarely needs monitoring or treatment. Significant chronic mitral regurgitation is classified as either primary (caused by disease of the valve leaflets) or secondary (due to disease of the left ventricle or atria). In high-income countries, the most common cause of primary MR is myxomatous valve degeneration, resulting in mitral valve prolapse [5, 10]. Less common etiologies include rheumatic heart disease, radiation, infective endocarditis, and connective tissue disorders. Primary MR and mitral valve prolapse are diagnosed more often in women, although surgical intervention is more often needed in men [28, 29]. Secondary MR typically is due to ischemic disease and cardiomyopathies, with prevalence of secondary MR mirroring the prevalence of those underlying disease processes in men and women [29, 30].

Clinical Presentation The morphology of mitral valve prolapse differs between women and men. While women have higher rates of bileaflet prolapse, they are less likely to have severe regurgitation or significant symptoms associated with mitral valve prolapse [28]. Women with severe MR are more likely to be older with more severe symptoms and greater comorbidities than men [31, 32].

Management Current guidelines recommend surgical intervention in patients with symptoms due to severe MR [10, 11]. In asymptomatic patients with severe mitral regurgitation, surgery is indicated in patients with an LV ejection fraction less than or equal to 60% or evidence of end-systolic dilation of the LV, defined as an end-systolic diameter of 40 mm or greater [10, 11]. Women with severe MR are less likely to meet the end-systolic dimension criteria for surgery than men when using non-indexed values, have lower rates of reduced LV ejection fraction [28, 29], and smaller effective regurgitant orifice areas (EROA) [32]. Whether this means that women do not yet need intervention or whether we should be using sex-specific criteria for timing of intervention is unclear. In patients with severe MR, symptoms are less likely to be attributed to the valve lesion in women, and women are less likely to be referred for mitral valve surgery [28, 31, 33]. Outcomes after mitral surgery are worse in women, compared to men, with higher 30-day mortality (2% vs. 1%; $P = 0.036$) [31], longer hospital stays (7 vs. 6 days; $P < 0.001$) [31], and higher rates of non-fatal postoperative complications (pacemaker placement, stroke, myocardial infarction) [32–34]. This may in part be due to higher rates of mitral valve replacement (26.8% vs. 10.7%) rather than valve repair, secondary to increased amounts of valve calcification in women presenting for mitral valve surgery than men [35]. When stratified by age, one study found this result is most accentuated in women ages 40–59, with 2–2.5× higher in-hospital mortality than age-matched males [33]. Worse outcomes postoperatively may also be explained by differences in LV remodeling in response to mitral valve disease. In a randomized trial of patients with severe ischemic mitral regurgitation, utilizing an EROA to LV end-diastolic volume ratio was proposed to characterize mitral regurgitation severity. This ratio was increased in women (0.24 ± 0.09 vs. 0.20 ± 0.09; P = 0.002), and higher values are associated with lower rates of reverse LV remodeling [30, 32].

Transcatheter edge-to-edge repair is an available treatment option for primary MR who are not ideal surgical candidates or those with secondary mitral regurgitation. Like those undergoing mitral valve surgery, women undergoing transcatheter intervention are older with more symptoms, higher LV ejection fraction, and significantly smaller LV size compared to men [36, 37]. There are no sex-specific differences in procedural success rates or mortality [36, 37], but women have higher rates of vascular and bleeding complications (10.1% vs. 5.7%; P = 0.021) [37] after transcatheter mitral valve intervention, likely due to smaller, more fragile, vessels for arterial access.

2.6 Tricuspid Valve Disease

Etiology Rheumatic tricuspid valve stenosis is a rare finding that can occur in tandem with rheumatic mitral valve disease [6]. No sex differences have been identified as data is scarce secondary to low prevalence, but tricuspid stenosis is likely more common in women due to its rheumatic etiology.

A small amount of tricuspid regurgitation (TR) is present in 90% of normal individuals. Significant TR is uncommon, most often secondary to pulmonary hypertension, either due to primary pulmonary disease, pulmonary vascular disease, or left-sided heart disease (particularly mitral stenosis or regurgitation). TR also can be due to primary disease of the valve leaflets with causes including rheumatic, myxomatous, carcinoid, and congenital. TR appears to be more common in women than in men [38, 39], and women with severe TR tend to be slightly older (72 [62 to 79] years compared to men with severe TR (70 [61 to 77] years, P = 0.003) [39] and with better biventricular function than men [39, 40]. Most often, significant TR in older women is associated with atrial fibrillation, although whether one causes the other remains unclear. Significant TR in older adults also may be related to the position of a pacemaker lead across the valve.

Clinical Presentation Symptom presentation in patients with severe TR differs in men and women. Women are less like to have ascites (20.3% vs. 32.1%; P < 0.01) and prior hospitalizations for right-sided heart failure (65.1% vs. 75.7%, P = 0.02) than men [39].

Management One study suggests women are more likely to undergo tricuspid valve surgery than men (38% vs. 32%; P = 0.010) [39], likely due to higher rates of primary TR or multivalve disease in women [39, 41]. Current guidelines do not recommend surgery to treat secondary TR; management should focus on treating underlying cardiomyopathy or pulmonary hypertension [10, 11]. Intervention to prevent TR is recommended in patients undergoing mitral valve surgery, particularly when rheumatic mitral valve disease is present [10].

No significant differences in mortality or outcomes have been reported between men and women who undergo tricuspid valve surgery [41]. Transcatheter edge-to-edge repair (TEER) is an emerging therapy for treating severe secondary TR. Current European guidelines recommend considering transcatheter tricuspid valve intervention in patients with severe secondary TR who are not operative candidates as a class IIb guideline [11]. This treatment is not yet included in the United States guidelines, which recommend medical therapy for treating severe secondary TR with evidence of either LV dysfunction or pulmonary hypertension [10]. A recent review of the Tricuspid Valve Therapies registry suggests that women with severe TR may undergo TEER less often than men (74.4% vs. 83.3%; $P < 0.01$) [40]. Women who underwent transcatheter intervention had fewer clips placed despite similarities in right ventricular size and function [40]. Survival rates after this procedure are similar between the two sexes [40].

2.7 Pulmonic Valve Disease

Pulmonic valve disease is rare in adults, although trace to mild pulmonary regurgitation (PR) is present in most people. Significant PR is most often caused by pulmonary hypertension, left-sided heart disease, or iatrogenic during valve intervention. However, an increasing number of patients with severe PR after tetralogy of Fallot repair are now seen as adults. Rates of pulmonic valve disease are similar in men and women [2], with little information available regarding sex-specific outcomes after pulmonic valve intervention.

3 Clinical Practice

3.1 Valvular Heart Disease in Pregnancy

Etiology With continued medical advances, patients with congenital heart disease are surviving well into their childbearing years. In addition, rheumatic valve disease typically affects women of childbearing age. Maternal VHD is associated with a 1% mortality rate during pregnancy, with approximately 17% developing heart failure symptoms during gestation [42]. Based on the World Health Organization (WHO) maternal risk score, severe AS and severe MS are categorized as Class IV with the recommendation to avoid pregnancy [43]. Other pre-pregnancy predictors of maternal mortality include NYHA class III to IV disease, reduced LV ejection fraction, pulmonary hypertension, and anticoagulant use [42].

Clinical Presentation and Outcomes Mild to moderate AS is generally well tolerated throughout pregnancy with low risk of maternal cardiac complication, with cardiac hospitalizations occurring in approximately 0–12.9% of women [44, 45]. Maternal and fetal morbidity is significantly higher in pregnant women with severe AS. One study found that 42% of patients with severe, symptomatic AS required hospitalization for a cardiac cause during pregnancy [45]. Pregnancy duration was significantly shorter in women with severe AS (37.9 [IQR: 35.2 to 39.0] weeks vs. 39.0 [IQR: 38.0 to 40.0] weeks; $P = 0.001$) with higher rates of Cesarean section (75.0% vs. 48.3%; $P = 0.008$) and lower fetal birthweight when compared to women with moderate AS [45].

Women with rheumatic mitral stenosis are often initially diagnosed during pregnancy as the normal hemodynamic changes of pregnancy lead to increased left atrial and pulmonary pressure, reduced forward cardiac output and clinical evidence of heart failure. Pregnancy represents a high-risk period for women with mitral stenosis, with one study reporting antenatal mortality rates of ~34% [6]. Moderate to severe regurgitant native valve disease is believed to be better tolerated than moderate to severe stenotic lesions [46]. However, there is still an increased risk of complications, with rates of adverse neonatal and fetal events occurring in 26–35% of pregnancies and rates of maternal cardiac events occurring in 4–15% of pregnancies depending on the valve lesion [46].

Not surprisingly, women with left-sided bioprosthetic valves with evidence of valve dysfunction had an increased rate of any cardiovascular event (47% vs. 5%; $P = 0.01$) in addition to a higher rate of fetal adverse events (60% vs. 16%; $P = 0.012$) than women without evidence of valve dysfunction [47].

Management of Valve Disease in Pregnancy Medical management of pregnant women with valvular heart disease can be challenging. Physiologically, pregnancy results in increased cardiac output, increased plasma volume, and decreased systemic vascular resistance.

Plasma volume expansion can exacerbate symptoms of valvular disease and heart failure. Additionally, many cardiac medications should be used with caution during pregnancy. Due to teratogenicity, statins, angiotensin-converting enzyme inhibitors, and angiotensin receptor blockers are contraindicated. Diuretics should be cautiously used, as dehydration may decrease placental blood flow [48]. Although maternal use of some beta-blockers is associated with lower fetal birth weight, beta-blockers are commonly used to allow a longer diastolic filling period, thus reducing heart failure symptoms, particularly when mitral stenosis is present [48].

Valve intervention before pregnancy is recommended for symptomatic valve disease or asymptomatic severe left-sided stenotic valve lesions. Mechanical valves should be avoided due to high rates of valve thrombosis, excess bleeding, and maternal and fetal death. Management of anticoagulation during pregnancy is challenging, as detailed in current guidelines [10, 49].

When severe MS is present, percutaneous mitral balloon commissurotomy may be needed during pregnancy in those with NYHA class III or IV symptoms despite optimum medical therapy [10, 11].

4 Conclusions

The pathophysiology of VHD is similar in women compared to men, but there are some important differences in clinical presentation and management as summarized in this chapter. In women with VHD who become pregnant, the hemodynamic changes of pregnancy may precipitate symptoms or lead to hemodynamic decompensation. Management during pregnancy of women with known VHD or a prosthetic valve can be challenging.

Key Issues

- Rheumatic heart disease remains the most prevalent cause of valve dysfunction in middle to low-income countries, with women accounting for the majority of cases.
- In high-income countries, degenerative valve conditions such as calcific aortic stenosis (AS) predominate, tending to occur in equal numbers of women and men, albeit women often are diagnosed later in life with more severe symptoms.
- The LV response to chronic pressure overload due to AS differs in women, compared to men, with a small LV chamber, relatively thicker walls and more severe diastolic dysfunction.
- The disease process in the aortic valve leaflets shows sex-specific differences with more calcification is more severe in men versus more fibrosis in women.
- Primary aortic regurgitation is less common in women with severity often underrecognized, due to smaller aortic and LV dimensions.
- Mitral stenosis (MS) is more prevalent in women and predominately caused by rheumatic heart disease, with rates of calcific MS increasing in high-income countries.
- Primary mitral regurgitation (MR) and mitral valve prolapse are more frequently diagnosed in women but less often require surgical intervention when compared to men
- Women requiring mitral valve surgery are more likely to undergo mitral valve replacement instead of repair due to higher rates of circumferential mitral annular calcification.
- Transcatheter valve interventions are associated with a high rate of vascular complications in women, but TAVI may offer a long-term survival benefit compared to SAVR in older women.
- As more clinical evidence is published, it may become possible to develop more nuanced sex-specific thresholds for disease severity, LV size and function, timing and choice of intervention in women with valvular heart disease.
- Pregnancy is a high-risk period for patients with severe valvular lesions due to changes in hemodynamics and circulating plasma volume.
- Intervention should be performed before pregnancy when severe AS or severe MS is present due to high rates of maternal morbidity and mortality, however mechanical valves should be avoided.

Questions and Answers

1. A 78-year-old woman is referred for evaluation of a murmur, described as a grade 2/6 ejection murmur at the cardiac base. Chest auscultation was clear and neck veins were not distended. She has been seen by multiple prior providers for symptoms of decreased exercise capacity. An echocardiogram revealed a calcified trileaflet aortic valve with reduced motion. Aortic valve area is 0.8 cm^2 with a maximum velocity of 3.4 m/s and mean pressure of 36 mmHg. Her ventricle is small with an LV ejection fraction of 58%. What is the next best step in evaluation?
   (A) Dobutamine stress echocardiogram
   (B) CT calcium score
   (C) Calculate stroke volume index
   (D) Exercise treadmill
   (E) No further evaluation required
   Comment: The best answer is C. The Doppler data in this older woman suggest only moderate AS based on an aortic velocity of 3.4 m/s and mean systolic gradient of 38 mmHg. However, a valve area less than 1.0 cm^2 suggests severe AS. Thus, additional evaluation is needed to determine if AS is severe, which might account for symptoms of reduced exercise tolerance. Her LV size and systolic function are normal so that a dobutamine stress echocardiogram is unlikely to result in an increase in transaortic stroke volume and thus is not recommended when ejection fraction is normal. Exercise treadmill testing would provide an objective measure of exercise capacity and determine whether blood pressure increases appropriately with exercise but would not distinguish exercise limitation due to AS from other cardiac causes. Although a CT calcium score can be helpful, using sex-specific cut-off values for women to define severe AS, the most appropriate next step at this point is to calculate the echocardiographic stroke volume index. A reduced stroke volume index (<35 mL/m^2) would be consistent with low-flow low-gradient severe AS and would warrant referral to a structural heart team for consideration of bioprosthetic SAVR or TAVI.
2. A 32-year-old woman is referred to your clinic with known rheumatic mitral stenosis. She has had worsening dyspnea with exertion over the past year. Physical exam revealed a soft diastolic murmur at the apex, clear lungs, normal carotid pulses and a normal jugular venous pressure. Medications include torsemide 20 mg and metoprolol succinate 25 mg daily. An echocardiogram reveals a mitral valve area of 1.0 cm^2 with mild mitral regurgitation, pulmonary artery systolic pressure of 32 mmHg, and LV ejection fraction of 56%. She desires pregnancy in the near future. What is the next best step in management?
   (A) Continue medical management
   (B) Mitral valve surgical repair
   (C) Bioprosthetic mitral valve replacement
   (D) Percutaneous mitral balloon commissurotomy
   (E) Mechanical mitral valve replacement
   Comments: The best answer is D. In this young woman with rheumatic mitral stenosis, echocardiographic imaging and Doppler hemodynamics are consistent with severe valve obstruction. Even though she currently is asymptomatic, the risk of pregnancy is high as the increased volume flow rate during pregnancy is likely to result in heart failure and adverse maternal and fetal outcomes. Intervention prior to pregnancy is recommended, with avoidance of a prosthetic valve if possible. Bioprosthetic valves are prone to degeneration, often accelerated during pregnancy, and management of anticoagulation in women with mechanical heart valves is challenging. Mitral regurgitation is only mild and valve anatomy is favorable so that the optimal intervention is a transcatheter mitral balloon commissurotomy. Surgical mitral valve repair would be considered only if significant mitral regurgitation was present or a transcatheter approach was not successful.
3. A 56-year-old woman who has been followed annually for mitral valve prolapse with moderate mitral regurgitation returns for annual follow-up. Her medical history is otherwise unremarkable. She is physically active and denies exertional symptoms. Exam shows a

BP 122/69 mmHg, a heart rate of 68 bpm, and a systolic murmur with no signs of heart failure. Her echocardiogram shows prolapse of the central scallop of the posterior leaflet with an eccentric anteriorly directed jet of mitral regurgitation with a vena contracta width is 8 mm and estimated regurgitant orifice area of 0.41 cm^2. Estimated pulmonary systolic pressure if 35 mm Hg, LV end-systolic diameter is 42 mm and LV ejection fraction is 57%. The next best step in management is:

(A) Begin an angiotensin converting enzyme inhibitor
(B) Mitral valve surgical repair
(C) Bioprosthetic mitral valve replacement
(D) Mitral transcatheter edge-to-edge repair
(E) Mechanical mitral valve replacement

Comment: The best answer is B.

This woman with mitral valve prolapse now has severe mitral regurgitation, based on the vena contracta width over 7 mm and regurgitant orifice area over 0.4 cm^2. Medical therapy is not effective for treatment of mitral regurgitation. Although she is asymptomatic, her LV ejection fraction less than 60% and end-systolic diameter greater than 40 mm are Class 1 indications for mitral valve intervention. Mitral valve repair is recommended in preference to valve replacement whenever possible and her valve anatomy is favorable for a repair procedure. Mitral transcatheter edge-to-edge repair would only be considered if her surgical risk was very high.

References

1. Preventza O, Critsinelis A, Simpson K, Olive JK, LeMaire SA, Cornwell LD, et al. Sex, racial, and ethnic disparities in U.S. cardiovascular trials in more than 230,000 patients. Ann Thorac Surg. 2021;112(3):726–35.
2. Andell P, Li X, Martinsson A, Andersson C, Stagmo M, Zöller B, et al. Epidemiology of valvular heart disease in a Swedish nationwide hospital-based register study. Heart. 2017;103(21):1696–703.
3. Singh A, Chan DCS, Greenwood JP, Dawson DK, Sonecki P, Hogrefe K, et al. Symptom onset in aortic stenosis. JACC Cardiovasc Imaging. 2019;12(1):96–105.
4. Bienjonetti-Boudreau D, Fleury MA, Voisine M, Paquin A, Chouinard I, Tailleur M, et al. Impact of sex on the management and outcome of aortic stenosis patients. Eur Heart J. 2021;42:2683.
5. Coffey S, Roberts-Thomson R, Brown A, Carapetis J, Chen M, Enriquez-Sarano M, et al. Global epidemiology of valvular heart disease. Nat Rev Cardiol. 2021;18(12):853–64.
6. Watkins DA, Beaton AZ, Carapetis JR, Karthikeyan G, Mayosi BM, Wyber R, et al. Rheumatic heart disease worldwide. J Am Coll Cardiol. 2018;72(12):1397–416.
7. Clavel MA, Messika-Zeitoun D, Pibarot P, Aggarwal SR, Malouf J, Araoz PA, et al. The complex nature of discordant severe calcified aortic valve disease grading. J Am Coll Cardiol. 2013;62(24):2329–38.
8. Simard L, Côté N, Dagenais F, Mathieu P, Couture C, Trahan S, et al. Sex-related discordance between aortic valve calcification and hemodynamic severity of aortic stenosis. Circ Res. 2017;120(4):681–91.
9. Thomassen HK, Cioffi G, Gerdts E, Einarsen E, Midtbø HB, Mancusi C, et al. Echocardiographic aortic valve calcification and outcomes in women and men with aortic stenosis. Heart. 2017;103(20):1619–24.
10. Otto CM, Nishimura RA, Bonow RO, Carabello BA, Erwin JP, Gentile F, et al. 2020 ACC/AHA guideline for the management of patients with valvular heart disease: a report of the American College of Cardiology/American Heart Association joint committee on clinical practice guidelines. Circulation. 2021;143(5):e72–227.
11. Vahanian A, Beyersdorf F, Praz F, Milojevic M, Baldus S, Bauersachs J, et al. 2021 ESC/EACTS guidelines for the management of valvular heart disease: developed by the task force for the management of valvular heart disease of the European Society of Cardiology (ESC) and the European Association for Cardio-Thoracic Surgery (EACTS). Eur Heart J. 2022;43(7):561–632.
12. Kong WKF, Regeer MV, Ng ACT, McCormack L, Poh KK, Yeo TC, et al. Sex differences in phenotypes of bicuspid aortic valve and aortopathy. Circ Cardiovasc Imaging. 2017;10(3):e005155.
13. Eveborn GW, Schirmer H, Heggelund G, Lunde P, Rasmussen K. The evolving epidemiology of valvular aortic stenosis. The Tromsø Study. Heart. 2013;99(6):396–400.
14. Vlastra W, Chandrasekhar J, García Del Blanco B, Tchétché D, de Brito FS, Barbanti M, et al. Sex differences in transfemoral transcatheter aortic valve replacement. J Am Coll Cardiol. 2019;74(22):2758–67.
15. Dobson LE, Fairbairn TA, Musa TA, Uddin A, Mundie CA, Swoboda PP, et al. Sex-related differences in left ventricular remodeling in severe aortic stenosis and reverse remodeling after aortic valve replacement: a cardiovascular magnetic resonance study. Am Heart J. 2016;175:101–11.
16. Tastet L, Kwiecinski J, Pibarot P, Capoulade R, Everett RJ, Newby DE, et al. Sex-related differences

in the extent of myocardial fibrosis in patients with aortic valve stenosis. JACC Cardiovasc Imaging. 2020;13(3):699–711.
17. Chandrasekhar J, Dangas G, Yu J, Vemulapalli S, Suchindran S, Vora AN, et al. Sex-based differences in outcomes with transcatheter aortic valve therapy: TVT registry from 2011 to 2014. J Am Coll Cardiol. 2016;68(25):2733–44.
18. O'Connor SA, Morice MC, Gilard M, Leon MB, Webb JG, Dvir D, et al. Revisiting sex equality with Transcatheter aortic valve replacement outcomes: a collaborative, patient-level meta-analysis of 11,310 patients. J Am Coll Cardiol. 2015;66(3):221–8.
19. Chaker Z, Badhwar V, Alqahtani F, Aljohani S, Zack CJ, Holmes DR, et al. Sex differences in the utilization and outcomes of surgical aortic valve replacement for severe aortic stenosis. J Am Heart Assoc. 2017;6(9):e006370.
20. Hernandez-Vaquero D, Rodriguez-Caulo E, Vigil-Escalera C, Blanco-Herrera O, Berastegui E, Arias-Dachary J, et al. Differences in life expectancy between men and women after aortic valve replacement. Eur J Cardiothorac Surg. 2021;60(3):681–8.
21. Eltchaninoff H, Bonaros N, Prendergast B, Nietlispach F, Vasa-Nicotera M, Chieffo A, et al. Rationale and design of a prospective, randomized, controlled, multicenter study to evaluate the safety and efficacy of transcatheter heart valve replacement in female patients with severe symptomatic aortic stenosis requiring aortic valve intervention (randomized researcH in womEn all comers wIth aortic stenosis [RHEIA] trial). Am Heart J. 2020;228:27–35.
22. Yang LT, Enriquez-Sarano M, Pellikka PA, Thapa P, Scott CG, Hung JW, et al. Sex differences in outcomes of patients with chronic aortic regurgitation: closing the mortality gap. Mayo Clin Proc. 2021;96(8):2145–56.
23. Yang LT, Michelena HI, Scott CG, Enriquez-Sarano M, Pislaru SV, Schaff HV, et al. Outcomes in chronic hemodynamically significant aortic regurgitation and limitations of current guidelines. J Am Coll Cardiol. 2019;73(14):1741–52.
24. Movahed MR, Ahmadi-Kashani M, Kasravi B, Saito Y. Increased prevalence of mitral stenosis in women. J Am Soc Echocardiogr. 2006;19(7):911–3.
25. Kato N, Padang R, Scott CG, Guerrero M, Pislaru SV, Pellikka PA. The natural history of severe calcific mitral stenosis. J Am Coll Cardiol. 2020;75(24):3048–57.
26. Davutoglu V, Yilmaz M, Soydinc S, Celen Z, Turkmen S, Sezen Y, et al. Mitral annular calcification is associated with osteoporosis in women. Am Heart J. 2004;147(6):1113–6.
27. Chehab O, Roberts-Thomson R, Bivona A, Gill H, Patterson T, Pursnani A, et al. Management of patients with severe mitral annular calcification: JACC state-of-the-art review. J Am Coll Cardiol. 2022;80(7):722–38.
28. Avierinos JF, Inamo J, Grigioni F, Gersh B, Shub C, Enriquez-Sarano M. Sex differences in morphology and outcomes of mitral valve prolapse. Ann Intern Med. 2008;149(11):787–94.
29. Namazi F, van der Bijl P, Vo NM, van Wijngaarden SE, Ajmone Marsan N, Delgado V, et al. Sex differences in prognosis of significant secondary mitral regurgitation. ESC Heart Fail. 2021;8(5):3539–46.
30. Chehab O, Roberts-Thomson R, Ling CNY, Marber M, Prendergast BD, Rajani R, et al. Secondary mitral regurgitation: pathophysiology, proportionality and prognosis. Heart. 2020;106(10):716–23.
31. Kislitsina ON, Zareba KM, Bonow RO, Andrei AC, Kruse J, Puthumana J, et al. Is mitral valve disease treated differently in men and women? Eur J Prev Cardiol. 2019;26(13):1433–43.
32. Giustino G, Overbey J, Taylor D, Ailawadi G, Kirkwood K, DeRose J, et al. Sex-based differences in outcomes after mitral valve surgery for severe ischemic mitral regurgitation. JACC Heart Fail. 2019;7(6):481–90.
33. Song HK, Grab JD, O'Brien SM, Welke KF, Edwards F, Ungerleider RM. Gender differences in mortality after mitral valve operation: evidence for higher mortality in perimenopausal women. Ann Thorac Surg. 2008;85(6):2040–5.
34. Kandula V, Kislitsina ON, Rigolin VH, Thomas JD, Malaisrie SC, Andrei AC, et al. Does gender bias affect outcomes in mitral valve surgery for degenerative mitral regurgitation? Interact Cardiovasc Thorac Surg. 2021;33(3):325–32.
35. Seeburger J, Eifert S, Pfannmüller B, Garbade J, Vollroth M, Misfeld M, et al. Gender differences in mitral valve surgery. Thorac Cardiovasc Surg. 2012;61(01):042–6.
36. Park SD, Orban M, Karam N, Lubos E, Kalbacher D, Braun D, et al. Sex-related clinical characteristics and outcomes of patients undergoing transcatheter edge-to-edge repair for secondary mitral regurgitation. JACC Cardiovasc Interv. 2021;14(8):819–27.
37. Werner N, Puls M, Baldus S, Lubos E, Bekeredjian R, Sievert H, et al. Gender-related differences in patients undergoing transcatheter mitral valve interventions in clinical practice: 1-year results from the German TRAMI registry. Catheter Cardiovasc Interv. 2020;95(4):819–29.
38. Singh JP, Evans JC, Levy D, Larson MG, Freed LA, Fuller DL, et al. Prevalence and clinical determinants of mitral, tricuspid, and aortic regurgitation (The Framingham Heart Study). Am J Cardiol. 1999;83(6):897–902.
39. Dietz MF, Prihadi EA, van der Bijl P, Fortuni F, Marques AI, Ajmone Marsan N, et al. Sex-specific differences in etiology and prognosis in patients with significant tricuspid regurgitation. Am J Cardiol. 2021;147:109–15.
40. Scotti A, Coisne A, Taramasso M, Granada JF, Ludwig S, Rodés-Cabau J, et al. Sex-related characteristics and short-term outcomes of patients undergoing transcatheter tricuspid valve intervention for tricuspid regurgitation. Eur Heart J. 2023;44(10):822–32.

41. Veen KM, Mokhles MM, Braun J, Versteegh MIM, Bogers AJJC, Takkenberg JJM. Male–female differences in characteristics and early outcomes of patients undergoing tricuspid valve surgery: a national cohort study in The Netherlands. Eur J Cardiothorac Surg. 2019;55(5):859–66.
42. Roos-Hesselink J, Baris L, Johnson M, De Backer J, Otto C, Marelli A, et al. Pregnancy outcomes in women with cardiovascular disease: evolving trends over 10 years in the ESC registry of pregnancy and cardiac disease (ROPAC). Eur Heart J. 2019;40(47):3848–55.
43. Thorne S, MacGregor A, Nelson-Piercy C. Risks of contraception and pregnancy in heart disease. Heart. 2006;92(10):1520–5.
44. Silversides CK, Colman JM, Sermer M, Farine D, Siu SC. Early and intermediate-term outcomes of pregnancy with congenital aortic stenosis. Am J Cardiol. 2003;91(11):1386–9.
45. Orwat S, Diller GP, van Hagen IM, Schmidt R, Tobler D, Greutmann M, et al. Risk of pregnancy in moderate and severe aortic stenosis: from the multinational ROPAC registry. J Am Coll Cardiol. 2016;68(16):1727–37.
46. Pfaller B, Dave Javier A, Grewal J, Gabarin N, Colman J, Kiess M, et al. Risk associated with valvular regurgitation during pregnancy. J Am Coll Cardiol. 2021;77(21):2656–64.
47. Wichert-Schmitt B, Grewal J, Malinowski AK, Pfaller B, Losenno KL, Kiess MC, et al. Outcomes of pregnancy in women with bioprosthetic heart valves with or without valve dysfunction. J Am Coll Cardiol. 2022;80(21):2014–24.
48. Halpern DG, Weinberg CR, Pinnelas R, Mehta-Lee S, Economy KE, Valente AM. Use of medication for cardiovascular disease during pregnancy. J Am Coll Cardiol. 2019;73(4):457–76.
49. Steinberg ZL, Dominguez-Islas CP, Otto CM, Stout KK, Krieger EV. Maternal and fetal outcomes of anticoagulation in pregnant women with mechanical heart valves. J Am Coll Cardiol. 2017;69(22):2681–91.

Stable Ischaemic Heart Disease, Including Obstructive CAD, INOCA and Coronary Vasomotor Disorders

Michael Lawless, Graziella Pompei, Mila Kovacevic, and Vijay Kunadian

Abstract

Ischaemic heart disease (IHD) is the leading cause of death in women worldwide. The presentation of chronic coronary syndrome (CCS) differs in men and women, which may be a function of different pathophysiological mechanisms. Classically, IHD was recognised as a consequence of decreased coronary perfusion secondary to atherosclerotic lesions, however this rhetoric has since been reconsidered as myocardial microcirculation may play a much wider role in the pathophysiology of angina than previously thought. Women are more likely to be diagnosed with angina secondary to non-obstructive coronary arteries and are at greater risk of coronary microvascular dysfunction. Unfortunately, most clinical trials have a male preponderance, which makes it challenging to extrapolate specific therapies for IHD in women. Most guidelines focus on such trials and thus there remain important knowledge gaps for the future of management of stable IHD in women.

Keywords

Stable angina · Myocardial ischaemia · Epicardial coronary artery disease · Coronary microvascular dysfunction · Percutaneous coronary intervention

Michael Lawless and Graziella Pompei have contributed equally to this work.

M. Lawless · V. Kunadian (✉)
Faculty of Medical Sciences, Translational and Clinical Research Institute, Newcastle University Medical School, Newcastle University, Newcastle upon Tyne, United Kingdom

Cardiothoracic Centre, Freeman Hospital, Newcastle upon Tyne Hospitals NHS Foundation Trust, Newcastle upon Tyne, United Kingdom
e-mail: michael.lawless@nhs.net; vijay.kunadian@newcastle.ac.uk

G. Pompei
Faculty of Medical Sciences, Translational and Clinical Research Institute, Newcastle University Medical School, Newcastle University, Newcastle upon Tyne, United Kingdom

Cardiovascular Institute, Azienda Ospedaliero-Universitaria di Ferrara, Cona, FE, Italy
e-mail: g.pompei2@newcastle.ac.uk

M. Kovacevic
Faculty of Medicine, University of Novi Sad, Novi Sad, Serbia

Institute of Cardiovascular Diseases of Vojvodina, Cardiology Clinic, Sremska Kamenica, Serbia

A. H.E.M. Maas, E. Gerdts (eds.), *Manual of Cardiovascular Disease in Women*,
https://doi.org/10.1007/978-3-031-65952-2_19

Test your learning and check your understanding of this book's contents: use the "Springer Nature Flashcards" app to access questions using ▶ https://sn.pub/51ny7m
To use the app, please follow the instructions in chapter 1.

1 Introduction

Women make up less than 30% of study populations in cardiovascular studies, however women are more likely to present to hospital with chest pain than men [1]. Ischaemic heart disease (IHD) has classically been considered a structural disease caused by obstructive coronary artery disease (CAD), however recently more emphasis has been on the investigation and management of patients with angina/ischaemia with non-obstructive coronary arteries (ANOCA/INOCA). This latter diagnosis is more common in women, however specific clinical trials to define and explore the diagnosis and management of women remain lacking.

IHD encompasses patients with CAD presenting with coronary ischaemia, however not all patients with angina and ischaemia have obstructive coronary arteries. Women are more likely to present with angina as a primary manifestation of cardiovascular disease [2], and frequently have worse outcomes then men following a diagnosis. Large scale registry data shows that female sex is a significant predictor of all-cause mortality at 30 days post percutaneous coronary intervention (PCI) for both chronic and acute coronary syndromes [3]. Furthermore, women are chronically underrepresented in clinical trials directed at management options for those with CAD, making their results less transferrable into this population [4], and despite equal treatment in women and men, differences in their health needs mean women are not being treated based on equity [5]. In this chapter, we will explore the differences in physiology, presentation, diagnosis, and management in women compared with men presenting with chronic coronary syndrome (CCS).

2 Ischaemic Heart Disease

Women frequently present with angina symptoms including chest pain at rest, pain during sleep, pain in the neck/shoulders, fatigue, emotional stress, dyspnoea, and general weakness [6]. Major epicardial coronary arteries act as conduit vessels to supply all areas of the myocardium with oxygen-rich blood. The heart's basal metabolic oxygen consumption is higher than all other major organs, approximately 10 mL O_2.min^{-1}.100 g^{-1}, which increases substantially during incremented cardiac activity. Coronary blood flow is thus tightly coupled to oxygen demand in an almost linear relationship to cardiac oxygen consumption. Aortic blood pressure is pulsatile in nature, resulting in coronary perfusion pressure flux with systole and diastole, however coronary circulation autoregulation maintains coronary flow rate despite these fluctuations in pressure. This system of autoregulation is determined by vasoactive mediators such as adenosine, nitric oxide, and the autonomic nervous system.

Myocardial ischaemia may occur through two main mechanisms:

1. Flow limiting epicardial CAD, obstructive CAD caused by atherosclerotic plaque formation.
2. Non-obstructive coronary artery causes such as arterial vasospasm or coronary microvascular dysfunction.

These mechanisms affect both men and women, with the latter often found to affect women more frequently.

3 Ischaemia with Obstructive Coronary Arteries (IOCA) in Women

The pathogenesis of atherosclerosis is believed to be ubiquitous between men and women. However, there do exist specific sex differences in the physiology of atherosclerotic plaque progression and instability, which, unfortunately, are yet not completely understood [7]. For females with IOCA, progression, severity, and symptoms may be directly affected by the differences in biology of female vasculature than male. Women are known to have smaller coronary arteries, and even those with less plaque burden were shown to have more obvious vessel stenosis, which may be related to either the overall vessel size or differences in the biology of vasculature remodelling in females versus males, a pathophysiological process which is poorly understood [8].

Women who present with symptoms of obstructive CAD are more commonly older than men presenting with the same condition. In the absence of evidence to suggest that the nature of the atherosclerotic process is different, we can extrapolate that other factors influence this sex-difference in the progression of IHD. There exist a number of differences in the risk factors for formation and progression of atherosclerosis between the sexes. These risk factors can be classified as traditional and sex-specific (Fig. 1).

3.1 Traditional Risk Factors

These risk factors are the ones clinicians would typically use to risk stratify IHD, such as Heart Score and QRisk score [9–11]. Such risk factors have been associated with increased prevalence of both stable and unstable IHD, and most studies show that they exist with more prevalence in men versus women.

1. **Hypertension:** Uncontrolled hypertension increases the risk of IHD in both men and women [12], however this risk is increased significantly in women who take oral hormonal contraceptive therapy or in women aged 60 years and over. Furthermore, women are shown to be consistently undertreated for hypertension [13].
2. **Dyslipidaemia:** Cholesterol and lipid metabolism are different for women and men, which in part is related to hormonal changes and imbalances. High total cholesterol and low-density lipoproteins (LDL), and low high-density lipoproteins (HDL) or lower total

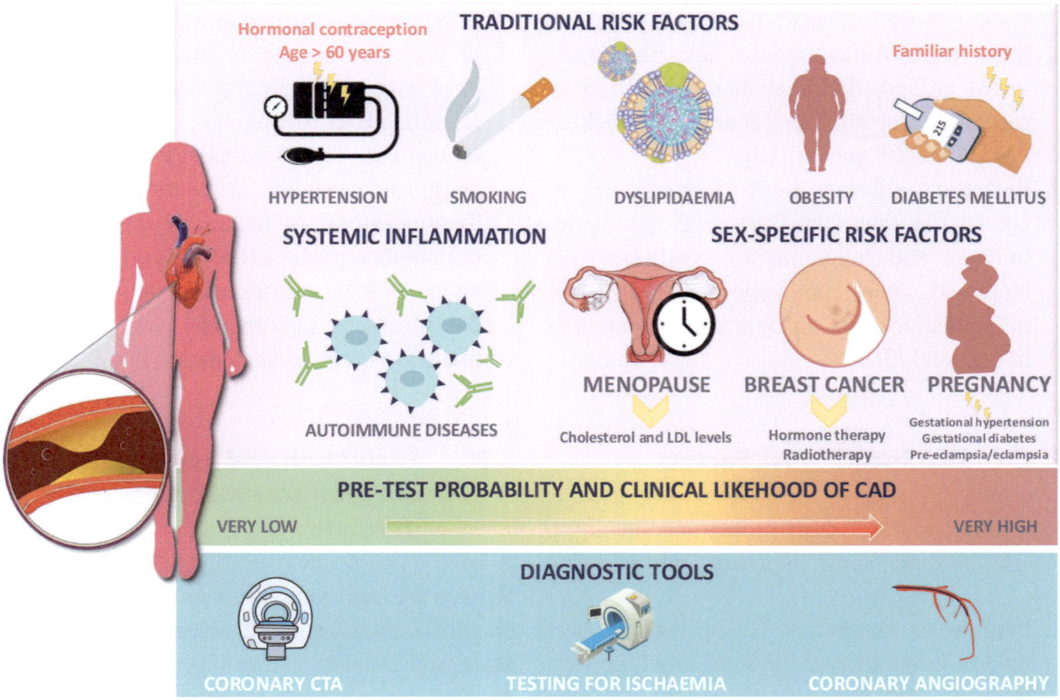

Fig. 1 IOCA in women: risk factors and diagnostic tools. *CAD,* coronary artery disease; *LDL,* low density lipoproteins

cholesterol/HDL ratio are associated with increased incidence of CAD in both men and women. Women are known to have higher levels of HDL across all ages, and premenopausal women have lower LDL levels than men. Moreover, premenopausal women have faster cholesterol metabolism than men of the same age [14]. Unfortunately for postmenopausal women, when oestrogen levels are lower and declining, total cholesterol and LDL levels consistently increase with female age [15], and in fact postmenopausal women are more likely to have greater chance of adverse cardiovascular events. This lends support to the hypothesis that sex hormones play an important role in the pathophysiology of atherosclerosis and IHD [16].

3. **Obesity, diabetes mellitus and metabolic syndrome:** The Framingham study showed that the excess risk of cardiovascular disease from obesity was significantly higher in women (64%) then men (46%) [17]. The relative risk of death from CAD was much greater in women with diabetes (women: risk 2.58, 95% confidence interval (CI) 2.05–3.26; men: 1.85, 95% CI 1.47–2.33, $p = 0.045$) [18].
4. **Smoking:** Women smoke less than men across all ages, however their excess risk of cardiovascular disease secondary to smoking is significantly greater [19].
5. **Systemic inflammation:** Women are at greater risk than men from developing autoimmune and inflammatory conditions. An increased level of widespread systemic inflammation may potentiate atherosclerosis in women [20].

3.2 Sex-Specific Risk Factors

This group of risk factors relates specifically to female biology, some represent unmodifiable risk.

1. **Female sex hormones:** The influence of hormones is paramount to female physiology. Females with hypertension are discouraged from combined hormonal contraception due to the almost 12-fold increased risk of myocardial infarction (MI) and are therefore encouraged to use progesterone-only alternatives [21]. The menopause is a good example of how changes in the female hormonal axis can influence their cardiovascular health, for example premature menopause increases the risk of cardiovascular disease [22], and hormone replacement therapy similarly increases these risks, especially in those older than 70 years [23]. Similarly, those patients who had a younger (<10 years) or older (>25 years) menarche have increased risk of future cardiovascular events [24].
2. **Pregnancy:** Pregnancy is a time when hormonal flux is particularly significant. Women may develop a number of pregnancy-related cardiovascular diseases, such as gestational hypertension or diabetes, pre-eclampsia/eclampsia [25]. Furthermore, if a woman experiences such disease states during pregnancy, her future cardiovascular risk is significantly increased [26]. Miscarriage, stillbirth, preterm birth, low birth weight babies, and hysterectomy are all independently associated with increased cardiovascular risk later in life [27]. Unfortunately, due to low involvement of pregnant women in clinical trials, there exist large gaps in the current knowledge regarding CAD in pregnancy.
3. **Breast cancer:** Breast cancer is a significant cause of mortality in women worldwide. Treatment options include hormone therapy or radiotherapy. It has been shown that there is an increase in cardiovascular events following breast cancer radiotherapy, which may be related to coronary endothelial injury [28].

3.3 Evaluation and Investigation of Coronary Artery Disease in Women

Women are less likely than men to be referred for diagnostic coronary artery assessment in both the acute and chronic setting [29]. Invasive testing involves coronary angiography with intravascular physiological and imaging assessment of coronary arteries. Non-invasive investigation strategies include coronary computed tomography angiography (CCTA) [30], cardiac magnetic resonance imaging (CMRI), single-photon emission computed tomography (SPECT), Dobutamine stress echocardiography, as well as exercise tolerance test (ETT). However, due to the reduced accuracy of ECG response to exercise testing in women and the greater frequency of non-obstructive CAD in women, these modalities are frequently suboptimal for female patients [29].

3.4 Management of Obstructive Coronary Artery Disease in Women

The mainstay of management for obstructive CAD in women remains the same as men—PCI with drug eluting stents and guideline-directed medical therapy. Most trials investigating the outcomes of patients who undergo revascularisation compared with optimal medical therapy for stable angina have shown reduction in anginal symptom burden, however no overall reduction in mortality or prevalence of MI [4]. Unfortunately, females make up less than 30% of the studied population of these trials and thus this important limitation means there is limited woman-directed information to provide sufficient evidence in support of specific guidelines for management in women. Recent evidence from large registries indicates that patients with stable CAD often gain symptoms relief with optimal medical therapy without the requirement for intervention [31]. Management should include full assessment and control of cardiovascular risk factors, alongside antianginal drug therapy.

4 Non-Obstructive Coronary Arteries in Women

Historically, IHD has inextricably been linked to the concept of obstructive CAD, leading to misdiagnosis, especially in women discharged without any medical treatment and referred to other physicians with a diagnosis of non-cardiac chest pain. Recently, large multicenter studies reported no evidence of obstructive CAD in approximately 40% of the patients undergoing coronary angiography because of suspected angina and/or positive stress test. This frequency is much higher among women (50–70%) compared to men (30–50%), and it is estimated that it will increase with the use of non-invasive imaging tests, as a high proportion of women traditionally refuse to undergo invasive assessment [32]. Similarly, almost two-thirds of women enrolled in the WISE study did not have significant obstructive stenosis at coronary angiography [33]. Until recently, diagnosis and management of stable angina has been guided by trials with a male predominance, leading to few specific management strategies for such patients with non-obstructive coronary arteries, particularly in women [34]. Nevertheless, clinical research in these scenarios has gained significant interest, leading to better definition, classification, and prognostic stratification according to the underlying pathophysiological mechanisms.

4.1 Angina with Non-Obstructive Coronary Arteries (ANOCA)

Women commonly present with angina, however, may have non-obstructive coronary arteries identified on coronary angiography (ANOCA) [35, 36]. ANOCA symptoms should not be automatically classified as non-cardiac in origin, considering that women have a much higher prevalence of non-obstructive coronary arteries than men, and it is associated with different clinical presentation. For example, epicardial coronary artery spasm is characterised by resting chest pain not associated with increased oxygen demand, chest pain with diurnal variation frequently at night or early morning. ANOCA is not a benign condition. Presentation with stable angina and non-obstructive coronary arteries is associated with greater future adverse cardiovascular outcomes, compared to those without IHD [37]. Women with ANOCA had a 2.5% annual increase in major adverse cardiovascular events (MACE) over a 5-year follow-up period, compared with men, and a threefold higher frequency than a control group of participants without [33]. Up to 50% of women with ANOCA have increased frequency of many of the traditional cardiovascular risk factors, including hypertension, dyslipidaemia, family history of CAD, diabetes mellitus and obesity [38, 39]. Furthermore, age is a significant risk factor, as there is a significantly higher prevalence in those aged 45–65 years of age [40]. To some extent, this effect may be explained by the protective role of oestrogen, which is known to reduce systemic inflammation and vasoconstriction.

4.2 Ischaemia with Non-Obstructive Coronary Arteries (INOCA)

Myocardial ischaemia stems from the mismatch between blood supply and myocardial oxygen demands, and in the absence of obstructive CAD it may be caused by coronary vasomotor disorders, consisting of coronary microvascular dysfunction (CMD) and vasospastic angina (VSA). The traditional hypothesis that non-obstructive CAD was a "benign syndrome" is clearly not correct. INOCA impacts women's lives, as shown by a recent quality-of-life survey. Most of the surveyed patients were women and 80% of them declared the condition affected their home and social life, and over 70% reported an impact on mental health. Patients reduced or stopped work completely approximately in 75% of cases [41]. Furthermore, strong evidence reports increased risk for major adverse outcomes in this population, mainly represented by hospitalisation for recurrent angina, heart failure, or both. The WISE study reported that the volume of repeat catheterizations or angina hospitalisations was 1.8-fold higher in women with non-obstructive CAD versus 1-vessel CAD at 1-year follow-up [42]. In the same manner, a recent study showed that INOCA patients with CMD showed a threefold higher risk of MACE compared with those without CMD [43]. Specifically, women with INOCA are at increased risk of MACE, most commonly heart failure with preserved ejection fraction (HFpEF) [44]. CMD has been associated with features of HFpEF such as diastolic dysfunction and elevated high-sensitivity cardiac troponin levels [45]. Interestingly, the higher incidence of CMD and abnormal myocardial perfusion imaging in INOCA patients may be implicated in the increased MACE [46]. Along with an adverse cardiovascular prognosis, the majority of INOCA patients also have a considerably impaired functional status and decreased exercise tolerance. When evaluation is performed in these patients, impaired left-ventricular relaxation either elevated left-ventricular end-diastolic pressure or echo-Doppler abnormalities are often detected. It had been previously reported that women with INOCA have diastolic dysfunction compared with healthy patients as assessed by CMRI. This concept has been expanded by demonstrating that subclinical diastolic dysfunction is frequently prevalent in women with INOCA, and associated with higher levels of systemic oxidative stress [47]. Also VSA is associated with major adverse events such as sudden cardiac death, MI, and syncope [48].

4.3 Sex-Related Risk Factors and Patients Characteristics

The role of cardiovascular risk factors in the pathogenesis of INOCA has not been well elucidated. Women with INOCA are younger, with a progressively decreasing prevalence after 70 years. This subset of patients is less likely to have traditional risk factors including hypertension, diabetes, or cigarette smoking [49]. Smoking is a risk factor for coronary spasm, unlike diabetes and hypertension, and the relationship with dyslipidaemia is unclear [50]. Smoking, age, diabetes, hypertension, and dyslipidaemia have been associated with CMD [51]. In women, novel risk factors such as pro-inflammatory markers seem to be involved [52]. The higher incidence of inflammatory diseases in postmenopausal women underlies the sex-differences in CMD. Moreover, psychosocial stress may play a crucial role. Recent findings suggest a greater contribution of the sympathetic nervous system to coronary flow. The greater coronary reactivity to cold pressure test observed in women with INOCA may reflect one or more non-endothelial dependent mechanisms increasing myocardial blood flow in response to sympathetic stress in non-obstructive CAD [53]. A recent study supported sex-related difference in the vasomotor response to provocative test, with a higher prevalence of microvascular spasm among women and epicardial spasm among men. Although ejection fraction did not differ between the groups, patients with microvascular spasm had significantly higher rates of diastolic dysfunction compared with patients with epicardial spasm. The greater burden of CMD in women is underpinned by several mechanisms, including smaller body size and myocardial mass. In addition, coronary arteries have a smaller diameter, thinner walls, and tortuous course (Fig. 2) [54].

4.4 Pathophysiology of INOCA

Myocardial ischaemia can arise from any part of the vascular structure. The epicardial vessels are characterised by a diameter >500 μm and serve

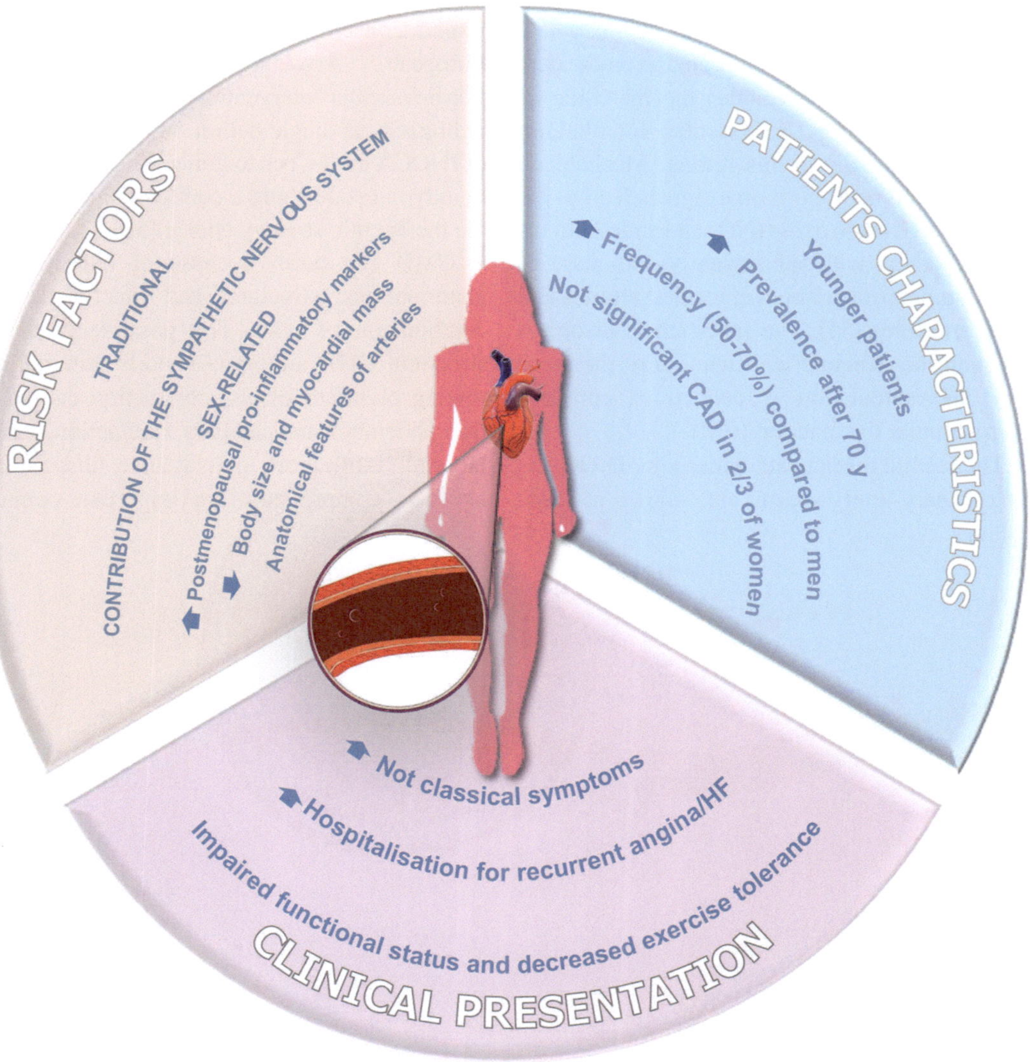

Fig. 2 INOCA in women: risk factors, patient characteristics and clinical presentation

as conduits with little resistance. The intermediate compartment consists of prearteriolar vessels (500 μm to 100 μm diameter) with measurable pressure drops due to the significant resistance. These can be further classified in two territories: the proximal (500 to 150 μm), more responsive to changes in flow, and the distal (150 to 100 μm), more sensitive to pressure variations. Finally, the distal segments are represented by intramural arterioles (<100 μm), more responsive to changes in the metabolites concentration. Pre-arterioles, arterioles, and capillaries compose the coronary microcirculation. The variation in smooth muscle tone of pre-arterioles and arterioles is responsible for the regulation and distribution of coronary blood flow (CBF) in the underlying capillary bed. When myocardial oxygen demand increases, arteriolar vasodilation enables the matching of these requirements. The vascular endothelium plays a central role in this setting. Mechanical, chemical, and neurohormonal signals lead to the production of nitric oxide (NO) and endothelium-derived factors with subsequent vasodilation of the smooth muscle of both epicardial arteries and small arterioles [55]. The spectrum of disorders affecting the structure and function of the coronary microcirculation is defined as coronary microvascular dysfunction (CMD).

The second mechanism underlying INOCA is the coronary artery spasm, also known as vasospastic angina (VSA), associated with a hyperreactive response of the epicardial segments to vasoconstrictive stimuli. Non-endothelial-dependent contraction of smooth muscle cells has been demonstrated in patients with epicardial artery spasm, but also endothelial dysfunction can be related to epicardial spasm. Coronary artery spasm can also occur at pre-arteriolar and arterioles level (microvascular spasm) due to an increased release of vasoconstrictive substances, exacerbated susceptibility of vascular smooth muscle cells, or an abnormal activation of sympathetic tone [35]. Microvascular spasm and CMD are often grouped together as underlying causes of microvascular angina (Fig. 3). In 2020 an Expert Consensus Document was drafted by the European Association of Percutaneous Cardiovascular Interventions with the aim of providing a clear single definition and classification of INOCA endotypes to guide the scientific community in establishing a correct diagnosis and in the therapeutic strategy choice [56].

CMD can occur because of two types of abnormalities: structural and functional, or a combination of both. The possible causes of structural CMD are represented by luminal narrowing of microvessels, obstruction caused by thromboembolism, capillary rarefaction, vascular wall infiltration, perivascular fibrosis, and extrinsic compression. An important common

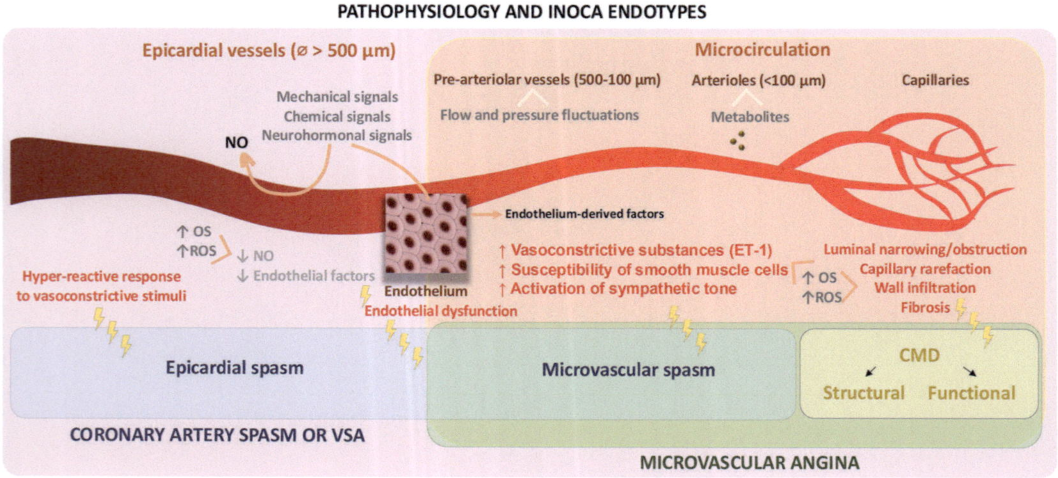

Fig. 3 Pathophysiologic mechanisms in INOCA. *NO,* nitric oxide; *OS,* oxidative stress; *ROS,* reactive oxygen species; *VSA,* vasospastic angina; *CMD,* coronary microvascular dysfunction

feature is the diffuse nature of 'microvascular remodeling'. The haemodynamic correlates of structural microcirculatory remodeling in response to a non-endothelium-dependent vasodilator (adenosine) are a reduced coronary flow reserve (CFR) and an increase in minimal (hyperaemic) microcirculatory resistance.

On the other hand, functional mechanisms may be related to the presence of an impaired dilation (vasodilator abnormalities) and/or an increased vasoconstriction of coronary microvessels (microvascular spasm). Impaired vasodilation may be, in turn, caused by endothelium-dependent and/or endothelium-independent mechanisms. Endothelial dysfunction is associated with impaired vasodilation and paradoxical vasoconstriction of upstream arteries and arterioles when myocardial oxygen demands increase. The reduced production and/or accelerated degradation of NO and other endothelial-derived relaxation factors are the main cause of a limited endothelium-dependent mechanism; a reduced response to papaverine, adenosine, or dipyridamole, suggest that endothelial-independent vasodilatation likely involves an impaired relaxation of vascular smooth muscle cells. Moreover, an increased release of vasoconstrictor agonists (i.e., endothelin-1—ET-1), an enhanced susceptibility of vascular smooth muscle cells to normal vasoconstrictor stimuli and an abnormal increase in sympathetic activity, may be other potential mechanisms. Conversely, endothelium-independent mechanisms are less understood. Microvascular spasm is part of the spectrum of vasomotor abnormalities seen in patients with CMD and it appears to be closely linked to endothelial dysfunction [57]. Some of the haemodynamic correlates of arteriolar dysregulation, observed during intracoronary acetylcholine test, are a limited vasodilatory response to the drug, a marked reduction in blood flow, without epicardial vessel spasm (denoting microvascular spasm) or the development of diffuse narrowing of distal epicardial vessels (epicardial spasm).

Oxidative stress (OS) with the consequent inflammatory response are considered key mechanisms driving the development of CMD. As a consequence, myocytes exhibit alterations in structure and function, increased collagen content, elevated passive myocyte stiffness, and increased left ventricular (LV) end-diastolic stiffness [47]. An increased concentration of intracellular reactive oxygen species (ROS) promotes the switching of the activity of endothelial NO synthetase, leading to an impairment of NO-mediated vasodilation and an enhanced ET-1 vasoconstriction activity through activation of Rho-kinase pathway. Furthermore, epigenetic modifications, commonly detected in ageing, further sustain OS by increasing ROS production [57].

A recent optical coherence tomography (OCT) analysis showed the correlation between CMD and changes in intracoronary morphology, demonstrating the prognostic links between coronary morphologies and functional abnormalities in INOCA patients. In particular, the quantified adventitial vasa vasorum (AVV) density was significantly greater in microvascular spasm patients as compared with the control group. Interestingly, a significant positive correlation between AVV and index of microvascular resistance (IMR) in microvascular spasm was noticed. Regarding the epicardial spasm, the study distinguished two groups of patients: a diffuse spasm ($\geq$2 segments) group and a focal spasm group. The first one exhibited the greatest AVV density, positively associated with IMR and positively correlated with Rho-kinase activation. Thus, a Rho-kinase inhibitor would hold promise for a risk-reduction strategy for diffuse spasm. Focal spasm had the worst outcome, remaining a poor prognostic factor compared with the other groups [58].

4.5 Non-invasive Evaluation

Since a diagnosis of INOCA requires both myocardial ischaemia and no evidence of obstruction in epicardial vessels, defining myocardial ischaemia represents the first step. In the latest ESC guidelines for CCS, a non-invasive imaging assessment is recommended as a first-line test [36]. Positron Emission Tomography (PET) is the gold standard for non-invasive assessment of CMD, albeit its use is restricted due to limited availability and high costs [59]. CMRI has also diagnostic and prognostic value in patients with suspected CMD, allowing the quantification of myocardial blood flow (MBF) at rest and during induced maximal hyperaemia. Semi-quantitative assessment of the first-pass perfusion images allow the calculation of the myocardial perfusion reserve index (MPRI) in response to vasodilator stress [60]. Similarly, myocardial first-pass dynamic computed tomography (CT) scan allows a (semi-) quantitative assessment of MBF and MPR [57].

Since non-invasive functional tests rely on detecting regional differences in myocardial perfusion or wall motion, their ability to diagnose CMD affecting the whole myocardium or VSA occurring in specific situations could be hampered. Moreover, most of the non-invasive modalities cannot provide anatomical information. Coronary computed tomography angiography (CCTA) is a non-invasive diagnostic tool able to rule out significant coronary stenosis with a very high negative predictive value. However, the presence of epicardial stenosis on CCTA does not exclude the possibility of INOCA. Nevertheless, CT imaging represents a promising technique that allows to combine CCTA and CT perfusion to exclude epicardial CAD and assess microvascular function.

The problem is that ischaemia related to CMD is often "patchy" and the aforementioned non-invasive modalities have been validated by comparison with obstructive CAD, where a relatively well perfused region is compared with a poorly perfused region. In patients with non-obstructive CAD on CCTA and/or no regional reversible ischaemia on functional testing, CMD or VSA may be the cause of symptoms, and in case of a significant burden of disease further invasive testing should be considered. A recent study classified stable patients from the international ILIAS registry, showing a diagnosis of INOCA based only on non-invasive test does not identify patients with higher risk of long-term cardiovascular events. Indeed, among patients with anginal symptoms and functionally non-obstructive CAD, 28.2% showed positive non-invasive test results and 45.3% had CMD. These findings support the current Experts Consensus Document, encouraging incorporating intracoronary physiologic assessment to the non-invasive tests for a better risk stratification and tailored management of INOCA patients depending on its endotypes [43].

Firstly, it is appropriate to distinguish the epicardial vessels from the microcirculation, as diagnostic and treatment are based on different approaches. The Coronary Vasomotor Disorders International Study (COVADIS) group drafted an updated standardization of diagnostic criteria for patients presenting with angina pectoris or ischaemia-like symptoms in the absence of flow-limiting CAD. According to the document, microvascular angina is defined as angina caused by dysfunction in the microcirculation, and VSA as angina precipitated by spasms of the epicardial domain [61].

Non-invasive modalities offer advantages related to their less invasive nature and ease of use. However, the integration of invasive testing provides comprehensive care in ANOCA/INOCA patients. Nowadays, in a precision medicine-based world, there is no reason for a patient with debilitating symptoms to be discharged without a complete assessment of the function of the coronary circulation (Fig. 4) [62].

4.6 Invasive Coronary Function Assessment

After exclusion of flow-limiting obstructive CAD, the assessment of microvascular function is needed to define CMD. Coronary flow reserve (CFR) is a physiological index of how coronary blood flow can be increased during a hyperaemic state compared with a resting state, and it is affected by both epicardial stenosis and microvascular function [63]. An invasive evaluation with either thermodilution or Doppler flow velocity modality is endorsed by the ESC CCS guidelines and the AHA/ACC Guidelines for the Evaluation and Diagnosis of Chest Pain, with a IIa recommendation in patients with persistent symptoms and angiographically normal coronary arteries [36, 64]. Invasive CFR can be measured

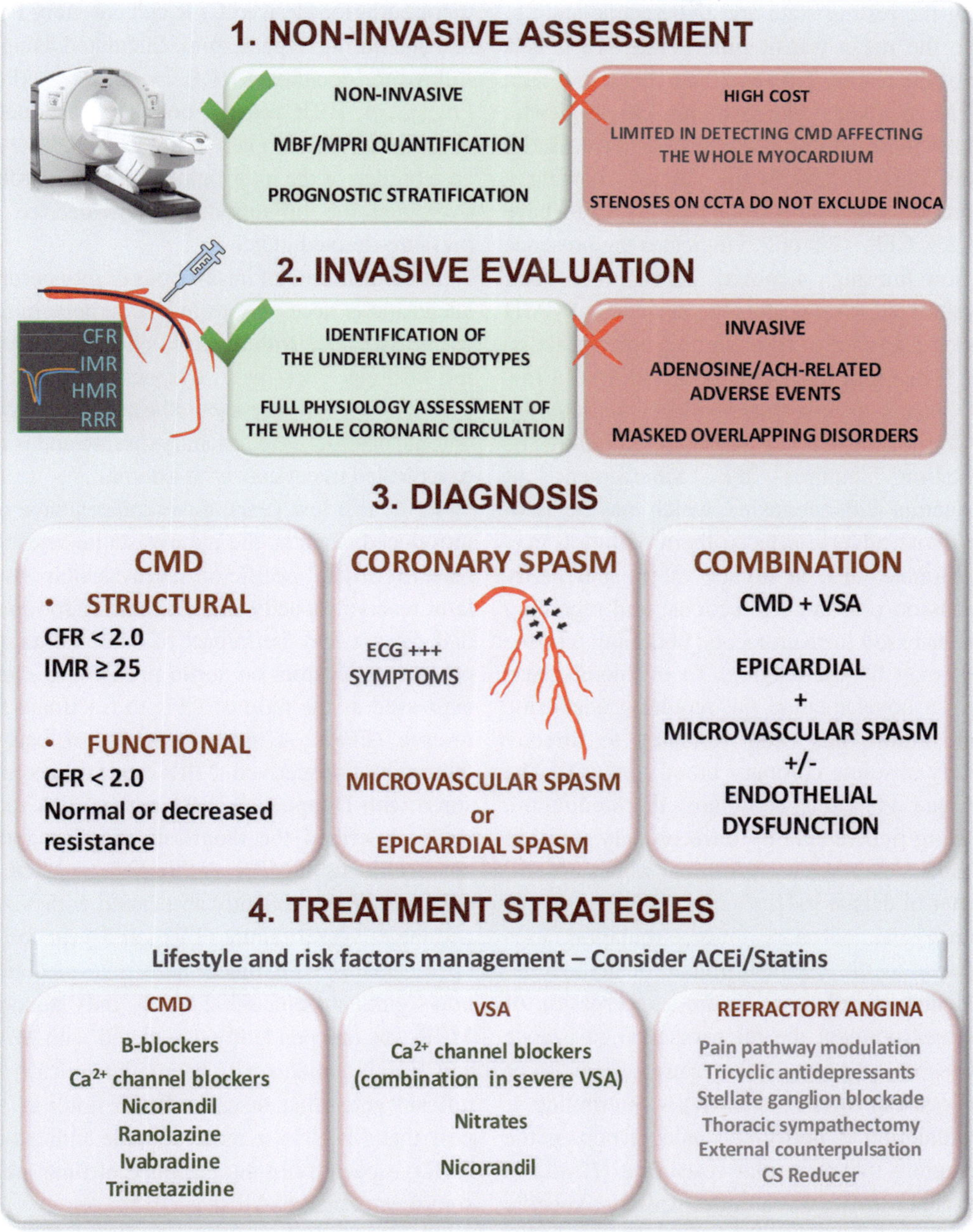

Fig. 4 Non-invasive and invasive assessment in INOCA. *ACEi,* angiotensin-converting enzyme inhibitors; *ACh,* acetylcholine; *CCTA,* coronary computed tomography angiography; *CMD,* coronary microvascular dysfunction; *CFR,* coronary flow reserve; *CS,* coronary sinus; *IMR,* index of microvascular resistance; *INOCA,* ischaemia with non-obstructive coronary arteries; *MPRI,* myocardial perfusion reserve index; *MBF,* myocardial blood flow; *VSA,* vasospastic angina

using a Doppler wire or a pressure-temperature sensor-equipped guidewire, usually in left anterior descending (LAD) artery. Using the Doppler wire, CFR can be obtained as the ratio of hyperaemic average peak coronary flow velocity (CFV) to resting average peak CFV. The thermodilution technique is used to calculate CFR via the saline bolus transit time, a surrogate marker of coronary blood flow. Thermodilution curves are obtained by 3 injections of 3–4 mL saline during the resting state and hyperaemic state to derive the mean transit time (Tmn). CFR is a ratio of the resting Tmn and the hyperaemic Tmn [65]. Most studies demonstrating the prognostic value of thermodilution-based CFR have used a cut-off value of 2.0, while studies showing a prognostic value of Doppler-based CFR have used 2.5. CFR $\leq$2.0 or 2.5 indicates the presence of flow-limiting stenosis, CMD, or both. Therefore, CFR represents the presence of CMD in case of absence of flow-limiting epicardial disease. Data from the WISE study showed a low CFR was a robust independent predictor of MACE [66]. CFR is not free from limitations: its calculation requires the achievement of hyperaemia with adenosine, which may be associated with adverse effects; thermodilution may overestimate CFR at higher values and partly depends on operator's injections; and regarding Doppler-based measurements, obtaining a stable signal may be challenging. To overcome these issues, a novel method not requiring adenosine administration has been validated to directly quantify absolute coronary blood flow (Q). The technique is based on continuous thermodilution, achieving hyperaemia by intracoronary infusion of saline. Nevertheless, its normal values are still a matter of debate [67].

Since the coronary microcirculation uses resistance as the key determinant of myocardial blood flow distribution, in the same session of CFR measurement the microvascular resistance is assessed: if thermodilution is used, the index of microvascular resistance (IMR) is determined, if the evaluation is performed using Doppler, the hyperaemic microvascular resistance (HMR) is calculated. IMR is a microvascular-specific index, less dependent on haemodynamic conditions. The uncorrected IMR is defined as distal coronary artery pressure multiplied by hyperaemic Tmn [68]. An IMR value >25 indicates the presence of microvascular dysfunction. HMR is defined as the ratio between the distal coronary artery pressure and maximal coronary flow velocity during hyperaemia. For the diagnosis of CMD, 2.5 mmHg/cm/s is used as the cut-off value for HMR [69]. The Resistive Reserve Ratio (RRR) is an integrated index that uses thermodilution-derived CFR and coronary Pd (at rest and during hyperaemia), calculated using the following equation: RRR = CFR × (Pd_{rest}/$Pd_{hyperaemia}$). RRR reflects both the vasodilatory capacity of the coronary circulation and the disease burden of the interrogated vessel, in order to overcome the limitations of flow-derived and pressure-derived indices.

Administration of intravenous or intracoronary adenosine is necessary to induce hyperaemia. Its use is associated with multiple side effects including flushing, chest pain, dyspnea, and atrioventricular blocks. Its use should be avoided in severe chronic obstructive pulmonary disease and is contraindicated in patients with asthma.

In the last few years, novel indices have been introduced, such as the microvascular resistance reserve (MRR) specific of microvascular vasodilator reserve capacity, and accounting for epicardial disease and the impact of administration of potent vasodilators on aortic pressure. It can be expressed as the ratio of CFR to fractional flow reserve (FFR). A strong correlation between thermodilution-derived MRR and values measured with Doppler has been reported. A recent study described the diagnostic and prognostic characteristics of MRR. Although both MRR and CFR were independently associated with MACE and target vessel failure (TVF) at 5-year follow-up in vessels with functionally intermediate or non-significant epicardial CAD, only abnormal MRR was independently associated with MACE and TVF in patients with haemodynamically significant epicardial disease. These findings suggest that MRR is a more reliable indicator of CMD, especially in the presence of functionally significant epicardial disease [70].

Finally, novel angiography-derived indices have been developed, starting from the IMR_{angio}. Angio-based IMR (aIMR) is another novel index that may explain ischaemia as detected by stress CMRI in INOCA patients [71]. Recently, the diagnostic performance of a wire- and adenosine-free index (angio-IMR) has been investigated in patients with suspected INOCA. These results open future possibility of providing important information for clinicians when investigating chest pain in INOCA patients [72].

4.7 Prognosis of Structural and Functional CMD

Structural CMD describes the traditional CMD endotype and is characterised by a reduced CFR in the presence of an increase in microvascular resistance (MR). This endotype is considered to represent architectural changes in the microvasculature which impair microcirculation under maximally vasodilated conditions. On the contrary, functional CMD is characterised by a reduced CFR in the presence of normal MR. This is considered related to an increased demand for myocardial oxygen or disordered coronary autoregulation, leading to increased coronary flow in resting conditions despite unaltered myocardial workload and normal microcirculation during maximally vasodilated conditions. Both endotypes have previously been related to a similar prevalence of inducible myocardial ischaemia, as well as to a similarly impaired prognosis during a 5-year follow-up period. Structural CMD tends to have a more traditional cardiovascular risk profile and an increased prevalence of hypertension. These patients benefit from targeted lifestyle interventions and treatment to improve afterload reduction and vascular remodeling, such as beta-blockers (BBs), angiotensin-converting enzyme inhibitors (ACEi) or statins [73]. In contrast, patients with diminished CFR and preserved MR (functional CMD) are characterised by a preserved maximal CBF, but an increased resting CBF, prognostically important in CCS. The elevated resting CBF can be explained by either impaired coronary autoregulation, or by increased myocardial oxygen demand at rest. Targeted therapy for these patients should aim to improve basic myocardial metabolism. However, scientific evidence for this subgroup is lacking and future research is needed [74].

4.8 Coronary Artery Spasm

If the specific mechanism of INOCA is not identified based on a comprehensive invasive physiologic assessment aimed at CMD diagnosis or if there are specific features of VSA, such as resting chest pain, diurnal variation, or a prompt response to nitroglycerin, a provocation test is needed to diagnose coronary artery spasm.

A recent meta-analysis has shown that coronary vasospasm is highly prevalent in patients with non-obstructive coronary arteries [75]. Women were more likely to suffer from microvascular spasm whereas men were more likely to have epicardial artery spasm. It is therefore important that a thorough evaluation and investigation is carried out in this context to establish the underlying phenotype to direct appropriate therapy. Women are known to be underrepresented in clinical trials, thus diagnostic pathways specifically for women are currently unavailable. The acetylcholine (ACh) provocation test is the most widely used method to confirm the presence of coronary artery spasm and is recommended by the ESC CCS guidelines [36]. ACh influences vascular tone via muscarinic receptors on endothelial and vascular smooth muscle cells. Normal healthy endothelial cells respond to ACh through liberation of vasoactive mediators inducing vasodilation. However, in the presence of a dysfunctional endothelium failing to produce such mediators, ACh directly stimulates muscarinic receptors in smooth muscle cells, inducing vasoconstriction. Constriction of epicardial vessels can be directly assessed with standard invasive coronary angiography. However, only dedicated intracoronary wires are able to measure constriction of the small arterioles and quantification of CBF [55]. A standard approach involves sequential infusion of ACh at progressively increasing concentrations. According to the COVADIS criteria, the test is considered positive if symptoms occur, accompanied by ischaemic ECG changes and an angiographic ≥90% reduction of the coronary lumen. If the lumen reduction is <90%, the diagnosis of microvascular spasm is made. After ACh, intracoronary nitroglycerin is administered to assess coronary vasodilatation and counter symptoms. The overall rate of complications associated with Ach use is quite low, including transient atrio-ventricular block (4.2%), sinus block (0.8%) and paroxysmal atrial fibrillation (3.5%). In a recent study, previous history of paroxysmal atrial fibrillation, moderate-to-severe

LV diastolic dysfunction, and higher QT dispersion at baseline ECG were the only predictors of complications during the test. Interestingly, the occurrence of complications during ACh test was not associated with a worse prognosis at a medium- to long-term follow-up [54].

Despite the intrinsic availability of information on endothelial function during ACh testing, its quantification is currently not incorporated in diagnostic assessment, leading to under diagnosis of vasomotor disorders in the form of endothelial dysfunction. Endothelial dysfunction is characterised by a blunted coronary vasodilator response to gradual intracoronary administration of low dose ACh, and is associated with impaired quality of life and a high incidence of adverse cardiovascular events. A recent study evaluated the diagnostic value of coronary endothelial function testing in addition to standard assessment. A reduced ACh-mediated vasodilator response to identify coronary endothelial dysfunction was defined as any reduction in epicardial coronary diameter and/or <50% increase in CBF in response to the last ACh infusion. The adoption of the additional endothelial function testing increased the diagnostic yield of standard functional testing (including only adenosine testing and spasm provocation) by 17% to 92% [76].

Similarly, the detection of the combination of both spasm disorders is currently limited to cases in which microvascular spasm occurs at lower ACh doses than epicardial spasm, whereas in others epicardial spasm may mask coexisting microvascular spasm. Thus, the frequency of coexisting mechanisms may be underestimated. The novel concept of rechallenging coronary arteries with ACh immediately after intracoronary administration of an antivasospastic substance (ACh rechallenge) has been introduced to detect coexisting different spasm endotypes. In a study enrolling a high percentage of women (69%), ACh rechallenge was systematically performed 3 minutes after intracoronary injection of nitroglycerin by readministration of the ACh provocation dose with the aim to assess the reinducibility of microvascular and epicardial spasm. ACh rechallenge proved to be useful to unmask combined spasm disorders. Moreover, in 48% of patients with epicardial spasm ACh rechallenge revealed coexisting nitroglycerin-persistent microvascular spasm. The study demonstrated that nitroglycerin is much more effective in preventing epicardial spasm than microvascular spasm, challenging current recommendations, and may pave the way towards a more tailored treatment of the two different forms [77].

4.9 Management of ANOCA/INOCA in Women

Current specific treatments for ANOCA/INOCA are limited by evidence based on small sample sizes, and a considerable proportion of patients report persistent symptoms and poor quality of life despite treatment. The aim of strict control of blood pressure is to prevent progression of microvascular remodeling and to reduce the frequency of angina. When epicardial spasm is suspected, triggers such as smoking or recreational drugs should be strongly discouraged. Combination of blood pressure medications depends on the predominant mechanism of anginal symptoms. The CorMicA trial [78], which included 74% of women, enrolled symptomatic patients without obstructive CAD and positive invasive testing. A stratified medical therapy was used, considering the measurements at coronary function testing, and the approach was shown to improve angina and quality of life at 6 months and 1 year. The intervention consisted of anti-ischaemic therapy using BBs and ACEi along with preventive care (statins) and lifestyle changes (Table 1).

The use of ACEis improves CFR in CMD and ACEi/angiotensin receptor blockade (ARB) can be easily combined with both calcium channel blockers (CCBs) and BBs. In CMD with predominantly resting symptoms, CCBs have been shown to be effective in both epicardial spasm and CMD, whereas BBs are recommended in patients with predominantly exercise-related symptoms. Statins, besides their lipid-lowering effect, have anti-inflammatory properties effective in reduced CFR and vascular spasm [84]. In patients with evidence of

Table 1 Evidence about INOCA from studies enrolling a high percentage of female patients

Reference	Patients (n)	Female patients (%)	Take home messages
Pepine et al. (2010) [66]	189	100%	• Lower CFR associated with increased risk for major adverse outcomes (HR 1.16, 95% CI 1.04 to 1.30; p = 0.009)
Jespersen et al. (2012) [39]	11 223	42%	• Higher prevalence of non-obstructive CAD in women (65%) compared to men (33%) • Elevated risk of MACE and all-cause mortality in patients with stable angina and normal coronaries or non-obstructive CAD compared with a reference population without IHD
Wei et al. (2012) [79]	293	100%	• In women undergoing coronary reactivity testing for suspected CMD, contemporary testing carries a relatively low risk compared to the MACE rate in these women
Sharaf et al. (2013) [33]	917	100%	• No significant obstructive stenosis in 62% of women
Aziz et al. (2017) [80]	1379	58%	• A pathological ACh test was more common in females (70% vs. 43%; p < 0.001) • In a multivariable logistic regression model, the sex difference was statistically significant with a female–male odds ratio for CMD and epicardial vasospasm of 4.2 (95% CI: 3.1 to 5.5; p < 0.001) and 2.3 (95% CI: 1.7 to 3.1; p < 0.001), respectively
CorMicA trial Ford et al. (2018) [78]	151	73.5%	• Mean improvement of 11.7 U in the SAQ summary score at 6 months (95% CI: 5.0 to 18.4; p ¼ 0.001) and in the mean quality-of-life score in the intervention group (stratified medical therapy) (EQ-5D index 0.10 U; 95% CI: 0.01 to 0.18; p 1/4 0.024)
Raad et al. (2020) [47]	75	100%	• Cystine levels correlates negatively with the peak filling rate ($r = -0.31$, $P = 0.007$) and positively with LVEDP ($r = 0.25$; $P = 0.038$), indicating that increased OS was associated with diastolic dysfunction, even after multivariate adjustment including multiple known risk factors for diastolic dysfunction and cardiovascular medications
AlBadri et al. (2020) [81]	263	100%	• Women with CMD had higher plasma u-hscTnI levels, suggesting that ischaemic cardiomyocyte injury in this setting contribute to adverse cardiovascular outcomes in these women
Aldiwani et al. (2022) [82]	56	100%	• Lower LVEF (P = 0.02) among the INOCA and HFpEF groups than reference controls after age adjustment • In addition, a graded reduction in MPRI in HFpEF vs. INOCA vs. reference controls (1.5 ± 0.3, 1.8 ± 0.3, 1.9 ± 0.3, P = 0.02), attenuated with age-adjustment
Feenstra et al. (2022) [76]	110	86%	• Additional endothelial function testing increases the diagnostic yield of coronary function testing that only incorporates adenosine testing and spasm provocation by 17%–92%. In patients with normal adenosine-mediated vasodilation and without inducible spasm, 68% had endothelial dysfunction
Montone et al. (2020) [83]	120	51.7%	• A clear sex-related difference in the vasomotor response to provocative test was demonstrated, with a higher prevalence of microvascular spasm among women and epicardial spasm among men
Gulati et al. (2023) [41]	297	91%	• CMD and coronary artery spasm found in 64.3% and 50.5% of survey respondents, respectively • Almost 2/3 of patients diagnosed between the ages of 40–60 years • Adverse impact on home life reported in 80.5% of cases, on social life reported in 80.1%, on mental health in 70.4%, on sex life in 55.9% • Approximately 3 of every 4 respondents reduced or stopped work completely

CFR coronary flow reserve, *CAD* coronary artery disease, *MACE* major adverse cardiovascular events, *IHD* ischemic heart disease, *CMD* coronary microvascular dysfunction, *LVEF* left ventricular ejection fraction, *HFpEF* heart failure with preserved ejection fraction, *MPRI* myocardial perfusion reserve index, *LVEDP* left ventricular end diastolic pressure, *OS* oxidative stress, *HR* hazard ratio, *CI* confidence interval, SAQ Seattle Angina Questionnaire.

either epicardial or microvascular spasm, the 2020 Consensus Document recommends CCBs as first-line therapy. The dosages may exceed commonly recommended dosages in severe VSA, or a combination of non-dihydropyridine with dihydropyridine may be needed [56]. The efficacy of short-acting nitrates may vary, and long-acting nitrates are frequently ineffective, poorly tolerated and may aggravate symptoms [56]. Nicorandil, a vasodilator agent acting via nitrate and potassium channel activation, has been shown to be effective for epicardial spasm and can be added if symptoms are insufficiently controlled. First-line therapy can also be combined with the use of ranolazine, an anti-anginal agent improving myocyte relaxation and ventricular compliance by decreasing sodium and calcium overload. Some patients with persistent symptoms may benefit from the use of ivabradine, which decreases heart rate both at rest and during exercise without affecting LV contractility. However, its efficacy in microvascular angina is poorly investigated and still controversial. Second-line medications include trimetazidine, an anti-ischaemic metabolic agent that improves myocardial glucose utilization with good results on angina and stress testing results. Moreover, the use of low-dose tricyclic antidepressants (imipramine) may mitigate anginal symptoms. Rho-kinase inhibitors reduce contractility in the vascular wall and are currently under investigation [85].

The role of aspirin is still unclear but might be considered based on modifiable risk factors and risk of adverse cardiovascular outcomes. However, bleeding risk in premenopausal women is increased as antiplatelet therapy can increase menstrual bleeding and must be considered in discussions regarding specific patient management. SGLT2 inhibitors have been shown to improve endothelial function [86]. Given the key role of inflammation in INOCA, agents attenuating inflammation (IL-6 signaling, IL-1a, IL-1b, TNF-α inhibitors) are of interest but still investigated [87].

Patients with microvascular disorders suffer from hyperalgesic responses to pain, irrespective of the presence of ischaemia. The hyperalgesic nociceptive pathway could arise from abnormalities at different levels. Therapeutic strategies modulating the pain pathway, by inhibiting nociceptive adenosine receptors, inhibiting afferent pain neurons, blocking pain transmission at the spinal cord level, or modulating cortical inputs, have been used in refractory angina [88].

Stellate ganglion blockade or thoracic sympathectomy have been shown to reduce symptoms and ischaemic ECG changes in patients with VSA. However, whether this approach reduces symptoms by inhibiting spasm or disrupting sympathetic pain afferents remains unclear. Other anti-ischaemic devices reported to improve symptoms include enhanced external counterpulsation and coronary sinus (CS) Reducer. The preliminary experience suggests that CS Reducer is safe and may have a role in the management of refractory angina, increasing back pressure and redistributing blood into ischaemic myocardium [89]. CS Reducer is particularly appealing in this setting, and future studies are needed to confirm its effect on myocardial perfusion in INOCA patients.

4.10 Ongoing Studies

It is evident that INOCA is not often correctly diagnosed and that, consequently, no tailored therapy is prescribed for these patients. There is an urgent need of large studies addressing this problem. The ongoing INOCAIT (NCT05164640) and DISCOVER INOCA (NCT05288361) studies will clarify the prevalence and patterns of overlapping mechanisms and their prognosis. Moreover, to date there are no disease-modifying therapies specific to women with INOCA. The ongoing WARRIOR study (NCT03417388) is currently enrolling subjects in a multicentre, prospective, randomised blinded outcome assessment, to evaluate intensive statin and ACEI/ARB therapy and usual care on MACE in symptomatic women with INOCA. Similarly, the ongoing iCorMicA study (NCT04674449) will provide answers to this issue for both men and women. Finally, with regards to the development of future therapies, the BIOPLATINO study (NCT05714241) was designed to evaluate if there is a unique signature of circulating biomarkers and/or platelet function tests able to discriminate between the multiple pathogenetic mechanisms of INOCA and it may pave the way for the identification of more specific pathophysiologic pathways.

5 Conclusion and Future Directions

Women are more likely to present with angina as a primary manifestation of cardiovascular disease, complaining of other symptoms compared to men. Thus, they are more likely to be misdiagnosed or discharged from follow-up earlier than men. Furthermore, women make up less than 30% of study populations, and large-scale registry data shows that female sex is a significant predictor of all-cause mortality at 30 days post-PCI for both stable and acute IHD.

Anginal symptoms are caused by decreased coronary perfusion, however morbidity may be secondary to both obstructive and non-obstructive CAD mechanisms. Cardiovascular risk in women is governed by risk factors both traditional and specific to female sex such as hormonal influences. Non-obstructive CAD is more frequently diagnosed in women and is not a benign condition. Presentation with stable angina and non-obstructive coronary arteries in women is associated with greater future adverse cardiovascular outcomes. The pathophysiology of ANOCA/INOCA has been investigated in the last years, and is secondary to coronary dysfunction including coronary artery vasospasm and microvascular dysfunction.

Concerningly, women are chronically underrepresented in clinical trials directed at management options for those with CAD, making their results less transferrable and limiting options for specific guideline-directed medical therapy. It is important that clinicians investigate the underlying cause of angina, particularly in those with suspected ANOCA/INOCA, in order to direct appropriate management and reduce sex-differences in adverse health outcomes.

Key Issues

- Stable IHD is a multifaceted disease, which burdens both men and women, yet women are disproportionately included in clinical trials which direct clinical guidelines for the investigation and management of this disease.
- Women are subject to the same traditional risk factors for IHD as men; however, they are at more exposed to sex-specific hormonal factors, which may further increase their risk of morbidity and mortality.
- Women are more likely to present with angina differently to men and are more likely to have non-obstructive coronary arteries. This may reduce the follow-up length and the rates of appropriate guideline-directed medical therapy due to the lack of clinical trials currently available.
- Angina and ischaemia with non-obstructive coronary arteries are more common in women and may be caused by coronary vasomotor disorders. Clinicians should further investigate the underlying cause in order to direct therapy in these patients and reduce morbidity and mortality.

Questions and Answers

1. Does the female sex play a role in the physiology of atherosclerotic plaque progression in IOCA?
   (A) Yes, younger women have greater risk of adverse cardiovascular events compared to men
   (B) Sex does not impact on obstructive CAD progression
   (C) Yes, women with obstructive CAD are older than men with the same condition
   (D) Yes, men have a lower risk of cardiovascular events compared to women

   Best answer: C

   Women who present with obstructive CAD are more commonly older than men with the same condition. Indeed, postmenopausal women have greater chance of adverse cardiovascular events, mainly linked to the drop in hormones levels and the consequent increase of total cholesterol and LDL levels associated with higher blood pressure.

2. Why is it important to establish a diagnosis of INOCA?
   (A) To proceed with PCI even in the absence of obstructive CAD
   (B) To establish that medical therapy optimization is not necessary
   (C) To refer patients to a psychiatrist specialist after exclusion of coronaries abnormalities
   (D) To prevent early discharge providing a correct diagnosis and optimal medical therapy

   Best answer: D

   INOCA is a cardiovascular disease impacting women's lives. Furthermore, strong evidence reports increased risk of major adverse outcomes in this setting, mainly represented by hospitalisation for recurrent angina, heart failure, or both. Along with an adverse cardiovascular prognosis, the majority of INOCA women also have a considerably impaired functional status and decreased exercise tolerance. Therefore, a correct evaluation prevents women from being discharged with an incorrect diagnosis without any medical treatment.

3. Which is the role of a complete intracoronary physiology assessment in INOCA?
   (A) To detect atherosclerotic plaques in the coronary microcirculation
   (B) To identify the underlying pathophysiological endotype responsible for coronary microvascular dysfunction and/or vasospasm
   (C) To detect coronary artery dissection
   (D) To locate spasmic coronary segments eligible to stent implantation

   Best answer: B

   Invasive assessment of coronary microvascular dysfunction or vasospasm (through adenosine and acetylcholine testing) guides physicians in detecting the specific underlying pathophysiological endotype to establish a correct diagnosis and choose the best therapeutic strategy.

References

1. Bairey Merz CN, Shaw LJ, Reis SE, Bittner V, Kelsey SF, Olson M, et al. Insights from the NHLBI-sponsored Women's ischemia syndrome evaluation (WISE) study: part II: gender differences in presentation, diagnosis, and outcome with regard to gender-based pathophysiology of atherosclerosis and macrovascular and microvascular coronary disease. J Am Coll Cardiol. 2006;47(3 Suppl):S21–9.
2. Canto JG, Rogers WJ, Goldberg RJ, Peterson ED, Wenger NK, Vaccarino V, et al. Association of age and sex with myocardial infarction symptom presentation and in-hospital mortality. JAMA. 2012;307(8):813–22.
3. Kunadian V, Qiu W, Lagerqvist B, Johnston N, Sinclair H, Tan Y, et al. Gender differences in outcomes and predictors of all-cause mortality after percutaneous coronary intervention (data from United Kingdom and Sweden). Am J Cardiol. 2017;119(2):210–6.
4. Cartlidge T, Kovacevic M, Navarese EP, Werner G, Kunadian V. Role of percutaneous coronary intervention in the modern-day management of chronic coronary syndrome. Heart. 2023;109:1429–35.
5. van Diemen J, Verdonk P, Chieffo A, Regar E, Mauri F, Kunadian V, et al. The importance of achieving sex- and gender-based equity in clinical trials: a call to action. Eur Heart J. 2021;42(31):2990–4.
6. Douglas PS, Ginsburg GS. The evaluation of chest pain in women. N Engl J Med. 1996;334(20):1311–5.
7. Norris CM, Yip CYY, Nerenberg KA, Clavel MA, Pacheco C, Foulds HJA, et al. State of the science in Women's cardiovascular disease: a Canadian perspective on the influence of sex and gender. J Am Heart Assoc. 2020;9(4):e015634.
8. Vakhtangadze T, Singh Tak R, Singh U, Baig MS, Bezsonov E. Gender differences in atherosclerotic vascular disease: from lipids to clinical outcomes. Front Cardiovasc Med. 2021;8:707889.
9. Backus BE, Six AJ, Kelder JC, Mast TP, van den Akker F, Mast EG, et al. Chest pain in the emergency room: a multicenter validation of the HEART score. Crit Pathw Cardiol. 2010;9(3):164–9.
10. Antman EM, Cohen M, Bernink PJ, McCabe CH, Horacek T, Papuchis G, et al. The TIMI risk score for unstable angina/non-ST elevation MI: a method for prognostication and therapeutic decision making. JAMA. 2000;284(7):835–42.
11. Bawamia B, Mehran R, Qiu W, Kunadian V. Risk scores in acute coronary syndrome and percutaneous coronary intervention: a review. Am Heart J. 2013;165(4):441–50.
12. Peters SA, Huxley RR, Woodward M. Comparison of the sex-specific associations between systolic blood pressure and the risk of cardiovascular disease: a systematic review and meta-analysis of 124 cohort studies, including 1.2 million individuals. Stroke. 2013;44(9):2394–401.

13. Lloyd-Jones DM, Evans JC, Levy D. Hypertension in adults across the age spectrum: current outcomes and control in the community. JAMA. 2005;294(4):466–72.
14. Matthan NR, Jalbert SM, Barrett PH, Dolnikowski GG, Schaefer EJ, Lichtenstein AH. Gender-specific differences in the kinetics of nonfasting TRL, IDL, and LDL apolipoprotein B-100 in men and premenopausal women. Arterioscler Thromb Vasc Biol. 2008;28(10):1838–43.
15. Virani SS, Smith SC, Stone NJ, Grundy SM. Secondary prevention for atherosclerotic cardiovascular disease: comparing recent US and European guidelines on dyslipidemia. Circulation. 2020;141(14):1121–3.
16. Orshal JM, Khalil RA. Gender, sex hormones, and vascular tone. Am J Physiol Regul Integr Comp Physiol. 2004;286(2):R233–49.
17. Wilson PW, D'Agostino RB, Sullivan L, Parise H, Kannel WB. Overweight and obesity as determinants of cardiovascular risk: the Framingham experience. Arch Intern Med. 2002;162(16):1867–72.
18. Lee WL, Cheung AM, Cape D, Zinman B. Impact of diabetes on coronary artery disease in women and men: a meta-analysis of prospective studies. Diabetes Care. 2000;23(7):962–8.
19. Huxley RR, Woodward M. Cigarette smoking as a risk factor for coronary heart disease in women compared with men: a systematic review and meta-analysis of prospective cohort studies. Lancet. 2011;378(9799):1297–305.
20. Young L, Cho L. Unique cardiovascular risk factors in women. Heart. 2019;105(21):1656–60.
21. Curtis KM, Mohllajee AP, Martins SL, Peterson HB. Combined oral contraceptive use among women with hypertension: a systematic review. Contraception. 2006;73(2):179–88.
22. Honigberg MC, Zekavat SM, Aragam K, Finneran P, Klarin D, Bhatt DL, et al. Association of premature natural and surgical menopause with incident cardiovascular disease. JAMA. 2019;322(24):2411–21.
23. Manson JE, Chlebowski RT, Stefanick ML, Aragaki AK, Rossouw JE, Prentice RL, et al. Menopausal hormone therapy and health outcomes during the intervention and extended poststopping phases of the Women's Health Initiative randomized trials. JAMA. 2013;310(13):1353–68.
24. Virani SS, Alonso A, Aparicio HJ, Benjamin EJ, Bittencourt MS, Callaway CW, et al. Heart disease and stroke Statistics-2021 update: a report from the American Heart Association. Circulation. 2021;143(8):e254–743.
25. Kramer CK, Campbell S, Retnakaran R. Gestational diabetes and the risk of cardiovascular disease in women: a systematic review and meta-analysis. Diabetologia. 2019;62(6):905–14.
26. Leon LJ, McCarthy FP, Direk K, Gonzalez-Izquierdo A, Prieto-Merino D, Casas JP, et al. Preeclampsia and cardiovascular disease in a large UK pregnancy cohort of linked electronic health records: a CALIBER study. Circulation. 2019;140(13):1050–60.
27. Peters SA, Woodward M. Women's reproductive factors and incident cardiovascular disease in the UK biobank. Heart. 2018;104(13):1069–75.
28. Venkatesulu BP, Mahadevan LS, Aliru ML, Yang X, Bodd MH, Singh PK, et al. Radiation-induced endothelial vascular injury: a review of possible mechanisms. JACC Basic Transl Sci. 2018;3(4):563–72.
29. Gaudino M, Di Franco A, Cao D, Giustino G, Bairey Merz CN, Fremes SE, et al. Sex-related outcomes of medical, percutaneous, and surgical interventions for coronary artery disease: JACC focus seminar 3/7. J Am Coll Cardiol. 2022;79(14):1407–25.
30. Investigators S-H. CT coronary angiography in patients with suspected angina due to coronary heart disease (SCOT-HEART): an open-label, parallel-group, multicentre trial. Lancet. 2015;385(9985):2383–91.
31. Orsini E, Marzilli M, Zito GB, Carbone V, Latina L, Oliviero U, et al. Clinical outcomes of newly diagnosed, stable angina patients managed according to current guidelines. The ARCA (Arca registry for chronic angina) registry: a prospective, observational, nationwide study. Int J Cardiol. 2022;352:9–18.
32. Pepine CJ. ANOCA/INOCA/MINOCA: open artery ischemia. Am Heart J Plus. 2023;26:26.
33. Sharaf B, Wood T, Shaw L, Johnson BD, Kelsey S, Anderson RD, et al. Adverse outcomes among women presenting with signs and symptoms of ischemia and no obstructive coronary artery disease: findings from the National Heart, Lung, and Blood Institute-sponsored Women's ischemia syndrome evaluation (WISE) angiographic core laboratory. Am Heart J. 2013;166(1):134–41.
34. Montalescot G, Sechtem U, Achenbach S, Andreotti F, Arden C, Budaj A, et al. 2013 ESC guidelines on the management of stable coronary artery disease: the task force on the management of stable coronary artery disease of the European Society of Cardiology. Eur Heart J. 2013;34(38):2949–3003.
35. Taqueti VR, Di Carli MF. Coronary microvascular disease pathogenic mechanisms and therapeutic options: JACC state-of-the-art review. J Am Coll Cardiol. 2018;72(21):2625–41.
36. Knuuti J, Wijns W, Saraste A, Capodanno D, Barbato E, Funck-Brentano C, et al. 2019 ESC guidelines for the diagnosis and management of chronic coronary syndromes. Eur Heart J. 2020;41(3):407–77.
37. Pepine CJ, Ferdinand KC, Shaw LJ, Light-McGroary KA, Shah RU, Gulati M, et al. Emergence of nonobstructive coronary artery disease: a Woman's problem and need for change in definition on angiography. J Am Coll Cardiol. 2015;66(17):1918–33.
38. Sara JD, Widmer RJ, Matsuzawa Y, Lennon RJ, Lerman LO, Lerman A. Prevalence of coronary microvascular dysfunction among patients with chest pain and nonobstructive coronary artery disease. JACC Cardiovasc Interv. 2015;8(11):1445–53.
39. Jespersen L, Hvelplund A, Abildstrøm SZ, Pedersen F, Galatius S, Madsen JK, et al. Stable angina pectoris with no obstructive coronary artery disease is associ-

ated with increased risks of major adverse cardiovascular events. Eur Heart J. 2012;33(6):734–44.
40. Shaw LJ, Shaw RE, Merz CN, Brindis RG, Klein LW, Nallamothu B, et al. Impact of ethnicity and gender differences on angiographic coronary artery disease prevalence and in-hospital mortality in the American College of Cardiology-National Cardiovascular Data Registry. Circulation. 2008;117(14):1787–801.
41. Gulati M, Khan N, George M, Berry C, Chieffo A, Camici PG, et al. Ischemia with no obstructive coronary artery disease (INOCA): a patient self-report quality of life survey from INOCA international. Int J Cardiol. 2023;371:28–39.
42. Shaw LJ, Merz CN, Pepine CJ, Reis SE, Bittner V, Kip KE, et al. The economic burden of angina in women with suspected ischemic heart disease: results from the National Institutes of Health—National Heart, Lung, and Blood Institute—sponsored Women's Ischemia Syndrome Evaluation. Circulation. 2006;114(9):894–904.
43. Lee SH, Shin D, Lee JM, van de Hoef TP, Hong D, Choi KH, et al. Clinical relevance of ischemia with nonobstructive coronary arteries according to coronary microvascular dysfunction. J Am Heart Assoc. 2022;11(9):e025171.
44. Bakir M, Nelson MD, Jones E, Li Q, Wei J, Sharif B, et al. Heart failure hospitalization in women with signs and symptoms of ischemia: a report from the women's ischemia syndrome evaluation study. Int J Cardiol. 2016;223:936–9.
45. Taqueti VR, Solomon SD, Shah AM, Desai AS, Groarke JD, Osborne MT, et al. Coronary microvascular dysfunction and future risk of heart failure with preserved ejection fraction. Eur Heart J. 2018;39(10):840–9.
46. Mohammed AA, Zhang H, Abdu FA, Liu L, Singh S, Lv X, et al. Effect of nonobstructive coronary stenosis on coronary microvascular dysfunction and long-term outcomes in patients with INOCA. Clin Cardiol. 2023;46(2):204–13.
47. Raad M, AlBadri A, Wei J, Mehta PK, Maughan J, Gadh A, et al. Oxidative stress is associated with diastolic dysfunction in women with ischemia with no obstructive coronary artery disease. J Am Heart Assoc. 2020;9(10):e015602.
48. Lanza GA, Sestito A, Sgueglia GA, Infusino F, Manolfi M, Crea F, et al. Current clinical features, diagnostic assessment and prognostic determinants of patients with variant angina. Int J Cardiol. 2007;118(1):41–7.
49. Reynolds HR, Diaz A, Cyr DD, Shaw LJ, Mancini GBJ, Leipsic J, et al. Ischemia with nonobstructive coronary arteries: insights from the ISCHEMIA trial. JACC Cardiovasc Imaging. 2023;16(1):63–74.
50. Sato K, Kaikita K, Nakayama N, Horio E, Yoshimura H, Ono T, et al. Coronary vasomotor response to intracoronary acetylcholine injection, clinical features, and long-term prognosis in 873 consecutive patients with coronary spasm: analysis of a single-center study over 20 years. J Am Heart Assoc. 2013;2(4):e000227.
51. Mygind ND, Michelsen MM, Pena A, Frestad D, Dose N, Aziz A, et al. Coronary microvascular function and cardiovascular risk factors in women with angina pectoris and no obstructive coronary artery disease: the iPOWER study. J Am Heart Assoc. 2016;5(3):e003064.
52. Schroder J, Mygind ND, Frestad D, Michelsen M, Suhrs HE, Bove KB, et al. Pro-inflammatory biomarkers in women with non-obstructive angina pectoris and coronary microvascular dysfunction. Int J Cardiol Heart Vasc. 2019;24:100370.
53. Wei J, Barsky LL, Jalnapurkar S, Zarrini P, Cook-Wiens G, AlBadri A, et al. Cold pressor testing and sympathetic nervous system contribution to ischemia with no obstructive coronary artery disease: results from the women's ischemia syndrome evaluation-coronary vascular dysfunction project. Am Heart J Plus. 2022;13:100080.
54. Montone RA, Rinaldi R, Del Buono MG, Gurgoglione F, La Vecchia G, Russo M, et al. Safety and prognostic relevance of acetylcholine testing in patients with stable myocardial ischaemia or myocardial infarction and non-obstructive coronary arteries. EuroIntervention. 2022;18(8):e666–e76.
55. Travieso A, Jeronimo-Baza A, Faria D, Shabbir A, Mejia-Renteria H, Escaned J. Invasive evaluation of coronary microvascular dysfunction. J Nucl Cardiol. 2022;29(5):2474–86.
56. Kunadian V, Chieffo A, Camici PG, Berry C, Escaned J, Maas A, et al. An EAPCI expert consensus document on ischaemia with non-obstructive coronary arteries in collaboration with European Society of Cardiology Working Group on Coronary Pathophysiology & Microcirculation Endorsed by Coronary Vasomotor Disorders International Study Group. Eur Heart J. 2020;41(37):3504–20.
57. Del Buono MG, Montone RA, Camilli M, Carbone S, Narula J, Lavie CJ, et al. Coronary microvascular dysfunction across the spectrum of cardiovascular diseases: JACC state-of-the-art review. J Am Coll Cardiol. 2021;78(13):1352–71.
58. Nishimiya K, Suda A, Fukui K, Hao K, Takahashi J, Matsumoto Y, et al. Prognostic links between OCT-delineated coronary morphologies and coronary functional abnormalities in patients with INOCA. JACC Cardiovasc Interv. 2021;14(6):606–18.
59. Ong P, Safdar B, Seitz A, Hubert A, Beltrame JF, Prescott E. Diagnosis of coronary microvascular dysfunction in the clinic. Cardiovasc Res. 2020;116(4):841–55.
60. Kotecha T, Martinez-Naharro A, Boldrini M, Knight D, Hawkins P, Kalra S, et al. Automated pixel-wise quantitative myocardial perfusion mapping by CMR to detect obstructive coronary artery disease and coronary microvascular dysfunction: validation against invasive coronary physiology. JACC Cardiovasc Imaging. 2019;12(10):1958–69.
61. Ong P, Camici PG, Beltrame JF, Crea F, Shimokawa H, Sechtem U, et al. International standardization

of diagnostic criteria for microvascular angina. Int J Cardiol. 2018;250:16–20.

62. De Bruyne B, Belmonte M, Jabbour RJ, Curzen N. Invasive functional testing in the cath lab as a routine investigation in INOCA: pros and cons. EuroIntervention. 2023;19(1):23–5.
63. Barbato E, Aarnoudse W, Aengevaeren WR, Werner G, Klauss V, Bojara W, et al. Validation of coronary flow reserve measurements by thermodilution in clinical practice. Eur Heart J. 2004;25(3):219–23.
64. Writing Committee M, Gulati M, Levy PD, Mukherjee D, Amsterdam E, Bhatt DL, et al. 2021 AHA/ACC/ASE/CHEST/SAEM/SCCT/SCMR guideline for the evaluation and diagnosis of CHEST pain: a report of the American College of Cardiology/American Heart Association joint Committee on clinical practice guidelines. J Am Coll Cardiol. 2021;78(22):e187–285.
65. Hwang D, Park SH, Koo BK. Ischemia with nonobstructive coronary artery disease: concept, assessment, and management. JACC Asia. 2023;3(2):169–84.
66. Pepine CJ, Anderson RD, Sharaf BL, Reis SE, Smith KM, Handberg EM, et al. Coronary microvascular reactivity to adenosine predicts adverse outcome in women evaluated for suspected ischemia results from the National Heart, lung and blood institute WISE (Women's ischemia syndrome evaluation) study. J Am Coll Cardiol. 2010;55(25):2825–32.
67. van't Veer M, Adjedj J, Wijnbergen I, Toth GG, Rutten MC, Barbato E, et al. Novel monorail infusion catheter for volumetric coronary blood flow measurement in humans: in vitro validation. EuroIntervention. 2016;12(6):701–7.
68. Fearon WF, Kobayashi Y. Invasive assessment of the coronary microvasculature: the index of microcirculatory resistance. Circ Cardiovasc Interv. 2017;10(12):e005361.
69. Williams RP, de Waard GA, De Silva K, Lumley M, Asrress K, Arri S, et al. Doppler versus Thermodilution-derived coronary microvascular resistance to predict coronary microvascular dysfunction in patients with acute myocardial infarction or stable angina pectoris. Am J Cardiol. 2018;121(1):1–8.
70. Boerhout CKM, Lee JM, de Waard GA, Mejia-Renteria H, Lee SH, Jung JH, et al. Microvascular resistance reserve: diagnostic and prognostic performance in the ILIAS registry. Eur Heart J. 2023;44:2862–9.
71. Milzi A, Dettori R, Lubberich RK, Burgmaier K, Marx N, Reith S, et al. Coronary microvascular dysfunction as assessed by angiography-derived index of microvascular resistance co-localizes with and may explain the presence of ischemia in stress-cardiac magnetic resonance imaging in the absence of coronary artery disease. Front Cardiovasc Med. 2022;9:1060764.
72. Faria D, Hennessey B, Shabbir A, Mejia-Renteria H, Wang L, Lee JM, et al. Functional coronary angiography for the assessment of the epicardial vessels and the microcirculation. EuroIntervention. 2023;19(3):203–21.
73. Rahman H, Demir OM, Khan F, Ryan M, Ellis H, Mills MT, et al. Physiological stratification of patients with angina due to coronary microvascular dysfunction. J Am Coll Cardiol. 2020;75(20):2538–49.
74. Boerhout CKM, de Waard GA, Lee JM, Mejia-Renteria H, Lee SH, Jung JH, et al. Prognostic value of structural and functional coronary microvascular dysfunction in patients with non-obstructive coronary artery disease; from the multicentre international ILIAS registry. EuroIntervention. 2022;18(9):719–28.
75. Woudstra J, Vink CEM, Schipaanboord DJM, Eringa EC, den Ruijter HM, Feenstra RGT, et al. Meta-analysis and systematic review of coronary vasospasm in ANOCA patients: prevalence, clinical features and prognosis. Front Cardiovasc Med. 2023;10:1129159.
76. Feenstra RGT, Boerhout CKM, Woudstra J, Vink CEM, Wittekoek ME, de Waard GA, et al. Presence of coronary endothelial dysfunction, coronary vasospasm, and adenosine-mediated vasodilatory disorders in patients with ischemia and nonobstructive coronary arteries. Circ Cardiovasc Interv. 2022;15(8):e012017.
77. Seitz A, Feenstra R, Konst RE, Martinez Pereyra V, Beck S, Beijk M, et al. Acetylcholine Rechallenge: a first step toward tailored treatment in patients with coronary artery spasm. JACC Cardiovasc Interv. 2022;15(1):65–75.
78. Ford TJ, Stanley B, Sidik N, Good R, Rocchiccioli P, McEntegart M, et al. 1-year outcomes of angina management guided by invasive coronary function testing (CorMicA). JACC Cardiovasc Interv. 2020;13(1):33–45.
79. Wei J, Mehta PK, Johnson BD, Samuels B, Kar S, Anderson RD, et al. Safety of coronary reactivity testing in women with no obstructive coronary artery disease: results from the NHLBI-sponsored WISE (Women's Ischemia Syndrome Evaluation) study. JACC Cardiovasc Interv. 2012;5(6):646–53. https://doi.org/10.1016/j.jcin.2012.01.023.
80. Aziz A, Hansen HS, Sechtem U, Prescott E, Ong P. Sex-related differences in vasomotor function in patients with angina and unobstructed coronary arteries. J Am Coll Cardiol. 2017;70(19):2349–235. https://doi.org/10.1016/j.jacc.2017.09.016.
81. AlBadri A, Wei J, Quesada O, Mehta PK, Xiao Y, Ko Y-A, et al. Coronary vascular function and cardiomyocyte injury: a report from the WISE-CVD. Arterioscler Thromb Vasc Biol. 2020;40(12):3015–21. https://doi.org/10.1161/ATVBAHA.120.314260.
82. Aldiwani H, Nelson MD, Sharif B, Wei J, Samuel TJ, Suppogu N, et al. Reduced myocardial perfusion is common among subjects with ischemia and no obstructive coronary artery disease and heart failure with preserved ejection fraction: a report from the WISE-CVD continuation study. Vessel Plus. 2022;6:16. https://doi.org/10.20517/2574-1209.2021.103.
83. Montone RA, Niccoli G, Russo M, Giaccari M, Del Buono MG, Meucci MC, et al. Clinical, angiographic and echocardiographic correlates of epicardial and microvascular spasm in patients with myocardial

ischaemia and non-obstructive coronary arteries. Clin Res Cardiol. 2020;109(4):435–43. https://doi.org/10.1007/s00392-019-01523-w.

84. Zhang X, Li Q, Zhao J, Li X, Sun X, Yang H, et al. Effects of combination of statin and calcium channel blocker in patients with cardiac syndrome X. Coron Artery Dis. 2014;25(1):40–4.
85. Shimokawa H, Sunamura S, Satoh K. RhoA/rho-kinase in the cardiovascular system. Circ Res. 2016;118(2):352–66.
86. Durante W, Behnammanesh G, Peyton KJ. Effects of sodium-glucose co-transporter 2 inhibitors on vascular cell function and arterial remodeling. Int J Mol Sci. 2021;22(16):8786.
87. Mehta PK, Huang J, Levit RD, Malas W, Waheed N, Bairey Merz CN. Ischemia and no obstructive coronary arteries (INOCA): a narrative review. Atherosclerosis. 2022;363:8–21.
88. Beltrame JF, Tavella R, Jones D, Zeitz C. Management of ischaemia with non-obstructive coronary arteries (INOCA). BMJ. 2021;375:e060602.
89. Giannini F, Baldetti L, Ielasi A, Ruparelia N, Ponticelli F, Latib A, et al. First experience with the coronary sinus reducer system for the management of refractory angina in patients without obstructive coronary artery disease. JACC Cardiovasc Interv. 2017;10(18):1901–3.

Acute Coronary Syndromes in Women Including MINOCA

Valeria Paradies, Giulia Botti, and Alaide Chieffo

Abstract

Among patients admitted to the emergency departments with suspected acute coronary syndrome (ACS), half of them are women and most likely present with non-ST-segment elevation myocardial infarction (NSTEMI) and unstable angina (UA).

Sex differences in pathophysiology, clinical presentation, diagnosis, and treatment have an important impact on clinical outcomes. Women with ACS may have traditional and/or sex-specific risk factors and more frequently than men have non-atherosclerotic involvement of coronary arteries.

Over the last decades, ACS mortality has dramatically decreased due to better treatment. However, women still have a higher short term mortality risk after successful percutaneous coronary intervention (PCI) compared with men. Women are less likely to undergo evidence-based and guideline-recommended diagnostic and revascularization pathways.

The scientific community hasn't adequately addressed gaps in knowledge in the diagnosis and treatment of women presenting with ACS.

Keywords

Sex specific considerations · Acute coronary syndromes · Prognosis

V. Paradies
Department of Cardiology, Maasstad Hospital, Rotterdam, The Netherlands
e-mail: paradiesV2@maasstadziekenhuis.nl

G. Botti · A. Chieffo (✉)
Interventional Cardiology Unit, IRCCS San Raffaele Scientific Institute, Milan, Italy

Vita-Salute San Raffaele University, Milan, Italy
e-mail: g.botti2@studenti.unisr.it; chieffo.alaide@hsr.it

A. H.E.M. Maas, E. Gerdts (eds.), *Manual of Cardiovascular Disease in Women*,
https://doi.org/10.1007/978-3-031-65952-2_20

Test your learning and check your understanding of this book's contents: use the "Springer Nature Flashcards" app to access questions using ▶ https://sn.pub/51ny7m
To use the app, please follow the instructions in chapter 1.

1 Sex-Specific Mechanisms in the Pathophysiology of Acute Coronary Syndromes

1.1 Plaque Erosion Versus Plaque Rupture

Despite a significant decline in cardiovascular mortality in women during the past several decades, sex differences associated with pathophysiology of ACS have not been fully elucidated. Sex-specific characteristics in atherosclerotic plaque burden and volume have been reported from largely observational studies, both in chronic and acute settings.

The natural progression of atherosclerosis comprises adaptive intimal thickening, pathologic intimal thickening, fibroatheroma and thin cap fibroatheroma (TCFA). In a sub-analysis of the "Providing Regional Observations to Study Predictors of Events in the Coronary Tree" (PROSPECT) study, women had fewer non-culprit lesions and showed less total necrotic core volume than men [1]. A higher incidence of fibroatheromas with larger plaque volumes and fewer fibrotic plaques was found in men aged <65 years as compared to women of the same age. Comparable differences in plaque characteristics were not found in the subgroup aged >65 years [2].

TFCA has been considered the immediate precursor of plaque rupture, being the non-thrombosed lesion that most resembles acute plaque rupture. The underlying etiologies of thrombotic lesions associated with sudden cardiac death have been attributed to plaque rupture (55–60%), plaque erosion (30–35%) and calcified nodule (2–7%) in postmortem studies [3]. Plaque rupture occurs frequently in the context of TCFA, when the overlying thin fibrotic cap discontinuity exposes a large lipid pool to the coronary lumen [4]. Plaque erosion is defined by endothelial discontinuity without signs of cap rupture. Both can ultimately result in thrombus formation and consequent partial or total occlusion of the vessel, superimposed coronary spasm or transient thrombosis with complete spontaneous resolution [3].

Plaque erosion seems to be more frequent in young women (under the age of 50 years) and represents most acute coronary thrombi in premenopausal women. In a subanalysis of ADAPT DES trial, plaque rupture was more common in men versus women (36.3 vs 23%; $p < 0.01$) [5]. These findings have been recently confirmed in a large population of 1368 patients where women ($n = 286$) showed an increasing prevalence of plaque rupture as well as a higher plaque vulnerability with age while the prevalence of plaque erosion decreased with age regardless of sex [6].

1.2 Non Obstructive Atherosclerosis

1.2.1 Coronary Thromboembolism

In approximately 6–15% of patients with an initial diagnosis of ACS, angiography shows non-obstructive coronary arteries. Myocardial infarction with no obstructive coronary disease (MINOCA) is defined as a myocardial infarction (MI) with elevated cardiac biomarkers, typically cardiac troponin >99th percentile of the upper reference level which can be attributed to ischemic mechanisms, in the context of no coronary artery stenosis ≥50% and in the absence of a specific alternate diagnosis for the clinical presentation. MINOCA subjects are younger, more often female (up to fivefold higher odds than men) and tend to have fewer traditional cardiovascular risk factors [7]. The underlying pathogenesis of MINOCA ranges from functional alterations at the level of epicardial coronary arteries to microvascular dysfunction. Previous studies have shown that plaque rupture and erosion may be identified in 47% of patients diagnosed with MINOCA [8].

Thromboembolism may be the consequence of plaque rupture/erosion or occur in the context of hereditary or acquired thrombotic disorders or other predisposing factors. Atrial fibrillation, valvular heart disease, cardiac tumors, auto-immune disorders, myeloproliferative neoplasms may determine a hypercoagulable status. Up to 14% of MINOCA patients may present with hereditary thrombophilia disorders such Factor V Leiden, elevated factor VIII/von Willebrand factor, Protein S and C deficiencies [9].

1.2.2 Vasospasm (Fig. 1)

Coronary artery spasm is defined as an intense epicardial vasoconstriction with compromised myocardial blood flow and represents the relevant pathogenetic mechanism in up to 27% of MINOCA patients [9]. The consensus from the Coronary Vasomotion Disorders International Study Group (COVADIS) defined a 90% diameter stenosis as the angiographic threshold to diagnose inducible spasm [10]. Coronary vasospasm is the result of hyperreactivity of vascular smooth muscles or spontaneous vasospasm due to disorders in coronary vasomotor tone. This may occur either in response to drugs or toxins (e.g., cocaine, fluorouracil). Episodes of vasospasm may be fortuitously documented but usually require intracoronary provocative testing which have been proved to be safe even when performed within 48 h after the index event in patients with MINOCA [11].

1.2.3 Microvascular Mechanisms

Previous studies showed that about 25% of patients with MINOCA have evidence of functional alterations at the level of coronary microcirculation [12]. The definition of an impaired microvascular system include all four following criteria: (1) Symptoms of myocardial ischemia, (2) Absence of obstructive CAD (3) Objective evidence of myocardial ischemia with documented ECG changes during chest pain or stress-induced chest pain and (4) evidence of impaired microvascular function based on impaired coronary flow reserve, reproduction of symptoms during acetylcholine test, impaired microvascular resistance indexes, impaired coronary blood flow, as measured with a corrected Thrombolysis in Myocardial Infarction (TIMI) frame count [13]. Microvascular dysfunction can be a cause

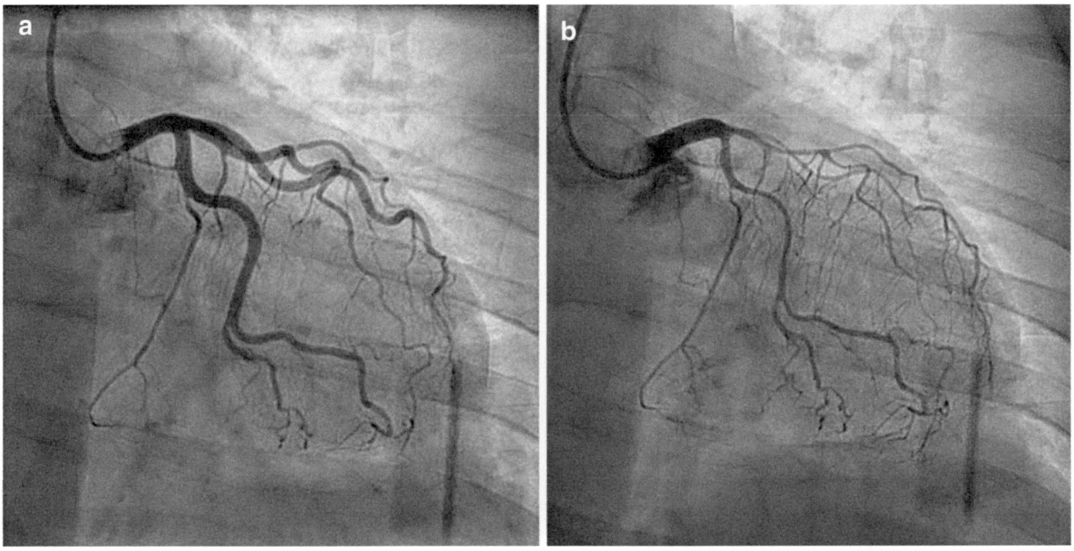

Fig. 1 (**a**) Coronary angiography shows non obstructive coronary artery disease. (**b**) Coronary angiography shows diffuse epicardial vasospasm (>90%) after administration of acetylcholine

of ischemia but can also be the consequence of myocardial injury of an ischemic or nonischemic origin making it challenging to identify the role of microvascular dysfunction in MINOCA.

1.2.4 SCAD

Spontaneous coronary artery dissection (SCAD) is a relatively uncommon nonatherosclerotic mechanism of ACS (about 1% of all ACS) but its prevalence can rise to 35% among young women [14–16].

The underlying mechanism of SCAD is a separation of the media and adventitial vascular walls which can be associated with intramural hematoma. Fibromuscular dysplasia or other vasculopathy may be present in other vascular beds in most cases of SCAD when screening is performed [17].

The angiographic images of a SCAD can vary from a near-normal coronary artery to contrast staining with multiple radiolucent lumens, tapering of the vessel or diffuse stenosis of varying severity.

2 Clinical Presentation of Acute Coronary Syndromes in Women

2.1 Sex Differences in Risk Profile

The risk profile of patients affected by acute coronary syndromes includes traditional risk factors, as well as sex-specific, and non-traditional and under-recognized factors. Moreover, the incidence of MINOCA is considerably higher in women than in men and is characterized by different pathophysiology and risk profile compared to obstructive coronary artery disease. Concerning traditional, mainly acknowledged risk factors, women tend to be older and more frequently affected by chronic kidney disease, hypercholesterolemia, hypertension, left ventricular heart failure or atrial fibrillation, but they are less frequently current smokers [18].

Sex-specific risk factors are associated with the various fluctuations of pro-thrombotic activity that women experience during their lifetime, which include pregnancy, use of oral contraceptives, menopause, and hormonal replacement therapy [19]. Menopause also induces metabolic changes that may be associated with the formation of lipid-rich increasingly vulnerable plaques, which rupture more frequently. Moreover, relatively rare conditions such as SCAD show a significant increase in incidence among pregnant women compared to the general population: SCAD is the main cause of pregnancy-associated ACS, accounting for 43% of cases [20].

Non-traditional risk factors, such as autoimmune diseases and rheumatic immune-mediated inflammatory diseases, which include systemic lupus erythematosus, rheumatoid arthritis, systemic sclerosis, dermatomyositis, or psoriasis are more frequent prevalent in females. The risk of developing cardiovascular disease in these patients is related not only to traditional cardiovascular risk factors but also to disease-specific factors, such as the degree of activity, autoantibodies, organ damage, and treatment. These patients tend to be younger and most frequently present with NSTEMI, with accelerated atherosclerosis being one of the main contributors to pathogenesis [21, 22]. Under-recognized risk factors have been more recently acknowledged as strong determinants of cardiovascular disease in women; these include depression - which might be due to mainly female psychosocial disadvantages, such as unemployment, chronic mental stress, insufficient social support, and bereavement or widowhood—indirect effects of physical and psychological abuse (increased likelihood to be heavy smokers and drinkers, and to avoid seeking medical care) and poor health literacy and access to education [23].

Finally, results from the "Variation in Recovery: Role of Gender on Outcomes of Young AMI Patients" (VIRGO) study report MINOCA to be more frequent in women than in men, and more prevalent in nonwhite compared to white patients. These patients are generally younger than those suffering obstructive CAD, and they present with significantly fewer traditional risk factors, whereas a hypercoagulable state is more frequently seen in

MINOCA patients. Conversely, affected women are less likely to be menopausal and to have experienced early menarche (<12 years) compared to women with obstructive CAD [24].

2.2 Sex Differences in Symptoms and Presentation

Multiple studies have established that chest pain, described as pain, pressure, tightness or discomfort, is the most common symptom in women and men diagnosed with ACS [7, 25, 26]. However, women are more likely to present with a cluster of multiple symptoms, such as epigastric symptoms, palpitations, and pain or discomfort in the jaw, neck, arms, or between the shoulder blades, in addition to conventional chest pain. These were formerly referred to as "atypical" chest pain symptoms. In the 2021 AHA/ACC Chest pain guideline the use of the term "atypical" is discouraged as it can be unclear if the term is being used to indicate angina without typical chest symptoms or describe symptoms that are noncardiac in origin which may therefore be misinterpreted as benign [27]. Conversely, women with an ST-segment–elevation ACS (STEMI) are more likely than men to present without chest pain [7] Clinical signs such as pulmonary oedema and pedal oedema are more common in women than in men [25]. Regarding the perception of symptoms, women are also more likely to believe that their discomfort might be due to stress or anxiety and therefore present later to medical facilities. According to data from the "International Registry of Acute Coronary Syndromes registry study in Transitional Countries" (ISACS-TC) registry, delay in ACS presentation was significantly higher in women and mainly due to a prolonged time between first medical contact and hospital admission. No differences in door-to-balloon time was reported in this cohort [28]. Moreover, although women seek medical care for comparable complaints more frequently than men, more than 50% of them report that their healthcare professional excludes cardiac involvement in their presenting complaints [29].

2.3 Young Women and Acute Myocardial Infarction

Although hospitalization rates for ACS have decreased substantially over the last 20 years when considering the overall population [30], worrisome data report that this cannot be said when the analysis is limited to young female patients. Data from the US documented a reduction in ACS hospitalizations from 1995 to 2014 among male community residents aged 35–54, whereas this decline was not observed for women aged 35–54. Conversely, a 3.6% mean annual increase in STEMI between 2004 and 2014 was reported [31]. Similar data have also been presented in a large French nationwide study performed from 2004 to 2014, in which rates of age-standardized admissions for ACS in patients younger than 65 years increased by 6.3%, with a strong association between smoking and obesity in STEMI in younger women [32]. Moreover, rates of mortality and adverse outcomes are higher in young women who suffer an ACS when compared to similar aged men: mortality in women is almost twofold than in men in the <50 age group, and the risk of death increases by 7% for every 5 years of decreasing age [33].

The increased incidence and mortality of ACS in young women has been associated with traditional risk factors such as severe obesity, diabetes, and smoking. However, lower income and education, and a higher prevalence of depression, post-traumatic stress disorders, and perceived mental stress have also been described in this population [34].

In this perspective, general underestimation of cardiovascular risk in women, especially in young women requires tackling via education of healthcare providers and women themselves, to guarantee early detection and treatment of established and emerging cardiovascular risk factors [23].

2.4 ACS Complicated by Cardiogenic Shock

Women have been described to more frequently present with acute myocardial infarction cardiogenic shock (AMI CS). Sex sub analyses of large trials such as "Culprit Lesion Only PCI versus Multivessel PCI in Cardiogenic Shock (CULPRIT SHOCK) trial and "Intraaortic Balloon Pump in Cardiogenic Shock II" (IABP SHOCK II) trial report that women who suffer AMICS are older and more frequently affected by diabetes and chronic kidney disease. Conversely, they have less often a history of prior ACS and smoking than men. They also present more often with ST-segment depression, non-anterior ST-segment elevation, and a culprit lesion in the right coronary artery. Adverse outcomes in women are mainly periprocedural and limited to the in-hospital time frame, and no significant sex differences in terms of mortality are reported at longer follow-up [35, 36].

Interestingly, results from a Spanish cohort of AMICS patients report lower rates of referral to tertiary care centers (revascularization capable hospitals or intensive cardiac care units) for female patients, consequently leading to minor accessibility to primary PCI and worse outcomes [37].

3 Impact of Female Sex in Diagnosis and Treatment of Acute Coronary Syndromes

3.1 Sex Differences in the Use of Intravascular Imaging (Fig. 2)

The role of intravascular imaging in the assessment of atheroma burden in ACS is well established. However, the low representation of women in randomized controlled trials (RCTs) and the cost associated with the use of intravascular imaging determine a gap in knowledge regarding sex differences in plaque morphology. In the workup diagnosis of MINOCA patients, one-third of cases can be ascribed to plaque rupture or erosion using intravascular modalities [38, 39]. Both Intravascular ultrasound (IVUS) and Optical Coherence Tomography (OCT) may help to identify SCAD when coronary angiogram is not conclusive [13].

Intravascular imaging is an adjuvant procedural tool to optimize PCI and current guidelines emphasize the added value of using these modalities in selected cases such as left main stenting, chronic total occlusion, long lesions and bifurcations [40]. Observational data from the British

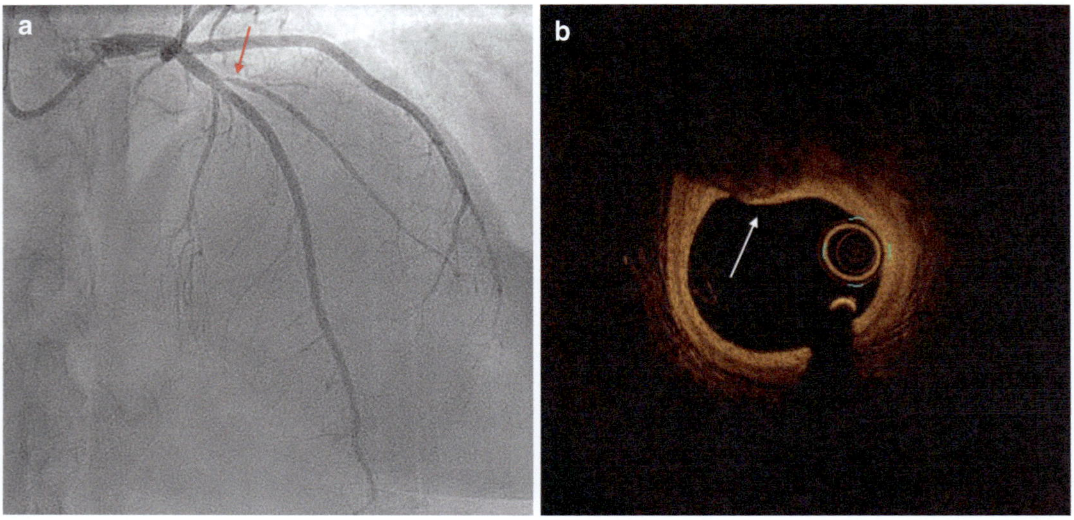

Fig. 2 (**a**) Coronary angiography shows non obstructive coronary artery disease at showing image of haziness in the mid segment of LAD (red arrow). (**b**) OCT cross section shows a thin cap fibroatheroma with a gap in the intima which may suggest plaque erosion (white arrow)

Cardiovascular Intervention Society (BCIS) registry of patients undergoing PCI between 2006 and 2019 showed that women are less likely to receive intracoronary imaging than their male counterparts (7.9% of the 255,862 women vs 8.4% of the 738,616 men; $p < 0.001$) [41].

3.2 Conservative vs Invasive Approach and Treatment Delay

Although major progress has been made in reducing cardiovascular disease mortality, women receive less frequently guideline-directed medical therapy and are more likely to receive conservative treatment than men [42, 43].

Overall primary PCI reperfusion rates have increased over the past two decades, however several barriers impact on the timely presentation and appropriate treatment of women with STEMI. Low awareness of personal risk and misinterpretation of symptoms impact on delayed presentation to hub centers [44–46]. The risk of being withheld primary PCI and evidence-based pharmacological treatment is higher among women; this may partially explain the sex-related mortality gap in STEMI patients [47–49]. Prehospital delay of longer than 1 h in women was associated with higher 30-day survival as compared to men [28].

An early revascularization appears to be beneficial in women presenting with NSTEMI as compared to conservative strategy [50]. However, women are less likely than men to undergo revascularization in this setting [51].

Despite adjustment for sex-related baseline differences, many studies have shown worse clinical outcomes, including two-fold higher mortality, in young women with ACS compared with similarly aged men [52].

3.3 Sex Specific Procedural Considerations

Female sex has been shown to be associated with worse clinical outcomes including in-hospital mortality following PCI. Women are more prone to spontaneous and procedure-related bleeds compared with men. The excess in bleeding complications in women cannot entirely be ascribed to their higher age and higher prevalence of risk factors for bleeding but is often driven by access site bleeds [53, 54]. Radial access is usually preferred, but sometimes not technically feasible because of smaller vessel size and increased likelihood of radial arterial spasm. As a consequence a higher use of femoral access has been reported. The use of ultrasound-guided femoral access during PCI may reduce the rates of bleeding and vascular complications [55].

Inappropriate dosing of antithrombotic drugs contributes to the higher bleeding risk. Current guidelines do not implement sex-based dosage recommendations for antithrombotic, therefore women, who generally have lower body volume, are more likely to receive excess doses then men [40, 56].

3.4 ACS Complicated by Cardiogenic Shock and Mechanical Circulatory Support

The delayed presentation and management of STEMI in women determine a higher risk of developing mechanical complications such as papillary muscle rupture, mitral regurgitation, and ventricular septal rupture [57].

Higher rate of CS and heart failure complicating STEMI in female patients might be partially explained by the prolonged untreated ischemia. However, women representation in STEMI trials complicated by CS only ranges from 20% to 30% [58]. The use of mechanical circulatory support (MCS) in STEMI patients has been associated with improved hemodynamics from unloading the left ventricle, reducing left ventricular end-diastolic volume, and lowering ventricular pressure and oxygen demand. The 2021 ACC/AHA and 2017 ESC guidelines give a class IIb recommendation to the use of MCS in select/refractory cases of STEMI complicated by CS [59, 60]. Acute and Chronic Heart Failure in the

2021 ESC guidelines gave a IIA recommendation to MCS in AMICS. A recent consensus document on percutaneous ventricular assist devices endorsed by the European Association of Percutaneous Cardiovascular Interventions (EAPCI) and the Association for Acute Cardiovascular Care (ACVC) indicates that Impella CP may be used as a short-term therapy in CS, in stage C and D with potentially reversible underlying cause [61]. The ultimate decisions on the use and the timing of MSC should be based on the severity of shock and the burden of comorbidities. No randomized data are currently available on pre-emptive unloading strategy in patients with high-risk ACS not complicated by CS; the DTU (Door to Unload) trial is currently enrolling patients and will shed light on this strategy.

Observational data suggest higher survival rates with device placement before revascularization than after in patients with ACS complicated by CS [62]. However, MCS devices remain underused in women with STEMI and CS, likely due to their smaller body and the peripheral vessel size. Currently, there are limited data on gender-specific outcomes of MCS in CS. Among 17,195 patients from the National Cardiovascular Data Registry presenting with ACS complicated by CS, women (37.3%) were less likely to receive MCS (25.4% vs 33.8%) and had a higher risk of in-hospital mortality (adjusted OR: 1.10; 95% CI: 1.02–1.19) and major bleeding (adjusted OR: 1.23; 95% CI: 1.12–1.34). No differences in 1 year mortality were reported [63]. A recent sub analysis of an Italian registry reported an increasing use of Impella in the female population presenting with CS. Among patients enrolled in the IMP-IT (IMPella mechanical circulatory support device in Italy), only 22.4% were women and 14.5% of them had a diagnosis of MINOCA. Of note, more women had PCI on the left main compared with men (65.5% vs 37.8%, $p = 0.002$) and significantly more women had rotational atherectomy (34.5% vs 16.9%, $p = 0.036$) with no significant difference in vascular complications [64]. Efforts are needed to tackle sex-disparities in initial care of patients in this setting.

4 Prognosis

4.1 Sex Related Outcomes in ACS

Women suffering ACS are reported to experience worse in-hospital and short-term mortality rates [28, 33, 47, 65, 66]. These outcomes have been partially attributed to the higher comorbidity burden that characterizes this group of patients; however, differences remains significant when adjusting for these confounders [36, 65].

Delay in presentation and delivery of care for women presenting with ACS has also been associated with overall worse outcomes; late access to reperfusion facilities, minor immediate eligibility for primary PCI and lower admission rate to tertiary-care centers have all been associated with increased mortality [28, 37, 44]. However, prolonged untreated ischemia also appears to be less tolerated by women than by men [28]. Moreover, post-MI management, guideline-directed medical therapy and referral to cardiac rehabilitation facilities are less consistently delivered to female patients [47].

Overall, women suffering STEMI and experience worse in-hospital outcomes, especially in the younger age groups and when including patients who did not undergo pPCI [67, 68]. Conversely, data on NSTEMI are more controversial concerning differences in mortality rates. However, it is suggested that men and high risk women derive comparable benefits from an invasive strategy, both experiencing a reduction in the composite end point of death, MI, or rehospitalization with ACS, whereas a conservative strategy in low-risk women showed better outcomes than in men and, therefore, might be beneficial in this patient group [50].

Regarding MINOCA, outcomes appear similar in men and women, and more benign than in obstructive coronary syndromes: patients experience lower mortality rates and reduced need for repeated revascularization [23, 69]. However, some studies report a lack of improvement in quality of life at 1-year follow-up [70]. To date, there is no standardized treatment protocol for MINOCA, and the management is strongly patient-tailored and etiology-based. In this perspective, outcomes for these patients are strongly dependent on the accurate identification and treatment of underlying causes [13].

4.2 Future Directions

Considering the overall improvement of outcomes for ACS patients, reaching equal outcomes in men and women is a priority. Acknowledgement by the scientific community has led to several initiatives which aim at identifying the gaps in management of female patients in the cardiovascular field. The main identified issues include poor understanding of sex-based dissimilarities, lack of management algorithms taking sex-related factors into account, but also underrepresentation in clinical trials and low number of initiatives towards gender-specific research [23]. In this perspective, numerous national and international societies of (interventional) cardiology have promoted initiatives which focus on addressing under-recognition and suboptimal treatment of CVD in women, on promoting sex-specific research and on encouraging projects led by female researchers and physicians.

Increasing the involvement of female patients in study populations would produce the data needed for gender-specific management protocols and potentially improve the outcomes of women suffering from ACS. On the other hand, educating healthcare providers and patients on the sex specific presentation of ACS in women could reduce misdiagnosis and minimize delay in presentation to equipped medical facilities. Ultimately, the aim of the medical community should be to close the gaps in knowledge and promote knowledge of ACS in women, to upscale up the quality of care and level the promising trends that are detected in the overall population.

Key Issues
Epidemiology and Treatment Disparities:

- About half of emergency department ACS admissions are women, often presenting with non-ST-segment elevation myocardial infarction (NSTEMI) and unstable angina.
- Despite improved ACS treatment, women face higher short-term mortality post-percutaneous coronary intervention (PCI), with lower adherence to recommended diagnostic and revascularization pathways.

Sex-Specific Mechanisms in Pathophysiology:

- Women exhibit differences in atherosclerotic plaque characteristics, with fewer non-culprit lesions and less total necrotic core volume.
- Plaque erosion, more common in young women, and plaque rupture contribute to thrombosis, affecting outcomes.

Clinical Presentation in Women:

- Women have unique risk factors like hormonal fluctuations and autoimmune diseases.
- Presentation of ACS in women includes atypical symptoms like epigastric discomfort and palpitations.
- Young women face higher ACS rates, associated with traditional and emerging risk factors.

ACS Complications in Women:

- Women are more prone to acute myocardial infarction complicated by cardiogenic shock (AMI CS).
- Access to tertiary care centers is lower for women, impacting outcomes in AMI CS.

Impact on Diagnosis and Treatment:

- Women receive less intravascular imaging during ACS diagnosis, affecting plaque assessment.
- Conservative approaches are more common in women, and delays in treatment contribute to worse outcomes.

Prognosis and Outcomes:

- Women experience higher in-hospital and short-term mortality in ACS.

- Delayed presentation, lower adherence to guideline-directed therapy, and underutilization of mechanical circulatory support contribute to worse outcomes.

Future Directions and Initiatives:

- Initiatives aim to address gaps in understanding sex-specific differences in ACS.
- Increasing female representation in research studies is crucial for developing gender-specific management protocols.

References

1. Lansky AJ, et al. Gender and the extent of coronary atherosclerosis, plaque composition, and clinical outcomes in acute coronary syndromes. JACC Cardiovasc Imaging. 2012;5(Suppl 3):S62–72. https://doi.org/10.1016/J.JCMG.2012.02.003.
2. Ruiz-García J, et al. Age-and gender-related changes in plaque composition in patients with acute coronary syndrome: the PROSPECT study. EuroIntervention. 2012;8(8):929–38. https://doi.org/10.4244/EIJV8I8A142.
3. Arbustini E, et al. Plaque erosion is a major substrate for coronary thrombosis in acute myocardial infarction. Heart. 1999;82(3):269–72. https://doi.org/10.1136/HRT.82.3.269.
4. Virmani R, Burke AP, Farb A, Kolodgie FD. Pathology of the vulnerable plaque. J Am Coll Cardiol. 2006;47(Suppl 8):C13–8. https://doi.org/10.1016/J.JACC.2005.10.065.
5. Wang L, et al. Differences in underlying culprit lesion morphology between men and women: an IVUS analysis from the ADAPT-DES study. JACC Cardiovasc Imaging. 2016;9(4):498–9. https://doi.org/10.1016/J.JCMG.2015.02.019.
6. Seegers LM, et al. Sex differences in culprit plaque characteristics among different age groups in patients with acute coronary syndromes. Circ Cardiovasc Interv. 2022;15(6):E011612. https://doi.org/10.1161/CIRCINTERVENTIONS.121.011612.
7. Lichtman JH, et al. Sex differences in the presentation and perception of symptoms among young patients with myocardial infarction: evidence from the VIRGO study (variation in recovery: role of gender on outcomes of young AMI patients). Circulation. 2018;137(8):781–90. https://doi.org/10.1161/CIRCULATIONAHA.117.031650.
8. Reynolds HR, et al. Coronary optical coherence tomography and cardiac magnetic resonance imaging to determine underlying causes of myocardial infarction with nonobstructive coronary arteries in women. Circulation. 2021;143(7):624–40. https://doi.org/10.1161/CIRCULATIONAHA.120.052008.
9. Pasupathy S, Air T, Dreyer RP, Tavella R, Beltrame JF. Systematic review of patients presenting with suspected myocardial infarction and nonobstructive coronary arteries. Circulation. 2015;131(10):861–70. https://doi.org/10.1161/CIRCULATIONAHA.114.011201.
10. Beltrame JF, et al. International standardization of diagnostic criteria for vasospastic angina. Eur Heart J. 2017;38(33):2565–8. https://doi.org/10.1093/EURHEARTJ/EHV351.
11. Montone RA, et al. Patients with acute myocardial infarction and non-obstructive coronary arteries: safety and prognostic relevance of invasive coronary provocative tests. Eur Heart J. 2018;39(2):91–8. https://doi.org/10.1093/EURHEARTJ/EHX667.
12. Mohri M, et al. Angina pectoris caused by coronary microvascular spasm. Lancet. 1998;351(9110):1165–9. https://doi.org/10.1016/S0140-6736(97)07329-7.
13. Tamis-Holland JE, et al. Contemporary diagnosis and management of patients with myocardial infarction in the absence of obstructive coronary artery disease: a scientific statement from the American Heart Association. Circulation. 2019;139(18):E891–908. https://doi.org/10.1161/CIR.0000000000000670.
14. Tweet MS, Hayes SN, Codsi E, Gulati R, Rose CH, Best PJM. Spontaneous coronary artery dissection associated with pregnancy. J Am Coll Cardiol. 2017;70(4):426–35. https://doi.org/10.1016/J.JACC.2017.05.055.
15. Saw J, et al. Spontaneous coronary artery dissection: clinical outcomes and risk of recurrence. J Am Coll Cardiol. 2017;70(9):1148–58. https://doi.org/10.1016/J.JACC.2017.06.053.
16. Hayes SN, et al. Spontaneous coronary artery dissection: current state of the science: a scientific statement from the American Heart Association. Circulation. 2018;137(19):e523–57. https://doi.org/10.1161/CIR.0000000000000564.
17. Saw J, et al. Spontaneous coronary artery dissection: association with predisposing arteriopathies and precipitating stressors and cardiovascular outcomes. Circ Cardiovasc Interv. 2014;7(5):645–55. https://doi.org/10.1161/CIRCINTERVENTIONS.114.001760.
18. Kuehnemund L, et al. Gender differences in acute myocardial infarction—a nationwide German real-life analysis from 2014 to 2017. Clin Cardiol. 2021;44(7):890–8. https://doi.org/10.1002/CLC.23662.
19. Renda G, et al. Thrombotic and hemorrhagic burden in women: gender-related issues in the response to antithrombotic therapies. Int J Cardiol. 2019;286:198–207. https://doi.org/10.1016/J.IJCARD.2019.02.004.
20. Elkayam U, et al. Pregnancy-associated acute myocardial infarction: a review of contemporary experience in 150 cases between 2006 and 2011. Circulation.

2014;129(16):1695–702. https://doi.org/10.1161/CIRCULATIONAHA.113.002054.
21. Melano-Carranza E, et al. Coronary artery disease in systemic lupus erythematosus: what do the facts say? Cureus. 2023;15(1):e33449. https://doi.org/10.7759/CUREUS.33449.
22. Wassif H, et al. Outcomes following acute coronary syndrome in patients with and without rheumatic immune-mediated inflammatory diseases. J Am Heart Assoc. 2022;11(18):26411. https://doi.org/10.1161/JAHA.122.026411.
23. Vogel B, et al. The Lancet women and cardiovascular disease Commission: reducing the global burden by 2030. Lancet. 2021;397(10292):2385–438. https://doi.org/10.1016/S0140-6736(21)00684-X.
24. Safdar B, et al. Presentation, clinical profile, and prognosis of young patients with myocardial infarction with nonobstructive coronary arteries (MINOCA): results from the VIRGO study. J Am Heart Assoc. 2018;7(13):e009174. https://doi.org/10.1161/JAHA.118.009174.
25. DeFilippis EM, et al. Women who experience a myocardial infarction at a young age have worse outcomes compared with men: the Mass General Brigham YOUNG-MI registry. Eur Heart J. 2020;41(42):4127–37. https://doi.org/10.1093/EURHEARTJ/EHAA662.
26. Ferry AV, et al. Presenting symptoms in men and women diagnosed with myocardial infarction using sex-specific criteria. J Am Heart Assoc. 2019;8(17):e012307. https://doi.org/10.1161/JAHA.119.012307.
27. Gulati M, et al. 2021 AHA/ACC/ASE/CHEST/SAEM/SCCT/SCMR guideline for the evaluation and diagnosis of chest pain: a report of the American College of Cardiology/American Heart Association Joint Committee on clinical practice guidelines. J Am Coll Cardiol. 2021;78(22):e187–285. https://doi.org/10.1016/J.JACC.2021.07.053.
28. Bugiardini R, et al. Delayed care and mortality among women and men with myocardial infarction. J Am Heart Assoc. 2017;6(8):e005968. https://doi.org/10.1161/JAHA.117.005968.
29. Kaur G, De Oliveira-Gomes D, Rivera FB, Gulati M. Chest pain in women: considerations from the 2021 AHA/ACC chest pain guideline. Curr Probl Cardiol. 2023;48:101697. https://doi.org/10.1016/J.CPCARDIOL.2023.101697.
30. Chi GC, et al. Trends in acute myocardial infarction by race and ethnicity. J Am Heart Assoc. 2020;9(5):e013542. https://doi.org/10.1161/JAHA.119.013542.
31. Arora S, et al. Twenty year trends and sex differences in young adults hospitalized with acute myocardial infarction. Circulation. 2019;139(8):1047–56. https://doi.org/10.1161/CIRCULATIONAHA.118.037137.
32. Gabet A, Danchin N, Juillière Y, Olié V. Acute coronary syndrome in women: rising hospitalizations in middle-aged French women, 2004-14. Eur Heart J. 2017;38(14):1060–5. https://doi.org/10.1093/EURHEARTJ/EHX097.
33. Vaccarino V, Parsons L, Every NR, Barron HV, Krumholz HM. Sex-based differences in early mortality after myocardial infarction. National registry of myocardial infarction 2 participants. N Engl J Med. 1999;341(4):217–25. https://doi.org/10.1056/NEJM199907223410401.
34. Vaccarino V, et al. Mental stress-induced-myocardial ischemia in young patients with recent myocardial infarction: sex differences and mechanisms. Circulation. 2018;137(8):794–805. https://doi.org/10.1161/CIRCULATIONAHA.117.030849.
35. Fengler K, et al. Gender differences in patients with cardiogenic shock complicating myocardial infarction: a substudy of the IABP-SHOCK II-trial. Clin Res Cardiol. 2015;104(1):71–8. https://doi.org/10.1007/S00392-014-0767-2.
36. Rubini Gimenez M, et al. Sex-specific management in patients with acute myocardial infarction and cardiogenic shock: a substudy of the CULPRIT-SHOCK trial. Circ Cardiovasc Interv. 2020;13(3):e008537. https://doi.org/10.1161/CIRCINTERVENTIONS.119.008537.
37. Sambola A, et al. Sex bias in admission to tertiary-care centres for acute myocardial infarction and cardiogenic shock. Eur J Clin Investig. 2021;51(7):e13526. https://doi.org/10.1111/ECI.13526.
38. Reynolds HR, et al. Mechanisms of myocardial infarction in women without angiographically obstructive coronary artery disease. Circulation. 2011;124(13):1414–25. https://doi.org/10.1161/CIRCULATIONAHA.111.026542.
39. Ouldzein H, et al. Plaque rupture and morphological characteristics of the culprit lesion in acute coronary syndromes without significant angiographic lesion: analysis by intravascular ultrasound. Ann Cardiol Angeiol (Paris). 2012;61(1):20–6. https://doi.org/10.1016/J.ANCARD.2011.07.011.
40. Collet JP, et al. 2020 ESC Guidelines for the management of acute coronary syndromes in patients presenting without persistent ST-segment elevation. Eur Heart J. 2021;42(14):1289–367. https://doi.org/10.1093/EURHEARTJ/EHAA575.
41. Rashid M, et al. Sex differences in use of intracoronary imaging in patients undergoing percutaneous coronary intervention. JACC Cardiovasc Interv. 2022;15(12):1290–2. https://doi.org/10.1016/J.JCIN.2022.03.034.
42. Mehta LS, et al. acute myocardial infarction in women: a scientific statement from the American Heart Association. Circulation. 2016;133(9):916–47. https://doi.org/10.1161/CIR.0000000000000351.
43. Pilgrim T, et al. Age- and gender-related disparities in primary percutaneous coronary interventions for acute ST-segment elevation myocardial infarction. PLoS One. 2015;10(9):e0137047. https://doi.org/10.1371/JOURNAL.PONE.0137047.
44. Kaul P, Armstrong PW, Sookram S, Leung BK, Brass N, Welsh RC. Temporal trends in patient and

treatment delay among men and women presenting with ST-elevation myocardial infarction. Am Heart J. 2011;161(1):91–7. https://doi.org/10.1016/J.AHJ.2010.09.016.
45. Kang SH, et al. Sex differences in management and mortality of patients with ST-elevation myocardial infarction (from the Korean Acute Myocardial Infarction National Registry). Am J Cardiol. 2012;109(6):787–93. https://doi.org/10.1016/J.AMJCARD.2011.11.006.
46. Dey S, et al. Sex-related differences in the presentation, treatment and outcomes among patients with acute coronary syndromes: the global registry of acute coronary events. Heart. 2009;95(1):20–6. https://doi.org/10.1136/HRT.2007.138537.
47. Hao Y, et al. Sex differences in in-hospital management and outcomes of patients with acute coronary syndrome. Circulation. 2019;139(15):1776–85. https://doi.org/10.1161/CIRCULATIONAHA.118.037655.
48. Jackson AM, et al. Healthcare disparities for women hospitalized with myocardial infarction and angina. Eur Heart J Qual Care Clin Outcomes. 2020;6(2):156–65. https://doi.org/10.1093/EHJQCCO/QCZ040.
49. Huded CP, et al. 4-Step protocol for disparities in STEMI care and outcomes in women. J Am Coll Cardiol. 2018;71(19):2122–32. https://doi.org/10.1016/J.JACC.2018.02.039.
50. O'Donoghue M, et al. Early invasive vs conservative treatment strategies in women and men with unstable angina and non-ST-segment elevation myocardial infarction: a meta-analysis. JAMA. 2008;300(1):71–80. https://doi.org/10.1001/JAMA.300.1.71.
51. Worrall-Carter L, McEvedy S, Wilson A, Rahman MA. Gender differences in presentation, coronary intervention, and outcomes of 28,985 acute coronary syndrome patients in Victoria, Australia. Womens Health Issues. 2016;26(1):14–20. https://doi.org/10.1016/J.WHI.2015.09.002.
52. Leifheit-Limson EC, et al. Sex differences in cardiac risk factors, perceived risk, and health care provider discussion of risk and risk modification among young patients with acute myocardial infarction: the VIRGO study. J Am Coll Cardiol. 2015;66(18):1949–57. https://doi.org/10.1016/J.JACC.2015.08.859.
53. Mason PJ, et al. An update on radial artery access and best practices for transradial coronary angiography and intervention in acute coronary syndrome: a scientific statement from the American Heart Association. Circ Cardiovasc Interv. 2018;11(9):e000035. https://doi.org/10.1161/HCV.0000000000000035.
54. Reifart J, et al. Acceptance and safety of femoral versus radial access for percutaneous coronary intervention (PCI): results from a large monitor-controlled German registry (QuIK). BMC Cardiovasc Disord. 2022;22(1):7. https://doi.org/10.1186/S12872-021-02283-0.
55. Neumann FJ, et al. 2018 ESC/EACTS guidelines on myocardial revascularization. Eur Heart J. 2019;40(2):87–165. https://doi.org/10.1093/EURHEARTJ/EHY394.
56. Cirillo P, et al. Optimal medical therapy on top of dual-antiplatelet therapy: 1-year clinical outcome in patients with acute coronary syndrome: the START Antiplatelet Registry. Angiology. 2020;71(3):235–41. https://doi.org/10.1177/0003319719895171.
57. Wong SC, et al. Absence of gender differences in clinical outcomes in patients with cardiogenic shock complicating acute myocardial infarction. A report from the SHOCK Trial Registry. J Am Coll Cardiol. 2001;38(5):1395–401. https://doi.org/10.1016/S0735-1097(01)01581-9.
58. Thiele H, et al. One-year outcomes after PCI strategies in cardiogenic shock. N Engl J Med. 2018;379(18):1699–710. https://doi.org/10.1056/NEJMOA1808788.
59. Lawton JS, et al. 2021 ACC/AHA/SCAI guideline for coronary artery revascularization: a report of the American College of Cardiology/American Heart Association Joint Committee on clinical practice guidelines. Circulation. 2022;145(3):E18–E114. https://doi.org/10.1161/CIR.0000000000001038.
60. Ibanez B, et al. 2017 ESC guidelines for the management of acute myocardial infarction in patients presenting with ST-segment elevation: the task force for the management of acute myocardial infarction in patients presenting with ST-segment elevation of the European Society of Cardiology (ESC). Eur Heart J. 2018;39(2):119–77. https://doi.org/10.1093/EURHEARTJ/EHX393.
61. Chieffo A, et al. Joint EAPCI/ACVC expert consensus document on percutaneous ventricular assist devices. Eur Heart J Acute Cardiovasc Care. 2021;10(5):570–83. https://doi.org/10.1093/EHJACC/ZUAB015.
62. O'Neill WW, et al. Analysis of outcomes for 15,259 US patients with acute myocardial infarction cardiogenic shock (AMICS) supported with the Impella device. Am Heart J. 2018;202:33–8. https://doi.org/10.1016/J.AHJ.2018.03.024.
63. Elgendy IY, et al. Sex differences in management and outcomes of acute myocardial infarction patients presenting with cardiogenic shock. JACC Cardiovasc Interv. 2022;15(6):642–52. https://doi.org/10.1016/J.JCIN.2021.12.033.
64. Beneduce A, et al. Multicenter registry of patients treated with Impella mechanical circulatory support device in Italy: sex subanalysis. JACC Cardiovasc Interv. 2023;16(1):124–6. https://doi.org/10.1016/J.JCIN.2022.10.042.
65. Bavishi C, Bangalore S, Patel D, Chatterjee S, Trivedi V, Tamis-Holland JE. Short and long-term mortality in women and men undergoing primary angioplasty: a comprehensive meta-analysis. Int J Cardiol. 2015;198:123–30. https://doi.org/10.1016/J.IJCARD.2015.07.001.
66. Berger JS, et al. Sex differences in mortality following acute coronary syndromes. JAMA. 2009;302(8):874–82. https://doi.org/10.1001/JAMA.2009.1227.
67. Cenko E, et al. Sex differences in outcomes after STEMI: effect modification by treatment strategy and

age. JAMA Intern Med. 2018;178(5):632–9. https://doi.org/10.1001/JAMAINTERNMED.2018.0514.
68. Alkhouli M, Alqahtani F, Jneid H, Al Hajji M, Boubas W, Lerman A. Age-stratified sex-related differences in the incidence, management, and outcomes of acute myocardial infarction. Mayo Clin Proc. 2021;96(2):332–41. https://doi.org/10.1016/J.MAYOCP.2020.04.048.
69. Williams MGL, et al. Sex differences in patients with acute coronary syndromes and non-obstructive coronary arteries: presentation and outcome. Int J Cardiol. 2023;372:15–22. https://doi.org/10.1016/J.IJCARD.2022.11.032.
70. Berg E, et al. Health-related quality-of-life up to one year after myocardial infarction with non-obstructive coronary arteries. Eur Heart J Qual Care Clin Outcomes. 2022;9:639–44. https://doi.org/10.1093/EHJQCCO/QCAC072.
71. Smilowitz NR, et al. Mortality of myocardial infarction by sex, age, and obstructive coronary artery disease status in the ACTION Registry-GWTG (acute coronary treatment and intervention outcomes network registry-get with the guidelines). Circ Cardiovasc Qual Outcomes. 2017;10(12):e003443. https://doi.org/10.1161/CIRCOUTCOMES.116.003443.
72. Potts J, et al. Persistent sex disparities in clinical outcomes with percutaneous coronary intervention: insights from 6.6 million PCI procedures in the United States. PLoS One. 2018;13(9):e0203325. https://doi.org/10.1371/JOURNAL.PONE.0203325.
73. Udell JA, et al. Sustained sex-based treatment differences in acute coronary syndrome care: insights from the American Heart Association Get With The Guidelines Coronary Artery Disease Registry. Clin Cardiol. 2018;41(6):758–68. https://doi.org/10.1002/CLC.22938.

SCAD in Acute and Chronic Phase and Work Up for FMD

Teresa Bastante, David del Val, and Fernando Alfonso

Abstract

Spontaneous coronary artery dissection (SCAD) is not longer an extremely rare and exceptional disease. Over the past 10 years, we have witnessed an exponential increase in the interest and attention devoted to this condition. The publication of large patient series, some of which were prospective studies, has provided us with invaluable insights into the clinical characteristics of SCAD. The widespread utilization of coronary angiograms and intracoronary imaging in the context of acute coronary syndrome (ACS) has enabled us to apply this newfound knowledge in practice. Hence, an increasing number of patients are now being recognized as suffering from SCAD, thus replacing the diagnosis of ACS with an unknown etiology in many cases. Moreover, although clinical trials are currently unavailable, we now understand that the management and prognosis of SCAD differ significantly from those of atherothrombotic ACS. As someone once stated, "if you do not consider SCAD, you cannot diagnose SCAD." Therefore, in this chapter, we will attempt to summarize the key aspects of SCAD: when it should be suspected, how to confirm the diagnosis, the expected outcomes and various management options, as well as the evaluation during the chronic phase.

Keywords

Spontaneous coronary artery dissection · Acute myocardial infarction · Acute coronary syndrome · Fibromuscular dysplasia · MINOCA

Test your learning and check your understanding of this book's contents: use the "Springer Nature Flashcards" app to access questions using ▶ https://sn.pub/51ny7m
To use the app, please follow the instructions in chapter 1.

T. Bastante · D. del Val · F. Alfonso (✉)
Hospital Universitario de La Princesa, Madrid, Spain

A. H.E.M. Maas, E. Gerdts (eds.), *Manual of Cardiovascular Disease in Women*,
https://doi.org/10.1007/978-3-031-65952-2_21

1 Introduction

Spontaneous coronary artery dissection (SCAD) has emerged in recent years as a new underlying substrate of acute coronary syndrome (ACS). First described in 1931 [1], for a long time it was believed to be very rare and limited to specific situations such as pregnancy, collagen-related disorders, or young women without cardiovascular risk factors. However, significant efforts have been made to enroll patients in prospective clinical registries [2–4]. These works have revealed that SCAD is a major cause of ACS in young women, with the peripartum period being a rare predisposing condition, and most patients with SCAD are middle-aged and not uncommonly have traditional cardiovascular risk factors. Furthermore, SCAD is a distinct condition from atherothrombotic ACS, with different pathophysiology and recommended management strategies. Therefore, our ability to recognize and appropriately manage SCAD is of paramount importance.

Although there are currently no randomized clinical trials available for the treatment of SCAD, significant conclusions and recommendations can be drawn from recent large series. Conservative management is the preferred approach, with the avoidance of high-intensity antithrombotic therapy, and is highly recommended the screening for extracoronary vascular anomalies, particularly fibromuscular dysplasia (FMD). The growing awareness and interest in this condition will provide us with more knowledge about this intriguing disease, including findings from ongoing randomized clinical trials that are currently enrolling patients [5].

2 Theory

SCAD is defined as the acute separation of the layers of the coronary artery wall by an intramural hematoma, with or without the presence of an intimal tear that connects the true and false lumens. This condition specifically excludes coronary artery dissections related to atherosclerotic disease, iatrogenic causes, or trauma [6, 7]. Two hypotheses have been proposed to explain the pathophysiology of SCAD. The "inside-out" mechanism suggests that the primary event is a disruption of the endothelial-intimal layer, allowing blood to enter from the lumen into the vessel wall. Conversely, the "outside-in" theory posits that spontaneous bleeding, likely from the *vasa vasorum* within the coronary artery wall, is the primary event. Recent studies based on optical coherence tomography (OCT) have provided supporting evidence for this hypothesis [8]: the presence of a coronary intramural hematoma without a connection between the lumen and the arterial wall could be the initial event. In certain cases, rising pressure within the vessel may lead to the development of an intimal tear, resulting in the formation of the typical false and true lumens. The ultimate consequence is limited coronary blood flow due to luminal compression, leading to myocardial ischemia and the full spectrum of signs and symptoms observed in ACS. The severity of clinical manifestations, ranging from mild elevation of cardiac enzymes to sudden death, depends on the extent of myocardial involvement by the dissected coronary artery.

Little is known about the ultimate cause of these series of phenomena. However, there is no doubt that hormones play a significant role, as evidenced by the well-established relationship between SCAD and pregnancy, hormone therapy, and female gender [6, 7, 9]. On the other hand, certain precipitating stressors have been described in approximately half of the patients, including emotional or physical stress [3, 4], as well as the Valsalva maneuver. Additionally, there are some predisposing conditions associated with SCAD, such as type IV Ehlers-Danlos syndrome and Marfan syndrome (although these are rare when a systematic genetic evaluation is conducted in SCAD patients, accounting for only 5% of cases [10]). In recent years, there have been notable advancements in understanding the genetic basis of SCAD. The PHACTR1-EDN1 genetic locus, which is associated with migraine and extracoronary arterial pathology, has been identified as a potential genetic substrate for SCAD [11]. However, the low prevalence of familial cases observed in large series of SCAD patients suggests that inheritance plays a limited role in the condition [12].

A consistent association has been found between SCAD and FMD. In over 50% of SCAD patients, these two rare conditions coexist [4, 13]. FMD is a noninflammatory and nonatherosclerotic vascular disease that primarily affects medium-large arteries. Similar to SCAD, FMD predominantly affects women, and its underlying pathophysiology and causes remain unclear. FMD is characterized by arterial stenosis, dissections, and aneurysms in various arterial beds, including the renal, iliac, splanchnic, and intracranial arteries. Although the exact connection between SCAD and FMD remains unexplained, it is unequivocal, and consensus documents from both sides of the Atlantic recommend universal screening for extracoronary vascular anomalies in SCAD patients [6, 7].

In summary, SCAD is the final event of a myriad of different compounds, probably affected by genetic susceptibility, hormone situation, precipitating factors and acquired conditions. Future investigations are needed to better understand this intriguing entity.

3 Clinical Scenario

Nowadays, we could define a comprehensive vision of SCAD patients. Valuable insights for this purpose have been obtained from large prospective series of patients that have undergone centralized evaluation with sufficient follow-up time [3, 4]. Figure 1 provides a summary of the crucial and well-established components that characterize the typical clinical scenario in SCAD.

Nearly 9 out of 10 cases of SCAD occur in women. Distinct differences have been established between SCAD in men and women [14, 15]. Men tend to be younger and less frequently present with depression and emotional stress as triggers. Conversely, physical stress triggers and recreational drug use are more commonly reported in men. It is noteworthy that men are less likely to have associated FMD. In terms of in-hospital and long-term follow-up, event rates are similar between men and women. Although the proportion of acute myocardial infarction (AMI) cases with SCAD as the underlying substrate is even smaller in men than in women, we should strive to avoid a "reverse gender bias" and consider SCAD as a possibility in men when the clinical and angiographic presentations are suggestive. If necessary, intracoronary imaging can be used to confirm the diagnosis and rule out atherosclerosis [16]. Figure 2 depicts a case of SCAD in a man, which was confirmed using OCT imaging.

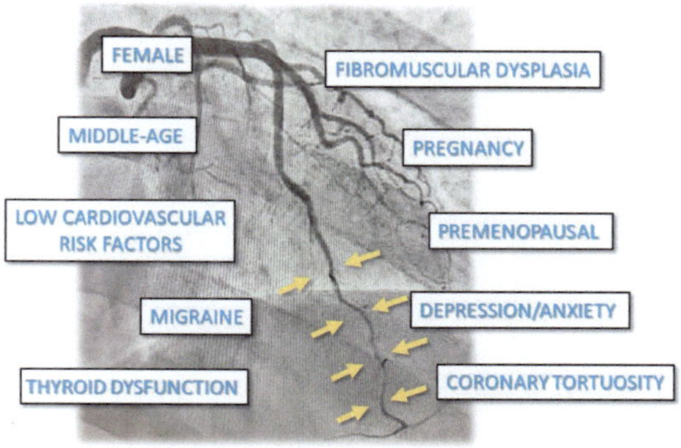

Fig. 1 Frequently associated conditions in SCAD patients and indicative scenarios for suspicion

SCAD has been documented across all stages of life, including neonates and elderly patients [17]. Figure 3 illustrates a case of SCAD in an octogenarian woman who also had FMD. However, the primary population affected by SCAD falls within the 50–55-year-old age range. In young women, SCAD accounts for approximately one-third of premenopausal women presenting with AMI [6, 7]. Therefore, the higher incidence of SCAD is concentrated in middle-aged women, but in the rare case of AMI in young woman, SCAD should feature strongly on the differential diagnosis.

Another paradigm that has been revised based on new data is the absence of traditional cardiovascular risk factors in SCAD patients: only one-third of patients do not have any of these. Furthermore, approximately 30% of patients have hypertension and dyslipidemia, and 10–30% were smokers at the time of diagnosis. Diabetes mellitus is rarely observed, affecting less than 5% of SCAD patients [3, 4]. Therefore, the presence of conventional cardiovascular risk factors should not discard the possibility of SCAD, unless a high concentration of these risk factors is uncommonly observed.

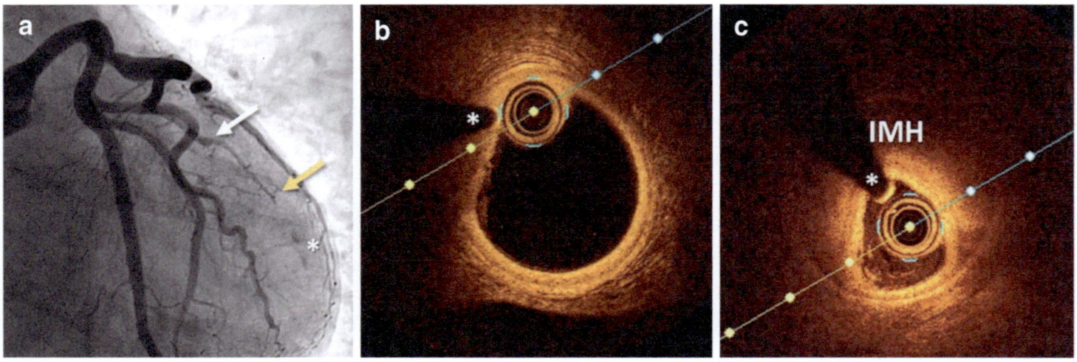

Fig. 2 72-year-old man. Hypertension being treated, admitted with non-ST segment elevation myocardial infarction. (**a**) Coronary angiogram revealed an obtuse marginal branch exhibiting an abrupt change in caliber (white arrow), followed by a long stenosis leading to final subocclusion (yellow arrow). A small amount of contrast media staining was observed (asterisk). (**b**) Optical coherence tomography demonstrated a normal coronary artery with a well-defined three-layer structure. (**c**) Distally, there was a clear separation between the media and adventitia layers, with compression of the lumen, indicating the presence of an intramural hematoma (IMH). * in (**b**) and (**c**) panel denotes wire artifact

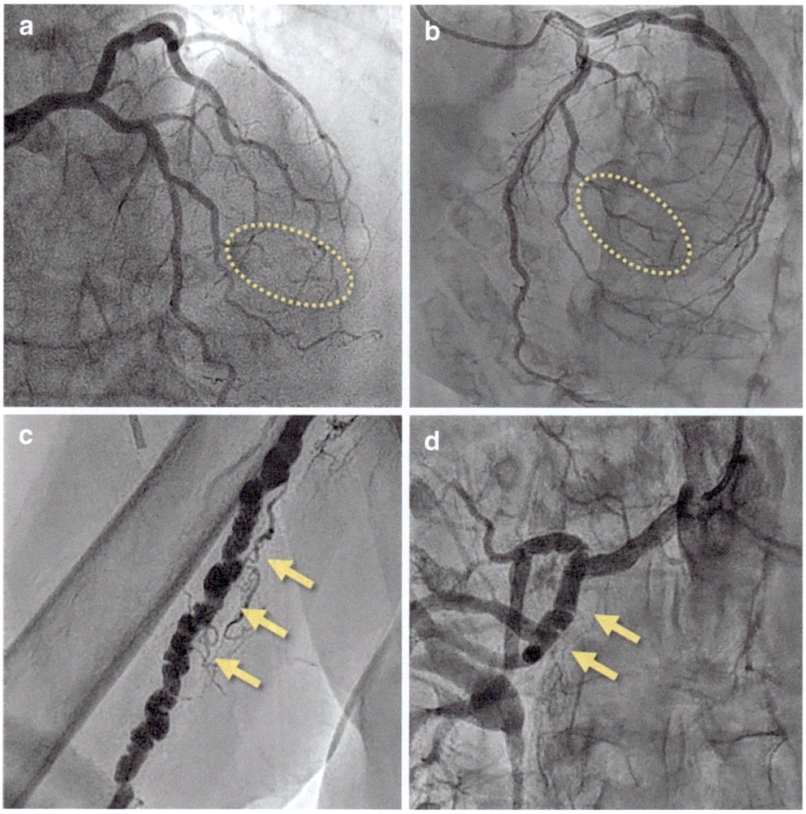

Fig. 3 88-year-old woman admitted for non-ST segment elevation myocardial infarction, without evident electrocardiographic abnormalities. (**a**) Coronary angiography showing a long stenosis suggestive of spontaneous coronary artery dissection in the diagonal branch (oval with dashed line). Conservative management was performed with satisfactory evolution. (**b**) Coronary angiography performed 4 years later as part of the pre-transcatheter aortic valve implantation evaluation for symptomatic degenerative aortic stenosis, revealing *restitutio ad integrum* of the diagonal branch (oval with dashed line). (**c**) and (**d**) Fibromuscular dysplasia of the right brachial and renal arteries (arrows), observed in the initial study, supporting the diagnosis of SCAD

A step forward in the connection between cardiovascular risk factors-atherosclerosis and SCAD is the coexistence of the two entities in the same patient. The contemporary definition of SCAD excludes coronary dissections related to atherosclerotic disease [6, 7] because they have distinct etiologies and management approaches. Furthermore, when describing the typical scenario for SCAD, it is often stated that "smooth vessels and otherwise healthy coronary arteries" are present. However, SCAD can occur in patients with concurrent atherosclerotic disease in segments unaffected by atherosclerotic plaques [18]. In this specific and uncommon scenario, intracoronary imaging can play a crucial role in reaching a definitive diagnosis. Figure 4 illustrates a case of a middle-aged woman with atherosclerotic coronary artery disease and SCAD-related AMI occurring in different segments of the same vessel. OCT was the key to unravel the pathophysiology of the ACS and changed the management, that was conservative with excellent outcome.

Migraine has emerged as a condition associated with SCAD. The connection remains poorly understood, but migraines are known to be influenced by the menstrual cycle and pregnancy, and a genetic locus has been implicated in linking the two entities [11]. History of migraine headaches is present in over one-third of SCAD patients. These patients appear to exhibit a distinct profile: they are younger at the time of SCAD episode, have a higher prevalence of depression and anxiety disorders, and, during the screening for extracoronary vascular anomalies, they are more likely to have aneurysms and dissections. There was no difference in SCAD recurrence during mid-term follow-up [19].

Thyroid disorders are common among patients with SCAD [20]. Although no association has

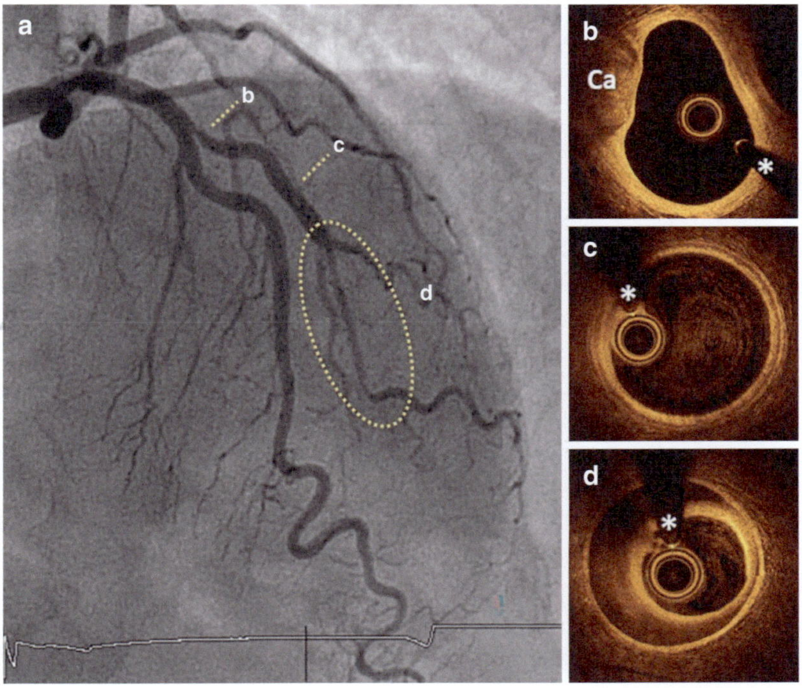

Fig. 4 A 63-year-old woman, former smoker, with hypertension, and dyslipidemia. Admitted for non-ST segment elevation myocardial infarction. (**a**) Coronary angiography revealed coronary arteries with mild atheromatosis and a long lesion, with an abrupt change in caliber in the diagonal branch, which also recovers abruptly distally (oval with dashed line). Optical coherence tomography imaging showed: (**b**) origin of the diagonal branch with a calcium nodule (Ca: calcium); (**c**) segment of a healthy artery, and (**d**) separation between layers of the coronary artery wall consistent with SCAD. * Denotes wire artifact

been found with thyroid functional status, approximately 13% of patients had a history of thyroid pathology, particularly hypothyroidism [3, 4]. It has even been suggested that these patients have a worse prognosis, with a higher rate of events during the disease [21].

Like other cardiac diseases that have a clear predominance in females (such as stress cardiomyopathy) and linking with the high prevalence of emotional triggers, it is common to find anxiety and/or depression disorders. In comparative studies with atherothrombotic AMI, scores obtained from validated anxiety and depression questionnaires showed significantly higher values among patients with SCAD [22].

Pregnancy has long been seen as the archetypal scenario. Pregnancy-associated SCAD is defined as one that occurs during pregnancy or within 12 months after delivery. Nowadays, we know that although the presence of an ongoing pregnancy, and particularly the postpartum period (with the highest incidence within 6 weeks after delivery), is a key factor for diagnosis, these cases account for less than 5% of all diagnosed SCAD [3, 4, 23].

4 Diagnosis

Invasive coronary angiography in a patient who has experienced an ACS remains the gold standard diagnostic test for SCAD. The typical angiographic image of intimal flap, with double lumen and contrast retention is actually rare, occurring in only 20–30% of cases. The description of other angiographic patterns in recent years, which are less evident but much more common, has led to an increase in the recognized cases. Initially, the use of intravascular imaging techniques was necessary to accurately demonstrate the separation between the layers of the artery, often without connection between the vessel lumen and the wall [24]. Nowadays, the presence of an abrupt change in vessel caliber, causing a long stenosis (>20 mm) with smooth edges, especially in an appropriate epidemiological context, can be considered diagnostic for SCAD due to intramural hematoma. There is consensus in using the classification described by Saw [25]. Figure 5 shows examples of the different angiographic patterns: in addition to the already described classic pattern with a double-lumen image (Type 1) and the pattern showing a long stenosis (Type 2; which can be subdivided into 2A: with distal recovery of vessel caliber, or 2B: without recovery), the presence of a focal stenosis (<20 mm) similar to that found in common atherosclerotic disease may correspond to SCAD (Type 3). The suspicion arises from a suggestive epidemiological context, but a definitive and unequivocal diagnosis can only be made through intravascular imaging techniques (IVUS—intravascular ultrasound and OCT). Intravascular imaging is not always feasible and/or may not have a favourable risk-benefit balance when used in arteries weakened by dissection. Therefore, the epidemiological context and key factors (such as pregnancy, the presence of FMD, or a history of previous SCAD) can provide a sufficiently high reliability for the diagnosis, despite a Type 3 angiographic pattern. Figure 6 proposes a diagnostic algorithm in this regard. OCT examples could be found in cases presented in Figs. 2 and 4 and IVUS example in Fig. 5.

Angiographic assessment of the coronary arteries in a suspected SCAD patient could be challenging: it usually affects more distal segments and small branches than atherosclerotic disease and pathological findings could be subtle. Coronary tortuosity could be a marker of SCAD. It is highly prevalent in the SCAD population and has been proposed a worse prognosis in terms of recurrent SCAD [3, 26], but the latter has not been confirmed in subsequent studies [21]. There are unique patterns described as looking like a "stick insect" or a "radish", produced by external true lumen compression by the intramural hematoma [27]. Another proposed clue pattern is "broken-line", defined as the development of sharp angles in a tortuous but smooth coronary artery segment, giving a "saw" line appearance [2, 28]. This finding is related with longer lesions and severe vessel tortuosity, but these patients have better coronary flow, received more frequently conservative medical management, and could be expected a better clinical out-

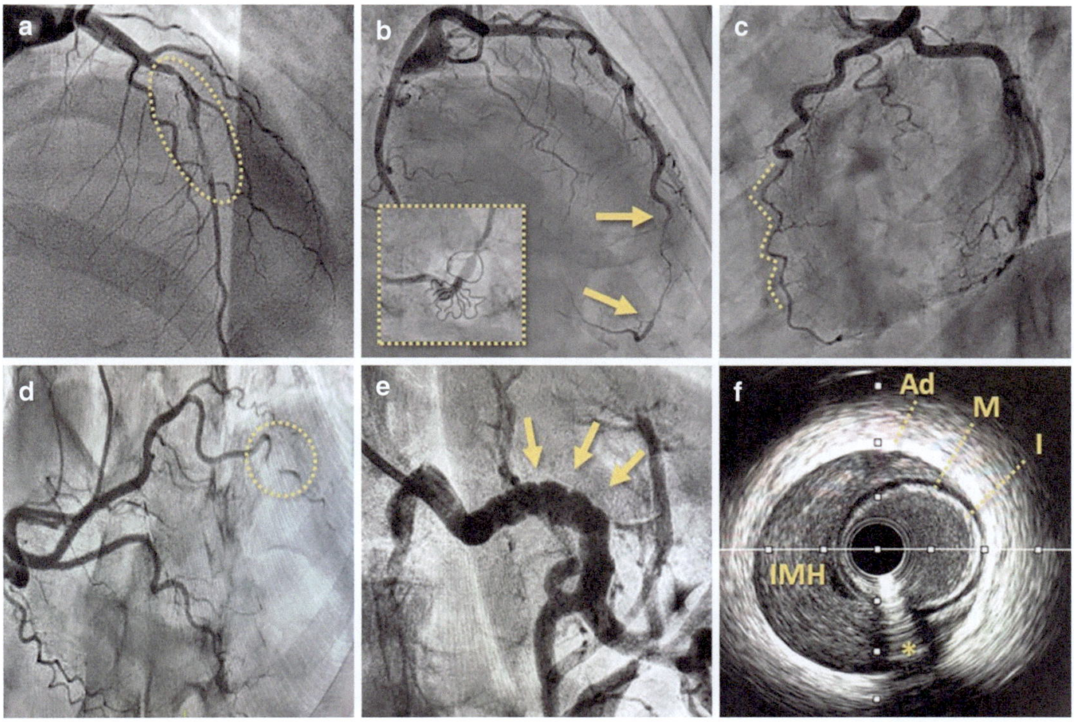

Fig. 5 Angiographic classification of SCAD, clue patterns, and typical IVUS imaging. (**a**) Type 1: Intimal flap image with double lumen and contrast retention in the mid-left anterior descending artery (yellow circle). (**b**) Type 2A: Abrupt caliber loss in the distal left anterior descending artery, with a long stenosis (arrows) and caliber recovery with a "radish-like" shape (zoomed image framed in yellow dashed line). (**c**) Type 2B: Long stenosis in the distal left anterior descending artery, without caliber recovery in the distal vessel; note the resulting "broken line" phenomenon in a tortuous artery (yellow dashed line). (**d**) Type 3: Focal stenosis in the posterolateral branch of the right coronary artery (yellow circle), resembling an atherosclerotic lesion. The diagnosis of SCAD was established based on the epidemiological context (44-year-old female smoker) and the presence of FMD in renal and iliac arteries. (**e**) Angiography of the left renal artery of the patient from (**d**), showing typical vascular wall irregularities in the form of a "string of beads". (**f**) IVUS image of intramural hematoma (IMH). Note the distinct differentiation between the adventitia (Ad), hypoechoic media (M), and intima (I) layers with separation between the first two. * Denotes wire artifact

come in late clinical follow-up [29]. Figure 5 shows examples of these clue patterns.

Invasive angiography carries risk in the context of SCAD and, in most cases, conservative management is possible, avoiding intervention [3, 4, 30]. Therefore, the possibility of non-invasive diagnosis with techniques such as coronary computed tomography angiography (CCTA) has been investigated. However, the limited spatial resolution of this technique and the fact that SCAD preferentially affects the mid-distal segments of the vessels, restricts its diagnostic capability in the acute context. In two different series, 20% of dissections were not identified by CCTA, despite invasive angiography images were used as a guide [31, 32]. Therefore, invasive coronary angiography remains the gold standard in the acute setting. On the other hand, CCTA has shown promising results during follow-up: to confirm healing and to rule out a new episode of dissection in future events with low pre-test probability [13, 33].

The role of cardiac magnetic resonance imaging (CMR) in the context of SCAD is also limited, although, as in any AMI of unknown cause, it can be crucial in confirming the presence and location of late gadolinium enhancement with an ischemic pattern. In an appropriate epidemiologi-

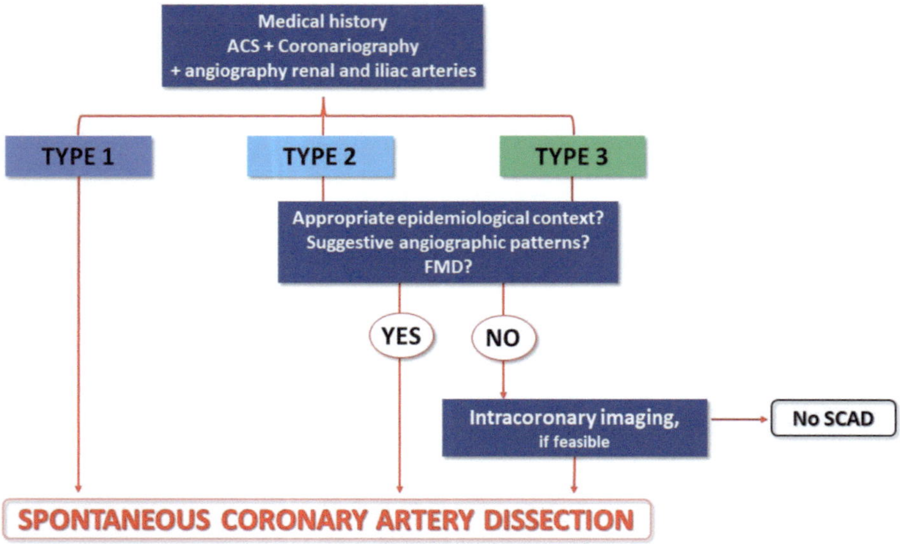

Fig. 6 Diagnosis algorithm for SCAD. After a careful assessment of coronary angiography images, in multiple views and following intracoronary nitroglycerin administration, renal and iliac angiography can be performed during the same procedure. In Type 2 SCAD, the presence of an epidemiological context and/or FMD is sufficient to conclude the diagnosis of SCAD with a high level of certainty. In Type 3 SCAD, the diagnosis should be much more cautious, always considering the use of intravascular imaging techniques for an unequivocal diagnosis. Overdiagnosis of SCAD could leave an unstable and untreated atherosclerotic lesion, with unpredictable consequences

cal context, with uncertain images of SCAD in invasive coronary angiography, affecting segments that are not accessible for assessment with intracoronary imaging and in the absence of FMD, the finding of ischemic late gadolinium enhancement in myocardial territory consistent with the suspected coronary artery can support the diagnosis of SCAD [34].

In a few cases, despite a comprehensive evaluation in the acute phase, the final diagnosis of SCAD can only be established at follow-up when coronary angiography shows the natural healing of the vessel [35]. The risk-benefit of the strategy of repeated invasive angiography should be individualized.

A different approach to achieve the elusive diagnosis of SCAD is through blood biomarkers: microRNAs have a differential expression in patients with SCAD compared to patients with atherothrombotic AMI. MicroRNAs are small fragments of non-coding RNA that regulate post-transcriptional gene expression by inhibiting the translation of messenger RNA into proteins. They can be determined in peripheral blood, and although preliminary, there are promising data supporting microRNAs as a potential biomarker with diagnostic utility in the context of SCAD [36].

5 Treatment

The recommended management for SCAD is conservative medical whenever possible [6, 7]. The natural history of the disease suggests that most lesions will heal completely within weeks. Once the diagnosis of SCAD is established, hemodynamic status, persistence of ischemic symptoms, coronary segment affected, myocardial involvement, and coronary flow should be evaluated and taken into consideration. Most patients can be managed without intervention, with supportive measures and close monitoring, resulting in good short- and long-term outcomes [3, 4]. Furthermore, treating specific arterial vessels or segments does not protect against the occurrence of a new episode of SCAD. Patients referred to bypass surgery show low long-term graft patency due to competitive flow from the native artery once it has healed [37]. In cases of clinical instability, the recommended option is revascularization with percutaneous coronary intervention (PCI).

PCI in the setting of SCAD is challenging, with lower success and higher complication rates compared to interventions in an atherosclerotic scenario [3, 37, 38]. In any case, the use of intracoronary imaging to guide the procedure is highly recommended as it provides valuable information, including confirmation of the diagnosis, proper positioning of the guidewire in the true lumen, accurate measurement of vessel caliber and affected segment, and assessment of the intervention result.

Multiple strategies have been proposed for PCI in SCAD, ranging from simple balloon angioplasty to the implantation of metallic stents and bioabsorbable scaffolds, as well as the fenestration of the hematoma to relieve pressure on the true lumen. The fenestration approach appears to be quite attractive and has shown good short- and medium-term results. This strategy avoids the implantation of a permanent device—a stent—in a coronary artery which no longer will need it, because it tends to heal once the acute phase has passed [39]. The "outside-in" theory suggests that the initial event is the intramural hematoma, which occasionally fenestrates naturally, relieving pressure and allowing the creation of a false lumen and true lumen. The presence of an intramural hematoma without natural fenestration seems to be associated with a higher rate of events [21, 40, 41]. Therefore, fenestration using a scoring balloon aims to transform an intramural hematoma into a true dissection, reducing the pressure of the wall on the vessel lumen and improving coronary flow, thereby decreasing the chances of reocclusion. Figure 7 illustrates an example of an unstable patient treated with fenestration.

Thus, in the context of SCAD, the conservative strategy is currently used in most patients (85–88%), with good medium to long-term results [4, 21]. The long-term outcome of patients who required PCI during the acute event does not significantly differ from patients managed conservatively [4, 42]. Therefore, when clinically needed, PCI is a useful therapeutic option to improve coronary flow and myocardial perfusion in the acute setting of SCAD.

Pharmacological treatment in SCAD has been based on general recommendations for patients with atherothrombotic AMI for years. However, the lack of data in this specific clinical context, along with the recent demonstration of a different pathophysiology, leads to the absence of clear recommendations for these patients [6, 7]. One of the most controversial aspects is antiplatelet therapy. In those patients requiring stent implantation during the acute event, there is a consensus that dual antiplatelet therapy (usually with aspirin and clopidogrel) should be maintained for 12 months, followed by indefinite use of a single antiplatelet agent. However, for those patients managed conservatively, there is no definitive data. The natural evolution of the dissected artery is towards *restitutio ad integrum* and, considering that the acute primary event could be an intraparietal vessel bleeding, there are reasonable doubts regarding the need for intense and/or long-lasting antiplatelet therapy. Patient series with low-intensity and limited-duration antiplatelet therapy after the event show favorable results [13]. In patients managed conservatively, single antiplatelet therapy even seems to be associated with a lower event rate than dual antiplatelet therapy at 12 months [21, 43].

Beta-blockers have been traditionally used systematically in patients with SCAD, probably as an assimilation of the existing data in the context of aortic dissection, in addition to the overall scenario of AMI. The scientific basis for this use is limited, relying on a retrospective case-control series in which an improved prognosis was observed in patients receiving beta-blockers as long-term treatment [44]. However, prospective data from the same expanded series (in terms of size and follow-up duration) have not confirmed the protective nature of beta-blockers against recurrences in the context of SCAD [4].

Currently, the first randomized clinical trial in SCAD (ClinicalTrials.gov: NCT04850417) is in an advanced stage of recruitment [5]. The

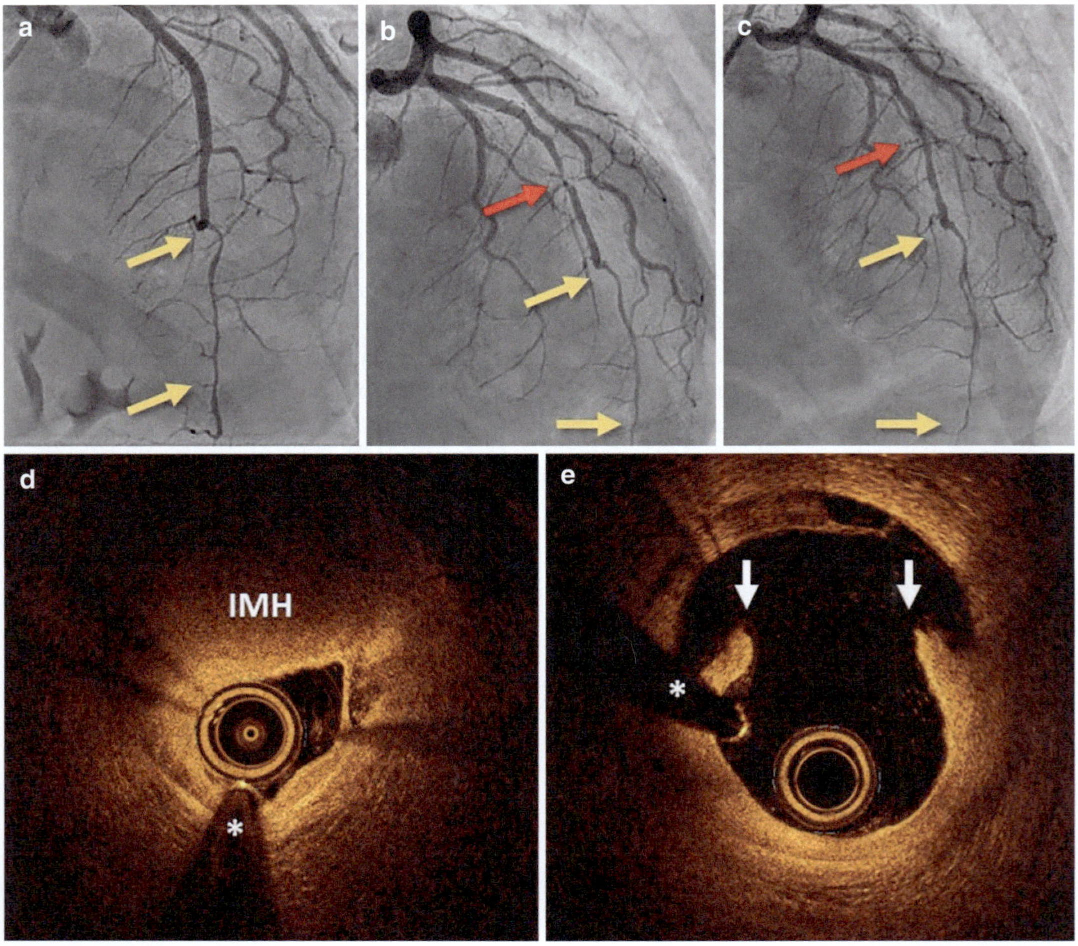

Fig. 7 Unstable SCAD patient treated with fenestration. (**a**) A 49-year-old female, former smoker, was admitted with non-ST segment elevation myocardial infarction and diagnosed with Type 2a SCAD in the distal left anterior descending artery (yellow arrows). Initial conservative management was followed by recurrent angina and an electrocardiogram showing ST elevation in the anterior region. (**b**) Repeat coronary angiography revealed a "de novo" critical stenosis (red arrow) proximal to the previously identified SCAD segment (yellow arrows). (**c**) The patient was successfully treated with fenestration using a scoring balloon (Angiosculpt® 3 mm, up to 14 bar). (**d**) Prior to treatment, OCT images displayed intramural hematoma (IMH) with critical luminal stenosis. (**e**) After fenestration, intimal-medial ruptures (white arrows) with new connection between the true lumen and the false lumen (arrows). * Denotes wire artifact

BA-SCAD (Betablockers and Antiplatelet agents in patients with SCAD) is a multicenter trial sponsored by the Spanish Society of Cardiology, pragmatic in nature, in which patients diagnosed with SCAD are randomized using a 2 × 2 factorial design. They are assigned to receive either 1 month of aspirin treatment or 12 months of dual antiplatelet therapy, and simultaneously, they may or may not receive beta-blocker treatment. Prior to inclusion, each case undergoes individualized assessment by a centralized Core Lab that confirms the diagnosis of SCAD. The primary endpoint is a combination of events at 1-year follow-up (death, myocardial infarction, stroke, coronary revascularization, recurrent SCAD, hospitalization due to acute coronary syndrome or heart failure). Undoubtedly, this study will substantially expand our knowledge regarding the optimal treatment of SCAD, marking a turning point in the quality of scientific evidence in this regard.

A small study suggested a higher risk of recurrent SCAD associated with statins treatment, which has not been confirmed in large prospective series [3, 4, 45]. In general, statin therapy should be reserved for patients who have an indication according to the general recommendations for primary prevention, concomitant atherosclerotic coronary artery disease or diabetes mellitus, regardless of the SCAD event [6, 7].

5.1 Prognosis and Follow-Up

The prognosis of SCAD is generally favorable [4, 21]. In-hospital events are low (6–8%), with in-hospital mortality rates in recent series ranging from 0.1% to 1.8%. Most events occur within the first 15 days of the evolution, and in the case of reinfarction, it is usually related to the extension of the previous dissection. It is rare to have a new dissection in another vessel and/or coronary segment during the acute phase. The recurrence of symptoms leading to readmissions, particularly in the early days after discharge, is also common. This supports the empirical recommendation to extend hospital stay beyond 3 days [6, 7]. Furthermore, adjusted comparative results derived from administrative databases suggest that there are no significant differences in terms of in-hospital mortality and readmission between patients with AMI due to SCAD and patients with atherothrombotic etiology [46].

Once the acute phase has passed and the healing process of the arterial wall has completed, the prognosis will largely be determined by the permanent myocardial damage resulting from the acute event. In this regard, patients with ventricular systolic dysfunction have a worse prognosis, with higher mortality and readmission rates due to heart failure [47].

Previous reports show a high risk of recurrence of SCAD: Kaplan-Meier estimated rate of 27% at 5 years [37]. Contemporary series have dramatically decreased this figure: at 3 years follow-up time, SCAD recurrences are only 2%. However, overall events are common (13–14%), indicating that these patients will require meticulous and specialized follow-up [4, 21]. It is highly frequent for patients to experience chest pain, either stable or as a visit to the emergency department. In addition to ruling out a new event, it is important to consider other possible causes of chest pain, including other coronary etiologies, especially the concomitant presence of microvascular dysfunction [48].

As mentioned before, to date, there is no treatment that has proven to prevent recurrences [6, 7]. Therefore, long-term treatment will be directed towards concomitant diseases and possible sequelae resulting from the primary event (stent implantation, systolic dysfunction, arrhythmias, etc.). Inclusion in cardiac rehabilitation programs has shown benefits in terms of chest pain symptoms, exercise capacity, and psychosocial well-being, which is of utmost importance in this condition with a high prevalence of anxiety and depression disorders and emotional triggers [49, 50].

Albeit not fully elucidated, given the stablished relationship between exogenous hormone exposure and SCAD, there is a consensus on discontinuation of hormone replacement therapy and avoidance of hormonal contraception. In this regard, barrier methods, surgical options (vasectomy and tubal ligation), and intrauterine devices with local progestogen release are the preferred choices [6, 7]. Much more controversial is the possibility of pregnancy after experiencing SCAD: although traditionally discouraged, such a significant decision in a woman's and her partner's life should be undertaken after careful and individualized counseling. Recently, encouraging data have been published in this regard. An Eurpean series of 37 pregnancies in patients with a history of SCAD has been reported, with three new episodes occurring (8%), but no related deaths [23]. Moreover, from the United States, in a large series of 636 surviving SCAD patients, recurrences related to new pregnancies (32 pregnancies) were analyzed, and no significant differences were found in the number of recurrences compared to those outside of pregnancy [51]. These new data should be taken into account and discussed with patients for informed and updated decision-making.

5.2 Fibromuscular Dysplasia Work Up

Systematic and comprehensive screening for FMD and other extracoronary vascular anomalies is recommended in every patient who has suffered SCAD [6, 7]. Pathological findings are observed in about 50% of patients, although series with complete and nearly universal screening report even higher figures [4, 13]. The clinical significance of these findings is unknown, often showing only mild vascular wall alterations, which should be considered mere 'stigma' of FMD, without functional repercussion [52]. In fact, extracardiac vascular events in the follow-up of patients appear to be uncommon [53], and, except for older age, no clinical, angiographic, or short-to-medium-term prognostic differences (1-year follow-up) have been observed between patients with SCAD and FMD and those without it [54]. So, why should we screen for FMD in patients with SCAD? Reasons for conducting the screening are: (a) the diagnosis of SCAD is often complex, and in cases of diagnostic doubt, the presence of FMD can be crucial in confirming it [55]; (b) knowledge of structural wall alterations can be useful for the diagnosis and treatment of potential future extracardiac vascular events; (c) the finding of intracranial aneurysms is not negligible (6–9% of patients in series with high rates of complete screening [4, 13, 53]), with the potential risk of morbidity and mortality that this condition may entail.

The screening can be initiated, if the clinical situation allows, during the initial invasive coronary angiography, by selective injection into both renal and iliac arteries. Invasive angiography has been shown to be more sensitive than computed tomography angiography [56]. However, the latter is the most used modality due to its non-invasive nature, the possibility of performing it at any stage of evolution, and the ability to study all territories in a single procedure, exploring intracranial vessels, supra-aortic trunks, renal arteries, splanchnic territory, and iliofemoral axis with a single scan [57]. Magnetic resonance imaging, due to its non-invasive nature and absence of ionizing radiation, is another attractive option. It has lower spatial resolution, which may explain why series in which it has been used for screening found a lower prevalence of FMD in patients with SCAD than previously described [53, 58]. Future research is needed to clarify whether this lower sensitivity is truly relevant in the management of these patients and whether it can be accepted to reduce radiation exposure.

6 Conclusions

SCAD is an emerging disease, a cause of AMI with distinct pathophysiology and treatments. With the current information, we should be able to recognize it and apply differential principles in its management. Future and ongoing research will provide crucial data, particularly regarding the treatment and follow-up of these patients.

Key Issues

- SCAD should always be considered as a differential diagnosis of any ACS, especially if the epidemiological context is appropriate.
- The diagnosis is multimodal: clinical presentation and baseline characteristics, angiographic findings, intravascular imaging, presence of extracoronary vascular anomalies, location of fibrosis patterns in magnetic resonance imaging, and even verification of healing in the follow-up.
- Conservative expectant management, if the clinical situation allows, usually yields good results. If intervention is necessary, PCI is the preferred option. In this setting, intracoronary imaging could be used, increasing safety and optimizing outcomes.
- To date, there is no clearly recommended pharmacological treatment option. The first randomized clinical trial in this regard is currently underway.
- The management following an episode of SCAD is multidisciplinary, not forgetting the high prevalence of associated anxiety and depressive disorders, as well as the psychosocial factors that may influence the course of the disease.

- Comprehensive and systematic screening for FMD and other extracoronary vascular anomalies is recommended for all patients.

Questions and Answers

1. Which of the following conditions is NOT commonly found in patients suffering from SCAD?
   (A) Migraine
   (B) Hypothyroidism
   (C) Fibromuscular dysplasia
   (D) Aortic aneurysm
   Correct answer: D
   It has been established, through multiple registries, that migraine, thyroid disorders (especially hypothyroidism), and fibromuscular dysplasia are more frequently observed than usual in SCAD patients. It is worth noting that fibromuscular dysplasia primarily affects medium-sized arteries (such as renal and iliac arteries) and is not typically associated with aortic aneurysms.
2. In the context of diagnosing SCAD, please identify the INCORRECT statement:
   (A) Invasive coronary angiography is the gold standard.
   (B) In SCAD Type 3 according to the Saw classification, the use of intracoronary imaging should be considered to ensure an unequivocal diagnosis.
   (C) The finding of renal and/or iliac fibromuscular dysplasia during coronary angiography can be crucial for diagnosis in cases of SCAD Type 2 with an unfavorable epidemiological background.
   (D) A highly sensitive and specific non-invasive alternative to coronary angiography is the performance of CCTA.
   Correct answer: D
   The role of CCTA has been explored in the acute context of SCAD, showing limited sensitivity (1 in 5 SCAD cases were not detected). Therefore, coronary angiography continues to be the gold standard in diagnosis. Performing selective renal and iliac angiography during the same procedure can be highly supportive in diagnosis, especially if fibromuscular dysplasia is found in doubtful cases. The role of intracoronary imaging is particularly relevant in SCAD Type 3 cases, those that by definition resemble atherosclerotic disease (focal lesions <20 mm), and definitive exclusion of atherosclerosis and confirmation of SCAD can only be achieved through OCT or IVUS.
3. In the treatment of SCAD, please select the CORRECT option:
   (A) Like any acute coronary syndrome, the role of dual antiplatelet therapy is well established and, unless contraindicated, should be maintained for at least 12 months in all patients.
   (B) Beta-blockers have been shown to be crucial in preventing further SCAD events.
   (C) In cases of hemodynamic instability, outcomes obtained through CABG revascularization are highly promising and sustained in the long term.
   (D) Most patients can be managed without intervention, through an expectant approach, with good short and long-term results.
   Correct answer: D
   The preferred approach in the context of SCAD is medical management with an expectant attitude, except in selected cases. This is because most patients have a good outcome, interventions in SCAD context have often suboptimal results and do not prevent future SCAD episodes. Really, CABG has shown a low long-term patency rate due to technical challenges in this context and competitive flow to the bypass from the native artery once it heals. To date, there are no clinical trials that have shown which pharmacological strategy is ideal in the SCAD context. In fact, there are some data suggesting that dual antiplatelet therapy may be associated with a higher rate of events.

References

1. Pretty H. Dissecting aneurysms of coronary artery in woman aged 42: rupture. BMJ. 1931;1:667.
2. Alfonso F, Bastante T. Spontaneous coronary artery dissection: novel diagnostic insights from large series of patients. Circ Cardiovasc Interv. 2014;7(5):638–41.

3. García-Guimaraes BT, Macaya F, et al. Spontaneous coronary artery dissection in Spain: clinical and angiographic characteristics, management, and in-hospital events. Rev Esp Cardiol (Engl Ed). 2021;74(1):15–23.
4. Saw J, Starovoytov A, Aymong E, et al. Canadian spontaneous coronary artery dissection cohort study: 3-year outcomes. J Am Coll Cardiol. 2022;80(17):1585–97.
5. Alfonso F, de la Torre Hernández JM, Ibáñez B, et al. Rationale and design of the BA-SCAD (beta-blockers and antiplatelet agents in patients with spontaneous coronary artery dissection) randomized clinical trial. Rev Esp Cardiol (Eng Ed). 2022;75(6):515–22.
6. Adlam D, Alfonso F, Maas A, et al. European Society of Cardiology, Acute Cardiovascular Care Association, SCAD Study Group: a position paper on spontaneous coronary artery dissection. Eur Heart J. 2018;39(36):3353–68.
7. Hayes SN, Kim CESH, Saw J, et al. Spontaneous coronary artery dissection: current state of the science: a scientific statement from the American Heart Association. Circulation. 2018;137(19):e523–57.
8. Jackson R, Al-Hussaini A, Joseph S, et al. Spontaneous coronary artery dissection. Pathophysiological insights from optical coherence tomography. JACC Cardiovasc Imaging. 2019;12:2475–88.
9. Tweet M, Miller V, Hayes S. The evidence of estrogen, progesterone and spontaneous coronary artery dissection. JAMA Cardiol. 2019;4(5):403–4.
10. Henkin S, Negrotto SM, Tweet MS, et al. Spontaneous coronary artery dissection and its association with heritable connective tissue disorders. Heart. 2016;102:876–81.
11. Adlam D, Olson TM, Combaret N, et al. Association of the PHACTR1/EDN1 genetic locus with spontaneous coronary artery dissection. J Am Coll Cardiol. 2019;73:58–66.
12. Goel K, Tweet M, Olson T, et al. Familial spontaneous coronary artery dissection. JAMA Intern Med. 2015;175(5):821–6.
13. Bastante T, García-Guimaraes M, Muñiz M, et al. Contemporary management of spontaneous coronary dissection. REC Interv Cardiol. 2020;2(4):247–55.
14. McAlister C, Alfadhel M, Samuel R, et al. Differences in demographics and outcomes between men and women with spontaneous coronary artery dissection. J Am Coll Cardiol Intv. 2022;15(20):2052–61.
15. Alvarado T, García-Guimaraes M, Nogales JM, et al. Spontaneous coronary artery dissection: are there differences between men and women? Arq Bras Cardiol. 2023;120(1):e20210550.
16. Alfonso F, Bastante T. Spontaneous coronary artery dissection in men. So rare? So different? J Am Coll Cardiol Intv. 2022;15(20):2062–5.
17. Bassi S, Gearhart A, Sanders S, et al. 2 Cases of spontaneous coronary artery dissection in neonates. JACC Case Rep. 2023;6:1–4.
18. Choi J, Yang C, Saw J. Atherosclerotic spontaneous coronary artery dissection. JACC Case Rep. 2023;10:1–6.
19. Kok S, Hayes S, Cutrer M, et al. Prevalence and clinical factors of migraine in patients with spontaneous coronary artery dissection. J Am Heart Assoc. 2018;7(24):e010140.
20. Camacho-Freire S, Díaz Fernández J, Luciana L, et al. Spontaneous coronary artery dissection and hypothyroidism. Rev Esp Cardiol (Engl Ed). 2019;72(8):625–33.
21. García-Guimaraes M, Masotti M, Sanz-Ruiz R, et al. Clinical outcomes in spontaneous coronary artery dissection. Heart. 2022;108:1530–8.
22. Murphy B, Rogerson M, Hesselson S, et al. Prevalence of anxiety, depression, and distress in SCAD and non-SCAD AMI patients. J Cardiopulm Rehabil Prev. 2023;43(5):338–45. https://doi.org/10.1097/HCR.0000000000000782.
23. Chan N, Premawardhana D, Al-Hussaini A, et al. Pregnancy and spontaneous coronary artery dissection: lessons from survivors and nonsurvivors. Circulation. 2022;146:69–72.
24. Alfonso F, Paulo M, Gonzalo N, et al. Diagnosis of spontaneous coronary artery dissection by optical coherence tomography. J Am Coll Cardiol. 2012;59(12):1073–9.
25. Saw J. Coronary angiogram classification of spontaneous coronary artery dissection. Catheter Cardiovasc Interv. 2014;84:115–1122.
26. Eleid M, Guddeti R, Tweet M, et al. Coronary artery tortuosity in spontaneous coronary artery dissection. Circ Cardiovas Interv. 2014;7:656–62.
27. Motreff P, Malcles G, Combaret N, et al. How and when to suspect spontaneous coronary artery dissection: novel insights from a single-centre series on prevalence and angiographic appearance. EuroIntervention. 2017;12:e2236–43.
28. Alfonso F. Spontaneous coronary artery dissection: new insights from the tip of the iceberg? Circulation. 2012;126:667–70.
29. Alfonso F, Sanz-Ruiz R, Sabate M, et al. Clinical implications of the "broken-line" angiographic pattern in patients with spontaneous coronary artery dissection. Am J Cardiol. 2022;185:1–9.
30. Prakash R, Starovoytov A, Heydari M, et al. Catheter-induced iatrogenic coronary artery dissection in patients with spontaneous coronary artery dissection. JACC Cardiov Interv. 2016;9(17):1851–7.
31. Pozo-Osinalde E, García-Guimaraes M, Bastante T, et al. Characteristics findings of acute spontaneous coronary artery dissection by cardiac computed tomography. Coron Artery Dis. 2020;31(3):293–9.
32. Tweet M, Akhtar N, Hayes S, et al. Spontaneous coronary artery dissection: acute findings on coronary computed tomography angiography. Eur Heart J Acute Cardiovasc Care. 2019;8(5):467–75.
33. Roura G, Ariza-Solé A, Rodriguez-Caballero IF, et al. Noninvasive follow-up of patients with spontaneous coronary artery dissection with CT angiography. JACC Cardiovasc Imaging. 2016;9:896–7.
34. Chandrasekhar J, Thakkar J, Starovoytov A. Characteristics of spontaneous coronary artery

dissection on cardiac magnetic resonance imaging. Cardiovasc Diagn Ther. 2020;10(3):636–8.
35. Kubota N, Ozaki K, Tanabe Y, et al. Usefulness of repeat angiography to establish spontaneous coronary artery dissection in small vessels. Circ Rep. 2020;2:739–43.
36. Lozano-Prieto M, Adlam D, et al. Differential miRNAs in acute spontaneous coronary artery dissection: pathophysiological insights from a potential biomarker. EBioMedicine. 2020;66:103338.
37. Tweet M, Eleid M, Best P, et al. Spontaneous coronary artery dissection: revascularization versus conservative therapy. Circ Cardiovasc Interv. 2014;7:777–86.
38. Saw J, Starovoytov A, Humphries K, et al. Canadian spontaneous coronary artery dissection cohort study: in-hospital and 30-day outcomes. Eur Heart J. 2019;40(15):1188–97.
39. Bastante T, Rivero F, Cuesta J, et al. Treatment of spontaneous coronary artery dissection with fenestration: clinical and angiographic follow-up. Rev Esp Cardiol (Engl Ed). 2022;75(2):177–9.
40. Waterbury T, Tweet M, Hayes S, et al. Early natural history of spontaneous coronary artery dissection. Circ Cardiovasc Interv. 2018;11:e006772.
41. Mori R, Macaya F, Giacobbe F, et al. Clinical outcomes by angiographic type of spontaneous coronary artery dissection. EuroIntervention. 2021;17:516–24.
42. García-Guimaraes M, Fuertes-Ferre G, Jiménez-Valero S, et al. Characteristics, acute results, an prognostic impact of percutaneous coronary interventions in spontaneous coronary artery dissection (from the Prospective Spanish Registry on SCAD [SR-SCAD]). Am J Cardiol. 2022;171:177–8.
43. Cerrato E, Giacobbe F, Quadri G, et al. Antiplatelet therapy in patients with conservatively managed spontaneous coronary artery dissection from the multicentre DISCO registry. Eur Heart J. 2021;42:3161–71.
44. Saw J, Humphries K, Aymong E, et al. Spontaneous coronary artery dissection. Clinical outcomes and risk of recurrence. J Am Coll Cardiol. 2017;70:1148–58.
45. Tweet MS, Hayes SN, Pitta SR, et al. Clinical features, management, and prognosis of spontaneous coronary artery dissection. Circulation. 2012;126:579–88.
46. Alfonso F, Fernández-Pérez C, García-Márquez M, et al. Spontaneous coronary artery dissection in Spain: a study using the minimum data set of the Spanish National Health System. Rev Esp Cardiol (Eng Ed). 2022;75(11):903–10.
47. Díez-Villanueva P, García-Guimaraes M, Sanz-Ruiz R, et al. Prognostic implications of left ventricular systolic dysfunction in patients with spontaneous coronary artery dissection. Eur Heart J Acute Cardiovasc Care. 2023;12(5):299–305.
48. Sedlak T, Starovoytov A, Humphries K, et al. Coronary flow reserve in patients with prior spontaneous coronary artery dissection and recurrent angina. J An Heart Assoc. 2020;9(16):e015834.
49. Chou AY, Prakash R, Rajala J, et al. The first dedicated cardiac rehabilitation program for patients with spontaneous coronary artery dissection. Can J Cardiol. 2016;32:554–60.
50. Krittanawong C, Tweet MS, Hayes SE, et al. Usefulness of cardiac rehabilitation after spontaneous coronary artery dissection. Am J Cardiol. 2016;117:1604–9.
51. Tweet MS, Young KA, Best PJM, et al. Association of pregnancy with recurrence of spontaneous coronary artery dissection among women with prior coronary artery dissection. JAMA Netw Open. 2020;3(9):e2018170.
52. Bastante T, Rivero F, Cuesta J, et al. Association of spontaneous coronary artery dissection with fibromuscular dysplasia. Rev Esp Cardiol (Engl Ed). 2015;68(8):719–20.
53. Persu A, Lopez-Sublet M, Al-Hussaini A, et al. Prevalence and disease spectrum of extracoronary arterial abnormalities in spontaneous coronary artery dissection. JAMA Cardiol. 2022;7(2):159–66.
54. Combaret N, Liabot Q, Deiri M, et al. Characteristics and prognosis of patients with fibromuscular dysplasia in a population of spontaneous coronary artery dissections (from the French Registry of Spontaneous Coronary Artery Dissections "DISCO"). Am J Cardiol. 2022;175:38–43.
55. Bastante T, García-Guimaraes M, Rivero F, et al. Isolated septal branch lesion as the only diagnostic clue for spontaneous coronary artery dissection. Coron Artery Dis. 2020;31:98–9.
56. Rayner-Harley E, Verma T, Sarovoytov A, et al. Catheter-based angiography versus CT angiography for the diagnosis of extracoronary fibromuscular dysplasia in patients with spontaneous coronary artery dissection. Cardiovasc Diagn Ther. 2021;11(1):142–5.
57. Liang JJ, Prasad M, Tweet MS, et al. A novel application of CT angiography to detect extracoronary vascular abnormalities in patients with spontaneous coronary artery dissection. J Cardiovasc Comput Tomogr. 2014;8:189–97.
58. Andrulakis E, Azzu A, Papagkikas P, et al. Spontaneous coronary artery dissection: insights from cardiac magnetic resonance and extracoronary arterial screening. Circulation. 2022;145:555–7.

Atrial Fibrillation in Women

Amelie H. Ohlrogge and Renate B. Schnabel

Abstract

Atrial fibrillation (AF) is the most prevalent clinically relevant cardiac arrhythmia in women and men. The disease is associated with increased morbidity, in particular due to ischemic stroke and heart failure, and mortality. AF incidence and prevalence are lower in women than in men. The lifetime risk of AF is estimated to be up to 30% and higher for both sexes. The evidence regarding underlying risk factors and relevant comorbidities of AF in women versus men is conflicting. Women with AF are more symptomatic and report a lower quality of life than men. Their risk for complications, in particular ischemic stroke, is higher in conjunction with comorbidities. The biological principles underlying these sex differences are insufficiently understood. Differences in treatment can be observed, e.g. less rhythm control treatment in women. Treatment should be guided by the ABC (**A**void stroke, **B**etter symptom management, **C**ardiovascular and comorbidity risk reduction) pathway. The higher ischemic stroke risk and higher symptom burden of women should be considered. In conclusion, physicians should be aware of sex differences between men and women in AF risk, manifestation, and treatment to appropriately address the specific needs and risks.

Keywords

Atrial fibrillation · Stroke · Heart failure · ABC pathway

Test your learning and check your understanding of this book's contents: use the "Springer Nature Flashcards" app to access questions using ▶ https://sn.pub/51ny7m To use the app, please follow the instructions in chapter 1.

A. H. Ohlrogge (✉) · R. B. Schnabel
Department of Cardiology, University Heart and Vascular Centre Hamburg, Hamburg, Germany

German Centre for Cardiovascular Research (DZHK), Partner Site Hamburg/Kiel/Lübeck, Hamburg, Germany
e-mail: a.ohlrogge@uke.de; r.schnabel@uke.de

A. H.E.M. Maas, E. Gerdts (eds.), *Manual of Cardiovascular Disease in Women*,
https://doi.org/10.1007/978-3-031-65952-2_22

1 Introduction

Atrial fibrillation (AF) is the most frequent clinically relevant arrhythmia in women and men. It is associated with increased morbidity, especially due to ischemic stroke and heart failure, and mortality. The prevalence has been steadily increasing over the past decades [1] and the lifetime risk is estimated to be up to 1 in 3 in women and men [2].

The underlying pathophysiology of AF is complex. In the often-used simplified model, initially, there are irregular electric signals from the pulmonary veins that cause fast and uncoordinated atrial activation with ineffective atrial contractions and consecutively irregular ventricular activation, which is seen in the electrocardiogram (ECG) as irregular R-R-intervals and absence of p-waves. Over time, this impairs the atria themselves in structure, contractility and electrophysiology, which is described by the term "atrial cardiomyopathy" [3]. In these remodelled atria the arrhythmia perpetuates itself. During this natural disease progression, the pattern of AF changes from paroxysmal (termination within 7 days) to persistent (sustained AF for ≥7 days) to long-standing persistent (sustained AF for ≥12 month). Adequate treatment has the potential to decelerate or halt this disease progression.

The following chapter is focused on AF in women. The evidence on such sex or gender differences is often conflicting for numerous reasons. Firstly, publication bias may be present, leading to a single-sided tendency in published reports. Secondly, some articles on sex-differences are sub-analyses from trials that–even when pre-specified–have limited statistical power to detect such differences and might thus be vulnerable for noise or non-significant results. Lastly, the differences between cohorts in observational studies are substantial, and such results therefore need to be carefully assessed. Furthermore, whereas sex differences have increasingly come into the focus of research, gender differences have been more commonly reported.

2 Theory

2.1 Epidemiology

Multiple cohort studies have consistently reported lower incidence and prevalence of AF in women compared to men, with an 50–100% lower relative risk, though the absolute numbers vary greatly depending on the examined cohort [4–8]. On average, women are older at the time of AF diagnosis than men, with the risk of AF increasing at the age of 50 years in men and at the age of 60 years in women [6, 9–14]. In the Framingham Heart Study, there was a lower AF lifetime risk for women overall and within all risk factor profiles [15]. However, due to longer life expectancy in women, the overall lifetime risk is often estimated to be similar for both sexes at up to 30% and higher [2, 16, 17].

2.2 Comorbidities and Risk Factors

The majority of AF patients has relevant comorbidities and risk factors [18, 19]. Typical comorbidities of atrial fibrillation include obesity, arterial hypertension, heart failure and sleep apnoea. Other lifestyle factors that are important include excessive alcohol consumption and lack of physical activity.

The evidence regarding the underlying risk factors and comorbidities of AF in women versus men is conflicting. Whereas some studies reported no significant differences between the prevalence of comorbidities [20], other studies have found different comorbidities and a higher risk factor burden in women with AF, especially for hypertension and renal impairment [9, 12, 21–23], but also valvular, particularly mitral valve disease [13, 24–27]. In contrast, other studies report more favourable risk factor profiles in women [2, 15, 28, 29]. Notably, coronary artery disease is commonly reported to be less prevalent among women with AF [2, 9, 21, 23, 27].

The lifetime risk of AF is lower for women that for men within identical risk factor profiles

[15]. Body mass index (BMI) has been found to be a stronger risk factor for incident AF in men than in women [2, 30], whereas the association between hypertension and AF is higher in women compared to men [31]. Among >25,000 participants (51% women) in the VITAL study, women were at a greater risk of incident AF compared to men when adjusting for weight and height instead of BMI, suggesting a large impact of differences in body size for the observed differences between men and women. In the REGARDS study, the observed differences of AF risk between men and women were explained by the differential distribution of risk factors [32]. For women, the increase in lifetime risk of AF by a worsening in risk factor profiles is smaller than for men [15]. Mixed findings have been reported regarding sex differences in the association between AF and different biomarkers [2, 30, 33].

2.3 Symptoms

Women have repeatedly been reported to be more often and more severely symptomatic from AF compared to men [14, 22, 28, 34–37]. In detail, the complaints that women with symptomatic AF report differ from men: They more often report symptoms such as fatigue, weakness and palpitations, but less often exercise intolerance or negative impact on sexual life [9, 13, 36, 37]. This could to some extend be explained by a higher heart rate and more tachycardic episodes in AF in women [8, 38, 39]. Also, heart failure, both heart failure with reduced ejection fraction (HFrEF) but especially heart failure with preserved ejection fraction (HFpEF) is more common amongst women than men with AF [13, 21, 23, 26, 40–43], though it should be noted that heart failure can be both a risk factor and a consequence of AF [44]. Overall, women with AF report a lower quality of life than men with AF, are more likely to be in a depressed mood and perceive their health to be lower [21, 23, 35, 36, 45, 46]. They are more likely to seek medical attention [39] and report a higher treatment burden brought on to them by AF [47].

2.4 Complications

Female sex is often described as a risk factor for developing ischemic stroke and thromboembolism (TE) in AF, especially in older women, and is prominently featured in the CHA_2DS_2-VASc-Score [9, 14, 40, 43, 48–50]. For details regarding the risk stratification and therapy to avoid ischemic stroke see Sect. 2.8 Treatment. AF is further associated with the risk of developing dementia, though evidence regarding sex differences is sparse and contradictory [51–54].

All-cause and cardiovascular mortality in women is often reported higher than in men, even after adjusting for comorbidities [40, 48, 55, 56]. Again, these findings are not unopposed, some studies show a similar [2, 57] or lower risk of mortality associated with AF in women [14, 58, 59]. A meta-analysis concluded on a higher risk of all-cause and cardiovascular mortality for women with AF [43].

2.5 Structural and Electrophysiological Changes

Women with AF and ischemic stroke had significantly higher rates of echocardiographic atrial enlargement than men [25]. Structural remodelling in the left atrium detected by echocardiography and MRI was also worse in women than in men [60]. In women undergoing catheter ablations, left atrium volume index was larger in women than in men [24, 27, 61, 62] with worse contractile dysfunction of the left atrial appendage [61]. Evidence on electrophysiological changes is more conflicting. While similar remodelling between sexes has been described [63], other studies in repeated ablation for AF found less pulmonary vein reconnections than in men, but more triggers outside the pulmonary veins and an elevated left atrial pressure [27, 64–67]. Women undergoing catheter ablation showed evidence of stronger electrophysiological remodelling in the left atrium [62, 68]. The pulmonary veins of women with longstanding persistent AF showed higher degrees of fibrosis than those in men [69].

2.6 Hormonal Differences, Pregnancy and Menopause

Though hormonal differences between men and women are often named to biologically explain the above observed differences in AF, the evidence on the influence of different sex hormones on the development of AF is relatively thin. While androgens are typically lower in women, oestrogens and progestins are higher and under the influence of the menstrual circle until menopause. The effect of each of these hormones on the cardiovascular system is complex and is further influenced by the levels of the other sex hormones [70].

AF is the most common arrhythmia during pregnancy [71]. It is rare among healthy women, though more common in the presence of pre-existing heart disease (0.3% in women without known heart disease and 2.2% in women with structural heart disease [72]). The risk further increases with maternal age. It is associated with increased rate of pregnancy complication as well as unfavourable maternal and fetal outcomes [73, 74]. Hypertensive pregnancy disorders increase the long-term risk of AF [75]. Details on the management of AF in pregnancy can be found in the ESC guideline for the management of cardiovascular diseases during pregnancy [76].

Menopausal age does not appear to affect AF risk [77, 78], but prolonged reproductive years during a women's life lowered AF risk [79]. Postmenopausal hormone replacement therapy (HRT) with oestrogen and progesterone, or oestrogen alone in patients with prior hysterectomy, was associated with a significantly increased risk of AF compared to placebo, which was mostly driven by oestrogen [80]. The risk increase by oestrogen monotherapy was confirmed in another, prospective study [78]. In a Danish observational register, HRT reduced the risk of AF in women after myocardial infarction [81], whereas prolonged HRT increased AF risk in a Korean database [79]. Two retrospective analyses of hormonal replacement therapies in Asian cohorts found a risk increase for conjugated equine oestrogens, but not for oestradiol [82, 83]. Though HRT has prothrombotic effects in other contexts, HRT did not increase adverse outcomes of AF such as ischemic stroke or systemic embolism [84].

Besides these studies examining HRT in postmenopausal women, there is little clinical evidence on the association between oestrogen and AF in women. Higher levels of plasma dehydroepiandrosterone sulfate, a precursor of both androgenic and oestrogenic sex hormones, were associated with a lower AF risk in the Rotterdam study and in an Italian cross sectional study among elderly [85, 86]. In a study only amongst men decreased levels of oestradiol were associated with an increased AF risk [87]. A protective effect an agonist of oestrogenic receptors which reduced the occurrence of Angiotensin II-induced atrial fibrosis and AF has been demonstrated in an animal model [88]. Other animal models have confirmed the influence of oestrogen on cardiac conduction [89, 90].

The effect of testosterone on the development of AF is similarly complex and not well understood. While higher levels of endogenous bioavailable testosterone increase risk of AF in men, a non-significant protective effect could be observed in women [91]. In contrast, an association of testosterone deficiency with AF in men ≥80 year was observed in the Framingham cohort [87], and testosterone replacement therapy decreases AF risk in men with low testosterone levels [92]. Women with polycystic ovary syndrome, who have raised levels of testosterone, have a doubled AF risk compared to women without polycystic ovary syndrome [93]. Individuals with either Turner syndrome (Karyotype X0) or Klinefelter syndrome (Karyotype XXY) have a higher incidence of AF than the control groups. Both syndromes are associated with decreased testosterone levels [94].

2.7 Genetic Risk

One part of the multifactorial risk for an individual to develop AF is genetically determined. In the majority of individuals these are polygenic variants that moderately increase the risk of AF. Only a minority of familial AF cases is caused by monogenic mutations. Some genes associated with AF are x-linked, which might contribute to the observed sex differences [95–97]. Several studies have tried to identify the differential risk increase depending on the sex of affected individuals in families with AF, though with either statistically non-significant or conflicting results [98–100].

2.8 Treatment

The Atrial fibrillation Better Care (ABC) pathway has been proposed to structure a holistic approach of AF treatment to reduce adverse events [101, 102], and is incorporated by the guidelines of the European Society of Cardiology [103]. It is composed of A—Anticoagulation/Avoid stroke, B—Better symptom management and C—Cardiovascular and comorbidity optimization (Fig. 1).

2.8.1 A—Anticoagulation/Avoid Stroke

AF is associated with an increased risk of ischaemic stroke and systemic thromboembolism. The annual ischemic stroke risk in patients with AF varies greatly, depending on other risk factors. To assess the risk of ischemic stroke in an individual with AF, healthcare professionals typically use the CHA_2DS_2-VASc-Score, which incorporates female sex as a risk factor of ischemic stroke. Challenging this established score, several recent studies showed either no increase in ischemic stroke risk for women [34, 59] or rather a risk modification for those at an already increased risk due to other risk factors or comorbidities. A low rate of ischemic stroke and systemic embolism in "truly low risk" women with no other risk factor besides the sex category have been demonstrated [104–107]. Thus, the CHA_2DS_2-VA-Score without sex has been proposed. It is recommended in the 2018 Australian AF Guidelines compared to the classical score [108] and may also be applied in clinical practice. Going even further, a statement from the American Heart Association and American Stroke Association calls for a women-specific risk score to close gaps in sex-specific ischemic stroke risk assessment [109].

The most common treatment option to reduce the risk of ischemic stroke in AF patients is oral anticoagulation. Vitamin K antagonists (VKA) such as warfarin were the gold standard until the introduction of direct oral anticoagulants (DOACs) more than a decade ago. DOACs have proven to be similarly efficient in stroke reduction at a lower bleeding rate in non-valvular AF, coming at higher treatment costs [110]. For patients with valvular AF (moderate or severe mitral stenosis) VKA are superior to DOACs [111]. The landmark trials that led to the approval of DOACs [112–115] showed similar efficacies (primary endpoint in all four trials was stroke or systemic embolism) in women and men, though this should be regarded cautiously, as these trials were underpowered to detect smaller sex-differences.

Several observational studies and registries have reported an underuse of adequate prescription and dosing of oral anticoagulation in women [12, 116–120], though again the evidence is inconsistent, and other reports did not detect sex differences in anticoagulation [13, 14, 121]. Temporal changes in prescription practice after the introduction of DOACs could explain these differences, one registry reported on significant improvements, closing the gap of anticoagulation prescription in women between 2011 and 2015 [122]. The residual risk of ischemic stroke for women even when prescribed anticoagulation has been reported to be higher [123–126], though other studies describe similar [127, 128] or lower [58] residual ischemic stroke risks for women on OACs. The most current meta-analysis, which was published in 2014, found the residual risk of ischemic stroke and systemic embolism in women only higher when on Vitamin-K-antagonists (VKA), not when treated with DOACs, though evidence on DOACs at that time was still sparse [129]. Women suffer from less major and intracranial bleeding under anticoagulation therapy than men [12, 124, 129].

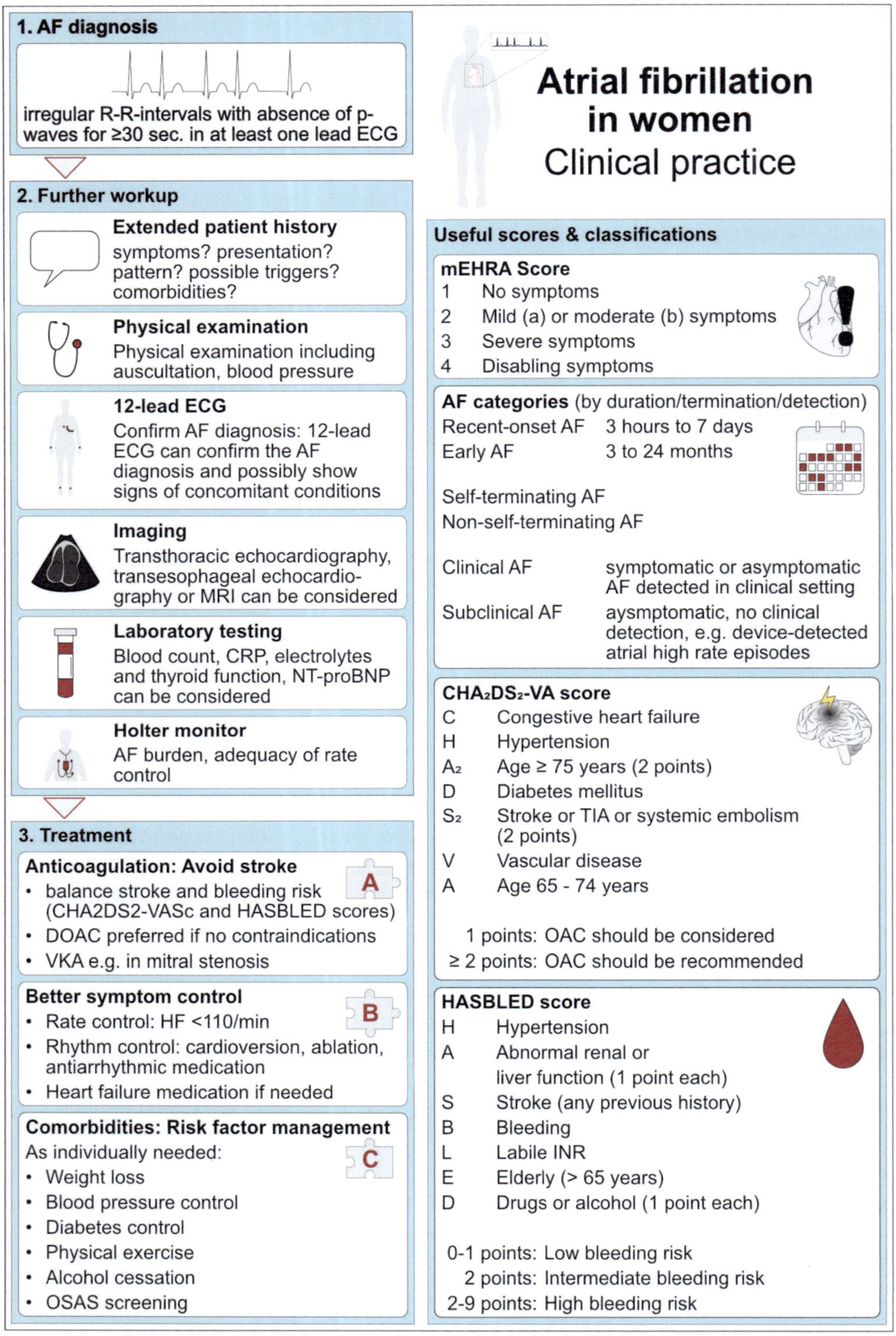

Fig. 1 Atrial fibrillation in women clinical practice

Further gaps of knowledge exist in sex differences in the pharmacokinetics of anticoagulants. On average, women significantly differ in aspects such as body weight and renal function but are underrepresented in many drug trials. When treated with a VKA, women have a lower time in therapeutic range and more over-anticoagulation episodes than men [130]. Reduced drug clearance of DOACs in women is reported inconsistently in pharmacokinetic studies, with a slightly (<25%) reduced clearance reported in a recent systematic meta-analysis [131].

2.8.2 B—Better Symptom Management

Better symptom control in AF is mainly achieved via one of two treatment strategies: rate or rhythm control. The first one usually is achieved medically, often with beta-blockers, but also calcium channel blockers and digitalis, while the latter can be achieved with antiarrhythmic medication, electrical cardioversion and/or catheter ablation. In rate control, a heart rate of below 110 beats per minute (bpm) should be targeted, lower target heart rates are not beneficial [132]. Several randomised studies have not been able detect any outcome differences between those two treatment strategies for many years [133–136]. Relatively recent results of the EAST-AFNET 4 trial showed a reduction of adverse cardiovascular events for the rhythm control group, an effect which the authors discuss to be attributable to both the early application of this strategy shortly after AF diagnosis and the synergistic effect of antiarrhythmic drugs and catheter ablation [137]. A sub-analysis of the EAST-AFNET 4 trial showed a larger benefit for patients with high comorbidity burden (CHA_2DS_2-VASc score ≥4), which had a larger proportion of women than the low comorbidity burden group (70 vs. 37%) [138]. The time window for the benefits of early rhythm control might be smaller for women than for men [139]. Catheter ablation has a benefit over medical antiarrhythmic or rate control therapy [140–142], with no differences between sexes in the CABANA trial [142], and it improves quality of life even with AF recurrence after ablation [143].

Many studies have reported on a trend towards more rate control and less rhythm control in women, especially lower rates of electrical cardioversion and catheter ablation [11, 13, 34, 35, 120, 144]. Women are referred to catheter ablation after a longer history of AF [10, 67]. Those women who undergo catheter ablation may have higher rates of procedure-related complications [22, 145–147], and they are typically older, have more comorbidities and larger atria [22, 24]. The majority of studies report higher rates of recurrence, both after first and repeated ablations for women [62, 64, 65, 67, 68, 145, 147]. This observation could be related to differences in structural and electrophysiological changes as discussed above, in particular higher rates of AF triggers originating from outside the pulmonary veins in women (see Sect. 2.5). The improvement in quality of life and cognitive function after ablation is reported similar for both sexes [10]. Women undergoing electrical cardioversion had higher cardiovascular morbidity and mortality compared with women who received rate control [148]. The use of antiarrhythmic drugs for medical rhythm control is similarly [149] or even more effective [65] in women, though there are reports of a higher proarrhythmic effect, including life threatening torsade de pointes arrhythmias [150, 151], bradyarrhythmia with need of pacemaker insertion [152] and amiodarone-induced hyperthyroidism [153]. The reasons for these observed differences in choice, complication rate and success of AF treatment are unknown, though the older age, later referral and high comorbidity burden of women could influence these outcomes. Referral bias on the side of the treating physicians and patient related biases, such as a higher unwillingness to undergo invasive procedures could also be hypothesized, though there is little evidence on this.

2.8.3 C—Cardiovascular and Comorbidity Optimization

As mentioned above, the data on the comorbidity burden between men and women with AF is conflicting. The presence of cardiovascular risk factors and comorbidities does not only affect the risk of an individual to develop AF, but also to suffer from AF progression and complications [18, 154, 155]. Obesity is associated with AF recurrence after ablation [156]. The comprehensive treatment of comorbidities can improve sinus rhythm maintenance in patients with persistent AF with or without ablation, though none of these studies reported on sex-differences [157–160].

The possibility of AF burden reduction by comorbidity management seems promising, especially since women are less likely to undergo rhythm control by medication, cardioversion or ablation, but are more symptomatic and have higher risks of complications. Reduction of blood pressure contributed largely to a reduction in AF incidence in women in the Tromsø Study [161]. As of now, there is no evidence on sex-specific benefits or downsides of this strategy.

3 Clinical Practice

3.1 AF Diagnosis

AF is diagnosed by an ECG showing irregular RR intervals at the absence of p-waves for 30 s or longer. Single-lead recordings of high quality are considered sufficient [103].

3.2 After AF Diagnosis

All patients—regardless of their sex—with a first diagnosis of AF should receive comprehensive and structured work-up to assess their (potentially reversible) causes and risk of complications. It includes a history of the symptoms, presentation, pattern and possible triggers of AF as well as comorbidities. The EHRA symptom scale can help to quantify the symptom burden (see Fig. 1). Patients should be educated about their condition. During physical examination, signs of valvular disease or heart failure can be detected. Blood pressure should be taken, if needed over 24 hours or in regular ambulatory intervals. A 12-lead ECG can confirm the AF diagnosis and possibly show signs of concomitant cardiac conditions such as coronary artery disease, left ventricular hypertrophy, or heart failure. Laboratory testing including blood count, C-reactive protein, electrolytes, and thyroid function can exclude causes such as infection, electrolyte imbalances or thyroid disorders. The natriuretic peptides can complement imaging technologies in the diagnosis of systolic or diastolic ventricular dysfunction. Lastly, transthoracic echocardiography is an important tool to understand cardiac function and structure, such as underlying valvular disease, atrial enlargement, or heart failure with reduced or preserved ejection fraction. Further investigations such as transoesophageal echocardiography, magnetic resonance imaging or computed tomography can provide additional information to this this basic assessment. Holter ECGs can be helpful in assessing AF burden and the adequacy of rate control, but also to confirm or exclude differential diagnoses.

Following the diagnostic assessment, therapeutic decisions along the ABC pathway need to be made. Female sex is a risk modifier for the occurrence of ischemic stroke and systemic embolism. There is evidence that women with no other risk factors are at a truly low risk of ischemic stroke [104–107], but the majority of patients does have such risk factors [18, 19]. The CHA_2DS_2-VA(Sc)-Score helps physicians to quantify stroke risk in AF patients, and the HASBLED score estimates the bleeding risk under anticoagulation in cases of complex decision making. Anticoagulation therapy should be considered at a CHA_2DS_2-VASc-Score of 2 and be recommended at a CHA_2DS_2-VASc-Score of ≥ 3 in women. Patients without contraindication (moderate to severe mitral stenosis or mechanical heart valves), which is the majority, should receive a DOAC due to the more favourable safety profile. Other valvular diseases besides mitral stenosis, bioprosthetic heart valves or valve repair do not pose a contraindication against DOAC use. [103].

In women, the higher symptom burden should be considered in clinical practice. AF ablation is more effective in improving quality of life than medical therapy with no significant differences between men and women [142], but as outlined above, observational studies repeatedly report less AF ablation rates in women. There is evidence of higher complication and recurrence rates for women undergoing ablation, which could be attributable to sex-specific differences in the electrophysiological changes in the atrium. From the existing evidence it is uncertain whether women would benefit from ablation therapy more often than it currently is clinical practice. Besides AF ablation, rate and rhythm control by cardioversion or antiarrhythmic medication remain valid therapeutic choices, though the short-term nature of cardioversion and the potential side effects of a long-term antiarrhythmic medication need to be considered, especially for class III antiarrhythmics like amiodarone. Heart failure medication should be started if needed.

Regardless of advanced therapeutic options, physicians should emphasize the need to address the optimal treatment of cardiovascular comorbidities and risk factors, which is best achieved in an integrated care setting.

4 Conclusions

Evidence on sex differences for AF is often conflicting, gender differences are hardly known. The lifetime risk of women to develop AF is high, though the incidence is often reported to be lower than in men. Women with AF are more symptomatic and suffer from a lower quality of life. The risk of ischemic stroke and systemic embolism in women with additional comorbidities is higher than in men. But female sex as an independent risk factor is debated. It is rather a risk modifier. The biological principles underlying these sex differences are insufficiently understood. Treatment differences, especially for rhythm control therapy can be observed. There is evidence of higher recurrence and complication rates for women undergoing cardioversion or AF ablation. How to address sex and gender differences in AF needs much more evidence. For now, all patients with AF, regardless of their sex, should undergo a comprehensive work-up and should be treated along the ABC pathway in an integrated care setting.

Key Issues

- Women have a high risk to develop AF during their lifetime, even though incidence and prevalence are lower than in men.
- Women are more symptomatic and suffer from a lower quality of life than men.
- Risk of ischemic stroke and systemic embolism is higher than in men.
- Female sex as an independent risk factor is debuted, rather a risk modifier.
- Biological principles behind these sex differences are insufficiently understood.
- Treatment differences can be observed.

Questions and Answers

1. A 58-year old woman presents with complaints of intermittent palpitations, shortness of breath and fatigue during these episodes. These episodes have been occurring for a few months and have been increasing in frequency and duration. She owns a smartwatch and has recorded a heart rate of up to 138 bpm during these episodes. This is the first time she seeks medical attention for this problem. You suspect that she has AF. Which of the following statements is correct regarding AF diagnoses?
   (A) The patient history is highly suspicious of AF, thus the diagnosis of AF should be made without further unnecessary diagnostic steps.
   (B) An irregular pulse during physical examination proofs the diagnosis of AF
   (C) If the mentioned smartwatch recording is a one-lead ECG of sufficient quality showing irregular RR intervals at the absence of p-waves for at least 30 s, the diagnoses of AF should be made.
   (D) A 12-lead ECG showing irregular RR intervals at the absence of p-waves for 30 s or longer is needed to proof the presence of AF, a one-lead ECG is not sufficient for the diagnosis of AF.

   Correct answer: C

   Neither patient history nor physical examination suffice to diagnose AF. Differential diagnoses like atrioventricular nodal re-entry tachycardia could also explain her complaints, and pulse irregularities can also be caused e.g. by atrial or ventricular premature beats. An ECG with irregular RR intervals at the absence of p-waves for at least 30 s is needed for the diagnosis of AF. However, according to the most recent 2020 ESC guidelines a single lead ECG recording suffices for AF diagnosis, if it is of high quality (see Sect. 3.1).

2. You indeed diagnose AF in this patient. It is time to consider further diagnostic work-up. Which of the following measures are least useful for a basic assessment in an AF patient?
   (A) Drawing blood samples to check for blood count, markers of inflammation, electrolytes, thyroid and kidney function.
   (B) Drawing blood samples for a hormonal status, including estrogen, progesterone and testosterone
   (C) Obtaining a 12-lead ECG to check for signs of possible concomitant conditions such as coronary artery disease.
   (D) Performing echocardiography to assess cardiac anatomy, ventricular functions and valve status.

   Correct answer: B

   A "routine" laboratory work-up ruling out acute infection, hyperthyroidism or kidney disease should be part of this initial work up, as well as an ECG and echocardiogram to assess concomitant conditions and underlying or consequential cardiac pathologies such as heart failure or valvular disease or detect atrial enlargement. Though imbalances of sexual hormones show association with AF in studies, they are not part of a basic assessment in AF patients. Even if hormonal imbalances were be detected, this would not lead to therapeutic consequences for the treatment of AF, as data on the effect of postmenopausal HRT on AF is sparse and conflicting (see Sects. 2.6 and 3.2).

3. Following AF diagnosis and basic diagnostic work-up, you plan your treatment along the ABC pathway, starting with "A–avoid stroke". The current patient reports a pre-existing hypertension, for which she is treated with ramipril, besides that there are no pre-existing medical conditions. How should she be treated with regards to ischemic stroke prevention?
   (A) She is at a very low risk of ischemic stroke, OAC should thus not be started to avoid bleeding complications.
   (B) She has an intermediately increased risk of ischemic stroke, OAC should be considered.
   (C) She has an intermediately increased risk of ischemic stroke, antiplatelet therapy should be recommended.
   (D) She is at a very high risk of ischemic stroke, OAC should be recommended.

   Correct answer: B

   The most commonly used score is the CHA_2DS_2-VASc-Score, which consists of Congestive heart failure (1 point), hypertension (1 point), Age $\geq$ 75 years (2 points), Diabetes mellitus (1 point), Stroke or TIA or systemic embolism (1 point), Vascular disease (Coronary or peripheral artery disease, aortic plaque, 1 point), Age 65–74 years (1 point), sex category (1 point for female sex). Anticoagulation therapy should be considered at a score of 2 and be recommended at a score of $\geq$3 in women. However, the criterion of female sex as an independent risk factor is debated, some argue that female sex is rather a risk modifier at the presence of other risk factors. Thus, the alternative CHA_2DS_2-VA-Score has been proposed. In either case, OAC should be considered as she has a CHA_2DS_2-VASc-Score of 2 (Hypertension, sex category) or a CHA_2DS_2-VA-Score of 1 (Hypertension). Antiplatelet therapy is not an alternative to OAC in patients with AF (see Sect. 2.8.1).

4. After avoiding stroke you want continue to improve your patient's symptoms, which is step "B–better symptom control" of the ABC pathway. Which of the following statements is true?
   (A) Rate and rhythm control should always be pursued simultaneously to ensure optimal symptom control for your patient.
   (B) In rate control strategy, the heart rate should be below 90 bpm at all times to

avoid consequential tachycardia-induced heart failure.
(C) Pulmonary vein isolation should be pursued in women more than in men, since women have higher success rates after ablation than men.
(D) Pulmonary vein isolation has benefits over medical therapy, though the complication rates in women are higher.

Correct answer: D

If rhythm control is successfully achieved, the patient is in sinus rhythm and usually does not require rate control anymore. Therefore, these strategies would not usually be applied simultaneously. However, exceptions exists and sequential combinations of both strategies may be useful in clinical practice, for example: A patient who has initially decided to choose rate control may be referred for rhythm control, if symptoms persist under this therapy; or a patient who is planned for rhythm control via ablation but is not eligible for medical antiarrhythmic therapy may be treated with rate control to bridge the waiting time for the procedure. If rate control is pursued, the goal is a heart rate below 110 bpm at rest, heart rate may be higher during exercise. Stricter heart rate targets do not show a benefit. Pulmonary vein isolation has lower success rates in women than in men, at higher rates of complications. Still, studies have shown a benefit over medical therapy (see Sect. 2.8.2).

5. Lastly, your treatment plan focuses on "C-Cardiovascular and comorbidity optimization". As mentioned before, your patient has known hypertension and is treated with ramipril. Further, she has a BMI of 31.6 kg/m^2 and reports intense snoring during her sleep and increase fatigue during daytime. Which of the following statements is least true?
(A) As the treatment burden of patients with newly diagnosed AF is already high, comorbidity treatment should be delayed to not overwhelm patients and improve adherence.
(B) Women with AF have on average a higher comorbidity burden than men.
(C) Work-up should include intensified blood pressure measurements and screening for obstructive sleep apnoea.
(D) Cardiovascular risk factors and comorbidities increase the risk of AF progression and complications.

Correct answer: A

Even though patients are confronted with a high treatment burden at the first diagnosis of AF, comorbidity treatment should not be disregarded. The comprehensive treatment of comorbidities can improve sinus rhythm maintenance in patients with persistent AF with or without ablation. The other three statements are true (see Sect. 2.8.3).

References

1. Chugh SS, Havmoeller R, Narayanan K, Singh D, Rienstra M, Benjamin EJ, et al. Worldwide epidemiology of atrial fibrillation: a global burden of disease 2010 study. Circulation. 2014;129(8):837–47.
2. Magnussen C, Niiranen TJ, Ojeda FM, Gianfagna F, Blankenberg S, Njølstad I, et al. Sex differences and similarities in atrial fibrillation epidemiology, risk factors, and mortality in community cohorts: results from the BiomarCaRE Consortium (Biomarker for Cardiovascular Risk Assessment in Europe). Circulation. 2017;136(17):1588–97.
3. Goette A, Kalman JM, Aguinaga L, Akar J, Cabrera JA, Chen SA, et al. EHRA/HRS/APHRS/SOLAECE expert consensus on atrial cardiomyopathies: definition, characterization, and clinical implication. EP Eur. 2016;18(10):1455–90.
4. Stewart S, Hart CL, Hole DJ, McMurray JJV. Population prevalence, incidence, and predictors of atrial fibrillation in the Renfrew/Paisley study. Heart. 2001;86(5):516.
5. Miyasaka Y. Secular trends in incidence of atrial fibrillation in Olmsted County, Minnesota, 1980 to 2000, and implications on the projections for future prevalence. Circulation. 2006;114(2):119–25.
6. Schnabel RB, Yin X, Gona P, Larson MG, Beiser AS, McManus DD, et al. 50 year trends in atrial fibrillation prevalence, incidence, risk factors, and mortality in the Framingham Heart Study: a cohort study. Lancet. 2015;386(9989):154–62.
7. Renoux C, Patenaude V, Suissa S. Incidence, mortality, and sex differences of non-valvular atrial fibrillation: a population-based study. J Am Heart Assoc. 2014;3(6):e001402.
8. Tan JL, Johnson L, Dziubinski M, Napiorkowski N, Witkowska O, Slusarczyk ME, et al. Sex differences in presentation of atrial fibrillation: findings

from 30-day ambulatory monitoring in real-world practice. Am Heart J Plus Cardiol Res Pract. 2022;22:100208.
9. Ball J, Carrington MJ, Wood KA, Stewart S, The SAFETY Investigators. Women versus men with chronic atrial fibrillation: insights from the standard versus atrial fibrillation spEcific managemenT studY (SAFETY). PLoS One. 2013;8(5):e65795.
10. Kloosterman M, Chua W, Fabritz L, Al-Khalidi HR, Schotten U, Nielsen JC, et al. Sex differences in catheter ablation of atrial fibrillation: results from AXAFA-AFNET 5. EP Eur. 2020;22(7):1026–35.
11. Noubiap JJ, Thomas G, Agbaedeng TA, Fitzgerald JL, Gallagher C, Middeldorp ME, et al. Sex differences in clinical profile, management, and outcomes of patients hospitalized for atrial fibrillation in the United States. Eur Heart J Qual Care Clin Outcomes. 2022;8(8):852–60.
12. Yong CM, Tremmel JA, Lansberg MG, Fan J, Askari M, Turakhia MP. Sex differences in oral anticoagulation and outcomes of stroke and intracranial bleeding in newly diagnosed atrial fibrillation. J Am Heart Assoc. 2020;9(10):e015689.
13. Lip GYH, Laroche C, Boriani G, Cimaglia P, Dan GA, Santini M, et al. Sex-related differences in presentation, treatment, and outcome of patients with atrial fibrillation in Europe: a report from the Euro Observational Research programme pilot survey on atrial fibrillation. EP Eur. 2015;17(1):24–31.
14. Piccini JP, Simon DN, Steinberg BA, Thomas L, Allen LA, Fonarow GC, et al. Differences in clinical and functional outcomes of atrial fibrillation in women and men: two-year results from the ORBIT-AF Registry. JAMA Cardiol. 2016;1(3):282–91.
15. Staerk L, Wang B, Preis SR, Larson MG, Lubitz SA, Ellinor PT, et al. Lifetime risk of atrial fibrillation according to optimal, borderline, or elevated levels of risk factors: cohort study based on longitudinal data from the Framingham Heart Study. BMJ. 2018;361:k1453.
16. Heeringa J, van der Kuip DAM, Hofman A, Kors JA, van Herpen G, Stricker BHC, et al. Prevalence, incidence and lifetime risk of atrial fibrillation: the Rotterdam study. Eur Heart J. 2006;27(8):949–53.
17. Lloyd-Jones DM, Wang TJ, Leip EP, Larson MG, Levy D, Vasan RS, et al. Lifetime risk for development of atrial fibrillation. Circulation. 2004;110(9):1042–6.
18. Kim EJ, Yin X, Fontes JD, Magnani JW, Lubitz SA, McManus DD, et al. Atrial fibrillation without comorbidities: prevalence, incidence and prognosis (from the Framingham Heart Study). Am Heart J. 2016;177:138–44.
19. LaMori JC, Mody SH, Gross HJ, daCosta DiBonaventura M, Patel AA, Schein JR, et al. Burden of comorbidities among patients with atrial fibrillation. Ther Adv Cardiovasc Dis. 2013;7(2):53–62.
20. Siddiqi HK, Vinayagamoorthy M, Gencer B, Ng C, Pester J, Cook NR, et al. Sex differences in atrial fibrillation risk: the VITAL Rhythm Study. JAMA Cardiol. 2022;7(10):1027–35.
21. Dagres N, Nieuwlaat R, Vardas PE, Andresen D, Lévy S, Cobbe S, et al. Gender-related differences in presentation, treatment, and outcome of patients with atrial fibrillation in Europe: a report from the Euro heart survey on atrial fibrillation. J Am Coll Cardiol. 2007;49(5):572–7.
22. Grecu M, Blomström-Lundqvist C, Kautzner J, Laroche C, Van Gelder IC, Jordaens L, et al. In-hospital and 12-month follow-up outcome from the ESC-EORP EHRA atrial fibrillation ablation long-term registry: sex differences. EP Eur. 2020;22(1):66–73.
23. Kloosterman M, Crijns HJGM, Mulder BA, Groenveld HF, Van Veldhuisen DJ, Rienstra M, et al. Sex-related differences in risk factors, outcome, and quality of life in patients with permanent atrial fibrillation: results from the RACE II study. EP Eur. 2020;22(11):1619–27.
24. Forleo GB, Tondo C, De Luca L, Russo AD, Casella M, De Sanctis V, et al. Gender-related differences in catheter ablation of atrial fibrillation. EP Eur. 2007;9(8):613–20.
25. Antonenko K, Paciaroni M, Agnelli G, Falocci N, Becattini C, Marcheselli S, et al. Sex-related differences in risk factors, type of treatment received and outcomes in patients with atrial fibrillation and acute stroke: results from the RAF-study (early recurrence and cerebral bleeding in patients with acute ischemic stroke and atrial fibrillation). Eur Stroke J. 2017;2(1):46–53.
26. Benjamin EJ, Levy D, Vaziri SM, D'Agostino RB, Belanger AJ, Wolf PA. Independent risk factors for atrial fibrillation in a population-based cohort: the Framingham Heart Study. JAMA. 1994;271(11):840–4.
27. Takigawa M, Kuwahara T, Takahashi A, Watari Y, Okubo K, Takahashi Y, et al. Differences in catheter ablation of paroxysmal atrial fibrillation between males and females. Int J Cardiol. 2013;168(3):1984–91.
28. Magnussen C, Ojeda FM, Wild PS, Sörensen N, Rostock T, Hoffmann BA, et al. Atrial fibrillation manifestations risk factors and sex differences in a population-based cohort (from the Gutenberg Health Study). Am J Cardiol. 2018;122(1):76–82.
29. Huxley RR, Lopez FL, Folsom AR, Agarwal SK, Loehr LR, Soliman EZ, et al. Absolute and attributable risks of atrial fibrillation in relation to optimal and borderline risk factors: the Atherosclerosis Risk in Communities (ARIC) Study. Circulation. 2011;123(14):1501–8.
30. Peters SAE, Woodward M. Established and novel risk factors for atrial fibrillation in women compared with men. Heart. 2019;105(3):226.
31. Sharashova E, Wilsgaard T, Ball J, Morseth B, Gerdts E, Hopstock LA, et al. Long-term blood pressure trajectories and incident atrial fibrillation

in women and men: the Tromsø Study. Eur Heart J. 2020;41(16):1554–62.
32. Bose A, O'Neal WT, Wu C, McClure LA, Judd SE, Howard VJ, et al. Sex differences in risk factors for incident atrial fibrillation (from the reasons for geographic and racial differences in stroke [REGARDS] Study). Am J Cardiol. 2019;123(9):1453–7.
33. De With RR, Artola Arita V, Nguyen BO, Linz D, Ten Cate H, Spronk H, et al. Different circulating biomarkers in women and men with paroxysmal atrial fibrillation: results from the AF-RISK and RACE V studies. EP Eur. 2022;24(2):193–201.
34. Schnabel RB, Pecen L, Ojeda FM, Lucerna M, Rzayeva N, Blankenberg S, et al. Gender differences in clinical presentation and 1-year outcomes in atrial fibrillation. Heart. 2017;103(13):1024–30.
35. Ikemura N, Kohsaka S, Kimura T, Ueda I, Katsumata Y, Nishiyama T, et al. Assessment of sex differences in the initial symptom burden, applied treatment strategy, and quality of life in Japanese patients with atrial fibrillation. JAMA Netw Open. 2019;2(3):e191145.
36. Blum S, Muff C, Aeschbacher S, Ammann P, Erne P, Moschovitis G, et al. Prospective assessment of sex-related differences in symptom status and health perception among patients with atrial fibrillation. J Am Heart Assoc. 2017;6(7):e005401.
37. Walfridsson U, Steen Hansen P, Charitakis E, Almroth H, Jönsson A, Karlsson LO, et al. Gender and age differences in symptoms and health-related quality of life in patients with atrial fibrillation referred for catheter ablation. Pacing Clin Electrophysiol. 2019;42(11):1431–9.
38. Dagres N, Clague JR, Breithardt G, Borggrefe M. Significant gender-related differences in radiofrequency catheter ablation therapy. J Am Coll Cardiol. 2003;42(6):1103–7.
39. Humphries KH, Kerr CR, Connolly SJ, Klein G, Boone JA, Green M, et al. New-onset atrial fibrillation. Circulation. 2001;103(19):2365–70.
40. Stewart S, Hart CL, Hole DJ, McMurray JJV. A population-based study of the long-term risks associated with atrial fibrillation: 20-year follow-up of the Renfrew/Paisley study. Am J Med. 2002;113(5):359–64.
41. Zakeri R, Morgan AD, Sundaram V, Bloom C, Cleland JGF, Quint JK. Under-recognition of heart failure in patients with atrial fibrillation and the impact of gender: a UK population-based cohort study. BMC Med. 2021;19(1):179.
42. Omar AM, Rahman MA, Rifaie O, Bella JN. Atrial fibrillation in heart failure with preserved left ventricular systolic function: distinct elevated risk for cardiovascular outcomes in women compared to men. J Cardiovasc Dev Dis. 2022;9(12):417.
43. Emdin CA, Wong CX, Hsiao AJ, Altman DG, Peters SA, Woodward M, et al. Atrial fibrillation as risk factor for cardiovascular disease and death in women compared with men: systematic review and meta-analysis of cohort studies. BMJ. 2016;352:h7013.
44. Wang TJ, Larson MG, Levy D, Vasan RS, Leip EP, Wolf PA, et al. Temporal relations of atrial fibrillation and congestive heart failure and their joint influence on mortality. Circulation. 2003;107(23):2920–5.
45. Silva RL, Guhl EN, Althouse AD, Herbert B, Sharbaugh M, Essien UR, et al. Sex differences in atrial fibrillation: patient-reported outcomes and the persistent toll on women. Am J Prev Cardiol. 2021;8:100252.
46. von Eisenhart Rothe A, Hutt F, Baumert J, Breithardt G, Goette A, Kirchhof P, et al. Depressed mood amplifies heart-related symptoms in persistent and paroxysmal atrial fibrillation patients: a longitudinal analysis—data from the German Competence Network on Atrial Fibrillation. EP Eur. 2015;17(9):1354–62.
47. Potpara TS, Mihajlovic M, Zec N, Marinkovic M, Kovacevic V, Simic J, et al. Self-reported treatment burden in patients with atrial fibrillation: quantification, major determinants, and implications for integrated holistic management of the arrhythmia. EP Eur. 2020;22(12):1788–97.
48. Friberg J, Scharling H, Gadsbøll N, Truelsen T, Jensen GB. Comparison of the impact of atrial fibrillation on the risk of stroke and cardiovascular death in women versus men (The Copenhagen City Heart Study). Am J Cardiol. 2004;94(7):889–94.
49. Marzona I, Proietti M, Farcomeni A, Romiti GF, Romanazzi I, Raparelli V, et al. Sex differences in stroke and major adverse clinical events in patients with atrial fibrillation: a systematic review and meta-analysis of 993,600 patients. Int J Cardiol. 2018;269:182–91.
50. Wu VCC, Wu M, Aboyans V, Chang SH, Chen SW, Chen MC, et al. Female sex as a risk factor for ischaemic stroke varies with age in patients with atrial fibrillation. Heart. 2020;106(7):534.
51. Ott A, Breteler MMB, de Bruyne MC, van Harskamp F, Grobbee DE, Hofman A. Atrial fibrillation and dementia in a population-based study. Stroke. 1997;28(2):316–21.
52. Wändell P, Carlsson AC, Sundquist J, Sundquist K. The association between relevant comorbidities and dementia in patients with atrial fibrillation. GeroScience. 2018;40(3):317–24.
53. Golive A, May HT, Bair TL, Jacobs V, Crandall BG, Cutler MJ, et al. The impact of gender on atrial fibrillation incidence and progression to dementia. Am J Cardiol. 2018;122(9):1489–95.
54. Rydén L, Zettergren A, Seidu NM, Guo X, Kern S, Blennow K, et al. Atrial fibrillation increases the risk of dementia amongst older adults even in the absence of stroke. J Intern Med. 2019;286(1):101–10.
55. Benjamin EJ, Wolf PA, D'Agostino RB, Silbershatz H, Kannel WB, Levy D. Impact of atrial fibrillation on the risk of death. Circulation. 1998;98(10):946–52.
56. Andersson T, Magnuson A, Bryngelsson IL, Frøbert O, Henriksson KM, Edvardsson N, et al. All-cause mortality in 272 186 patients hospitalized with incident atrial fibrillation 1995–2008: a Swedish nation-

wide long-term case–control study. Eur Heart J. 2013;34(14):1061–7.
57. Nabauer M, Oeff M, Gerth A, Wegscheider K, Buchholz A, Haeusler KG, et al. Prognostic markers of all-cause mortality in patients with atrial fibrillation: data from the prospective long-term registry of the German Atrial Fibrillation NETwork (AFNET). EP Eur. 2021;23(12):1903–12.
58. Penttilä T, Lehto M, Niiranen J, Mehtälä J, Khanfir H, Lassila R, et al. Differences in the risk of stroke, bleeding events, and mortality between female and male patients with atrial fibrillation during warfarin therapy. Eur Heart J Cardiovasc Pharmacother. 2019;5(1):29–36.
59. Inoue H, Atarashi H, Okumura K, Yamashita T, Origasa H, Kumagai N, et al. Impact of gender on the prognosis of patients with Nonvalvular atrial fibrillation. Am J Cardiol. 2014;113(6):957–62.
60. Kuppahally SS, Akoum N, Badger TJ, Burgon NS, Haslam T, Kholmovski E, et al. Echocardiographic left atrial reverse remodeling after catheter ablation of atrial fibrillation is predicted by preablation delayed enhancement of left atrium by magnetic resonance imaging. Am Heart J. 2010;160(5):877–84.
61. Yu HT, Lee JS, Kim T, Uhm J, Joung B, Hong G, et al. Advanced left atrial remodeling and appendage contractile dysfunction in women than in men among the patients with atrial fibrillation: potential mechanism for stroke. J Am Heart Assoc. 2016;5(7):e003361.
62. Yu HT, Yang PS, Kim TH, Uhm JS, Kim JY, Joung B, et al. Poor rhythm outcome of catheter ablation for early-onset atrial fibrillation in women—mechanistic insight. Circ J. 2018;82(9):2259–68.
63. Pfannmüller B, Boldt A, Reutemann A, Duerrschmidt N, Krabbes Graube S, Mohr FW, Dhein S. Gender-Specific Remodeling in Atrial Fibrillation? Thorac Cardiovasc Surg. 2013;61(01):066–73.
64. Pak HN, Park JW, Yang SY, Kim M, Yu HT, Kim TH, et al. Sex differences in mapping and rhythm outcomes of a repeat atrial fibrillation ablation. Heart. 2021;107(23):1862.
65. Park YJ, Park JW, Yu HT, Kim TH, Uhm JS, Joung B, et al. Sex difference in atrial fibrillation recurrence after catheter ablation and antiarrhythmic drugs. Heart. 2022;109:519–26. https://doi.org/10.1136/heartjnl-2021-320601.
66. Lee SH, Tai CT, Hsieh MH, Tsao HM, Lin YJ, Chang SL, et al. Predictors of non-pulmonary vein ectopic beats initiating paroxysmal atrial fibrillation. J Am Coll Cardiol. 2005;46(6):1054–9.
67. Patel D, Mohanty P, Di Biase L, Sanchez JE, Shaheen MH, Burkhardt JD, et al. Outcomes and complications of catheter ablation for atrial fibrillation in females. Heart Rhythm. 2010;7(2):167–72.
68. Wong GR, Nalliah CJ, Lee G, Voskoboinik A, Chieng D, Prabhu S, et al. Sex-related differences in atrial remodeling in patients with atrial fibrillation: relationship to ablation outcomes. Circ Arrhythm Electrophysiol. 2022;15(1):e009925.
69. Li Z, Wang Z, Yin Z, Zhang Y, Xue X, Han J, et al. Gender differences in fibrosis remodeling in patients with long-standing persistent atrial fibrillation. Oncotarget. 2017;8(32):53714–29.
70. Arnold AP, Cassis LA, Eghbali M, Reue K, Sandberg K. Sex hormones and sex chromosomes cause sex differences in the development of cardiovascular diseases. Arterioscler Thromb Vasc Biol. 2017;37(5):746–56.
71. Vaidya VR, Arora S, Patel N, Badheka AO, Patel N, Agnihotri K, et al. Burden of arrhythmia in pregnancy. Circulation. 2017;135(6):619–21.
72. Chokesuwattanaskul R, Thongprayoon C, Bathini T, O'Corragain OA, Sharma K, Prechawat S, et al. Incidence of atrial fibrillation in pregnancy and clinical significance: a meta-analysis. Adv Med Sci. 2019;64(2):415–22.
73. Salam AM, Ertekin E, van Hagen IM, Al Suwaidi J, Ruys TPE, Johnson MR, et al. Atrial fibrillation or flutter during pregnancy in patients with structural heart disease: data from the ROPAC (Registry on Pregnancy and Cardiac Disease). JACC Clin Electrophysiol. 2015;1(4):284–92.
74. Lee M, Chen W, Zhang Z, Duan L, Ng A, Spencer HT, et al. Atrial fibrillation and atrial flutter in pregnant women—a population-based study. J Am Heart Assoc. 2016;5(4):e003182.
75. Scantlebury DC, Kattah AG, Weissgerber TL, Agarwal S, Mielke MM, Weaver AL, et al. Impact of a history of hypertension in pregnancy on later diagnosis of atrial fibrillation. J Am Heart Assoc. 2018;7(10):e007584.
76. Regitz-Zagrosek V, Roos-Hesselink JW, Bauersachs J, Blomström-Lundqvist C, Cífková R, De Bonis M, et al. 2018 ESC guidelines for the management of cardiovascular diseases during pregnancy: the task force for the management of cardiovascular diseases during pregnancy of the European Society of Cardiology (ESC). Eur Heart J. 2018;39(34):3165–241.
77. Magnani JW, Moser CB, Murabito JM, Nelson KP, Fontes JD, Lubitz SA, et al. Age of natural menopause and atrial fibrillation: the Framingham Heart Study. Am Heart J. 2012;163(4):729–34.
78. Wong JA, Rexrode KM, Sandhu RK, Moorthy MV, Conen D, Albert CM. Menopausal age, postmenopausal hormone therapy and incident atrial fibrillation. Heart. 2017;103(24):1954.
79. Yang S, Kwak S, Kwon S, Lee HJ, Lee H, Park JB, et al. Association of total reproductive years with incident atrial fibrillation, and subsequent ischemic stroke in women with natural menopause. Circ Arrhythm Electrophysiol. 2019;12(11):e007428.
80. Perez MV, Wang PJ, Larson JC, Virnig BA, Cochrane B, Curb JD, et al. Effects of postmenopausal hormone therapy on incident atrial fibrillation. Circ Arrhythm Electrophysiol. 2012;5(6):1108–16.
81. Bretler DM, Hansen PR, Lindhardsen J, Ahlehoff O, Andersson C, Jensen TB, et al. Hormone replacement therapy and risk of new-onset atrial fibrillation

after myocardial infarction—a nationwide cohort study. PLoS One. 2012;7(12):e51580.
82. Tsai WC, Haung YB, Kuo HF, Tang WH, Hsu PC, Su HM, et al. Hormone replacement therapy and risk of atrial fibrillation in Taiwanese menopause women: a nationwide cohort study. Sci Rep. 2016;6(1):24132.
83. Lee J, Kim Y, Park H, Kim C, Cho S, Kim J. Clinical impact of hormone replacement therapy on atrial fibrillation in postmenopausal women: a nationwide cohort study. J Clin Med. 2021;10(23):5497.
84. Apostolakis S, Sullivan RM, Olshansky B, Lip GYH. Hormone replacement therapy and adverse outcomes in women with atrial fibrillation. Stroke. 2014;45(10):3076–9.
85. Krijthe BP, de Jong FH, Hofman A, Franco OH, Witteman JC, Stricker BH, et al. Dehydroepiandrosterone sulfate levels and risk of atrial fibrillation: the Rotterdam Study. Eur J Prev Cardiol. 2014;21(3):291–8.
86. Ravaglia G, Forti P, Maioli F, Sacchetti L, Nativio V, Scali CR, et al. Dehydroepiandrosterone-sulfate serum levels and common age-related diseases: results from a cross-sectional Italian study of a general elderly population. Exp Gerontol. 2002;37(5):701–12.
87. Magnani JW, Moser CB, Murabito JM, Sullivan LM, Wang N, Ellinor PT, et al. Association of sex hormones, aging, and atrial fibrillation in men. Circ Arrhythm Electrophysiol. 2014;7(2):307–12.
88. Liu D, Zhan Y, Ono K, Yin Y, Wang L, Wei M, et al. Pharmacological activation of estrogenic receptor G protein-coupled receptor 30 attenuates angiotensin II-induced atrial fibrosis in ovariectomized mice by modulating TGF-β1/smad pathway. Mol Biol Rep. 2022;49(7):6341–55.
89. Nakajima T, Iwasawa K, Oonuma H, Morita T, Goto A, Wang Y, et al. Antiarrhythmic effect and its underlying ionic mechanism of 17β-estradiol in cardiac myocytes. Br J Pharmacol. 1999;127(2):429–40.
90. Chen YJ, Lee SH, Hsieh MH, Hsiao CJ, Yu WC, Chiou CW, et al. Effects of 17β-estradiol on tachycardia-induced changes of atrial refractoriness and cisapride-induced ventricular arrhythmia. J Cardiovasc Electrophysiol. 1999;10(4):587–98.
91. O'Neal WT, Nazarian S, Alonso A, Heckbert SR, Vaccarino V, Soliman EZ. Sex hormones and the risk of atrial fibrillation: the Multi-Ethnic Study of Atherosclerosis (MESA). Endocrine. 2017;58(1):91–6.
92. Sharma R, Oni OA, Gupta K, Sharma M, Sharma R, Singh V, et al. Normalization of testosterone levels after testosterone replacement therapy is associated with decreased incidence of atrial fibrillation. J Am Heart Assoc. 2017;6(5):e004880.
93. Oliver-Williams C, Vassard D, Pinborg A, Schmidt L. Polycystic ovary syndrome as a novel risk factor for atrial fibrillation: results from a national Danish registry cohort study. Eur J Prev Cardiol. 2021;28(12):e20–2.
94. Cho JH, Choi EK, Moon IK, Jung JH, Han KD, Choi YJ, et al. Chromosomal abnormalities and atrial fibrillation and ischemic stroke incidence: a nationwide population-based study. Sci Rep. 2020;10(1):15872.
95. Ravn LS, Hofman-Bang J, Dixen U, Larsen SO, Jensen G, Haunsø S, et al. Relation of 97T polymorphism in KCNE5 to risk of atrial fibrillation. Am J Cardiol. 2005;96(3):405–7.
96. Karst ML, Herron KJ, Olson TM. X-linked nonsyndromic sinus node dysfunction and atrial fibrillation caused by emerin mutation. J Cardiovasc Electrophysiol. 2008;19(5):510–5.
97. Brcic L, Underwood JF, Kendall KM, Caseras X, Kirov G, Davies W. Medical and neurobehavioural phenotypes in carriers of X-linked ichthyosis-associated genetic deletions in the UK Biobank. J Med Genet. 2020;57(10):692.
98. Øyen N, Ranthe MF, Carstensen L, Boyd HA, Olesen MS, Olesen SP, et al. Familial aggregation of lone atrial fibrillation in young persons. J Am Coll Cardiol. 2012;60(10):917–21.
99. Chen LY, Herron KJ, Tai BC, Olson TM. Lone atrial fibrillation: influence of familial disease on gender predilection. J Cardiovasc Electrophysiol. 2008;19(8):802–6.
100. Zöller B, Ohlsson H, Sundquist J, Sundquist K. High familial risk of atrial fibrillation/atrial flutter in multiplex families: a nationwide family study in Sweden. J Am Heart Assoc. 2012;2(1):e003384.
101. Lip GYH. The ABC pathway: an integrated approach to improve AF management. Nat Rev Cardiol. 2017;14(11):627–8.
102. Proietti M, Romiti GF, Olshansky B, Lane DA, Lip GYH. Improved outcomes by integrated care of anticoagulated patients with atrial fibrillation using the simple ABC (atrial fibrillation better care) pathway. Am J Med. 2018;131(11):1359–1366.e6.
103. Hindricks G, Potpara T, Dagres N, Arbelo E, Bax JJ, Blomström-Lundqvist C, et al. 2020 ESC guidelines for the diagnosis and management of atrial fibrillation developed in collaboration with the European Association for Cardio-Thoracic Surgery (EACTS). Eur Heart J. 2021;42(5):373–498.
104. Tomasdottir M, Friberg L, Hijazi Z, Lindbäck J, Oldgren J. Risk of ischemic stroke and utility of CHA2DS2-VASc score in women and men with atrial fibrillation. Clin Cardiol. 2019;42(10):1003–9.
105. Nielsen PB, Skjøth F, Overvad TF, Larsen TB, Lip GYH. Female sex is a risk modifier rather than a risk factor for stroke in atrial fibrillation. Circulation. 2018;137(8):832–40.
106. Tomita H, Okumura K, Inoue H, Atarashi H, Yamashita T, Origasa H, et al. Validation of risk scoring system excluding female sex from CHA2DS2-VASc in Japanese patients with nonvalvular atrial fibrillation—subanalysis of the J-RHYTHM Registry. Circ J. 2015;79(8):1719–26.
107. Arnson Y, Hoshen M, Berliner Senderey A, Reges O, Balicer R, Leibowitz M, et al. Comparing

management and outcomes in men and women with Nonvalvular atrial fibrillation: data from a population-based cohort. JACC Clin Electrophysiol. 2018;4((5)):604–14.
108. Brieger D, Amerena J, Attia J, Bajorek B, Chan KH, Connell C, et al. National heart foundation of Australia and the cardiac society of Australia and New Zealand: Australian clinical guidelines for the diagnosis and management of atrial fibrillation 2018. Heart Lung Circ. 2018;27(10):1209–66.
109. Bushnell C, McCullough LD, Awad IA, Chireau MV, Fedder WN, Furie KL, et al. Guidelines for the prevention of stroke in women. Stroke. 2014;45(5):1545–88.
110. López-López JA, Sterne JAC, Thom HHZ, Higgins JPT, Hingorani AD, Okoli GN, et al. Oral anticoagulants for prevention of stroke in atrial fibrillation: systematic review, network meta-analysis, and cost effectiveness analysis. BMJ. 2017;359:j5058.
111. Connolly SJ, Karthikeyan G, Ntsekhe M, Haileamlak A, El Sayed A, El Ghamrawy A, et al. Rivaroxaban in rheumatic heart disease–associated atrial fibrillation. N Engl J Med. 2022;387:978–88. https://doi.org/10.1056/NEJMoa2209051.
112. Connolly SJ, Ezekowitz MD, Yusuf S, Eikelboom J, Oldgren J, Parekh A, et al. Dabigatran versus warfarin in patients with atrial fibrillation. N Engl J Med. 2009;361(12):1139–51.
113. Granger CB, Alexander JH, McMurray JJV, Lopes RD, Hylek EM, Hanna M, et al. Apixaban versus warfarin in patients with atrial fibrillation. N Engl J Med. 2011;365(11):981–92.
114. Patel MR, Mahaffey KW, Garg J, Pan G, Singer DE, Hacke W, et al. Rivaroxaban versus warfarin in nonvalvular atrial fibrillation. N Engl J Med. 2011;365(10):883–91.
115. Giugliano RP, Ruff CT, Braunwald E, Murphy SA, Wiviott SD, Halperin JL, et al. Edoxaban versus warfarin in patients with atrial fibrillation. N Engl J Med. 2013;369(22):2093–104.
116. Tsadok MA, Jackevicius CA, Rahme E, Humphries KH, Behlouli H, Pilote L. Sex differences in stroke risk among older patients with recently diagnosed atrial fibrillation. JAMA. 2012;307(18):1952–8.
117. Thompson LE, Maddox TM, Lei L, Grunwald GK, Bradley SM, Peterson PN, et al. Sex differences in the use of oral anticoagulants for atrial fibrillation: a report from the national cardiovascular data registry (NCDR®) PINNACLE Registry. J Am Heart Assoc. 2017;6(7):e005801.
118. Sur NB, Wang K, Di Tullio MR, Gutierrez CM, Dong C, Koch S, et al. Disparities and temporal trends in the use of anticoagulation in patients with ischemic stroke and atrial fibrillation. Stroke. 2019;50(6):1452–9.
119. Essien UR, Magnani JW, Chen N, Gellad WF, Fine MJ, Hernandez I. Race/ethnicity and sex-related differences in direct oral anticoagulant initiation in newly diagnosed atrial fibrillation: a retrospective study of Medicare data. J Natl Med Assoc. 2020;112(1):103–8.
120. Bhave PD, Lu X, Girotra S, Kamel H, Vaughan Sarrazin MS. Race- and sex-related differences in care for patients newly diagnosed with atrial fibrillation. Heart Rhythm. 2015;12(7):1406–12.
121. Lip GYH, Rushton-Smith SK, Goldhaber SZ, Fitzmaurice DA, Mantovani LG, Goto S, et al. Does sex affect anticoagulant use for stroke prevention in Nonvalvular atrial fibrillation? Circ Cardiovasc Qual Outcomes. 2015;8(2_suppl_1):S12–20.
122. Loikas D, Forslund T, Wettermark B, Schenck-Gustafsson K, Hjemdahl P, von Euler M. Sex and gender differences in thromboprophylactic treatment of patients with atrial fibrillation after the introduction of non–vitamin K oral anticoagulants. Am J Cardiol. 2017;120(8):1302–8.
123. Albertsen IE, Rasmussen LH, Overvad TF, Graungaard T, Larsen TB, Lip GYH. Risk of stroke or systemic embolism in atrial fibrillation patients treated with warfarin. Stroke. 2013;44(5):1329–36.
124. Proietti M, Cheli P, Basili S, Mazurek M, Lip GYH. Balancing thromboembolic and bleeding risk with non-vitamin K antagonist oral anticoagulants (NOACs): a systematic review and meta-analysis on gender differences. Pharmacol Res. 2017;117:274–82.
125. Pan Y, Li Z, Li J, Jin A, Lin J, Jing J, et al. Residual risk and its risk factors for ischemic stroke with adherence to guideline-based secondary stroke prevention. J Stroke. 2021;23(1):51–60.
126. Carlisle MA, Shrader P, Fudim M, Pieper KS, Blanco RG, Fonarow GC, et al. Residual stroke risk despite oral anticoagulation in patients with atrial fibrillation. Heart Rhythm O2. 2022;3((6, Part A)):621–8.
127. Maeda T, Nishi T, Funakoshi S, Tada K, Tsuji M, Satoh A, et al. Residual risks of ischaemic stroke and systemic embolism among atrial fibrillation patients with anticoagulation: large-scale real-world data (F-CREATE project). Heart. 2021;107(3):217.
128. Ding WY, Lane DA, Gupta D, Huisman MV, Lip GYH. Incidence and risk factors for residual adverse events despite anticoagulation in atrial fibrillation: results from phase II/III of the GLORIA-AF Registry. J Am Heart Assoc. 2022;11(15):e026410.
129. Pancholy SB, Sharma PS, Pancholy DS, Patel TM, Callans DJ, Marchlinski FE. Meta-analysis of gender differences in residual stroke risk and major bleeding in patients with nonvalvular atrial fibrillation treated with oral anticoagulants. Am J Cardiol. 2014;113(3):485–90.
130. Barcellona D, Schirru P, Mameli A, Cornacchini S, Fenu L, Marongiu F. Over-anticoagulation by vitamin K antagonists and gender differences. Int J Cardiol. 2022;362:147–51.
131. Terrier J, Gaspar F, Guidi M, Fontana P, Daali Y, Csajka C, et al. Population pharmacokinetic models for direct oral anticoagulants: a systematic review and clinical appraisal using exposure simulation. Clin Pharmacol Ther. 2022;112(2):353–63.

132. Van Gelder IC, Groenveld HF, Crijns HJGM, Tuininga YS, Tijssen JGP, Alings AM, et al. Lenient versus strict rate control in patients with atrial fibrillation. N Engl J Med. 2010;362(15):1363–73.
133. Van Gelder IC, Hagens VE, Bosker HA, Kingma JH, Kamp O, Kingma T, et al. A comparison of rate control and rhythm control in patients with recurrent persistent atrial fibrillation. N Engl J Med. 2002;347(23):1834–40.
134. Wyse DG, Waldo AL, DiMarco JP, Domanski MJ, Rosenberg Y, Schron EB, et al. A comparison of rate control and rhythm control in patients with atrial fibrillation. N Engl J Med. 2002;347(23):1825–33.
135. Carlsson J, Miketic S, Windeler J, Cuneo A, Haun S, Micus S, et al. Randomized trial of rate-control versus rhythm-control in persistent atrial fibrillation. J Am Coll Cardiol. 2003;41(10):1690–6.
136. Roy D, Talajic M, Nattel S, Wyse DG, Dorian P, Lee KL, et al. Rhythm control versus rate control for atrial fibrillation and heart failure. N Engl J Med. 2008;358(25):2667–77.
137. Kirchhof P, Camm AJ, Goette A, Brandes A, Eckardt L, Elvan A, et al. Early rhythm-control therapy in patients with atrial fibrillation. N Engl J Med. 2020;383(14):1305–16.
138. Rillig A, Borof K, Breithardt G, Camm AJ, Crijns HJGM, Goette A, et al. Early rhythm control in patients with atrial fibrillation and high comorbidity burden. Circulation. 2022;146(11):836–47.
139. Kang DS, Kim D, Jang E, Yu HT, Kim TH, Pak HN, et al. Sex difference in effectiveness of early rhythm-over rate-control in patients with atrial fibrillation. J Clin Med. 2022;11(17):4991.
140. Di Biase L, Mohanty P, Mohanty S, Santangeli P, Trivedi C, Lakkireddy D, et al. Ablation versus amiodarone for treatment of persistent atrial fibrillation in patients with congestive heart failure and an implanted device. Circulation. 2016;133(17):1637–44.
141. Marrouche NF, Brachmann J, Andresen D, Siebels J, Boersma L, Jordaens L, et al. Catheter ablation for atrial fibrillation with heart failure. N Engl J Med. 2018;378(5):417–27.
142. Mark DB, Anstrom KJ, Sheng S, Piccini JP, Baloch KN, Monahan KH, et al. Effect of catheter ablation vs medical therapy on quality of life among patients with atrial fibrillation: the CABANA randomized clinical trial. JAMA. 2019;321(13):1275–85.
143. Mantovan R, Macle L, De Martino G, Chen J, Morillo CA, Novak P, et al. Relationship of quality of life with procedural success of atrial fibrillation (AF) ablation and postablation AF burden: substudy of the STAR AF randomized trial. Can J Cardiol. 2013;29(10):1211–7.
144. Purmah Y, Proietti M, Laroche C, Mazurek M, Tahmatzidis D, Boriani G, et al. Rate vs. rhythm control and adverse outcomes among European patients with atrial fibrillation. EP Eur. 2018;20(2):243–52.
145. Zylla MM, Brachmann J, Lewalter T, Hoffmann E, Kuck KH, Andresen D, et al. Sex-related outcome of atrial fibrillation ablation: insights from the German Ablation Registry. Atr Fibrillation. 2016;13(9):1837–44.
146. Elayi CS, Darrat Y, Suffredini JM, Misumida N, Shah J, Morales G, et al. Sex differences in complications of catheter ablation for atrial fibrillation: results on 85,977 patients. J Interv Card Electrophysiol. 2018;53(3):333–9.
147. Cheng X, Hu Q, Gao L, Liu J, Qin S, Zhang D. Sex-related differences in catheter ablation of atrial fibrillation: a systematic review and meta-analysis. EP Eur. 2019;21(10):1509–18.
148. Rienstra M, Van Veldhuisen DJ, Hagens VE, Ranchor AV, Veeger NJGM, Crijns HJGM, et al. Gender-related differences in rhythm control treatment in persistent atrial fibrillation. J Am Coll Cardiol. 2005;46(7):1298–306.
149. Russo AM, Zeitler EP, Giczewska A, Silverstein AP, Al-Khalidi HR, Cha YM, et al. Association between sex and treatment outcomes of atrial fibrillation ablation versus drug therapy. Circulation. 2021;143(7):661–72.
150. Makkar RR, Fromm BS, Steinman RT, Meissner MD, Lehmann MH. Female gender as a risk factor for torsades de pointes associated with cardiovascular drugs. JAMA. 1993;270(21):2590–7.
151. Lehmann MH, Hardy S, Archibald D, Quart B, MacNeil DJ. Sex difference in risk of torsade de pointes with d,l-sotalol. Circulation. 1996;94(10):2535–41.
152. Essebag V, Reynolds MR, Hadjis T, Lemery R, Olshansky B, Buxton AE, et al. Sex differences in the relationship between amiodarone use and the need for permanent pacing in patients with atrial fibrillation. Arch Intern Med. 2007;167(15):1648–53.
153. Zhong B, Wang Y, Zhang G, Wang Z. Environmental iodine content, female sex and age are associated with new-onset amiodarone-induced hypothyroidism: a systematic review and meta-analysis of adverse reactions of amiodarone on the thyroid. Cardiology. 2016;134(3):366–71.
154. Blum S, Aeschbacher S, Meyre P, Zwimpfer L, Reichlin T, Beer JH, et al. Incidence and predictors of atrial fibrillation progression. J Am Heart Assoc. 2019;8(20):e012554.
155. Tsang TSM, Barnes ME, Miyasaka Y, Cha SS, Bailey KR, Verzosa GC, et al. Obesity as a risk factor for the progression of paroxysmal to permanent atrial fibrillation: a longitudinal cohort study of 21 years. Eur Heart J. 2008;29(18):2227–33.
156. Liu F, Song T, Hu Q, Zhu X, Zhao H, Tan Z, et al. Body mass index and atrial fibrillation recurrence post ablation: a systematic review and dose-response meta-analysis. Front Cardiovasc Med. 2023;9:999845. https://www.frontiersin.org/articles/10.3389/fcvm.2022.999845.
157. Rienstra M, Hobbelt AH, Alings M, Tijssen JGP, Smit MD, Brügemann J, et al. Targeted therapy of underlying conditions improves sinus rhythm maintenance in patients with persistent atrial fibril-

lation: results of the RACE 3 trial. Eur Heart J. 2018;39(32):2987–96.

158. Pathak RK, Middeldorp ME, Lau DH, Mehta AB, Mahajan R, Twomey D, et al. Aggressive risk factor reduction study for atrial fibrillation and implications for the outcome of ablation. J Am Coll Cardiol. 2014;64(21):2222–31.
159. Middeldorp ME, Pathak RK, Meredith M, Mehta AB, Elliott AD, Mahajan R, et al. PREVEntion and regReSsive Effect of weight-loss and risk factor modification on atrial fibrillation: the REVERSE-AF study. EP Eur. 2018;20(12):1929–35.
160. Pathak RK, Middeldorp ME, Meredith M, Mehta AB, Mahajan R, Wong CX, et al. Long-term effect of goal-directed weight management in an atrial fibrillation cohort. J Am Coll Cardiol. 2015;65(20):2159–69.
161. Sharashova E, Gerdts E, Ball J, Espnes H, Jacobsen BK, Kildal S, et al. Sex-specific time trends in incident atrial fibrillation and the contribution of risk factors: the Tromsø Study 1994-2016. Eur J Prev Cardiol. 2023;30(1):72–81.

Stroke in Women

Virginia Cancelloni, Ilaria Leone de Magistris, and Valeria Caso

Abstract

Stroke is a major global health issue, ranking as the second-leading cause of death and the third-leading cause of disability. Unfortunately, even today, disparities in stroke diagnosis and treatment persist, particularly concerning ethnicity and gender. Women are disproportionately affected by stroke, often experiencing more adverse outcomes. In addition to the well-established stroke causes and risk factors, there are sex-specific stroke mechanisms to consider, such as hormonal contraception, pregnancy-related stroke, and menopause. This chapter delves into the comprehensive diagnostic process for ischaemic stroke, covering various neuroimaging techniques and their applicability, with a specific focus on addressing the unique requirements of pregnant women. The treatment of acute ischemic stroke has seen significant advancements, with intravenous thrombolysis and mechanical thrombectomy now recognized as major milestones. We will provide detailed information on reperfusion therapies and discuss the challenges associated with stroke during pregnancy, emphasizing the necessity for evidence-based guidelines.

After surviving a stroke, effective secondary prevention strategies are crucial to reduce the risk of recurrence. These strategies include antithrombotic therapy, lifestyle modifications, and physical activity. For women, managing stroke risk during pregnancy and the postpartum period presents unique challenges, compounded by the impact of post-stroke depression and the need for personalized rehabilitation programs. This text offers a comprehensive exploration of the ischaemic stroke domain, covering its clinical characteristics, epidemiology, risk factors, diagnostic processes, acute treatments, and secondary prevention. Throughout, we emphasize addressing the distinctive considerations that women face, particularly during pregnancy and the postpartum period.

Keywords

Stroke · Time-dependent · Disparities

V. Cancelloni (✉) · I. L. de Magistris · V. Caso
Stroke Unit, Department of Emergency and Vascular Medicine, Santa Maria della Misericordia Hospital, University of Perugia, Perugia, Italy

A. H.E.M. Maas, E. Gerdts (eds.), *Manual of Cardiovascular Disease in Women*,
https://doi.org/10.1007/978-3-031-65952-2_23

Test your learning and check your understanding of this book's contents: use the "Springer Nature Flashcards" app to access questions using ▶ https://sn.pub/51ny7m
To use the app, please follow the instructions in chapter 1.

1 Introduction

Most stroke events occur in women, who tend to experience worse outcomes, as well as a higher overall mortality rate when compared to men. However, it is the preponderance of women in older age groups that most clearly elucidates this pattern. Despite this, the frequency of strokes is higher in men. On the whole, stroke rates are decreasing, with a more pronounced decline in men [1]. Consequently, the surplus number of strokes occurring in women is projected to increase in the (near) future [2].

Differences in risk factors emerge between men and women. For instance, among women, rates of atrial fibrillation and hypertension are higher, while rates of smoking or heavy alcohol consumption are more prevalent among men. Additionally, some risk factors, such as diabetes or smoking, confer a higher risk for women than men. The benefits are comparable between genders with regard to treatment realms where adequate data is available, such as intravenous thrombolysis and mechanical thrombectomy [3]. These intervention benefits might even be more pronounced in women due to the longer life expectancy of women. Unique female risk factors, including pregnancy or the use of sex hormone therapy, are infrequent causes of stroke, especially in high-income countries. Nonetheless, these specific stroke events often occur early in life and significantly impact individual families. Unfortunately, there is limited evidence regarding stroke care in these circumstances, underscoring an urgent requirement for more comprehensive data, including prospective observational data, that would offer better guidance to healthcare providers. Furthermore, there is a pressing need for specific data on women with strokes to ascertain whether gender might unduly influence treatment and care decisions in specific scenarios.

In this chapter, we will give an overview of clinical stroke presentation, epidemiology, aetiologies risk factors, acute stroke treatment, secondary prevention and rehabilitation.

2 Theory

2.1 Definition and Clinical Characteristics of Ischaemic Stroke

According to the 1970 World Health Organization definition, ischaemic stroke was first defined as a clinical entity, that is "rapidly developing signs of focal (or global) disturbance of cerebral function, with symptoms lasting 24 h or longer, or leading to death, with no apparent cause other than of vascular origin" [4]. Recently, a new tissue-based concept of ischaemic stroke was introduced by AHA/ASA [5], stating that it is an "episode of neurological dysfunction attributable to objective evidence of permanent brain, spinal cord, or retinal cell infarction due to a vascular aetiology, based on pathological, neuroimaging, or other objective evidence".

Ischaemic stroke typically presents with a sudden onset of neurological dysfunction with signs and symptoms depending on brain areas affected by decreased blood flow. In the case of anterior circulation infarction, patients can present with contralateral motor and/or sensory disturbances, speech difficulty (dysarthria and/or aphasia), neglect, personality change, and executive dysfunction. When posterior circulation is involved, patients can display hypersomnolence, visual field defects, ataxia, vertigo, nausea, vomiting, oropharyngeal dysfunction, abnormal oculomotor findings, and somatosensory and/or motor disturbances. Other less common signs and symptoms connected to specific aetiologies include Horner syndrome (unilateral miosis, ptosis, and face anhidrosis) in the case of artery dissection, and headache, seizures, and decreased level of consciousness, in the case of cerebral venous thrombosis [6].

The clinical presentation and the course of neurological deficits can sometimes suggest the underlying aetiology of ischaemic stroke [6]. Embolic strokes most often occur suddenly, with neurological deficits usually being maximal at the onset. Rapid recovery also favours embolism. Thrombosis-related ischemia and small vessel diseases often cause symptoms that fluctuate or progress in a stepwise or stuttering fashion with some periods of improvement. Penetrating artery disease usually causes symptoms that develop during short periods of time, hours, or at most a few days, compared with large artery-related brain ischemia, which can evolve over a longer period.

Sex-related differences may distinguish clinical characteristics of an ischaemic stroke. A recent meta-analysis pooling eight population-based stroke incidence studies, for a total of 6343 cases [7], evaluated factors contributing to sex-dependent differences in severity of acute ischemic and haemorrhagic stroke according to the NIHSS scale. In this paper, it was reported that women were more likely to have more severe stroke defined as a National Institutes of Health Stroke Scale/Score (NIHSS) >7. However, adjustment for age, pre-stroke dependency, and atrial fibrillation decreased this sex-dependent difference in severity, but it remained statistically significant.

Women have been reported to have significantly higher odds of presenting with non-focal neurological symptoms during acute stroke compared to men [8]. These non-focal symptoms include confusion, impaired consciousness, headache, light-headedness, and atypical symptoms such as chest pain, palpitations, nausea, and generalized weakness. Non-focal symptoms could mistakenly be interpreted as conversion disorder, migraine attack, or even stroke mimics, a diagnosis received more frequently for women than men with similar symptomatology [9]. It is important to point out that women with stroke have a higher mortality rate and a worse functional outcome compared with men [9]. It has been hypothesized that this could be in part explained by the more frequent misdiagnosis of stroke mimics in women with consequent delays to or even deferral of acute or secondary preventive treatment.

2.2 Epidemiology of Ischaemic Stroke in Women

Globally, stroke is reported to be the second-leading cause of death worldwide (11.6% of total deaths) and the third-leading cause of death and disability combined. From a systematic analysis conducted between 1990 and 2019 [10], the absolute number of incident strokes increased by 70%, prevalent strokes increased by 85%, deaths from stroke increased by 43%, and disability-adjusted life-years due to stroke increased by 32%. Among people younger than 70 years, prevalence and incidence rates increased by 22% and 15%, respectively. Stroke-related mortality and disability rates were reported to be almost 4 times higher in low-income countries than in high-income ones. Over the last few decades, high-income countries have shown decreases in mortality rates by an average of 55%, case-fatality rates by 40%, and stroke event rates by 20%. These benefits have been due to the implementation of stroke units and the adoption of overall better stroke prevention and acute management.

Behind these global data, hidden disparities exist between sexes, and frequently at the expense of women [11–13]. In the United States of America (USA) in 2019, stroke was the third leading cause of death in women, compared with the fifth in men [14]. All available data from past years show the same trends over time: beyond the age of 75 years, women have a higher stroke incidence than men [15]. Below this age, this tendency has always been considered indeed reversed, with a lower stroke incidence in younger women. However, more recent studies have identified important variations in stroke incidence by sex and age. Two important retrospective cohort studies of 5.8 and 9.3 million adults from Canada [16] and USA [17], observed lower stroke rates in men than in women, in persons aged under 30 and 44 years respectively, suggesting a causative role of vascular risk factors in women even at a younger age.

Stroke is more likely to be the first manifestation of cardiovascular disease in women, whereas in men coronary heart disease is more common [14]. The social context for women who experience stroke is important as well. Age at onset of stroke is on average 4–6 years older in women than men. Moreover, when compared to men, women are more likely to be widowed, unmarried, or living alone. All these factors, and considering that women tend to have also more severe strokes, lead to a higher degree of disability in their activities of daily living and a less favourable outcome [18].

Regional differences and disparities by race/ethnicity also matter, with the highest lifetime risks for women in Eastern Europe and East Asia (36.5% and 36.3%, respectively). In the Northern Manhattan Study (NOMAS), Black and Hispanic women aged 70 and older had a 76–77% higher risk of stroke than Caucasian women after adjusting for age, education, and insurance status, a difference not seen in men [19]. The intersectionality of these factors and multiple dimensions of marginalization, e.g., race/ethnicity, sex, age, and socioeconomic factors are determining factors in stroke risk and outcome.

2.3 Aetiologies and Risk Factors for Ischaemic Stroke in Women

Considering stroke aetiologies, three principal pathophysiological mechanisms of brain hypoperfusion can be considered: artery thrombosis of a brain-supplying vessel (both large or small vessels) with subsequently reduced blood flow distally or artery-to-artery embolism, embolism from a distant source (such as cardiac or aortic embolism) or systemic hypoperfusion due to cardiac pump failure, reduced cardiac output or hypoxemia.

The TOAST classification system [20] was introduced for the categorization of subtypes of ischemic stroke mainly based on aetiology and using clinical features in association with diagnostic studies (neuroimaging, cardiac and laboratory studies). This classification includes five categories of stroke mechanism: large-artery atherosclerosis, cardioembolism (due to atrial fibrillation (AF) and other arrhythmias, valvular pathologies, intracardiac thrombus or mass, left ventricle ejection fraction <35%, endocarditis, patent foramen ovale), small-vessel disease (with concomitant lacunar deep infarctions, severe leukoaraiosis, and microbleeds), stroke of other determined aetiology (less frequent causes such as haematological or rheumatological diseases, Fabry's disease, cerebral inflammatory or infectious angiitis, Moyamoya disease, hypercoagulability states due to cancer or genetic conditions), and stroke of undetermined aetiology (defined when two or more causes are identified, or a negative/incomplete evaluation is performed).

Among stroke aetiologies, cardiac pathologies account for almost 20% of all ischaemic strokes, with AF being the most frequent cardioembolic source. The incidence of AF doubles with every 10-year increase in age, which is particularly important in women, as they have a higher life expectancy. Indeed, female sex is an independent predictor of stroke in patients with AF. The attributable risk of stroke due to AF increases with age, from 1.5% for those aged 50–59 years to nearly 25% for those aged ≥80 years [21, 22]. Because of this, the female sex has been incorporated into risk stratification tools (e.g., CHA_2DS_2-VASc score) used in the decision-making for anticoagulation prophylaxis [23].

Major risk factors for ischemic stroke can be divided into modifiable (hypertension, dyslipidaemia, diabetes mellitus, smoking, alcohol abuse, physical inactivity, obesity) and non-modifiable (older age, race and ethnicity, sex, family history, and genetic disorders) [24]. Among stroke patients, women are more likely to have hypertension and diabetes mellitus, when compared to men. Although different studies have shown that obesity, abdominal adiposity, and metabolic syndrome are independent risk factors for stroke in both men and women, the prevalence of obesity is higher in women than men, especially in the premenopausal period [22].

Apart from conventional vascular risk factors and aetiologies, we need to consider unconventional stroke risk factors and mechanisms that are specific for women.

Cerebral venous thrombosis makes up 0.5–1% of all strokes but it is the stroke type that is associated with the most prominent differential sex prevalence, with the majority of affected individuals being women, especially those aged 31–50 years [22]. Beyond well-established risk factors for cerebral venous thrombosis (inherited or acquired thrombophilia, cancer, infection, hematologic and autoimmune conditions), two major risk factors are female-specific: oral contraceptive use and pregnancy/puerperium period.

Hormonal contraception is common, and its use is increasing, especially in developed countries. Different studies have demonstrated that combined hormonal contraception increased the risk of stroke; low-dose oestrogen was associated with reduced stroke risk, whereas the type of progestin was not associated with stroke risk. However, hormonal contraception is a very rare cause of ischaemic stroke and should be considered as such in clinical care [11].

During the peripartum (2 days before to 1 day after delivery) and postpartum (2 days to 6 weeks after delivery), hemodynamic changes, hypercoagulable state, hypertensive disorders, and their complications contribute to the increased risk for both ischemic and haemorrhagic stroke [25]. Different studies have reported that preeclampsia/eclampsia and gestational hypertension account for up to 48% of all pregnancy-related strokes [26]. Major complications of pregnancy (preeclampsia, gestational diabetes, and gestational hypertension) seem to be associated with a higher risk for future cardiovascular and renal disease, chronic hypertension, diabetes mellitus, and stroke beyond the childbearing years, compared to women without these disorders. Another two conditions common in postpartum stroke are the reversible cerebral vasospasm syndrome and the posterior reversible vasospasm syndrome, which are often concurrent with preeclampsia/eclampsia. Both of these conditions share underlying features of endothelial dysfunction and failure of cerebrovascular autoregulation [27].

The burden of risk factors for vascular diseases increases in women after menopause, presumably due to a postmenopausal decrease in oestrogen, a hormone with vasoprotective properties. Early menopause (<45 years) has been reported to increase the relative risks of overall coronary heart disease, stroke, cardiovascular and all-cause mortality [28]. However, a recent analysis including six randomized controlled clinical trials reported that hormone replacement therapy (HRT) does not reduce the risk of ischaemic stroke. However, due to the overall low number of studies available, the general quality of evidence was rated as very low, highlighting the need that more data are needed [29].

With a high worldwide prevalence, migraine affects four times more women than men. The absolute risk of migraine-associated stroke is relatively low. However, migraine with aura is associated with double the risk for ischaemic stroke; this association is stronger for women, women aged <45 years, use of oral contraceptives, smoking habits, and active migraine. These women generally show a better prognosis because of the association between migraine and non-disabling strokes and TIAs [30, 31]. People with migraine can also suffer from migrainous infarction, often asymptomatic, with white matter changes seen on neuroimaging modalities. The exact pathogenesis of migrainous infarct is not known, but it has been hypothesized that the duration of cortical spreading depression may be a key factor. Other factors contributing to migrainous infarction may include inflammation, endothelial dysfunction, patent foramen ovale, as well as vasoconstriction from triptans, which is commonly used to treat migraine [32].

Depression and psychosocial stress have been reported as sequelae of stroke but also can be associated with an increased risk of stroke incidence for both sexes. Even if a sex difference in stroke risk was not reported, these conditions affect more frequently women than men [33]. Depression has been hypothesized to be associated with an increased risk of stroke through a variety of mechanisms, such as neuroendocrine and inflammatory effects or poor health behaviours (isolation, physical inactivity, smoking, unhealthy diet) [11]. Table 1 reports stroke risk factors and aetiology on the basis of gender specificity.

Table 1 Stroke risk factors and aetiologies with gender specificity

	Sex-specific risk factors	Risk factors more prevalent in women	Risk factors with similar prevalence in women and men
Age			X
Atherosclerotic disease			X
Dyslipidemia			X
Smoking			X
Physical inactivity			X
Alcohol abuse			X
Atrial fibrillation		X	
Obesity		X	
Hypertension		X	
Diabetes mellitus		X	
Migraine with aura		X	
Cerebral venous thrombosis	X		
Hormonal contraception	X		
Pregnancy	X		
Preeclampsia	X		
Gestational diabetes	X		
Gestational hypertension	X		
Post-menopausal period	X		
Hormone replacement therapy	X		
Depression and psychosocial stress	X		

3 Clinical Practice

3.1 Ischaemic Stroke Diagnostic Work-Up

During the acute phase of an ischaemic stroke, performing a CT scan is of utmost importance (Fig. 1a–c). This diagnostic procedure serves two critical purposes: firstly, it helps rule out the presence of haemorrhage, and secondly, it assesses the extent of an ongoing infarction. This is particularly crucial because both haemorrhage and ongoing infarction are contraindications for reperfusion treatments, even if the patient seeks treatment within 4.5 h of experiencing stroke symptoms.

Furthermore, in cases where there is suspicion of a large vessel occlusion based on clinical symptoms, it is highly advisable to conduct a CT angiography. This specialized scan can provide valuable insights into the efficiency of collateral circulation. If the site of arterial occlusion is evidenced through this procedure, it may indicate a need for endovascular treatment via mechanical thrombectomy.

For patients who present with stroke symptoms beyond the initial 4.5-h window or those who experience symptoms upon awakening, more advanced radiological techniques become necessary. These include MRI with DWI/FLAIR mismatch analysis and perfusion imaging. These methods are employed to determine the presence of potentially salvageable cerebral tissue.

It is worth noting that there is a gap in the study of sex differences related to access to imaging modalities in stroke diagnosis. Additionally, pregnant women are generally not considered ideal candidates for radiation-based diagnostic procedures. When these procedures are deemed necessary, it is advisable to employ lead shielding to protect the foetus. During pregnancy, non-contrast MRI is the preferred imaging modality, and there is currently no evidence to suggest harm to the foetus from exposure to magnetic fields up to 3 T.

While the use of contrast agents is typically avoided during pregnancy, there are exceptions. In cases where the use of iodinated contrast can significantly impact the choice of therapy, such as in CT angiography or CT perfusion for suspected large vessel occlusion stroke, it can be considered an option [34, 35].

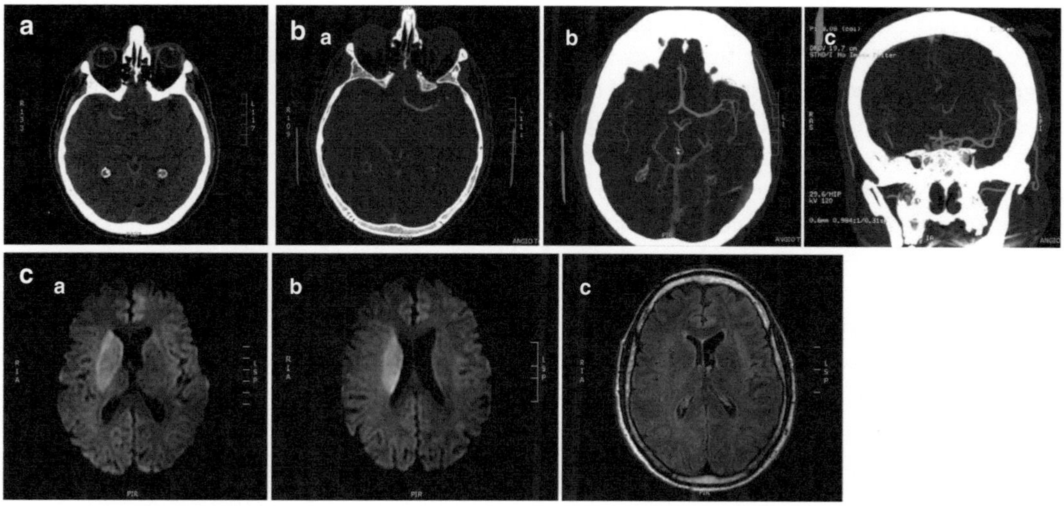

Fig. 1 Neuroimaging modalities in a 43-year-old patient with acute onset of dysarthria and left hemiparesis. (**a**): Upon admission, the initial CT scan showed no signs of acute intraparenchymal lesions but revealed a hyperdense area within the M1 segment of the right MCA. (**b**) (Panels A–C): AngioCT confirmed the M1 occlusion of the right MCA. (**c**) (Panels A–C): The MRI scan unveiled a subcortical acute ischaemic lesion on the right side. This lesion was visible in the DWI sequences but remained negative in the FLAIR sequences, indicating the presence of a DWI/FLAIR mismatch

3.2 Acute Ischaemic Stroke Treatment

Hyperacute/acute ischaemic stroke management consists of reperfusion strategies with intravenous thrombolysis, mechanical thrombectomy, and in selected cases, catheter-based thrombolysis. Eligibility for each treatment is time-dependent and varies according to the selected method [36, 37]. Based upon international guidelines, intravenous thrombolysis with alteplase is recommended to improve functional outcomes for patients with acute ischaemic stroke within 4.5 h after symptom onset at a dosage of 0.9 mg/kg. This time window can be extended further in stroke patients upon awakening, who had been seen in good condition beyond 4.5 h and who have MRI DWI-FLAIR mismatch. Mechanical thrombectomy, combined or not with fibrinolysis, is also recommended in cases of large vessel occlusion of the anterior circulation within 6 h after symptom onset. Late-presenting patients can still be treated for up to 24 h using perfusion-weighted imaging selection, according to criteria selection proposed by the DAWN and DEFUSE 3 trial results [38, 39]. Conversely, the efficacy of endovascular treatment in patients with posterior circulation stroke has not been demonstrated [40, 41]. Nevertheless, recent studies have suggested that its therapeutic efficacy might be maximized by reducing futile recanalization through the identification of prognostic factors and an optimal selection of endovascular procedures [42, 43].

Acute ischaemic stroke during pregnancy and during the post-partum period poses great challenges regarding the best therapeutic regimen to adopt. Pregnancy-associated stroke is rare but is the first cause of maternal mortality and morbidity worldwide, with a three-fold higher risk when compared to non-pregnant women. Moreover, the incidence of cerebrovascular events has been reported to vary according to the time from delivery: it is generally higher within the first 6 weeks and lower, but still present, 12 weeks post-partum [44]. However, data on the efficacy and safety of reperfusion strategies in this population is lacking, as current trial criteria do not allow pregnant women to be included in studies focused on the efficacy and safety of thrombolysis and thrombectomy [36, 37]. International guidelines highlight the lack of data driving the decision-making process in the hyperacute ischaemic stroke phase among pregnant women. Only recently have regulatory agencies supported the idea of enrolling pregnant/post-partum women in randomized clinical trials (RCTs) with the aim of better identifying an optimal diagnostic work-up, acute treatment and secondary prevention. The Stroke in Pregnancy and Postpartum (SiPP) [45] study is an ongoing observational, non-interventional, multidisciplinary, registry-based study on pregnancy-related cerebrovascular disease. This large-scale international investigation aims to collect data to solve the unmet needs to manage these uncommon conditions. A sub-study assessing bio-bank molecular and genetic data is planned in order to identify any biomolecular and genetic markers. Based on currently available evidence, intravenous thrombolysis and endovascular thrombectomy should be delivered more often to women with disabling symptoms who would be otherwise eligible for treatments. International guidelines recommend an early and appropriate assessment of the benefit/risk profile. Alteplase (tPA), and more recently tenecteplase (TNK), are the most widely used and effective recombinant tissue plasminogen activators for cerebral reperfusion: however, both are classified as pregnancy category C among drugs that cause or are suspected of causing potentially reversible, non-malformation, harmful effects to the foetus or newborn [46]. This is despite the fact that TNK and tPA do not cross the placenta. The reported adverse events after reperfusion/recanalisation treatment include vaginal and systemic bleeding (defined as life-threatening when requiring more than three transfused units of blood), miscarriage and haemorrhagic transformation of the index cerebral infarct. Given so, guidelines recommend thrombolysis to treat moderate to severe stroke during pregnancy and during the post-partum period (at least 10 days after delivery) whenever the benefits are deemed to outweigh the risks. Specifically, the risk of bleeding has been reported to be higher in the peripartum and post-partum periods, which have been associated with a high risk of strokes (40% and 50%) [47, 48]. In cases of disabling symptoms caused by large vessel occlusion, mechanical thrombectomy should be considered within 6 h of symptom onset or in the presence of salvageable brain tissue on diagnostic imaging (MRI, CT perfusion) according to international guidelines (Fig. 2a–c). This proce-

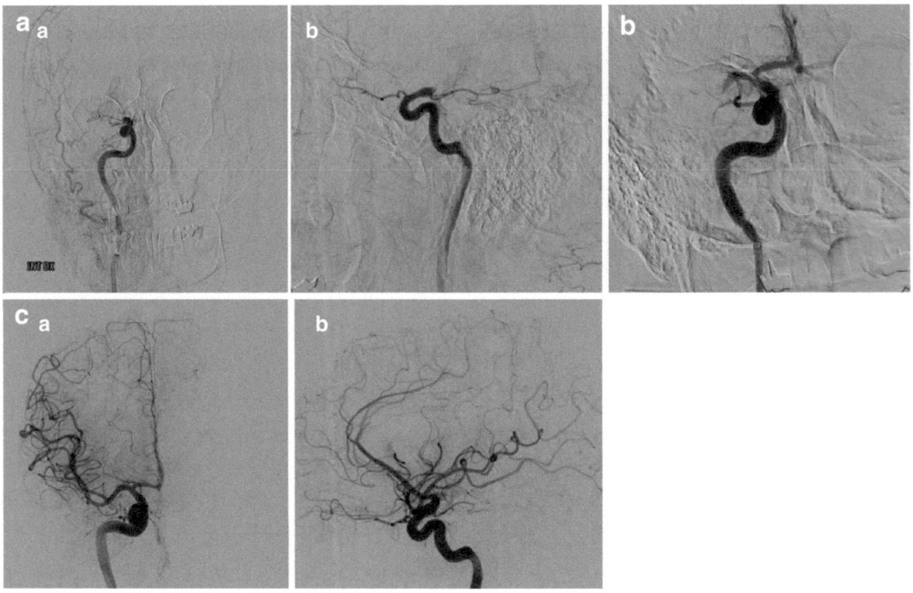

Fig. 2 Digital subtraction angiography (DSA) and mechanical thrombectomy were both performed on the same patient. (**a**) (Panels A and B): DSA confirmed M1 occlusion of the right arteria cerebri media (ACM) in both anterior-posterior and lateral-lateral projections. (**b**): DSA control, conducted after the initial attempt at thrombus aspiration, revealed a partial revascularization of the right M1 segment. (**c**) (Panels A and B): The final DSA control was performed after complete ACM revascularization in anterior-posterior and lateral-lateral projections

dure carries a negligible risk of systemic bleeding complications and the use of lead shielding minimizes foetal radiation exposure. If the risk of bleeding is deemed unacceptable, endovascular recanalization should be preferred over both systemic thrombolysis and bridging therapy. The USA Get with The Guidelines (GWTG) Stroke Registry compared outcomes following intravenous thrombolysis, catheter-based thrombolysis, mechanical thrombectomy or any combination of these treatments in pregnant/postpartum and non-pregnant/non-postpartum women [49]. Outcomes after reperfusion therapy in the two subgroups were comparable. However, in both pregnant and post-partum women a trend towards increased symptomatic intracranial haemorrhage was observed, along with a longer hospitalization.

3.3 Secondary Prevention and Rehabilitation

Following ischaemic stroke, the best medical therapy and intensive vascular risk factor management remain the cornerstone of stroke recurrence prevention [50]. Secondary prophylaxis treatment depends on the underlying aetiology and stroke subtype. Antithrombotic therapy, including antiplatelet or anticoagulant agents, is strongly recommended for patients without contraindications. Whereas short-term dual antiplatelet therapy is indicated in cases of non-cardioembolic minor stroke and high-risk transient ischemic attack or severe symptomatic intracranial stenosis. Oral anticoagulants should be prescribed for cardioembolic aetiology due to AF, preferring NOACs to warfarin in non-valvular forms. Patients with large artery atherosclerosis may instead benefit from surgical or endovascular correction (carotid endarterectomy or carotid artery stenting, respectively) based on comorbidities and anatomical features. In addition, lipid-lowering therapy with high-dose statins is often indicated in order to reduce stroke recurrence risk. Available data do not show sex differences regarding the efficacy of antithrombotic drugs. Concerning cardio-embolic stroke, women have been reported to be undertreated with oral anticoagulants compared to men [51]. Overall, guidelines highlight the need to identify evidence for secondary prevention in women in more vulnerable periods of their lifetime. Among pregnant and post-partum women, daily use of low-dose aspirin is generally considered safe. At the same time, there is limited data to corroborate the use of other antiplatelet therapies, like thienopyridines, which should be prescribed on a case-by-case assessment. When anticoagulants are indicated, low molecular weight heparin should be preferred. Conversely, warfarin is contraindicated for its well-established teratogenic effect, while there is insufficient data to recommend the use of direct oral anticoagulants, considering their ability to cross the placenta [22, 29, 52]. Statins are also contraindicated during pregnancy because of their reported teratogenicity; this is possibly due to an interruption of cholesterol synthetization. However, the safety of statin use during pregnancy has been questioned: a recent retrospective cohort study investigating the foetal outcomes of maternal statin exposure has evidenced an association between low birth weight (<2500 g) and preterm labour, in the absence of increased risk of congenital anomalies among offspring [53]. Conversely, as suggested by the FUTURE study [54] among the Dutch population, first-ever childbearing age stroke represents a higher risk condition for nulliparous women to develop severe complications in subsequent pregnancies, including hypertensive disorders, haemolysis, elevated liver enzymes, low platelet count syndrome and early preterm delivery. In these cohorts, nulliparous and multiparous were also exposed to a higher risk of miscarriage.

In the post-acute phase, early rehabilitation and non-pharmacological strategies were seen to improve long-term patient outcomes and prevent stroke recurrence compared to medical therapy alone [55]. Adopting a healthy lifestyle, including regular physical activity, prevents cerebrovascular disease and promotes medium-long-term recovery. It has been demonstrated that regularly practising sports can reduce the risk of stroke by acting favourably on blood pressure and body weight, optimizing glycolipid metabolism and improving endothelial function through the reduction of platelet aggregation, the viscosity of blood and the process of atherogenesis. Moreover, stroke survivors who had been regularly engaged in physical activity showed more resilience and a greater chance of good functional recovery [52, 56]. Approximately 48% of stroke survivors receive post-acute care rehabilitation in different settings, from inpatient rehabilitation facilities to outpatient offices, based on the individual's physical abilities, stroke severity, bed availability, and universal coverage of the National Healthcare Service [56]. Gender does not seem to discriminate in the access to rehabilitation facilities. However, it has been shown that women have less favourable functional outcomes because of older age at stroke onset and more severe strokes. In addition, women more frequently develop post-stroke depression and therefore often perceive a low quality of life [54]. Pregnancy-associated stroke among women of childbearing age is the most common cause of morbidity and severe long-term disability in this cohort. Recent studies have suggested that pregnant stroke patients have a higher hazard of death and readmission rates compared with pregnant patients without stroke at 1-year follow-up, and this finding persisted for a decade after delivery [57].

4 Conclusion

Stroke remains the second-leading cause of death worldwide and one of the main causes of long-term disability. Stroke pathophysiological mechanisms and risk factors are now well-established. However, particular aetiologies and risk factors can be considered female sex-specific or more prevalent in women, when compared to men. Moreover, women are disproportionately affected by stroke, often experiencing more adverse outcomes and high rates of mortality.

Clinical presentations of ischaemic stroke depend on the brain area affected by the hypoperfusion, but clinical characteristics may be distinguished by sex-related differences. Women often present with non-focal neurological symptoms (such as confusion, impaired consciousness, headache, light-headedness, and atypical symptoms), which often could mistakenly be misinterpreted.

In the acute phase of an ischaemic stroke, neurological and correct neuroradiological evaluation is mandatory, in order to candidate the patient for reperfusion therapies. Unfortunately, even today, disparities in stroke diagnosis and management still exist, particularly concerning ethnicity and gender. In particular, acute ischemic stroke during pregnancy and during the post-partum period poses great challenges regarding the best diagnostic and therapeutic regimen to adopt. Pregnant women are generally not considered ideal candidates for radiation-based diagnostic procedures, so non-contrast MRI is the preferred imaging modality. Based on currently available evidence, reperfusion therapies should be administered to women with disabling symptoms, with an early and appropriate assessment of the benefit/risk profile. After an ischaemic stroke, secondary prevention with aetiology-based secondary prophylaxis and intensive risk factor management is mandatory. These strategies include antithrombotic therapy, lifestyle modifications, and physical activity. Current guidelines highlight the need to identify evidence for secondary prevention in women in more vulnerable periods of their lifetime, such as pregnancy. Indeed, warfarin and statins are contraindicated for their established teratogenic effect.

Finally, gender disparities do not seem to exist regarding access to rehabilitation services. However, women experience less favourable functional outcomes because of older age and more severe strokes. In addition, women more frequently develop post-stroke depression and therefore often perceive a low quality of life.

Key Issues

- Stroke is the second-leading cause of death worldwide and the third-leading cause of long-term disability.
- When compared to men, women experience more severe strokes and consequently worse functional outcomes.
- Clinical characteristics may be distinguished by sex-related differences, with women presenting more often with non-focal neurologi-

cal or atypical symptoms, which often could mistakenly be misinterpreted.

- Apart from conventional stroke risk factors and aetiologies, unconventional risk factors and mechanisms that are sex-specific have to be considered and investigated in women.
- Eligibility for revascularisation therapies is time-dependent and varies according to time window and patient contraindications.
- Disparities in stroke diagnosis and management still exist, particularly concerning ethnicity and gender.
- Stroke in pregnant women represents an issue regarding acute diagnostic workup and management.
- In the post-acute phase, secondary prevention is mandatory, with personalized strategies regarding female sex.

Questions and Answers

1. Which of the following risk factors for ischaemic stroke appears to have similar prevalence in men and women and is not considered a female-specific factor?
   (A) Atrial fibrillation
   (B) Hypertension
   (C) Pregnancy
   (D) Hormone replace treatment
   (E) Atherosclerotic disease
   Correct answer: E
   Different risk factors for ischaemic stroke are well recognized. Among these, atrial fibrillation, obesity, hypertension and diabetes mellitus have been demonstrated to be more prevalent in women than in men. On the other hand, age, dyslipidaemia, atherosclerotic disease, smoking, physical inactivity and alcohol abuse appear to have the same prevalence in men and women. Apart from conventional vascular risk factors, women can present sex-specific unconventional stroke risk factors, such as hormone replace treatment, pregnancy and related disorders and the post-menopausal period.
2. A 75-year-old woman was admitted to the Emergency Department due to the sudden onset of aphasia and right-sided weakness occurring at approximately 8 a.m. A neurological examination was conducted at 10:30 a.m. and revealed aphasia, right hemiparesis with the left eye and gaze deviation, and global aphasia. A CT scan showed no significant abnormalities except a left M1 hyperdensity of the arteria cerebri media (ACM). The Angio-CT scan confirmed an occlusion the M1. What would be the most appropriate diagnostic and therapeutic course of action for this patient?
   (A) Perform a brain MRI to investigate the presence of the diffusion/FLAIR mismatch before proceeding to reperfusion therapies (intravenous thrombolysis or mechanical thrombectomy);
   (B) Perform only intravenous thrombolysis after excluding contra-indications;
   (C) Admit the patient to a Stroke Unit without performing acute revascularization therapies;
   (D) Proceed directly to reperfusion therapies (both intravenous thrombolysis and mechanical thrombectomy) after considering contraindications;
   (E) Perform an advanced neuroimaging (CT perfusion) to evaluate the extension of the ischaemic core and penumbra and then consider reperfusion therapies.
   Correct answer: D
   The patient was admitted to the Emergency Department for an acute and severe neurological focal syndrome arising approximately 2.5 h earlier. CT scan excluded acute intracerebral haemorrhages. According to the current guidelines, in the absence of any contraindication, the patient is a direct candidate to receive intravenous thrombolysis because symptom onset falls within the treatment time window of <4.5 h. Moreover, Angio-CT scan showed the presence of an intracranial large vessel occlusion, making treatment with mechanical thrombectomy also indicated.
3. Which of the following reperfusion strategies are recommended for the treatment of acute ischemic stroke within specific time windows, taking into account the management of pregnant and postpartum women?

(A) Intravenous thrombolysis with alteplase at a dosage of 0.9 mg/kg within 4.5 h after symptom onset for eligible patients, with considerations for pregnant and postpartum women.
(B) Mechanical thrombectomy for large vessel occlusion of the anterior circulation within 48 h after symptom onset, including pregnant and postpartum women.
(C) Endovascular recanalization for posterior circulation stroke within 24 h after symptom onset, considering pregnancy-related factors.
(D) Catheter-based thrombolysis for all acute ischemic stroke patients regardless of time since symptom onset, with a special focus on pregnant and postpartum women.

Correct answer: A

Based on European Stroke Guidelines on acute management of ischaemic stroke in pregnant women, intravenous thrombolysis should be administered at the dosage of 0.9 mg/kg within 4.5 h after symptom onset. Mechanical thrombectomy should be administered in all patients with a confirmed large vessel occlusion within 6 h after symptom onset. Administration of reperfusion therapies in the extended time window (4.5 h for intravenous thrombolysis and 6 h for mechanical thrombectomy) should be based on advanced neuroimaging (CT/MRI perfusion).

4. Which of the following strategies regarding secondary stroke prevention is **not** indicated in order to reduce the risk of future ischaemic events?
   (A) Short-term dual antiplatelet therapy in the case of minor stroke and high-risk transient ischemic attack;
   (B) Antiplatelet agent (aspirin) in the case of a 93-year-old patient with acute stroke, with a history of AF, mild renal impairment, high risk of falls and moderate atherosclerotic disease;
   (C) Adequate vascular risk factors control, such as antihypertensive treatment, dyslipidemia control, stop smoking, and screening for diabetes;
   (D) Anticoagulation treatment in a 50-year-old man with a new diagnosis of AF and without a history of hypertension, diabetes, or any other medical problem;
   (E) Anticoagulation with apixaban at the dosage of 2.5 bid in the case of an 81-year-old woman, with previously known AF and a recent ischaemic stroke, without renal impairment, with an estimated weight of 55 kg.

   Correct answer: B

   Antiplatelet treatment is contraindicated as a secondary prevention strategy in the case of a patient with AF and recent ischaemic stroke based on current European Society of Cardiology Guidelines.
5. A 43-year-old woman, 4 weeks after giving birth to a healthy baby, presented to the hospital with severe and progressively worsening headaches accompanied by nausea and vomiting. Her pregnancy and delivery had been uneventful. The headaches had initially begun 2 weeks after childbirth and had since become unbearable. Upon examination, the patient was visibly distressed due to the severity of her headaches. Neurological examination did not reveal any focal deficits. Her vital signs were stable, and there were no signs of infection or fever. The medical team took note of her recent childbirth, which is a risk factor for clot formation. CT scan in the Emergency Room is reported below (Fig. 3).
   (A) What do you think should not be part of the correct subsequent diagnostic and therapeutic approach for this patient?
   (B) Perform an Angio-CT/MRI with vein sequences in order to exclude a cerebral venous sinus thrombosis;
   (C) Consider eligibility for acute revascularization therapies, such as intravenous thrombolysis with rt-PA and mechanical thrombectomy;
   (D) Perform laboratory examination, assessing the patient's blood clotting profile, coagulation factors, and D-dimer levels and also genetic predispositions to clotting disorders;

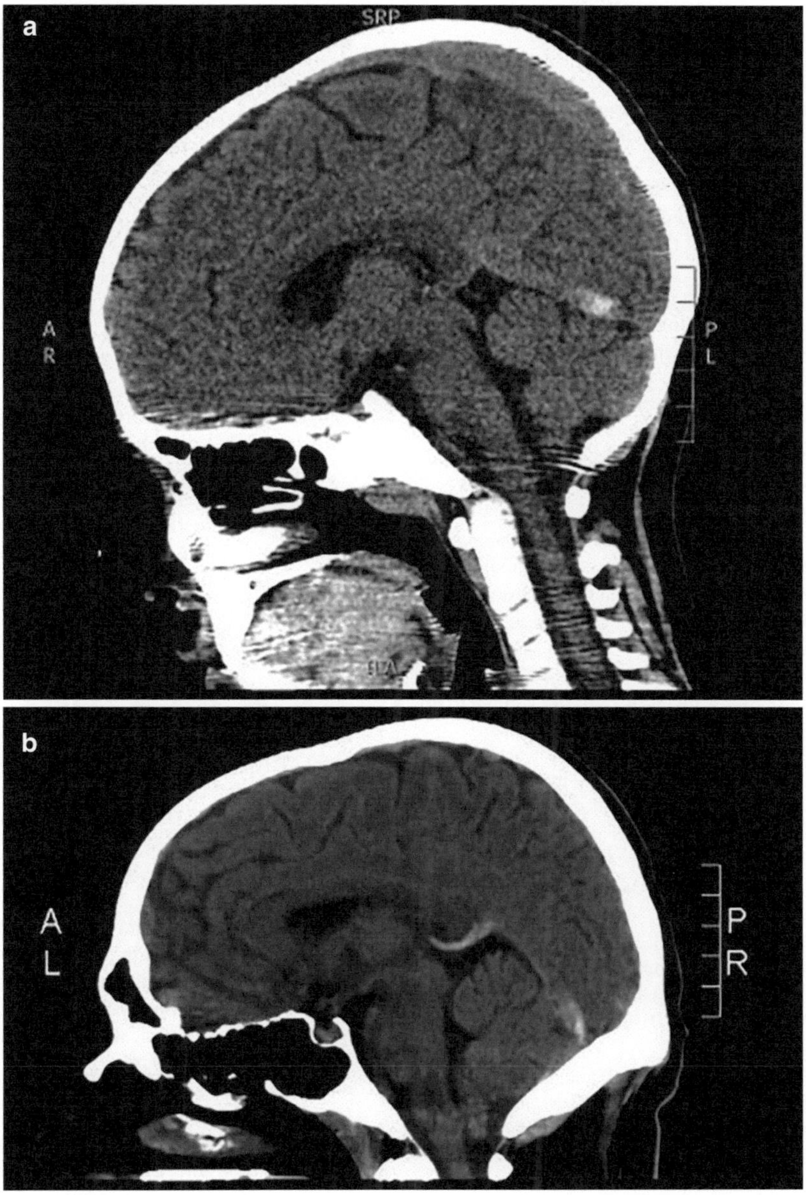

Fig. 3 CT scan in the emergency room in a woman 4 weeks postpartum (panels A and B)

(E) Promptly start of anticoagulation therapy with subcutaneous heparin at a therapeutic dose, despite the presence of an acute ischaemic venous lesion with a haemorrhagic component;

(F) Switch from heparin to warfarin 1 week after the diagnosis to maintain an INR (International Normalized Ratio) within the therapeutic range of 2–3, for 3 months.

Correct answer: C

The patient's clinical history, coupled with the predisposing factor of the post-partum period, strongly points toward a diagnosis of cerebral venous sinus thrombosis. The CT scan has revealed a thrombus within the transverse sinus, indicating an acute thrombotic event. According to current guidelines, the recommended approach for managing cerebral venous thrombosis does not involve acute revascularization therapies, but rather the initiation of appropriate anticoagulation therapy.

References

1. Persky RW, Turtzo LC, LD MC. Stroke in women: disparities and outcomes. Curr Cardiol Rep. 2010;12:6–13. https://doi.org/10.1007/s11886-009-0080-2.
2. Yoon CW, Bushnell CD. Stroke in women: a review focused on epidemiology, risk factors, and outcomes. J Stroke. 2023;25:2–15. https://doi.org/10.5853/jos.2022.03468.
3. Tsivgoulis G, Katsanos AH, Caso V. Underrepresentation of women in stroke randomized controlled trials: inadvertent selection bias leading to suboptimal conclusions. Ther Adv Neurol Disord. 2017;10:241–4. https://doi.org/10.1177/1756285617699588.
4. Aho K, et al. Cerebrovascular disease in the community: results of a WHO collaborative study. Bull World Health Organ. 1980;58:113–30.
5. Sacco RL, Kasner SE, Broderick JP, et al. An updated definition of stroke for the 21st century: a statement for healthcare professionals from the American heart association/American stroke association. Stroke. 2013;44(7):2064–89.
6. Pare JR, Kahn JH. Basic neuroanatomy and stroke syndromes. Emerg Med Clin North Am. 2012;30:601–15. https://doi.org/10.1016/j.emc.2012.05.004.
7. Phan HT, et al. Sex differences in severity of stroke in the INSTRUCT study: a meta-analysis of individual participant data. J Am Heart Assoc. 2019;8(1):e010235.
8. Ali M, et al. Sex differences in presentation of stroke: a systematic review and meta-analysis. Stroke. 2022;53:345–54. https://doi.org/10.1161/STROKEAHA.120.034040.
9. Yu AYX, et al. Sex differences in presentation and outcome after an acute transient or minor neurologic event. JAMA Neurol. 2019;76:962–8. (American Medical Association)
10. Feigin VL, et al. Global, regional, and national burden of stroke and its risk factors, 1990–2019: a systematic analysis for the Global Burden of Disease Study 2019. Lancet Neurol. 2021;20:795–820.
11. Cordonnier C, et al. Stroke in women - from evidence to inequalities. Nat Rev Neurol. 2017;13:521–32. https://doi.org/10.1038/nrneurol.2017.95.
12. Vyas MV, et al. Stroke incidence by sex across the lifespan. Stroke. 2021;52:447–51.
13. Leppert MH, et al. Young women had more strokes than young men in a large. United States claims sample. Stroke. 2020;51:3352–5.
14. Ekker MS, et al. Association of Stroke among adults aged 18 to 49 years with long-term mortality. JAMA. 2019;321:2113–23.
15. Barker-Collo S, et al. Sex differences in stroke incidence, prevalence, mortality and disability-adjusted life years: results from the global burden of disease study 2013. Neuroepidemiology. 2015;45:203–14.
16. Romain G, et al. Long-term relative survival after stroke: the Dijon Stroke Registry. Neuroepidemiology. 2020;54:498–505.
17. Rexrode KM, et al. The impact of sex and gender on stroke. Circ Res. 2022;130:512–28.
18. Petrea RE, et al. Gender differences in stroke incidence and poststroke disability in the Framingham Heart Study. Stroke. 2009;40(4):1032–7.
19. Gardener H, et al. Race and ethnic disparities in stroke incidence in the northern Manhattan Study. Stroke. 2020;51(4):1064–9.
20. Adams HP, et al. Classification of subtype of acute ischemic stroke definitions for use in a multicenter clinical trial. Stroke. 1993;24(1):35–41.
21. Chugh SS, et al. Worldwide epidemiology of atrial fibrillation: a global burden of disease 2010 study. Circulation. 2014;129:837–47.
22. Bushnell C, et al. Guidelines for the prevention of stroke in women: a statement for healthcare professionals from the American Heart Association/American Stroke Association. Stroke. 2014;45:1545–88.
23. Siddiqi TJ, et al. Utility of the CHA2DS2-VASc score for predicting ischaemic stroke in patients with or without atrial fibrillation: a systematic review and meta-analysis. Eur J Prev Cardiol. 2022;29(4):625–31.
24. Feigin VL, Forouzanfar MH, Krishnamurthi R, et al. Global and regional burden of stroke during 1990–2010: findings from the Global Burden of Disease Study 2010. Lancet. 2014;383:245–54.
25. Bushnell CD, et al. Sex differences in stroke: challenges and opportunities. J Cereb Blood Flow Metab. 2018;38:2179–91. https://doi.org/10.1177/0271678X18793324.
26. Sharshar T, Lamy C, Mas JL. Incidence and causes of strokes associated with pregnancy and puerperium. A study in public hospitals of Ile de France. Stroke in Pregnancy Study Group. Stroke. 1995;26(6):930–6.
27. Miller EC, et al. Clinical practice mechanisms and outcomes of stroke during pregnancy and the postpartum period. A cross-sectional study. Neurol Clin Pract. 2016;6(1):29–39.
28. Muka T, et al. Association of age at onset of menopause and time since onset of menopause with cardiovascular outcomes, intermediate vascular traits, and all-cause mortality: a systematic review and meta-analysis. JAMA Cardiol. 2016;1:767–76.
29. Kremer C, et al. European Stroke Organisation guidelines on stroke in women: management of menopause, pregnancy and postpartum. Eur Stroke J. 2022;7(2):I–XIX.
30. Schürks M, et al. Migraine and cardiovascular disease: systematic review and meta-analysis. BMJ (Online). 2009;339:1015.
31. Øie LR, et al. Migraine and risk of stroke. J Neurol Neurosurg Psychiatry. 2020;91:593–604. https://doi.org/10.1136/jnnp-2018-318254.
32. Zhang Y, Parikh A, Qian S. Migraine and stroke. Stroke Vasc Neurol. 2017;2:160–7. https://doi.org/10.1136/svn-2017-000077.

33. Zhang H, et al. Risk factors for ischaemic and intracerebral haemorrhagic stroke in 22 countries (the INTERSTROKE study): a case-control study. Lancet. 2010;376(9735):112–23.
34. Kapral MK, Bushnell C. Stroke in women. Stroke. 2021;52:726–8. https://doi.org/10.1161/STROKEAHA.120.033233.
35. Bushnell CD, Kapral MK. Advances in stroke: stroke in women. Stroke. 2022;53:605–7.
36. Berge E, et al. European Stroke Organisation (ESO) guidelines on intravenous thrombolysis for acute ischaemic stroke. Eur Stroke J. 2021;6:I–LXII.
37. Turc G, et al. European Stroke Organisation (ESO)—European Society for Minimally Invasive Neurological Therapy (ESMINT) guidelines on mechanical thrombectomy in acute ischemic stroke. J Neurointerv Surg. 2023;15:e8.
38. Albers GW, et al. Thrombectomy for stroke at 6 to 16 hours with selection by perfusion imaging. N Engl J Med. 2018;378:708–18.
39. Nogueira RG, et al. Thrombectomy 6 to 24 hours after stroke with a mismatch between deficit and infarct. N Engl J Med. 2018;378:11–21.
40. LCM L, et al. Endovascular therapy for stroke due to basilar-artery occlusion. N Engl J Med. 2021;384:1910–20.
41. Liu X, et al. Endovascular treatment versus standard medical treatment for vertebrobasilar artery occlusion (BEST): an open-label, randomised controlled trial. Lancet Neurol. 2020;19:115–22.
42. Jovin TG, et al. Trial of thrombectomy 6 to 24 hours after stroke due to basilar-artery occlusion. N Engl J Med. 2022;387:1373–84.
43. Tao C, et al. Trial of endovascular treatment of acute basilar-artery occlusion. N Engl J Med. 2022;387:1361–72.
44. Kamel H, et al. Risk of a thrombotic event after the 6-week postpartum period. Obstet Gynecol Surv. 2014;69:375–6.
45. Lorenzano S, et al. SiPP (Stroke in Pregnancy and Postpartum): a prospective, observational, international, multicentre study on pathophysiological mechanisms, clinical profile, management and outcome of cerebrovascular diseases in pregnant and postpartum women. Eur Stroke J. 2020;5:193–203.
46. Wang X, et al. Worse prognosis in women, compared with men, after thrombolysis: an individual patient data pooling study of Asian acute stroke registries. Int J Stroke. 2021;16:784–91.
47. O'Neal MA, Feske SK. Stroke in pregnancy: a case-oriented review. Pract Neurol. 2016;6(1):23–34. https://doi.org/10.1136/practneurol.
48. Eriksson M, Åsberg S, Sunnerhagen KS, Von Euler M. Sex differences in stroke care and outcome 2005–2018: observations from the Swedish Stroke Register. Stroke. 2021;52:3233–42. https://doi.org/10.1161/STROKEAHA.120.033893.
49. Leffert LR, et al. Treatment patterns and short-term outcomes in ischemic stroke in pregnancy or postpartum period. Presented at the American Heart Association/American Stroke Association 2015 International Stroke Conference, Nashville, TN, February 11–12, 2014. Am J Obstet Gynecol. 2016;214:723.e1–11.
50. Dawson J, et al. European Stroke Organisation (ESO) guideline on pharmacological interventions for long-term secondary prevention after ischaemic stroke or transient ischaemic attack. Eur Stroke J. 2022;7:I–II.
51. Kostopoulou A, et al. Atrial fibrillation-related stroke in women: evidence and inequalities in epidemiology, mechanisms, clinical presentation, and management. Clin Cardiol. 2020;43:14–23. https://doi.org/10.1002/clc.23284.
52. Acciarresi M, et al. Secondary stroke prevention in women. Womens Health. 2011;7:391–7. https://doi.org/10.2217/whe.11.20.
53. Chang JC, et al. Perinatal outcomes after statin exposure during pregnancy. JAMA Netw Open. 2021;4(12):e2141321.
54. Synhaeve NE, et al. Women have a poorer very long-term functional outcome after stroke among adults aged 18–50 years: the FUTURE study. J Neurol. 2016;263:1099–105.
55. Krishnan S, Hay CC, Pappadis MR, Deutsch A, Reistetter TA. Stroke survivors' perspectives on post-acute rehabilitation options, goals, satisfaction, and transition to home. J Neurol Phys Ther. 2019;43:160–7.
56. Joundi RA, et al. Age-specific and sex-specific trends in life-sustaining care after acute stroke. J Am Heart Assoc. 2021;10:e021499.
57. Liu S, et al. Stroke and cerebrovascular disease in pregnancy: incidence, temporal trends, and risk factors. Stroke. 2019;50:13–20.

Heart Failure in Women

Tiny Jaarsma, Joanna-Maria Papageorgiou, and Anna Strömberg

Abstract

There are important differences in epidemiology, pathophysiology, heart failure (HF) type, prognosis, and treatment. Women with HF have a higher incidence of HF with preserved ejection fraction (HFpEF) but in general treatment recommendation for guideline directed therapy are similar for men and women. There are still gaps in the management of women with HF. Self-care behaviour is vital for optimal outcomes for patients with HF and although there is no difference in the content of self-care advice, the challenges for optimal self-care might be different for women. A person-centred approach to treat and support women with HF is needed to attain optimal outcomes.

Keywords

Heart failure · Self-care · Diagnosis · Treatment · Heart failure clinics

Test your learning and check your understanding of this book's contents: use the "Springer Nature Flashcards" app to access questions using ▶ https://sn.pub/51ny7m To use the app, please follow the instructions in chapter 1.

T. Jaarsma (✉)
Department of Health, Medicine and Caring Sciences, Linköping University, Linköping, Sweden

Department of Cardiology, University Medical Center Utrecht, Utrecht, The Netherlands
e-mail: tiny.jaarsma@liu.se

J.-M. Papageorgiou
Department of Cardiology, Linköping University, Linköping, Sweden
e-mail: joanna-maria.papageorgiou@liu.se

A. Strömberg
Department of Health, Medicine and Caring Sciences, Linköping University, Linköping, Sweden

Department of Cardiology, Linköping University, Linköping, Sweden
e-mail: anna.stromberg@liu.se

A. H.E.M. Maas, E. Gerdts (eds.), *Manual of Cardiovascular Disease in Women*,
https://doi.org/10.1007/978-3-031-65952-2_24

1 Theory

1.1 Epidemiology

The age-adjusted incidence of heart failure (HF) for men and women is declining in most developing countries, presumably reflecting better management of cardiovascular disease in general and HF management in particular. Still the overall incidence of HF is increasing, mainly due to the aging of the population. Currently, the incidence of HF in Europe is about 5/1000 person-years in adults [1, 2]. The current chapter gives an overview of HF in women.

The overall lifetime risk of HF is quite comparable between the sexes; estimated at 21% for men and 20% for women at the age of 40 years in the Framingham Heart Study, and 33% for men and 29% for women at age of 55 years in the Rotterdam Study [3].

The prevalence of HF is different for men and women across the ejection fraction spectrum. HF with preserved ejection fraction (HFpEF) is about double in women than in men and it is higher at any given age [4]. In HF with reduced ejection fraction (HFrEF) men have a higher risk than women and this has been attributed to their higher tendency to coronary artery disease and myocardial infarction among men. This can be contrasted with microvascular dysfunction of the coronary circulation that may play a major role in HFpEF [5].

In a recent registry study including 42,987 patients, 37% were women (55% with HFpEF, 39% HFmrEF (HF with mid-range EF), and 29% with HFrEF. Women were older and more symptomatic and more likely to have hypertension and kidney disease but less likely to have diabetes and ischemic heart disease [6].

1.2 Aetiology and Diagnosis

HF has multifactorial aetiology. Causes, in both genders, are coronary artery disease, hypertension, idiopathic dilated cardiomyopathy, arrhythmias and valvular disease. Sex differences in aetiology are present, as sex hormones including oestrogen, progesterone and testosterone modify some of the pathophysiological processes promoting HF progression in women [7]. Premenopausal women do not frequently present with coronary artery disease, but once they develop it, the risk of HF is high [8]. Women are more likely to be affected by HFpEF [9]. The pathophysiological mechanisms are not completely revealed but hypothesized to be related to sex differences in inflammation and microvascular dysfunction along with traditional risk factors such as hypertension, diabetes and obesity [10].

Other aetiologies of HF in women include peripartum cardiomyopathy, inflammatory or infiltrative myocardial disease, metabolic diseases, genetic cardiomyopathies as well as cardiotoxicity due to chemotherapy with doxorubicin, trastuzumab or radiation towards the chest with the heart placed in the radiation field [11]. Takotsubo cardiomyopathy has a predilection for postmenopausal women with the main driver being emotional stress. It is usually a reversible cause of HF with better prognosis and long-term outcomes then HF with other underlying aetiology [12].

The diagnosis of HF requires the presence of symptoms and/or signs of HF and even objective evidence of cardiac dysfunction [2]. Symptoms and signs of HF are similar in both genders. Most common symptoms are breathlessness, reduced exercise tolerance, ankle swelling and fatigue. Patients often present with signs of elevated jugular venous pressure, laterally displaced apical impulse and third heart sound, so called gallop rhythm. However, women present often with exertional dyspnea, oedema, and exercise difficulties. The initial assessment of patients in both sexes with suspected HF includes:

- An electrocardiogram (ECG). A lot of information can be gathered from ECG, as for example if there are signs of arrhythmias, presence of Q-waves, signs of LV (left ventricular) hypertrophy. A normal ECG makes the diagnosis of HF unlikely.

- Measurement of natriuretic peptides (NP). A plasma concentration of B-type natriuretic peptide (BNP) <35 pg/ml or N-terminal pro-B-type natriuretic peptide (NT-ProBNP) <125 pg/ml make a diagnosis of HF unlikely.
- Echocardiography is recommended as the gold standard for diagnosing HF. It determines LVEF, and provides information on other parameters, as chamber size, regional wall motion abnormalities, signs of pulmonary hypertension, markers of diastolic dysfunction or valvular function.
- More specialized diagnostic tests like cardiac magnetic resonance (CMR), Fluorodeoxyglucose positron emission tomography (FDG-PET), diphosphono-1,2-propanodicarboxylic acid scintigraphy (DPD-scint)) may be taken into consideration for detection of reversible or treatable causes of HF, as for example sarcoidosis, Fabry disease, and amyloidosis.

1.3 Treatment

Guideline-directed medical therapies in HF show no differences in the overall recommendations for medical therapy between men and women [2, 13, 14], but there are differences depending on the HF phenotype. Medical therapy for HFrEF is proven to reverse LV-remodeling, improve quality of life, reduce HF hospitalizations and reduce mortality [8].

The cornerstones of pharmacotherapy in HFrEF include ACEI (Angiotensin converting enzyme inhibitor)/ARNI (Angiotension receptor blocker and neprilysine inhibitor), SGLT2-I (sodium-glucose co-transporter 2 inhibitor), beta-blocker and MRA (mineralocorticoid receptor antagonist). Regarding HFmrEF, there are no specific trials on this patient population, but all drugs used in HFrEF treatment algorithm can be considered in treating patients with HFmrEF. Finally, patients with HFpEF are recommended to be treated with SGLT2-I [9], but no other treatment has been shown to convincingly reduce mortality and morbidity in HFpEF patients. Treatment of underlying conditions should be prioritized.

Cardiac rhythm management of HFrEF include implantable cardioverter-defibrillator (ICD) both for secondary and primary prevention of sudden cardiac death, as well as cardiac resynchronization therapy (CRT). ICD, as secondary prevention, is recommended in patients who have recovered from a ventricular arrhythmia causing hemodynamic instability and who have an expected survival of >1 year with good functional status and in the absence of reversible causes. As a primary prevention, ICD is recommended in patients in NYHA II-III and an LVEF<35% despite 3 months optimal medical treatment, with an expected survival >1 year with good functional status. CRT is recommended for symptomatic patients with LBBB QRS morphology in ECG, QRS-duration >150 ms and LVEF <35% despite optimal medical treatment and must be considered in those with QRS duration of 130–150 ms.

Understanding of sex differences in therapy response is limited by retrospective and post-hoc subgroup analyses of landmark HF clinical trials that often have under-representation of women [15]. Review of these trials suggest that not all HF medications have the same benefit in men and women [16]. For example, a meta-analysis of 12 large RCT of ACEI could not prove a definitive benefit of ACEI in women [17]. Sex hormones may be responsible for some of these observed differences in HF medical therapies, as ACE activity, aldosterone secretion and vascular response to angiotensin II are decreased by oestrogen and increased by androgens. In conditions such as HF, oestrogen stimulates increased Angiotensin II type 2 receptor expression and activation leading to a more pronounced inhibitory effect of angiotensin receptor blocker in women than men, which may be able to explain the greater effect of angiotensin receptor blockers, and subsequently ARNIs, relative to ACE inhibitors in women.

There are sex differences in the utilization, outcomes and adverse events with ICD. There are several studies showing that women who are eligible for ICD are less likely to receive one [18]. Similar differences in CRT utilization is observed, although women are more likely to benefit from CRT with improvement of quality of life, reducing of HF-related hospitalizations and mortality, as shown in MASCOT study and meta-analysis of REVERSE, MADIT-CRT and RAFT studies.

It is of importance to point out that oestrogen has protective effect on the cardiovascular system, but the abrupt loss with menopause can potentially contribute to HFpEF development and activation of the renin-angiotensin-aldosterone system.

Last but not least, there are specific situations, as for example in pregnancy, where the management of heart failure needs modification. Potentially teratogenic drugs need to be avoided (ACEI, ARNI, MRA, SGLT2-I) and treatment should be continued with beta-blockers and diuretics. As soon as the mother has delivered, there is no concern about foetal maturity or eventually teratogenicity of medications and they should be reinitiated [19].

Advanced HF represents a threatening stage of HF, where conventional treatment are no longer effective and patients should be evaluated for more advanced therapies, as for example Left Ventricular Assist Device (LVAD) or heart transplantation. According to the International Society of Heart and Lung Transplantation (ISHLT) there is a clear shorter survival in women treated with LVAD, but the reason is most likely that women are hospitalized while in more severe clinical condition [19]. In a recent study analysing data from an international database including 2066 women with continuous flow LVAD women had higher risk of mortality during the first 4 months after LVAD implantation compared to men and died mainly due to neurological complications [20, 21]. Women are even less frequently referred to heart transplantation [22].

2 Clinical Practice

2.1 Follow Up at Heart Failure Clinics

It is emphasized in all guidelines [2, 23] that patients with HF should receive follow up at a heart failure clinic since it has been shown to reduce mortality and morbidity. The component of follow up in HF clinics are self-care education and skill building, psychosocial support, assessment of symptom signs and HF status as well as and optimization and up titration of medications. The setting for HF clinics with a multidisciplinary team, often led by specialist HF nurses is most often a hospital. HF clinics are rarely located in primary care despite that most elderly persons with HF receive most of the care in primary care.

A recent scoping review concluded that men were more frequently referred to an outpatient HF clinic compared to women [24]. In a large “real world” sample of >40,000 patient from the Swedish HF registry (SWEDEHF) it was found that 39% of all patients with HF in the registry had access to follow up at a nurse-led HF clinic. Independent predictors of follow up at a HF clinic were being male, having more severe HF, having fewer comorbidities and living with someone [25]. The last two factor are also more prominent in women. Those followed at the HF clinic received recommended HF treatment to a higher extent. This gender inequality regarding structured follow up and access to a multidisciplinary team is likely to affect survival negatively in women. A future development of more HF clinics available closer to the patients’ home e.g. organized in primary care would probably increase the number of women with HF receiving this evidence-based and structured form of follow up. Previous research has shown that HF clinics in primary care decrease hospitalisations and increase the number of persons with optimal HF treatment [26].

2.2 Lifestyle Changes and Self-Care

In addition to optimal medical treatment, self-care is essential for patients with HF irrespective of sex. Self-care can be defined as a process of maintaining health through health promoting and preventive practices. Self-care is overarching concept built from the three key concepts of self-care maintenance (e.g., taking medication as prescribed), self-care monitoring (e.g. observe signs and symptoms), and self-care management (e.g., change diuretic dose in response to symptoms) [27].

For patients with HF, it might be necessary to regulate and adapt self-care during the course of the illness, for example during deterioration, if co-morbidities occur, or in case of specific advanced treatment. Patients with HF who have better self-care have better quality of life and lower mortality and readmission rates than those with lower levels of self-care.

Some studies show that gender is related to self-care, with no consistency on directions and other studies did not find consistent gender-specific differences in self-care behaviours [28–31]. In other words if women have better or worse self-care. One study demonstrated that self-care maintenance in general was poor, but slightly better in women, [32] and another study found that males were more than four times as likely to have inadequate self-care maintenance compared to females [33].

But even with no clear gender difference in self-care itself, there are specific barriers and challenges to self-care that are gender specific and need tailoring of education and support.

For example, social support, knowledge, perceived control and confidence to do self-care influence self-care maintenance and these might differ between man and women [32, 34].

In men, perceived control and knowledge are found to be important factors affecting their self-care behaviours, while self-care confidence and functional status were important factors affecting women's self-care behaviours [35]. To provide effective interventions to improve self-care behaviours in patients with HF, men and women's unique situation should be considered [34].

Gender differences need to be contextualised to the patients' cultural norms. In some cultures men are more likely to undertake independent decisions about their self-care management, while women have higher self-care maintenance [33].

2.3 Unreflective Sufficient Self-Care

Both reflection and decision making play a vital role in self-care and these might need a different approach for men and women (Fig. 1). Some patients perform self-care activities but do not reflect about it. For example, a patient might take medications without knowing why they have been prescribed. Other patients dutifully monitor themselves, but do not know what to do with the information they gather.

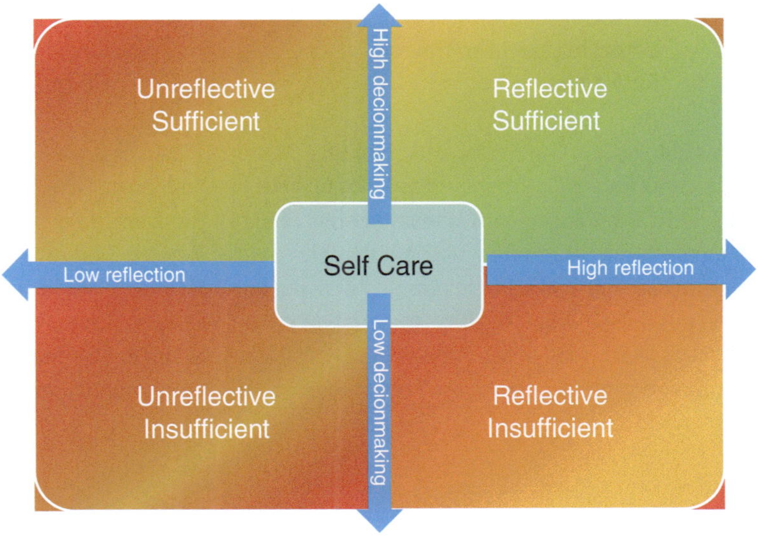

Fig. 1 Both reflection and decision making play a vital role in self-care

Both women and men have exhibited a lack of knowledge regarding reasons to perform their HF self-care. Women have been reported to have less knowledge about HF, for example attributing daily weights to measuring the amount of weight gain from adipose tissue, not fluid overload relative to HF exacerbation [36]. Another example that was described in a study in women with diastolic heart failure was that when oedema occurred, it was not typically recognized as a symptom of HF and was not considered important until dyspnea became a problem [35].

2.4 Reflective Sufficient Self-Care

Some patients have reflective and sufficient and reasoned self-care. They are knowledgeable about the self-care needed for their condition. They consciously monitor their symptoms and their condition and know what to do if signs or symptoms are abnormal. They have a total picture of their HF, treatment and lifestyle and make deliberate choices, for example to exercise daily or take medication.

A previous study found that there were distinct gender differences in the decisions made in interpreting and responding to symptoms [29]. The men were better than the women at interpreting their symptoms as being related to HF and in initiating treatment. These differences were associated with differences in self-care confidence, social support, and mood.

2.5 Unreflective Sufficient Self-Care

If patients do not have enough knowledge about their condition and the self-care needed and if they have a poor in-depth understanding of the rationale for self-care they will not be able to do appropriate self-care. For example, if a person does not know what healthy food is or never reflected about that or why medication can help to improve symptom she/he will not be motivated do good self-care. A supportive environment is important to learn about self-care and to reflect what choices to make. Women and men might have a different need and access to social support. While women saw a supportive relationships as being based on having someone to talk to they also frequently report that they do not have another close person they could rely on to even help with activities of daily living [37] Conversely, men report having more tangible support with family members being involved in supporting their HF self-care [37]. With the assistance of family, men had more confidence in interpreting symptoms of HF and self-care [37].

2.6 Reflective Insufficient Self-Care

Sometimes patients are reflective, but actively choose not to engage in self-care. They might have the knowledge and understanding of the self-care needed for their condition, but after reflection and perhaps a personal cost-benefit analysis, they make an informed choice not to perform the recommended self-care.

Sometimes persons deliberately will not do self-care because they do not want to burden others with a change in diet, going to the gym for exercise or spending money on medication or transportation to a clinic. In a review it was found that compared to men women worried more over a lack of money, not being able to care for others or of being dependent on others to do self-care [37].

3 Conclusions

Heart failure is an important cause of mortality and morbidity in women and with a different prevalence of HF is different for men and women across the ejection fraction spectrum. HFpEF is about twice as common in women as in men. Overall treatment and lifestyle advice is similar for men and women. However, women are generally underrepresented in clinical trials for HF. Barriers for lifestyle changes and self-care might also differ and a person-centred approach is needed to address gender specific issues.

Key Issues

- There are important differences in epidemiology, pathophysiology, HF type, prognosis, and treatment.
- Treatment recommendation for guideline directed therapy are similar for men and women but there are still gaps in the management of women with HF.
- Challenges for optimal self-care might be different for women and women.

Questions and Answers

1. What is the most common HF type in women with Heart failure?
   (A) Heart Failure with preserved ejection fraction (HFpEF)
   (B) Heart Failure with reduced ejection fraction (HFrEF)
   (C) Heart Failure with mid range ejection fraction (HFmrEF)
   (D) All types are equally prevalent in women.
   Correct answer: A
   The prevalence of HF is different for men and women across the ejection fraction spectrum. HF with preserved ejection fraction (HFpEF) is about double in women than in men and it is higher at any given age. In HF with reduced ejection fraction (HFrEF) men have a higher risk than women and this has been attributed to their higher tendency to coronary artery disease and myocardial infarction among men. This can be contrasted with microvascular dysfunction of the coronary circulation that may play a major role in HFpEF.
2. How would you evaluate the following two statements?
   1. Guidelines have no different recommendations for medical therapy between men and women,
   2. Women are more likely to benefit from CRT with improvement of quality of life, reducing of HF-related hospitalizations and mortality
   (A) Both statements are incorrect
   (B) 1 is correct and 2 is incorrect
   (C) 1 is incorrect and 2 is correct
   (D) Both statements are correct
   Correct answer: D
   Statement 1 is correct: Professional guidelines recommend similar treatment for men and women, but there are differences depending on the HF phenotype.
   Statement 2 is correct: There are sex differences in the utilization, outcomes and adverse events with ICD. There are several studies showing that women who are eligible for ICD are less likely to receive one. Similar differences in CRT utilization is observed, although women are more likely to benefit from CRT with improvement of quality of life, reducing of HF -related hospitalizations and mortality, as shown in MASCOT study and meta-analysis of REVERSE, MADIT-CRT and RAFT studies.
3. The best model of follow up care for women with HF has been shown to be
   (A) Hospital based heart failure clinic
   (B) Home based heart failure program
   (C) Hybrid model of home based an hospital based programs
   (D) There not a specific superior model of care for women with HF
   Correct answer: D
   It is emphasized in guidelines that patients with HF should receive follow up at a heart failure management program such as a HF clinic, home based program or hybrid model. There are no studies that show superiority of one model of the other for specific groups.
4. What is self-care management?
   (A) Those behaviours used by patients with a chronic illness to maintain physical and emotional stability
   (B) Adherence to medical treatment
   (C) The response to signs and symptoms when they occur
   (D) All of the above

Correct answer: C

Self-care is overarching concept built from the three key concepts of self-care maintenance taking medication as prescribed), self-care monitoring (e.g. observe signs and symptoms), and self-care management (e.g., change diuretic dose in response to symptoms).

References

1. Shahim B, Kapelios CJ, Savarese G, Lund LH. Global public health burden of heart failure: an updated review. Card Fail Rev. 2023;9:e11. https://doi.org/10.15420/cfr.2023.05.
2. McDonagh TA, Metra M, Adamo M, Gardner RS, Baumbach A, Böhm M, et al. 2021 ESC guidelines for the diagnosis and treatment of acute and chronic heart failure: developed by the task force for the diagnosis and treatment of acute and chronic heart failure of the European Society of Cardiology (ESC) with the special contribution of the Heart Failure Association (HFA) of the ESC. Eur Heart J. 2021;42(36):3599–726.
3. Arcopinto M, Valente V, Giardino F, Marra AM, Cittadini A. What have we learned so far from the sex/gender issue in heart failure? An overview of current evidence. Intern Emerg Med. 2022;17(6):1589–98. https://doi.org/10.1007/s11739-022-03019-4.
4. Dunlay SM, Roger VL, Redfield MM. Epidemiology of heart failure with preserved ejection fraction. Nat Rev Cardiol. 2017;14(10):591–602. https://doi.org/10.1038/nrcardio.2017.65.
5. Samuel RS, Hausdorff JM, Wei JY. Congestive heart failure with preserved systolic function: is it a woman's disease? Womens Health Issues. 1999;9(4):219–2. https://doi.org/10.1016/S1049-3867(99)00008-0.
6. Stolfo D, Uijl A, Vedin O, Strömberg A, Faxén UL, Rosano GMC, Sinagra G, Dahlström U, Savarese G. Sex-based differences in heart failure across the ejection fraction spectrum: phenotyping, and prognostic and therapeutic implications. JACC Heart Fail. 2019;7(6):505–15. https://doi.org/10.1016/j.jchf.2019.03.011. Erratum in: JACC Heart Fail. 2020;8(4):345–6.
7. Ebong IA, DeFilippis EM, Hamad EA, Hsich EM, Randhawa VK, Billia F, et al. Special considerations in the care of women with advanced heart failure. Front Cardiovasc Med. 2022;9:890108.
8. Lloyd-Jones DM, Larson MG, Leip EP, Beiser A, D'agostino RB, Kannel WB, et al. Lifetime risk for developing congestive heart failure: the Framingham Heart Study. Circulation. 2002;106(24):3068–72.
9. Hogg K, Swedberg K, McMurray J. Heart failure with preserved left ventricular systolic function: epidemiology, clinical characteristics, and prognosis. J Am Coll Cardiol. 2004;43(3):317–27.
10. Kaur G, et al. Sex differences in heart failure with preserved ejection fraction: from traditional risk factors to sex-specific risk factors. Womens Health (Lond). 2022;18:17455057221140209.
11. Canale ML, Bisceglia I, Gallucci G, Russo G, Camerini A, Di Fusco SA, et al. Women at heart: introducing gender cardio-oncology. Front Cardiovasc Med. 2022;9:974123.
12. Murakami T, Komiyama T, Kobayashi H, Ikari Y. Gender differences in takotsubo syndrome. Biology. 2022;11(5):653.
13. Bozkurt B, Khalaf S. Heart failure in women. Methodist Debakey Cardiovasc J. 2017;13(4):216.
14. McDonagh TA, Metra M, Adamo M, Gardner RS, Baumbach A, Böhm M, Burri H, Butler J, Čelutkienė J, Chioncel O, Cleland JGF, Crespo-Leiro MG, Farmakis D, Gilard M, Heymans S, Hoes AW, Jaarsma T, Jankowska EA, Lainscak M, Lam CSP, Lyon AR, McMurray JJV, Mebazaa A, Mindham R, Muneretto C, Francesco Piepoli M, Price S, Rosano GMC, Ruschitzka F, Skibelund AK, ESC Scientific Document Group. 2023 Focused update of the 2021 ESC guidelines for the diagnosis and treatment of acute and chronic heart failure. Eur Heart J. 2023;44(37):3627–39. https://doi.org/10.1093/eurheartj/ehad195.
15. Mentzer G, Hsich EM. Heart failure with reduced ejection fraction in women: epidemiology, outcomes, and treatment. Heart Fail Clin. 2019;15(1):19–27.
16. DeFilippis EM, Beale A, Martyn T, Agarwal A, Elkayam U, Lam CS, et al. Heart failure subtypes and cardiomyopathies in women. Circ Res. 2022;130(4):436–54.
17. Shekelle PG, Rich MW, Morton SC, Atkinson CSW, Tu W, Maglione M, et al. Efficacy of angiotensin-converting enzyme inhibitors and beta-blockers in the management of left ventricular systolic dysfunction according to race, gender, and diabetic status: a meta-analysis of major clinical trials. J Am Coll Cardiol. 2003;41(9):1529–38.
18. Al-Khatib SM, Hellkamp AS, Hernandez AF, Fonarow GC, Thomas KL, Al-Khalidi HR, et al. Trends in use of implantable cardioverter-defibrillator therapy among patients hospitalized for heart failure: have the previously observed sex and racial disparities changed over time? Circulation. 2012;125(9):1094–101.
19. Bright RA, Lima FV, Avila C, Butler J, Stergiopoulos K. Maternal heart failure. J Am Heart Assoc. 2021;10(14):e021019.
20. Weymann A, Patil NP, Sabashnikov A, Mohite PN, García Sáez D, Amrani M, et al. Gender differences in continuous-flow left ventricular assist device therapy as a bridge to transplantation: a risk-adjusted comparison using a propensity score-matching analysis. Artif Organs. 2015;39(3):212–9.
21. Nayak A, Hu Y, Ko Y-A, Mehta A, Liu C, Pennington J, et al. Gender differences in mortality after left ventricular assist device implant: a causal mediation analysis approach. ASAIO J. 2021;67(6):614–21.

22. Hsich EM. Sex differences in advanced heart failure therapies. Circulation. 2019;139(8):1080–93. https://doi.org/10.1161/CIRCULATIONAHA.118.037369.
23. Heidenreich PA, Bozkurt B, Aguilar D, Allen LA, Byun JJ, Colvin MM, Deswal A, Drazner MH, Dunlay SM, Evers LR, Fang JC, Fedson SE, Fonarow GC, Hayek SS, Hernandez AF, Khazanie P, Kittleson MM, Lee CS, Link MS, Milano CA, Nnacheta LC, Sandhu AT, Stevenson LW, Vardeny O, Vest AR, Yancy CW. 2022 AHA/ACC/HFSA guideline for the management of heart failure: a report of the American College of Cardiology/American Heart Association Joint Committee on clinical practice guidelines. Circulation. 2022;145(18):e895–e1032.
24. Chan E, Rooprai J, Rodger J, Visintini S, Rodger N, Philip S, Mielniczuk L, Sun LY. Sex-based differences in referral of heart failure patients to outpatient clinics: a scoping review. ESC Heart Fail. 2022;9(6):3702–12. https://doi.org/10.1002/ehf2.14143.
25. Savarese G, Lund LH, Dahlström U, Strömberg A. Nurse-led heart failure clinics are associated with reduced mortality but not heart failure hospitalization. J Am Heart Assoc. 2019;8(10):e011737. https://doi.org/10.1161/JAHA.118.011737.
26. Liljeroos M, Strömberg A. Introducing nurse-led heart failure clinics in Swedish primary care settings. Eur J Heart Fail. 2019;21(1):103–9. https://doi.org/10.1002/ejhf.1329.
27. Riegel B, Jaarsma T, Strömberg A. A middle-range theory of self-care of chronic illness. ANS Adv Nurs Sci. 2012;35(3):194–204. https://doi.org/10.1097/ANS.0b013e318261b1ba.
28. Graven LJ, Abbott L, Dickey SL, Schluck G. The influence of gender and race on heart failure self-care. Chronic Illn. 2021;17(2):69–80. https://doi.org/10.1177/1742395319843163.
29. Riegel B, Dickson VV, Kuhn L, Page K, Worrall-Carter L. Gender-specific barriers and facilitators to heart failure self-care: a mixed methods study. Int J Nurs Stud. 2010;47(7):888–95. https://doi.org/10.1016/j.ijnurstu.2009.12.011.
30. Jonkman NH, Westland H, Groenwold RH, Ågren S, Atienza F, Blue L, Bruggink-André de la Porte PW, DeWalt DA, Hebert PL, Heisler M, Jaarsma T, Kempen GI, Leventhal ME, Lok DJ, Mårtensson J, Muñiz J, Otsu H, Peters-Klimm F, Rich MW, Riegel B, Strömberg A, Tsuyuki RT, van Veldhuisen DJ, Trappenburg JC, Schuurmans MJ, Hoes AW. Do self-management interventions work in patients with heart failure? An individual patient data meta-analysis. Circulation. 2016;133(12):1189–98. https://doi.org/10.1161/CIRCULATIONAHA.115.018006.
31. Sedlar N, Lainscak M, Mårtensson J, Strömberg A, Jaarsma T, Farkas J. Factors related to self-care behaviours in heart failure: a systematic review of European Heart Failure Self-Care Behaviour Scale studies. Eur J Cardiovasc Nurs. 2017;16(4):272–82. https://doi.org/10.1177/1474515117691644.
32. Mei J, Tian Y, Chai X, Fan X. Gender differences in self-care maintenance and its associations among patients with chronic heart failure. Int J Nurs Sci. 2018;6(1):58–64. https://doi.org/10.1016/j.ijnss.2018.11.008.
33. Dellafiore F, Conte G, Baroni I, Magon A, Pittella F, Casole L, Caruso R. Gender differences in heart failure self-care behaviors: do we know enough? Minerva Med. 2018;109(5):401–3. https://doi.org/10.23736/S0026-4806.18.05579-9.
34. Heo S, Moser DK, Lennie TA, Riegel B, Chung ML. Gender differences in and factors related to self-care behaviors: a cross-sectional, correlational study of patients with heart failure. Int J Nurs Stud. 2008;45(12):1807–15. https://doi.org/10.1016/j.ijnurstu.2008.05.008.
35. Stamp KD. Women with heart failure: do they require a special approach for improving adherence to self-care? Curr Heart Fail Rep. 2014;11(3):307–13. https://doi.org/10.1007/s11897-014-0199-3.
36. Dickson VV, Buck H, Riegel B. Multiple comorbid conditions challenge heart failure self-care by decreasing self-efficacy. Nurs Res. 2013;62(1):2–9.
37. Thomas JR, Clark AM. Women with heart failure are at high psychosocial risk: a systematic review of how sex and gender influence heart failure self-care. Cardiol Res Pract. 2011;2011:918973.

Takotsubo Syndrome

Anenta Ratneswaren and Juan Carlos Kaski

Abstract

Takotsubo syndrome (TTS) has captured the imagination of the medical community and the public alike since it was first described three decades ago. Also known as 'broken heart syndrome' or 'stress cardiomyopathy', TTS predominantly affects older women. Whilst the presentation of TTS mimics an acute coronary syndrome, the natural history of TTS is more in keeping with an acute heart failure syndrome. Characteristically, albeit not exclusively, TTS patients present with a clinical history of a preceding negative emotional stress, unobstructed coronary arteries on angiography, and apical ballooning of the left ventricle on cardiac imaging.

This chapter discusses TTS epidemiology, pathophysiology, clinical presentation, and outcomes. Sex differences are also discussed but as a smaller proportion of TTS patients are men, comparisons between sexes are challenging. Current evidence suggests that neurohormonal mechanisms and the sympathetic system are involved in the pathogenesis of TTS with a catecholamine surge being a key pathogenic player in TTS. The female preponderance in TTS has been attributed to an increased susceptibility of older women to the effects of physiological stress on the heart-brain axis and lower levels of oestrogen during menopause.

Keywords

Takotsubo syndrome · Acute cardiomyopathy Stress · Neuro-hormonal system · Sympathetic nervous system · Broken heart syndrome · Takotsubo cardiomyopathy

A. Ratneswaren
National Heart and Lung Institute, Imperial College London, London, UK

Cardiology Clinical Academic Group, St George's University Hospitals NHS Trust, London, UK

J. C. Kaski (✉)
Molecular and Clinical Sciences Research Institute, St. George's, University of London, London, UK

Cardiology Clinical Academic Group, St. George's University Hospitals NHS Trust and Royal Brompton Hospital, London, UK
e-mail: jckaski@professorkaski.com

A. H.E.M. Maas, E. Gerdts (eds.), *Manual of Cardiovascular Disease in Women*,
https://doi.org/10.1007/978-3-031-65952-2_25

Test your learning and check your understanding of this book's contents: use the "Springer Nature Flashcards" app to access questions using ▶ https://sn.pub/51ny7m
To use the app, please follow the instructions in chapter 1.

1 Introduction

Takotsubo Syndrome (TTS) is an acute condition mimicking acute coronary syndrome (ACS) and typically involving the apex of the left ventricle. TTS was first described in 1990 by Sato and colleagues [1] who reported a series of five cases in Japan. Since then, TTS has been described consistently in populations across the world. Today, TTS is a widely recognised cardiovascular condition. Synonyms for TTS include 'broken heart syndrome', 'stress cardiomyopathy', 'apical ballooning syndrome' and 'Takotsubo cardiomyopathy'.

TTS presents as an ACS, with symptoms of chest pain, electrocardiographic (ECG) abnormalities reflecting myocardial ischaemia, and mildly elevated troponin concentrations. A diagnosis of ACS or myocardial infarction is often given, leading to urgent invasive coronary angiography and transthoracic echocardiography. Coronary arteries are typically found to be unobstructed, and a characteristic apical ballooning of the left ventricle may be observed during systole on left ventriculography or echocardiography. It is this characteristic shape of the ballooning left ventricle that provided the inspiration for the name 'Takotsubo', taken from the Japanese word for a style of pot used by Japanese fishermen to trap octopuses. In recent years several different forms of left ventricular abnormalities have been described in TTS patients [2].

TTS is characterised by the presence of an acute and significant stressor, either emotional or physical, and by the resolution of clinical features within just a few weeks. Although the pathogenesis of the condition remains elusive the sympathetic nervous system is involved in the pathophysiology of TTS, with a marked albeit transient surge of catecholamines playing an important role. An intriguing and poorly understood feature of TTS is its tendency to affect post-menopausal women.

There have been various attempts to provide diagnostic criteria and categorisation of TTS, but there remains ambiguity. The Fourth Universal Definition of Myocardial Infarction [3] considers TTS to be a mimic of a myocardial infarction. There has been debate over the inclusion of TTS in the diagnosis of Myocardial Infarction with Non-obstructed Coronary Arteries (MINOCA). Nearly a fifth of patients with a suspected MINOCA diagnosis have TTS [4].

2 Epidemiology: High Prevalence in Women

One of the most striking features of TTS is its marked tendency to affect older women (see Fig. 1). A national study involving hospitalised patients in the United States found that 90% of patients with TTS were over 55 years of age and 90% of the patients in the trial were women [5]. Women had 4.8 times higher risk of having TTS if they were over 55 years of age, and women over 55 years of age were 10.7 times more likely to have a diagnosis of TTS compared to men of a similar age.

Amongst all patients presenting with ACS, it is estimated that 2% are subsequently found to have TTS [6–8]. This figure rises significantly to 5–6% for female patients presenting with an ACS.

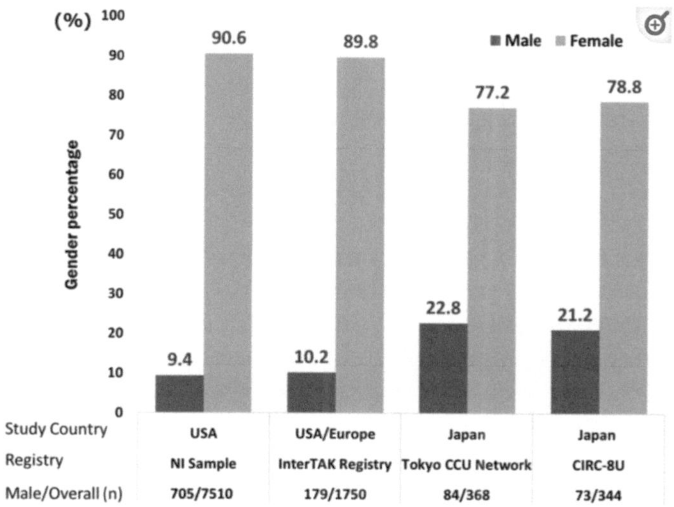

The gender differences in TTS in Japan, Europe, and the United States of America (USA). NI Sample, Nationwide Inpatient Sample; InterTAK Registry, The International Takotsubo Registry; CCU, Cardiovascular Care Unit; CIRC-8U, the Cardiovascular Research Consortium-8 Universities.

Fig. 1 Gender differences in TTS. From Murakami T, Komiyama T, Kobayashi H, Ikari Y. Gender Differences in Takotsubo Syndrome. *Biology (Basel).* 2022 Apr 24;11 [5]:653.Copyright © 2022 by the authors. Licensee MDPI, Basel, Switzerland. This article is an open access article distributed under the terms and conditions of the Creative Commons Attribution (CC BY) license (https://creativecommons.org/licenses/by/4.0/)

3 Pathophysiology

Myocardial biopsy studies of TTS have consistently shown inflammatory changes within the interstitium, the presence of contraction bands, and, only occasionally, necrotic changes. These pathological changes led researchers to characterise TTS as a cardiomyopathy that however differs from ischaemic and fibrotic cardiomyopathies. TTS' histological findings are in keeping with the pathological effects of the catecholamine surge observed during sympathetic stress (see Fig. 2).

It is widely understood that the sympathetic system plays a central role in TTS [9]. Evidence of microvascular dysfunction in TTS suggests that that the coronary microcirculation is another key mediator alongside the nervous system. Various mechanisms have been suggested, but the evidence-base to support any one of these mechanisms is limited. There is even greater uncertainty around the role of sex and gender in the onset and the development of the condition. Human [10] and experimental animal studies [11] suggest a possible role of oestrogen in the pathogenesis of TTS and may explain the high prevalence of TTS in older women.

3.1 A Cardiovascular Response to Stress

A captivating feature of TTS is that its onset is often marked by a sudden emotional stressor, such as bereavement or bad news. Other common triggers are fear, anger, and surprise. Stress is a physiological response that is mediated by the central nervous system, the sympathetic nervous system, and by the interplay between the two. Raised catecholamines and stress-related circulating neuropeptides have been associated in TTS. Sympathetic over-stimulation is a central pathway in TTS. Sympathetic nerve endings and beta-1 adrenoceptors are more densely found in the base of the left ventricle [12], whilst the apex of the left ventricle has a greater density of beta-2 adrenoceptors. This provides a plausible explanation for the classical pattern of apical hypokinesia and basal hypercontractility. Myocardial calcium

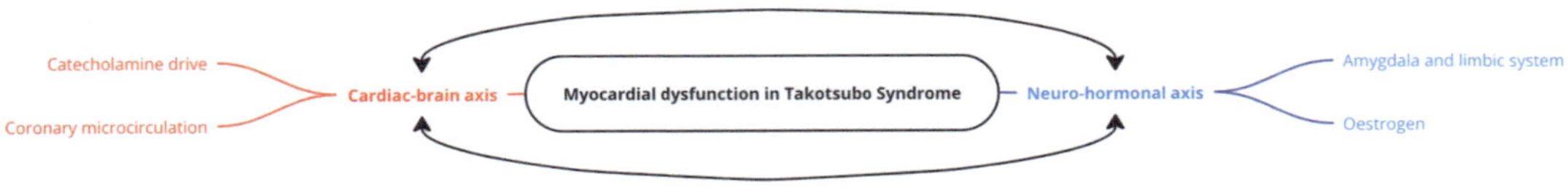

Fig. 2 Key mechanistic influences in TTS

handling may also be affected by adrenoceptor overstimulation in TTS and in turn contributed to altered myocardial contraction [13].

3.2 Catecholamine Mediation

Stress reactions produce a biological 'fight-or-flight' response, which is largely mediated by catecholamines such as epinephrine, norepinephrine, and dopamine. During the acute phase of TTS, circulating catecholamine levels are high, and far higher compared to the levels seen in the acute phase of myocardial infarction [14]. After the 'storm' of catecholamines, levels may be raised for a period beyond the acute presentation. Whilst the catecholamine storm activates adrenoceptors in a systemic fashion, there is also a localised production and release of catecholamines into synaptic clefts directly within the myocardium. In addition, epinephrine is synthesised by the myocardium itself, and interestingly, epinephrine-producing enzymes have a distribution localised to the apex of the left ventricle [15].

At low and moderate levels, catecholamines have a positive ionotropic effect on the left ventricle myocardium. At the very high levels seen in TTS, epinephrine leads to a reversible inhibitory effect and a resulting negative ionotropic effect. The high levels of epinephrine have an anti-apoptotic effect on the left ventricle. The localised, or direct, catecholamine excess is thought to have a greater impact than the systemic catecholamine excess on the myocardium. Further emphasising the localised catecholamine response is the observation that excess norepinephrine from cardiac sympathetic synapses can decrease myocardial viability and is associated with the histological finding of contraction band necrosis in TTS [16].

3.3 The Effect of Oestrogen

It has been suggested that sex-related differences in oestrogen and sympathetic system mediation may hold the answer to the higher incidence in women, particularly since catecholamine vasoconstriction is further modulated by oestrogen [17]. Certainly, the catecholamine storm or direct catecholamine toxicity alone are not sufficient an explanation for the acute onset of TTS nor the epidemiological pattern. Supporting this notion, cardiac magnetic resonance imaging has effectively demonstrated that TTS is subtly different from other excess catecholamine-mediated cardiomyopathies such as seen in phaeochromocytoma-induced myocarditis [18].

Lower levels of oestrogen, as seen in menopause, lead to increased sympathetic drive and endothelial dysfunction. Thus, a reduction in oestrogen has been proposed to explain the higher prevalence of TTS in older women. Importantly, it has been shown that oestrogen supplementation can attenuate the effect of the central nervous system sympathetic activation of the heart and even prevent LV apical ballooning [11]. Oestrogen supplementation also upregulates cardioprotective neuropeptides such as atrial natriuretic peptide [11].

Endothelial dysfunction due to oestrogen down-regulation may represent another important link between the stress-activated limbic system and the reversible myocardial dysfunction seen in TTS [18]. Endothelial dysfunction can be considered a common final pathway for impaired coronary flow, increased vagal tone, reduced cardioprotective neuropeptides, and moreover is associated with the neurological, psychiatric, and other comorbidities that are associated with TTS [19].

3.4 The Cardiac-Brain Axis

The importance of the cardiac-brain axis in both myocardial infarction and heart failure is increasingly recognised. Thus, is it unsurprising that the neurohormonal system can be implicated in TTS. Structural and neural connectivity studies of the brain in TTS have shown significantly reduced connectivity in the limbic system, particularly among several components of the autonomic-nervous system [20].

Moreover, recent research has shown that the neurohormonal system, particularly the amygdala and insular cortex, may influence the sympathetic system and the hypothalamic-pituitary-adrenal axis in TTS. Specifically, the amygdala is a core neural structure for processing fearful and threatening stimuli, and it has a direct impact on cortical autonomic nervous system dysregulation. Chronically reduced amygdala activity may either predispose individuals to TTS when exposed to stressful stimuli [21] or instead it may mediate an exaggerated neurohormonal response to stress. If the former, amygdala mediation may be a potential therapeutic target. Positron emission tomography (PET) imaging of metabolic activity with 18-F-FDG demonstrated increased stress activity of the amygdala in older women [22]. Further sex-related differences have been found for baseline sympathetic, parasympathetic, and vagal activity [23]. Besides, or alongside, oestrogen deficiency, differential dysregulation of the limbic system may be implicated in the sex-based differences seen in TTS.

3.5 The Coronary Microcirculation

Alongside sympathetic nervous system activation and excess catecholamine levels, the coronary microcirculation may play a key role in the development of TTS. Myocardial contrast echocardiography techniques confirm reversible microvascular perfusion defects in TTS [24]. The temporal pattern of reversibility is consistent with the acute but fully recoverable signs of myocardial ischaemia seen in TTS.

Another potential pathological mechanism that has been suggested to play a role in TTS is multivessel epicardial spasm. Some of the left ventricular abnormalities reported in TTS are somewhat consistent with this mechanism. In TTS, temporary epicardial artery occlusion, healthy coronary vessel wall on intravascular imaging, and the multi-territorial distribution of myocardial dysfunction are features that have been observed and are consistent with macrovascular spasm. However, spontaneous macrovascular spasm has not been consistently observed across populations. Even in case series' where coronary spasm has been provoked by pharmacological agents, only between 10–40% of patients demonstrate vasospasm [25, 26], and certainly, most patients do not have vasospasm evident on invasive angiography.

4 Clinical Practice

4.1 Clinical Presentation

TTS was originally associated with negative emotional events, hence the synonym 'broken heart syndrome' (see Table 1). However, the association with positive emotional events have increasingly been recognised [27]. This author recalls taking a 90-year-old female to the coronary cath lab in the middle of the night after the patient experienced typical angina on walking up a hill to her 90th birthday celebration meal with family visiting from abroad. She was found to have unobstructed coronary arteries and was given a diagnosis of 'happy heart syndrome' [28].

Interestingly, a higher prevalence of men and atypical mid-ventricular ballooning have been observed when the preceding emotions are positive, compared to negative emotions. Whilst the rate of TTS due to positive emotions is likely to be under-reported, it is still less than 5% of TTS registry cases [29] and it is difficult to draw definitive conclusions from these observations. There is no signal that positive and negative stressors are associated with variations in mortality outcome.

Table 1 Identified triggers of TTS

1. Emotional stress
(a) Grief or loss
(b) Panic or anxiety
(c) Fear
(d) Interpersonal conflict
(e) Anger
(f) Financial/employment loss
2. Physical stress
(a) Acute respiratory failure
(b) Subarachnoid haemorrhage
(c) Pancreatitis
(d) Cholecystitis
(e) Pheochromocytoma
(f) Stroke
(g) Malignancy
(h) Post-fracture
(i) Myocardial infarction
(j) Psychiatric or mood disease
3. Iatrogenic
(a) Chemotherapy or radiotherapy
(b) Electroconvulsive therapy
(c) Dobutamine stress echocardiography
(d) Drugs
(i) Sympathomimetic drugs e.g. epinephrine, metaraminol, atropine
(ii) Other drugs e.g. levothyroxine, 5-flurouracil

Emotional stressors may overlap with physiological stressors. Physical stressors range from physical activities to a range of causes for hospital admission. Commonly observed triggering medical conditions include acute exacerbation of asthma, stroke, and seizure, but surgical, psychiatric, and obstetric causes of hospital admission have also been associated with TTS. Cases of TTS developing in the context of another physical disease presentation and hospital admission, are classified as secondary TTS. The prognosis when TTS presents in medical, surgical, obstetric, or psychiatric in-patients appears to be worse than for classical or primary TTS.

Men and younger women are more likely than older women to describe a physical stress preceding TTS. Whether a sociocultural influence on age- and gender-based differences on vulnerability to TTS or the triggers of TTS is unknown. Drugs and other iatrogenic causes of TTS have also been described and in up to a third of cases, no triggering factors are reported [30, 31].

The symptoms, ECG abnormalities, and troponin elevations in TTS are similar to those seen in ACS. Chest pain and dyspnoea are commonly reported, whilst the more severe presentations of ACS, such as cardiogenic shock or cardiac arrest, are rare. ECG abnormalities, which are often transient, include ST-segment elevation in the precordial leads, and, or, diffuse T wave inversion. Prolonged corrected QT interval is another relatively common ECG abnormality in patients with TTS.

Whilst TTS, at presentation, mimics an ACS, ultimately the natural history of the syndrome is in keeping with an acute heart failure syndrome. Clinical scores have been developed to aid differentiation of TTS and ACS at presentation but are yet to be validated prospectively.

Arrhythmias maybe another complicating feature in a small proportion of patients with TTS. Case studies have described of both atrial and ventricular arrhythmias, and in some cases, permanent pacemaker systems have been implanted. However, it has also been suggested that the arrhythmia, or perhaps the symptom burden of the arrhythmia, maybe considered a trigger for TTS, rather than a consequence [31].

4.2 Diagnosis

Diagnosis of TTS requires a carefully taken clinical history, characterisation of the myocardium, particularly the left ventricle, assessment of the epicardial coronary arteries, a 12-lead ECG, troponin measurements and assessment of N-terminal pro-B-type natriuretic peptide (BNP) levels. Hospital admission for careful patient monitoring and ongoing clinical assessment is required.

Presenting symptoms of TTS are often indistinguishable from symptoms of ACS, and most commonly include acute chest pain and dyspnoea. Syncope may also be present. It is important to consider that patients with TTS may also present with less typical symptoms, such as tachycardia and hypotension. Particularly in the elderly, with less obvious symptoms, findings on blood tests or the ECG are often the first diagnostic clues available. These atypical presentations are more commonly found in men and those admitted with another primary medical condition.

Whilst cardiac troponin and BNP are raised in TTS, BNP is found to be significantly higher in TTS compared to that in patients with acute myocardial infarction [32, 33]. Perhaps an oversimplification, but the high NT-proBNP/TnT ratio in TTS is in keeping with the myocardial stretch or 'ballooning' of the left ventricle and the lack of necrotic myocardial ischaemia [34].

Imaging of the left ventricle, either with ventriculography, echocardiography or cardiovascular magnetic resonance (CMR) demonstrates circumferential left ventricle apical hypokinesia and basal hypercontractility in up to 80% of cases [35]. However, the inverse of this classical pattern, instead with basal hypokinesia and apical hypercontractility is a recognised variant (see Fig. 3). Further and much rarer variants include mid-ventricular hypokinesia with basal and apical hypercontractility and focal forms. In up to a

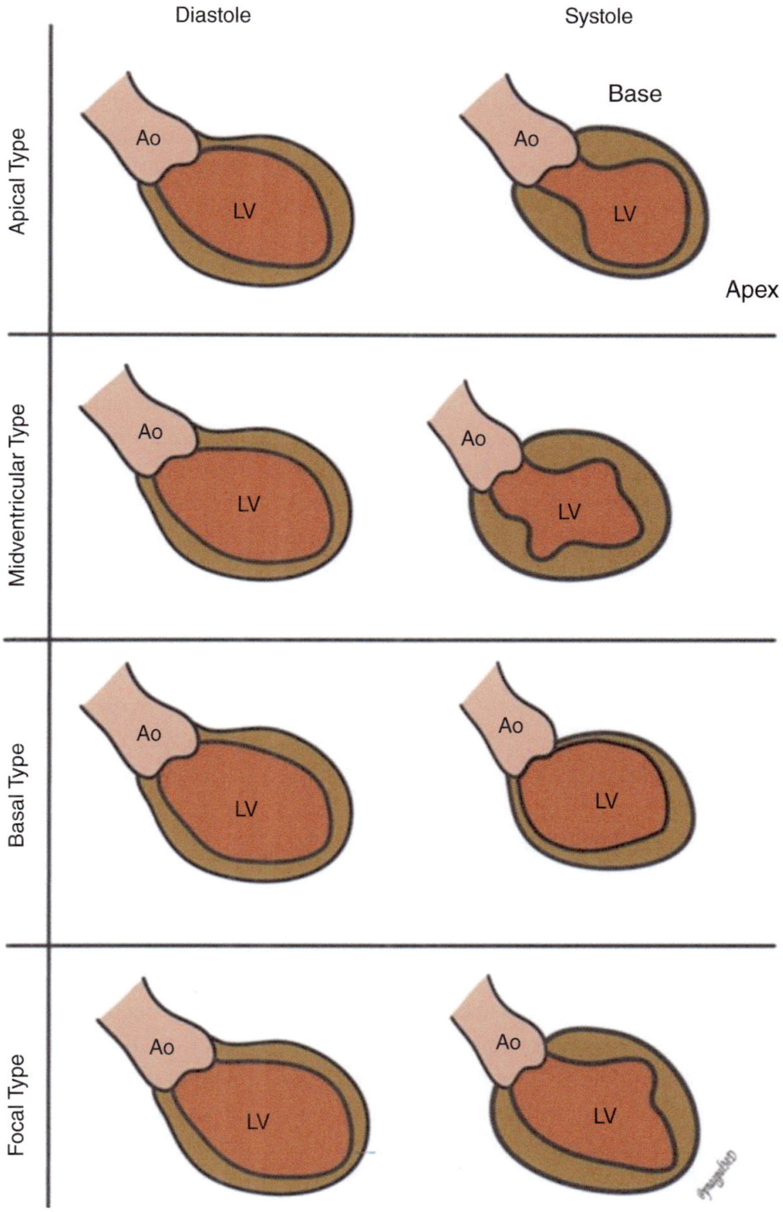

Fig. 3 Anatomic variants of TTS. Sarv Priya, Prashant Nagpal, Tanya Aggarwal, James Huynh, Kanika Khandelwal, Ashish Khandelwal, Review of multi-modality imaging update and diagnostic work up of Takotsubo cardiomyopathy, Clinical Imaging, 2021;80, Pages 334–347, ISSN 0899-7071, https://doi.org/10.1016/j.clinimag.2021.08.027. (https://www.sciencedirect.com/science/article/pii/S0899707121003612)

third of cases there is also involvement of the right ventricle [2]. No sex-related differences in the incidence or mechanisms of anatomical TTS variants have been observed.

Invasive coronary angiography may demonstrate bystander coronary artery disease, but no culprit lesions. Intravascular imaging maybe performed to aid a MINOCA diagnosis, and in TTS, no plaque rupture is identified [36]. CMR can also be used to investigate a MINOCA diagnosis, and a finding of fibrosis on late gadolinium enhancement can be used to identify acute myocardial infarction and myocarditis. In contrast, TTS rarely demonstrates fibrosis. However, a thin band of fibrosis may be seen at the junction of the hyperkinetic base and dyskinetic apex in TTS [37].

Several diagnostic criteria have been proposed but none have been robustly validated or reached routine clinical practice as yet. The most recently proposed criteria are the InterTAK Diagnostic Criteria for the identification of TTS prior to angiography and for risk stratification [38] and the Heart Failure Association diagnostic criteria [39]. These criteria commonly highlight that significant coronary artery disease is not a contraindication to TTS, that there are a range of triggers, including neurologic disorders, phaeochromocytoma, ACS itself, and even an absence of an identified trigger. Bystander coronary artery disease is found in up to 10% of TTS patients [30], and the implication of this on individual prognosis is unknown.

4.3 Treatment

Current management strategies for TTS reflect the fact that TTS is considered to be an acute cardiomyopathy. Reduced LV function is managed with known pharmacotherapeutic agents for heart failure. In the acute phase of the disease, cardiogenic shock may manifest due to the catecholamine surge, and requires supportive treatment with Extra-Corporeal Membrane Oxygenation (ECMO) or Left Ventricular Assist Device (LVAD) as a bridge to recovery.

Cardiac arrest is also possible in TTS, as is malignant ventricular arrhythmia due to LV structural and functional changes and the often-observed prolonged QTc interval in these patients. Atrial arrhythmias such as atrial fibrillation may also occur, which may require antiarrhythmic medication and anticoagulation for stroke risk reduction.

A further structural complication of dyskinetic or akinetic segments is the development of left ventricular thrombi. Distal thromboembolic events have been reported in the context of left ventricular thrombus in TTS. Therefore, clinicians should be vigilant of both echocardiography and CMR findings, and potentially consider prophylactic anticoagulation [40].

Follow-up cardiac imaging studies have shown that LV function recovers around 3–6 months after acute TTS presentation. Recurrent episodes of TTS have been reported. Echocardiography or cardiac MRI with late gadolinium enhancement are helpful modalities for LV ejection fraction assessment, as well as LV morphology, LV thrombus assessment, and differential diagnosis. At present, there is little evidence to guide the duration of heart failure therapy in patients with TTS.

Whilst the pathogenesis, clinical course and outcomes vary between men and women, there is currently no evidence to support the need for differential treatment for men and women. In addition to cardiovascular pharmacological agents, treatment may include psychological support therapies concomitant with cardiac rehabilitation. This may be of greater benefit in those patients with TTS triggered by an emotional event and/or patients with an underlying psychiatric or mood disorder.

4.4 Outcomes

Previously considered a benign disease, TTS has a mortality and morbidity that is higher than previously recognised. Mortality during the acute phase of the disease approaches 5%, which is comparable to that of STEMI [30]. The similarity between outcomes for TTS and ACS patients remains across age and sex groups.

Beyond the acute episode, most patients make a recovery within days to weeks, as measured by resolution of left ventricular function [14]. However, elevated BNP levels may persist for several months, and CMR studies have shown that inflammatory changes can last for at least 5 months despite resolution of symptoms [41]. Recurrence of TTS is uncommon, but it can occur as soon as 3-months after the first episode and the risk of recurrence within 5 years approaches 10% [38].

Evidence suggests that women and men experience a different trajectory once they develop TTS. Since the data are limited, the true significance of these observed trends is unknown. However, current data suggest that men experience worse both short-term and long-term outcomes. Specifically, cardiogenic shock, in-hospital mortality and long-term mortality are higher in men than women [42]. Although men with TTS tend to be younger that women with TTS, they have higher rates of comorbidity which may contribute to the three times higher rate of death and major adverse cardiovascular events compared with women [42]. This trend in sex difference persists over the longer term follow-up, with male sex, along with clinical severity of heart failure and diabetes mellitus, predicting poorer long-term mortality over 4 years [27].

Poor prognostic clinical features of TTS include high troponin levels and low ejection fraction [30]. Evidence is emerging for significantly different 30-day and 5-year mortality based on the classification of cause of TTS. If TTS is diagnosed in a patient admitted to hospital for another cause, mortality is at least double than for those admitted with TTS as the primary diagnosis [43]. Mortality rates are higher if TTS is triggered by a neurological disease or physical stressors, and it has been reported that an TTS related to an emotional stressor is associated with the most favourable long-term outcome [38].

5 Conclusions

TTS is considered to represent an acute form of LV cardiomyopathy with features that mimic ACS on presentation. The pathogenesis and prognosis of TTS remain to be fully elucidated. The heart-brain axis has been implicated in the onset and natural history of TTS, and this may provide a causal pathway for the marked sex-based variation in incidence, natural history, and prognosis of TTS. Using a sex- and gender-based approach to TTS research may yield insight into the interplay between sociocultural and biological mechanisms in TTS and more widely in cardiovascular disease.

Key Issues

- TTS is an acute heart failure syndrome often triggered by a negative emotional stress and characterised by a clinical presentation akin to acute coronary syndrome with unobstructed coronary arteries, and LV apical ballooning.
- TTS predominantly affects older women, and both the phenotype and prognosis is variable across age and sex. Generally, spontaneous resolution of TTS occurs within weeks.
- It is widely believed that a catecholamine surge, and neurohormonal and sympathetic responses, mediate the onset and development of the disease.
- The role of sex and gender in the pathophysiology of the disease is not fully known, but the heart-brain axis has been implicated.

Questions and Answers

1. What is the prevalence of TTS in women who present with an acute coronary syndrome?
   (A) 1–2%
   (B) 2–3%
   (C) 5–6%
   (D) Variable geographically
   Correct answer: C

   TTS accounts for 2% of all patients presenting with an acute coronary syndrome, but this rises to greater than 5% for female patients presenting with an acute coronary syndrome. Registry and observational data suggest that the incidence of TTS is consistent across geographical populations.

2. Which of the following is not a recognised early complication of TTS?
   (A) Bradycardia
   (B) Left ventricular thrombus
   (C) Coronary plaque rupture
   (D) Hypotension
   Correct answer: C

   Hypotension is a common early complication of TTS, and maybe further accompanied by cardiogenic shock due to left ventricular failure. Bradycardia and left ventricular are recognised complications that clinicians must be observant of. Coronary artery disease may be co-existent with TTS, but plaque rupture is not a recognised early complication of TTS.
3. Treatment for TTS includes which of the following?
   (A) Norepinephrine
   (B) Nitrates
   (C) ACE inhibitors
   (D) Warfarin
   Correct answer: C

   Exogenous catecholamines such as norepinephrine should be avoided as they may worsen TTS. Hypotension is better served by aggressive fluid resuscitation. Nitrates should also be avoided since they may worsen left ventricular outflow tract obstruction, but there may be a role for nitrates in treating pulmonary oedema. There is no evidence to support routine anticoagulation in all patients with TTS, but patients with LV thrombus identified on cardiac imaging should be anticoagulated for a minimum of 3 months. Though evidence is limited, ACE inhibitors form part of the optimal medical therapy for the recovery of left ventricular function in TTS. Duration of treatment reflects on-going assessment of left ventricular function and clinical judgement.

References

1. Sato H, Tateishi H, Uchida T, Dote K, Ishihara M. Tako-tsubo-like left ventricular dysfunction due to multivessel coronary spasm. In: Clinical aspect of myocardial injury: from ischemia to heart failure. Tokyo: Kagakuhyoronsha Publishing Co; 1990. p. 56–64.
2. Haghi D, Athanasiadis A, Papavassiliu T, Suselbeck T, Fluechter S, Mahrholdt H, et al. Right ventricular involvement in takotsubo cardiomyopathy. Eur Heart J. 2006;27(20):2433–9.
3. Thygesen K, Alpert JS, Jaffe AS, Chaitman BR, Bax JJ, Morrow DA, et al. Fourth universal definition of myocardial infarction (2018). J Am Coll Cardiol. 2018;72(18):2231–64.
4. Pasupathy S, Tavella R, Beltrame JF. Myocardial infarction with nonobstructive coronary arteries (MINOCA): the past, present, and future management. Circulation. 2017;135(16):1490–3.
5. Deshmukh A, Kumar G, Pant S, Rihal C, Murugiah K, Mehta JL. Prevalence of takotsubo cardiomyopathy in the United States. Am Heart J. 2012;164(1):66–71.e1.
6. Prasad A, Lerman A, Rihal CS. Apical ballooning syndrome (tako-tsubo or stress cardiomyopathy): a mimic of acute myocardial infarction. Am Heart J. 2008;155(3):408–17.
7. Kurowski V, Kaiser A, von Hof K, Killermann DP, Mayer B, Hartmann F, et al. Apical and midventricular transient left ventricular dysfunction syndrome (tako-tsubo cardiomyopathy): frequency, mechanisms, and prognosis. Chest. 2007;132(3):809–16.
8. Akashi YJ, Goldstein DS, Barbaro G, Ueyama T. Takotsubo cardiomyopathy: a new form of acute, reversible heart failure. Circulation. 2008;118(25):2754–62.
9. Pelliccia F, Kaski JC, Camici PG. Takotsubo syndrome's pathophysiology: still a mystery? Eur Heart J. 2019;40(24):1989.
10. Lyon AR, Rees PSC, Prasad S, Poole-Wilson PA, Harding SE. Stress (takotsubo) cardiomyopathy—a novel pathophysiological hypothesis to explain catecholamine-induced acute myocardial stunning. Nat Clin Pract Cardiovasc Med. 2008;5(1):22–9.
11. Ueyama T, Ishikura F, Matsuda A, Asanuma T, Ueda K, Ichinose M, et al. Chronic estrogen supplementation following ovariectomy improves the emotional stress-induced cardiovascular responses by indirect action on the nervous system and by direct action on the heart. Circ J. 2007;71(4):565–73.
12. Kawano H, Okada R, Yano K. Histological study on the distribution of autonomic nerves in the human heart. Heart Vessel. 2003;18(1):32–9.
13. Pérez-Treviño P, Sepúlveda-Leal J, Altamirano J. Simultaneous assessment of calcium handling and contractility dynamics in isolated ventricular myocytes of a rat model of post-acute isoproterenol-induced cardiomyopathy. Cell Calcium. 2020;86:102138.
14. Wittstein IS, Thiemann DR, Lima JAC, Baughman KL, Schulman SP, Gerstenblith G, et al. Neurohumoral features of myocardial stunning due to sudden emotional stress. N Engl J Med. 2005;352(6):539–48.
15. Ancona F, Bertoldi LF, Ruggieri F, Cerri M, Magnoni M, Beretta L, et al. Takotsubo cardiomyopathy and neurogenic stunned myocardium: similar albeit different. Eur Heart J. 2016;37(37):2830–2.
16. Basso C, Thiene G. The pathophysiology of myocardial reperfusion: a pathologist's perspective. Heart. 2006;92(11):1559–62.

17. Riedel K, Deussen AJ, Tolkmitt J, Weber S, Schlinkert P, Zatschler B, et al. Estrogen determines sex differences in adrenergic vessel tone by regulation of endothelial β-adrenoceptor expression. Am J Physiol-Heart Circ Physiol. 2019;317(2):H243–54.
18. Pelliccia F, Kaski JC, Crea F, Camici PG. Pathophysiology of takotsubo syndrome. Circulation. 2017;135(24):2426–41.
19. Pelliccia F, Greco C, Vitale C, Rosano G, Gaudio C, Kaski JC. Takotsubo syndrome (stress cardiomyopathy): an intriguing clinical condition in search of its identity. Am J Med. 2014;127(8):699–704.
20. Hiestand T, Hänggi J, Klein C, Topka MS, Jaguszewski M, Ghadri JR, et al. Takotsubo syndrome associated with structural brain alterations of the limbic system. J Am Coll Cardiol. 2018;71(7):809–11.
21. Radfar A, Abohashem S, Osborne MT, Wang Y, Dar T, Hassan MZO, et al. Stress-associated neurobiological activity associates with the risk for and timing of subsequent takotsubo syndrome. Eur Heart J. 2021;42(19):1898–908.
22. Haider A, Bengs S, Diggelmann F, Epprecht G, Etter D, Beeler AL, et al. Age- and sex-dependent changes of resting amygdalar activity in individuals free of clinical cardiovascular disease. J Nucl Cardiol. 2021;28(2):427–32.
23. Rossi A, Mikail N, Bengs S, Haider A, Treyer V, Buechel RR, et al. Heart–brain interactions in cardiac and brain diseases: why sex matters. Eur Heart J. 2022;43(39):3971–80.
24. Galiuto L, De Caterina AR, Porfidia A, Paraggio L, Barchetta S, Locorotondo G, et al. Reversible coronary microvascular dysfunction: a common pathogenetic mechanism in apical ballooning or tako-tsubo syndrome. Eur Heart J. 2010;31(11):1319–27.
25. Kurisu S, Sato H, Kawagoe T, Ishihara M, Shimatani Y, Nishioka K, et al. Tako-tsubo-like left ventricular dysfunction with ST-segment elevation: a novel cardiac syndrome mimicking acute myocardial infarction. Am Heart J. 2002;143(3):448–55.
26. Tsuchihashi K, Ueshima K, Uchida T, Oh-mura N, Kimura K, Owa M, et al. Transient left ventricular apical ballooning without coronary artery stenosis: a novel heart syndrome mimicking acute myocardial infarction. Angina pectoris-myocardial infarction investigations in Japan. J Am Coll Cardiol. 2001;38(1):11–8.
27. Stiermaier T, Moeller C, Oehler K, Desch S, Graf T, Eitel C, et al. Long-term excess mortality in takotsubo cardiomyopathy: predictors, causes and clinical consequences. Eur J Heart Fail. 2016;18(6):650–6.
28. Ghadri JR, Sarcon A, Diekmann J, Bataiosu DR, Cammann VL, Jurisic S, et al. Happy heart syndrome: role of positive emotional stress in takotsubo syndrome. Eur Heart J. 2016;37(37):2823–9.
29. Stiermaier T, Walliser A, El-Battrawy I, Pätz T, Mezger M, Rawish E, et al. Happy heart syndrome: frequency, characteristics, and outcome of takotsubo syndrome triggered by positive life events. JACC Heart Fail. 2022;10(7):459–66.
30. Templin C, Ghadri JR, Diekmann J, Napp LC, Bataiosu DR, Jaguszewski M, et al. Clinical features and outcomes of takotsubo (stress) cardiomyopathy. N Engl J Med. 2015;373(10):929–38.
31. Nyman E, Mattsson E, Tornvall P. Trigger factors in takotsubo syndrome—a systematic review of case reports. Eur J Intern Med. 2019;63:62–8.
32. Madhavan M, Borlaug BA, Lerman A, Rihal CS, Prasad A. Stress hormone and circulating biomarker profile of apical ballooning syndrome (takotsubo cardiomyopathy): insights into the clinical significance of B-type natriuretic peptide and troponin levels. Heart Br Card Soc. 2009;95(17):1436–41.
33. Randhawa MS, Dhillon AS, Taylor HC, Sun Z, Desai MY. Diagnostic utility of cardiac biomarkers in discriminating takotsubo cardiomyopathy from acute myocardial infarction. J Card Fail. 2014;20(1):2–8.
34. Fröhlich GM, Schoch B, Schmid F, Keller P, Sudano I, Lüscher TF, et al. Takotsubo cardiomyopathy has a unique cardiac biomarker profile: NT-proBNP/myoglobin and NT-proBNP/troponin T ratios for the differential diagnosis of acute coronary syndromes and stress induced cardiomyopathy. Int J Cardiol. 2012;154(3):328–32.
35. Ono R, Falcão LM. Takotsubo cardiomyopathy systematic review: pathophysiologic process, clinical presentation and diagnostic approach to takotsubo cardiomyopathy. Int J Cardiol. 2016;209:196–205.
36. Haghi D, Roehm S, Hamm K, Harder N, Suselbeck T, Borggrefe M, et al. Takotsubo cardiomyopathy is not due to plaque rupture: an intravascular ultrasound study. Clin Cardiol. 2010;33(5):307–10.
37. Singh T, Khan H, Gamble DT, Scally C, Newby DE, Dawson D. Takotsubo syndrome: pathophysiology, emerging concepts, and clinical implications. Circulation. 2022;145(13):1002–19.
38. Ghadri JR, Wittstein IS, Prasad A, Sharkey S, Dote K, Akashi YJ, et al. International expert consensus document on takotsubo syndrome (part I): clinical characteristics, diagnostic criteria, and pathophysiology. Eur Heart J. 2018;39(22):2032–46.
39. Lyon AR, Bossone E, Schneider B, Sechtem U, Citro R, Underwood SR, et al. Current state of knowledge on takotsubo syndrome: a position statement from the Taskforce on Takotsubo Syndrome of the Heart Failure Association of the European Society of Cardiology. Eur J Heart Fail. 2016;18(1):8–27.
40. Bratis K. Cardiac magnetic resonance in takotsubo syndrome. Eur Cardiol Rev. 2017;12(1):58–62.
41. Scally C, Abbas H, Ahearn T, Srinivasan J, Mezincescu A, Rudd A, et al. Myocardial and systemic inflammation in acute stress-induced (takotsubo) cardiomyopathy. Circulation. 2019;139(13):1581–92.
42. Natale E, Mistrulli R. Takotsubo syndrome: more frequent in women, more dangerous in men. Eur Heart J Suppl J Eur Soc Cardiol. 2023;25(Suppl B):B119–22.
43. Isogai T, Yasunaga H, Matsui H, Tanaka H, Ueda T, Horiguchi H, et al. Out-of-hospital versus in-hospital takotsubo cardiomyopathy: analysis of 3719 patients in the diagnosis procedure combination database in Japan. Int J Cardiol. 2014;176(2):413–7.

Peripartum Cardiomyopathy

Milos Kubanek and Tereza Schimerova

Abstract

Peripartum cardiomyopathy (PPCM) is defined as non-ischemic systolic dysfunction of the left ventricle (ejection fraction <45%) manifested towards the end of a pregnancy or in the early postpartum period when no other cause of heart failure is identified. The pathophysiology of PPCM seems to be related to complex interaction of genetic background with hormonal and vascular milieu of late pregnancy. Disease management should be tailored based on the hemodynamical status of the mother and the prognosis of the foetus within a multidisciplinary team. Importantly, PPCM patients with severe acute heart failure or cardiogenic shock should be transferred to centres with available mechanical circulatory support and scheduled for early delivery by a caesarean section. There are important differences in the pharmacotherapy of heart failure in the antepartum and postpartum periods. Preventive anticoagulation should be considered in left ventricular ejection fraction <35% and also during treatment with bromocriptine. Bromocriptine might be effective in severe forms of PPCM to facilitate left ventricular recovery. Women with PPCM considering a subsequent pregnancy should be counselled and monitored by physicians familiar with this disease.

Keywords

Peripartum cardiomyopathy · Heart failure · Pregnancy · Genetics · Prolactin

Test your learning and check your understanding of this book's contents: use the "Springer Nature Flashcards" app to access questions using ▶ https://sn.pub/51ny7m
To use the app, please follow the instructions in chapter 1.

M. Kubanek (✉) · T. Schimerova
Department of Cardiology, Institute for Clinical and Experimental Medicine, Prague, Czech Republic
e-mail: milos.kubanek@ikem.cz

A. H.E.M. Maas, E. Gerdts (eds.), *Manual of Cardiovascular Disease in Women*,
https://doi.org/10.1007/978-3-031-65952-2_26

1 Introduction

Peripartum cardiomyopathy (PPCM) is defined as non-ischemic systolic dysfunction of the left ventricle (ejection fraction <45%) manifested towards the end of a pregnancy or in the early postpartum period when no other cause of heart failure is identified [1]. Despite intensive research of this disease in the last decades, the aetiology of PPCM has not been fully elucidated and causal treatment of the disease is missing. We aimed to summarize the most recent information regarding the epidemiology, pathophysiology and clinical aspects of PPCM.

1.1 History

The first description of cases compatible with PPCM comes from the German pathologist Virchow, who noticed a post-mortem association between heart failure and puerperium in 1880. The first clinical reports of severe heart failure in the last month before delivery were authored by Gouley et al. (7 cases) and Hull et al. (80 cases), in 1937 and 1938 respectively. The term PPCM was introduced into clinical terminology by Demakis in 1971 [2]. The contemporary definition is based on an expert consensus from the 1990s, which includes manifestation of heart failure in the last month of pregnancy or within 5 months postpartum in the absence of another cause of heart failure. PPCM is thus a diagnosis per exclusion [3]. A subsequent study by Elkayam et al. demonstrated in a group of 123 women with non-ischemic cardiomyopathy manifested in pregnancy or postpartum, that 19% of cases became apparent during the 17th–26th week of pregnancy and had similar clinical and prognostic characteristics to classical PPCM cases [4]. The contemporary definition describes PPCM as an idiopathic cardiomyopathy leading to left ventricular systolic dysfunction (ejection fraction lower than 45%) and heart failure with present or absent left ventricular dilatation. The typical time frame for manifestation of PPCM are the last months of the pregnancy up to the sixth month postpartum [1].

1.2 Epidemiology and Risk Factors

Major epidemiologic data regarding PPCM come from the USA, the Republic of South Africa, Nigeria, and Haiti. The estimated incidence of PPCM varies in different studies from 1:100 in Nigeria to 1:20,000 in Japan. PPCM registries from the USA revealed an increase in the incidence of the disease from 1:1181 in 2004 to 1:849 in 2011 [5]. These findings were explained by an improvement in PPCM diagnostics, the average higher age of mothers, a higher incidence of pre-eclampsia and a higher proportion of multiple pregnancies. In addition, there is a trend towards increased cardiovascular risk in the general population related to the rising prevalence of arterial hypertension, diabetes, and obesity [6]. Another risk factor is African-American origin. In some countries like Haiti or Nigeria, an extremely high incidence of PPCM was reported, which was related to genetic background and also to acquired factors. For example, there is a description of increased salt intake and hot baths during ritual procedures in puerperium in Nigeria related to PPCM. Maternal age is another independent risk factor. Mothers older than 30 years have a 1.7–1.8 times higher risk of PPCM than younger females [7]. Not surprisingly, as pre-eclampsia and PPCM share some common pathophysiological mechanisms, there is a strong link between this hypertensive pregnancy disorder and the increased prevalence of PPCM. The 2013 meta-analysis of studies on PPCM revealed a prevalence of pre-eclampsia of 22% in this population, which was more than 4 times higher than in the general population [8]. A similar result provided by the PPCM registry EURObservational Research Programme identified pre-eclampsia in 22.8% of 411 women enrolled [9].

2 Theory

2.1 Inflammatory Hypothesis

The first pathophysiological concepts of PPCM linked the disease to viral and autoimmune myocarditis. However, a later comparison of results of endomyocardial biopsies in PPCM and other cardiomyopathies demonstrated a similar occurrence of viral genomes in myocardium of both groups. Inflammatory infiltrates were found in biopsies of PPCM patients with variable frequency, but rarely fulfilled the criteria of myocarditis [10]. Therefore, myocarditis does not seem to be the main cause of PPCM.

2.2 Genetic Contributors

Currently, most authors suggest a double hit theory. The interaction of genetic background with vascular and endocrine abnormalities in late pregnancy and puerperium seems to be the most important determinant of PPCM pathophysiology (Fig. 1). The familial occurrence of PPCM and manifestation PPCM in pedigrees with familial dilated cardiomyopathy inspired molecular-genetic studies in this field. In 2012, enrichment of titin truncating variants among patients with dilated cardiomyopathy was reported to reach 25% in familial and 18% in sporadic cases in comparison with 1% in hypertrophic cardiomyopathy patients and 3% in healthy controls [11]. Subsequently, in 2016, an assessment of 43 genes associated with dilated cardiomyopathy documented in 15% of 172 subjects with PPCM truncating variants in eight genes. Similarly, truncating variants were identified in 17% of the control group with dilated cardiomyopathy. Two thirds of identified truncating variants were in titin, as seen in 10% of the PPCM patients and in 1.4% of the reference population. The presence of titin truncating variants was significantly correlated with a lower left ventricular ejection fraction at 1-year follow-up [12]. Subsequent research was focused on composition titin isoforms in myocardial samples of patients with dilated cardiomyopathy [13–16] with data absent for PPCM. The enrichment of pathogenic and likely-pathogenic genetic variants in PPCM suggests the modifying effect of the genetic background on the pathophysiology of PPCM. However, in the majority of cases it remains unexplained.

2.3 Interaction of Free Oxygen Radicals and Prolactin

The important acquired determinants of PPCM pathophysiology seem to be an increased oxidative stress and hypersecretion of prolactin, a 23 kDa hormone synthetized in adenohypophysis (Fig. 1). Pregnancy has been associated with a gradual increase of oxidative stress, which returns to normal levels after delivery [17]. These abnormalities are counterbalanced by increased activity of antioxidative systems, which are preserved after pregnancy. Cardiomyocytes are protected against the oxidative stress by STAT3 (signal

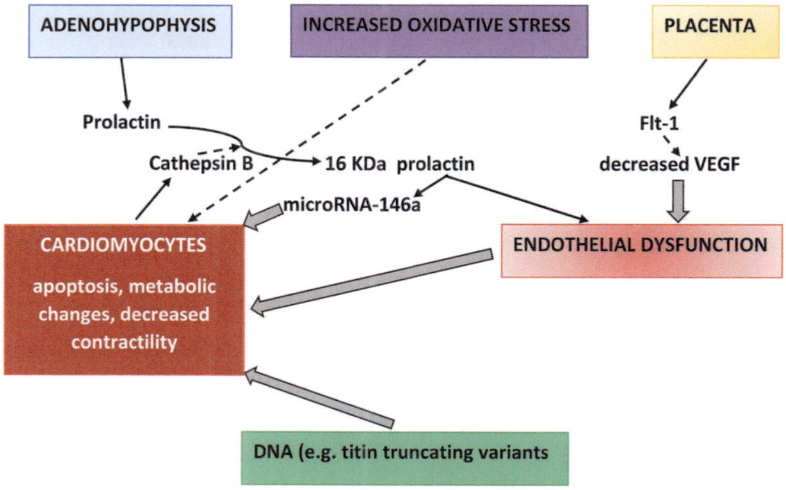

Fig. 1 The contemporary pathophysiological concept of peripartum cardiomyopathy. *DNA* deoxyribonucleic acid, *Flt-1* fms-like tyrosine kinase-1, *RNA* ribonucleic acid, *VEGF* vascular endothelial growth factor

transducer and activator of transcription 3). This transcription factor increases production of manganese superoxide dismutase, an antioxidative enzyme useful for the inactivation of free oxygen radicals [18]. Expression of STAT3 is enhanced in cardiomyocytes of pregnant and postpartum females physiologically. A mouse model with an increased myocardial expression of STAT3 showed favourable resistance against anthracycline cardiotoxicity mediated in a large proportion by free oxygen radicals. Oxidative stress increases by an unknown mechanism production of cathepsin D in cardiomyocytes. Cathepsin D cleaves prolactin into a 16 kDa fragment with a deleterious effect on cardiomyocytes and microvascular bed. It may cause an apoptosis of endothelial cells with subsequent rarefication of the capillary vascular bed. A mouse model with reduced expression of STAT3 showed in pregnancy (in comparison with wild-type mice) an increased proportion of cleaved prolactin to the 16 kDa fragment and more frequently developed the phenotype of PPCM. Manifestation of PPCM was inhibited by bromocriptine in this mouse model. In addition, an increased expression of the 16 kDa fragment of prolactin achieved by an adenoviral vector replicated in non-pregnant mice the phenotype of PPCM [17, 18]. Reduced expression of STAT 3 was also found in human cardiomyocytes from biopsies or explanted hearts with PPCM. It was accompanied by increased oxidative stress, high levels of cathepsin D and 16 kDa fragment of prolactin also in the serum of PPCM females as compared with healthy controls [17, 18].

The 16 kDa fragment of prolactin upregulates production of microRNA-146a, which mediates its cardiotoxic effects. MicroRNA146a blocks some metabolic pathways in cardiomyocytes, decreases their metabolic activity and may contribute to the development of the PPCM phenotype. Women with PPCM had a higher concentration of microRNA-146a than controls with DCM, which was normalized by bromocriptine. In an experimental model, administration of antisense oligonucleotide targeting microRNA-146a improved depletion of the capillary vessel bed and fibrosis in myocardium and led to improvement in left ventricular ejection fraction. MicroRNA146a thus could serve both as a biomarker and treatment target in PPCM patients [19]. In addition, upregulation of microRNA-199a-5p was found in subjects with PPCM. This finding may lead to decreased consumption of glucose in cardiomyocytes, increased production of free oxygen radicals, and cell death. Further effects of this microRNA included impairment of the ubiquitin-proteasome system with disorganisation of sarcomeres and increased production of the asymmetrical dimethyl arginine leading to reduced production of nitric oxide and endothelial dysfunction [20].

2.4 Pre-eclampsia Related Hypothesis

The high prevalence of pre-eclampsia in women with PPCM suggests common pathophysiological mechanisms of both diseases (Fig. 1). The placenta is the source for the production of the antiangiogenic protein called soluble fms-like tyrosine kinase-1 (sFlt-1), which rises exponentially during the pregnancy. sFlt1 decreases the beneficial effects of the vascular endothelial growth factor (VEGF) and placental growth factor (PlGF). An imbalance of these mediators is considered to be the main cause of arterial hypertension and endothelial dysfunction in pre-eclampsia. Importantly, the plasma level of sFlt1 indirectly correlates with reduced global longitudinal strain and directly with increased left ventricular mass in women with pre-eclampsia. Mouse models suggest that sFlt-1 may also play a role in the pathogenesis of PPCM [21]. This process may be mediated by peroxisome proliferator-activated receptor-γ coactivator 1-α (PGC-1α), a transcriptional coactivator able to up-regulate mitochondrial biogenesis, respiratory capacity, oxidative phosphorylation, and fatty acid β-oxidation with the final aim of providing a more efficient pathway for aerobic energy production. It is also involved in angiogenesis and increases expression of manganese superoxide dismutase. Mouse models with deletion of PGC-1α in cardiomyocytes developed dilated cardiomyopathy in pregnancy. This mouse strain was also prone to developing dilated cardiomyopathy after administration of Flt-1 even in the absence of pregnancy. Combined administration of bromocriptine and VEGF fully normalized left ventricular function in this model. Interestingly, administration of one of the abovementioned substances led to a partial effect on the left ventricular systolic function [22]. The plasma level of sFlt-1 falls rapidly in healthy women after delivery because its source is the placenta. On the other hand, women with PPCM had a slower decrease of sFlt-1 than healthy subjects. The source of sFlt-1 production after delivery is unknown. In a study group of patients with PPCM, plasma level of sFlt-1 positively correlated with NYHA class. The role of placental hormones in the pathogenesis of PPCM is not completely understood [22].

3 Clinical Practice

3.1 Clinical Manifestation

Women with PPCM usually report typical signs of congestion. They may experience progressive exercise dyspnoea, leg oedema or typical paroxysmal nocturnal dyspnoea with intolerance of horizontal position. Another presentation of PPCM is cardiogenic shock with a necessity of inotropic support or implantation of mechanical circulatory support. Less frequently, subjects with PPCM complain of palpitations or syncope. In addition, the diagnosis of PPCM should also be considered in women with a systemic embolism or jaundice during the last trimester of pregnancy or in the early post-partum period.

Physical examination may reveal signs of cardiomegaly left sided congestion like pulmonary rales, or right sided congestion including increased filling of jugular veins, hepatomegaly, ascites, or swollen lower extremities. The third heart sound is a non-specific finding in a pregnant woman as it may be present physiologically. Electrocardiography may show normal findings. However, abnormalities of the ST segment are frequent with a predominance of left ventricular strain. In clinically unstable patients, a chest X-ray may be performed, which can reveal signs of pulmonary congestion, pleural effusions and/or cardiomegaly. Otherwise, examinations with a radiation exposure should be performed in the postpartum period. Plasma levels of B-type natriuretic peptide and of N-terminal pro-B-type natriuretic peptide are usually markedly elevated. Nevertheless, mild elevation of both peptides may be physiological in the advanced stages of pregnancy [5].

3.2 Differential Diagnosis

Heart failure symptoms of PPCM patients may remain unrecognized as mild breathlessness and mild leg oedema may occur physiologically in advanced stages of pregnancy. Differential diagnosis includes pre-existing cardiomyopathy, myocarditis, cardiomyopathy induced by toxins or drugs, severe valve disease, congenital heart disease, or pulmonary arterial hypertension. Pregnancy leads to an increased volume of circulating blood and to an increase in cardiac output by more than 50% until the end of the second trimester. Consequently, heart failure in women with pre-existing heart disease usually manifests in the first two trimesters, earlier than PPCM [5]. An acute myocardial infarction may be caused in pregnant women either by a rupture of atherosclerotic plaque or by spontaneous coronary dissection. The risk of acute myocardial infarction is increased in the peripartum period 3–4 times in comparison with comparable non-pregnant women [23]. Other important diseases to consider in the differential diagnosis are acute thromboembolic pulmonary embolism and acute embolism of the amniotic fluid. The risk of pulmonary embolism is increased in pregnancy and puerperium 5–10 times as compared with the general population [23].

3.3 Therapeutic Decision Making

Therapeutic decision making should be done in a team including a cardiologist, an obstetrician, a neonatologist, an anaesthesiologist and possibly a cardiac surgeon. Based on the hemodynamical status of the mother and prognosis of the foetus, delivery should be planned. Patients in cardiogenic shock or who are dependent on inotropes should be transferred to facilities with an available mechanical circulatory support team. Induction of lung maturation in viable foetuses of gestational age >23 weeks + 5 days should be initiated [24]. Hemodynamically unstable women with PPCM are treated as acute heart failure syndrome. Their management includes optimalisation of preload and afterload (using diuretics and nitrates), adequate oxygenation, treatment of low cardiac output syndrome (inotropes, vasopressors, mechanical circulatory support in refractory cases), anticoagulation and planning of urgent delivery (caesarean section). Treatment with bromocriptine may be considered [24]. Stable patients with PPCM are treated as follows.

3.4 Treatment

3.4.1 Standard Treatment of Heart Failure with Reduced Ejection Fraction

Pharmacotherapy of PPCM follows recommendations for treatment of heart failure with reduced ejection fraction (HFREF) with a modification in pregnant women, who should not receive teratogenic drugs [24–27]. In pregnant women, angiotensin converting enzyme inhibitors (ACEi), angiotensin receptor blockers (ARBs), angiotensin receptor/neprilysin inhibitors (ARNi), mineralocorticoid receptor antagonists (MRAs), sodium-glucose transporter 2 inhibitors (SGLT2i), ivabradine, and vericiguat should not be administered because of significant risks of foetal harm [27]. Sodium restriction followed by the use of loop diuretics are recommended in individuals with hypervolaemia and congestion. Importantly, severe hypovolaemia and hypotension should be prevented as they may impair placental and foetal perfusion. In haemodynamically stable patients, treatment with beta-blockers should be started, preferably with cardio-selective beta-blockers like metoprolol succinate. Hydralazine and nitrates are allowed vasodilators in pregnant women with PPCM. Digoxin may also be used in pregnancy [5, 24–27].

Table 1 Pharmacotherapy of heart failure and its use during pregnancy and lactation

Drug	Pregnancy	Lactation
Furosemide, torasemide	Compatible	Compatible
Beta-blockers	Compatible	Compatible
Angiotensin converting enzyme inhibitors and angiotensin receptor blockers	Incompatible	Compatible: Captopril, enalapril, quinapril, benazepril
Spironolactone, eplerenone	Incompatible	Compatible
Sacubitril-valsartan	Incompatible	Missing data
Hydralazine and nitrates	Compatible	Compatible
Sodium-glucose transporter 2 inhibitors	Not recommended	Missing data
Ivabradin	Not recommended	Missing data
Digoxin	Compatible	Compatible
Vericiguat	Not recommended	Missing data
Heparin (unfractionated or low molecular weight)	Compatible	Compatible
Warfarin, phenprocoumon	Not recommended	Compatible
Direct oral anticoagulants	Incompatible	Missing data

On the other hand, ACEi, ARBs, ARNi, MRA, SGLT2i, ivabradine, and vericiguat can be used only postpartum. Some beta-blockers and ACEi can be used together with furosemide and MRA even during lactation after consultation with the paediatric team (Table 1). Sudden cardiac death may be prevented in outpatients with severe systolic dysfunction in the early period by wearable cardioverter-defibrillators, later by implantable cardioverter-defibrillators in patients with absent left ventricular recovery [24, 27].

3.4.2 Anticoagulation

Pregnancy is associated with a hypercoagulable state which, together with blood stasis in dysfunctional left ventricle, predisposes women with PPCM to formation of intracardiac thrombi. The incidence of intracardiac thrombi during acute heart failure caused by PPCM has been reported to be 16–17% [27] with 9% thromboembolic events in two separate cohorts [27]. Guidelines of the American Heart Association (AHA) therefore recommend considering anticoagulation in women with severely depressed left ventricular ejection fraction (LVEF) (<30%) in the setting of acute heart failure caused by PPCM, especially in the first 6–8 weeks postpartum, when hypercoagulability is most pronounced. In addition, anticoagulation is also recommended in postpartum women with PPCM treated with bromocriptine and having LVEF <35% [27]. Unfractionated or low molecular weight heparin may be used in pregnant women with PPCM. Warfarin is the anticoagulant of choice postpartum to prevent intracardiac thrombosis. It might also be administered during lactation [27].

3.4.3 Bromocriptine

Bromocriptine inhibits production of prolactin, a major hormone involved in the regulation of lactation markedly elevated postpartum. The rationale for administration of bromocriptine in PPCM was derived from experimental models showing formation of a 16 kDa fragment of prolactin with strong antiangiogenic and proapoptotic activity, possibly involved in the pathophysiology of PPCM [17]. A pilot open-label randomized controlled study in South Africa suggested that the addition of bromocriptine to optimal heart failure therapy was associated with greater LVEF improvement and a lower rate of the composite endpoint at 6 months [28]. Among 96 women with acute PPCM in Burkina Faso, 4-week treatment with bromocriptine was associated with LVEF recovery and lower mortality (16.6% versus 29.1%; $P < 0.001$) [29]. A multicentre German study randomized 63 patients to 1 versus 8 weeks of bromocriptine (with absent placebo group). The authors reported LVEF recovery ≥50% in 52% and 68% of the 1- and 8-week groups, respectively, and no deaths [30]. Some retrospective studies also suggested a benefit from bromocriptine [31]. A randomized double-blind, placebo control study (REBIRTH) to investigate the effect of bromocriptine on myocardial recovery and clinical outcome of 200 women with PPCM in the United States and Canada is under evaluation [32].

The 2018 ESC guidelines provide a weak recommendation (Class IIb, Level of Evidence: B) for the use of bromocriptine [24]. The latest AHA Heart failure guidelines [27] also provide a weak recommendation for administration of bromocriptine in women with severe PPCM with either LVEF <25% or cardiogenic shock. This treatment should be accompanied by anticoagulation, to prevent hypercoagulability [27]. The risks of discouraging breastfeeding should be considered mainly in countries with a low socioeconomic standard and poor access to artificial nutrition.

3.5 Prognosis

Mortality of PPCM depends on racial groups, geographical region, and duration of follow-up. At 1-year follow-up, mortality rates in the United States ranged from 4% in the IPAC study [33] to 11% in a population of African-American women [34]. Less data are available for long-term outcomes (>5 years), but U.S. mortality estimates have ranged from 7% to 20% (mean follow-up 6.3–8.6 years) [35–38].

PPCM has been associated with a higher rate of recovery than other cases of HFREF [39], and recovery frequently occurs within the first 3–6 months [4, 33, 40]. However, delayed recovery can also occur up to 2 years following diagnosis. Of the 100 prospectively enrolled women in the IPAC study, 72% recovered to LVEF >50% at 12 months [33]. A lower recovery rate was found in study groups with a predominance of African-American women. A recent retrospective analysis of 59 women reported 43% recovered to LVEF of ≥50% by 12 months with a median time to recovery of 8 months [38].

3.6 Recommendations for a Subsequent Pregnancy

The largest study on subsequent pregnancy in women with PPCM was published in 2001. The study was retrospective and included 44 women, 16 of them with persistent left ventricular systolic dysfunction. The new pregnancy was associated with a significant decrease in LVEF (49.9 ± 12% vs. 42 ± 13%, $P < 0.001$). Women with normalized LVEF did not experience any cardiac deaths. On the contrary, women with persistent left ventricular systolic dysfunction had a mortality rate of 19% [41]. A more recent prospective study enrolled 34 women with PPCM from Germany, Scotland and the Republic of South Africa. The relapse of PPCM was defined as a decrease in LVEF under 50% or death from cardiac causes. It was documented after the subsequent pregnancy in 56%. Importantly, 12% of the study participants died, all with a persistent left ventricular systolic dysfunction [42]. Long-term outcomes of subsequent pregnancies in 45 PPCM patients showed a recent report [43], 80% of individuals were of African American descent and 76% from a low socioeconomic background. Subjects with left ventricular recovery represented 67% of the study group. Importantly, at a median follow-up of 8 years there was a similar mortality around 20% both in the recovery and non-recovery group [43]. Therefore, the normalization of LV systolic function does not guarantee a favourable outcome in subsequent pregnancies. Women considering a subsequent pregnancy should be counselled and monitored by physicians familiar with PPCM.

4 Conclusions

The pathogenesis of PPCM has not been fully elucidated, but it seems to be related to a complex interaction of genetics with vascular and hormonal milieu of late pregnancy. Despite advances in the PPCM disease management, there are important gaps in the evidence regarding administration of bromocriptine, optimal anticoagulation and prevention of sudden cardiac death. An important issue is the appropriate counselling of PPCM women regarding a subsequent pregnancy.

Key Issues

- PPCM is defined as non-ischemic systolic dysfunction of the left ventricle (ejection fraction <45%) manifested towards the end of a pregnancy or in the early postpartum period when no other cause of heart failure is identified.
- Although not fully elucidated, the pathophysiology of PPCM seems to be related to complex interaction of genetic background with hormonal and vascular milieu of late pregnancy.
- Disease management should be tailored based on the hemodynamic status of the mother and the prognosis of the foetus within a multidisciplinary team.
- PPCM patients with severe acute heart failure or cardiogenic shock should be transferred to centres with available mechanical circulatory support and scheduled for early delivery by a caesarean section.
- There are important differences in the pharmacotherapy of heart failure in the antepartum and postpartum period. Anticoagulation should be considered in most cases. Bromocriptine might be effective in severe forms of PPCM.
- Women with PPCM considering a subsequent pregnancy should be counselled and monitored by physicians familiar with this disease.

Questions and Answers

1. What is the typical time frame for manifestation of PPCM?
   Correct answer: The last trimester of pregnancy and 5 months postpartum are the most typical periods for PPCM manifestation.
2. What heart failure pharmacotherapy is allowed in women with PPCM with a viable foetus in the antepartum period?
   Correct answer: Nitrates, hydralazine, furosemide, and digoxin are allowed in this period.

3. When is anticoagulation indicated in PPCM?
   Correct answer: Anticoagulation should be administered either in PPCM patients with established intracardiac thrombosis, or in LVEF<35% or during treatment with bromocriptine.
4. What stages of PPCM should be treated with bromocriptine?
   Correct answer: The evidence for treatment with bromocriptine is modest. It may be considered in severe cases of PPCM with LVEF<25% or cardiogenic shock.

Acknowledgement The project was supported by the Ministry of Health of the Czech Republic, the research grant [NV19-08-00122], MH CZ—DRO ("Institute for Clinical and Experimental Medicine—IKEM, IN 00023001").

References

1. Sliwa K, Hilfiker-Kleiner D, Petrie MC, Mebazaa A, Pieske B, Buchmann E, et al. Current state of knowledge on aetiology, diagnosis, management, and therapy of peripartum cardiomyopathy: a position statement from the Heart Failure Association of the European Society of Cardiology Working Group on peripartum cardiomyopathy. Eur J Heart Fail. 2010;12(8):767–78.
2. Demakis JG, Rahimtoola SH, Sutton GC, Meadows WR, Szanto PB, Tobin JR, et al. Natural course of peripartum cardiomyopathy. Circulation. 1971;44(6):1053–61.
3. Elkayam U. Clinical characteristics of peripartum cardiomyopathy in the United States: diagnosis, prognosis, and management. J Am Coll Cardiol. 2011;58(7):659–70.
4. Elkayam U, Akhter MW, Singh H, Khan S, Bitar F, Hameed A, et al. Pregnancy-associated cardiomyopathy: clinical characteristics and a comparison between early and late presentation. Circulation. 2005;111(16):2050–5.
5. Honigberg MC, Givertz MM. Peripartum cardiomyopathy. BMJ. 2019;364:1–14.
6. Kolte D, Khera S, Aronow WS, Palaniswamy C, Mujib M, Ahn C, et al. Temporal trends in incidence and outcomes of peripartum cardiomyopathy in the United States: a nationwide population-based study. J Am Heart Assoc. 2014;3(3):1–13.
7. Kao DP, Hsich E, Lindenfeld JA. Characteristics, adverse events, and racial differences among delivering mothers with peripartum cardiomyopathy. JACC Heart Fail. 2013;1(5):409–16.
8. Bello N, Rendon ISH, Arany Z. The relationship between pre-eclampsia and peripartum cardiomyopathy: a systematic review and meta-analysis. J Am Coll Cardiol. 2013;62(18):1715–23.
9. Sliwa K, Mebazaa A, Hilfiker-Kleiner D, Petrie MC, Maggioni AP, Laroche C, et al. Clinical characteristics of patients from the worldwide registry on peripartum cardiomyopathy (PPCM): EURObservational Research Programme in conjunction with the Heart Failure Association of the European Society of Cardiology Study Group on PPCM. Eur J Heart Fail. 2017;19(9):1131–41.
10. Bültmann BD, Klingel K, Näbauer M, Wallwiener D, Kandolf R. High prevalence of viral genomes and inflammation in peripartum cardiomyopathy. Am J Obstet Gynecol. 2005;193(2):363–5.
11. Herman DS, Lam L, Taylor MR, Wang L, Teekakirikul P, Christodoulou D, et al. Truncations of titin causing dilated cardiomyopathy. N Engl J Med. 2012;366(7):619–28. https://doi.org/10.1056/NEJMoa1110186.
12. Ware JS, Li J, Mazaika E, Yasso CM, De Souza T, Cappola TP, et al. Shared genetic predisposition in peripartum and dilated cardiomyopathies. N Engl J Med. 2016;374(3):233–41.
13. Makarenko I, Opitz CA, Leake MC, Neagoe C, Kulke M, Gwathmey JK, et al. Passive stiffness changes caused by upregulation of compliant titin isoforms in human dilated cardiomyopathy hearts. Circ Res. 2004;95(7):708–16.
14. Fukuda N, Wu Y, Farman G, Irving TC, Granzier H. Titin isoform variance and length dependence of activation in skinned bovine cardiac muscle. J Physiol. 2003;553(1):147–54.
15. Granzier H, Labeit S. Cardiac titin: an adjustable multi-functional spring. J Physiol. 2002;541(2):335–42.
16. Van Spaendonck-Zwarts KY, Posafalvi A, Van Den Berg MP, Hilfiker-Kleiner D, Bollen IAE, Sliwa K, et al. Titin gene mutations are common in families with both peripartum cardiomyopathy and dilated cardiomyopathy. Eur Heart J. 2014;35(32):2165–73.
17. Hilfiker-Kleiner D, Kaminski K, Podewski E, Bonda T, Schaefer A, Sliwa K, et al. A cathepsin D-cleaved 16 kDa form of prolactin mediates postpartum cardiomyopathy. Cell. 2007;128(3):589–600.
18. Negoro S, Kunisada K, Fujio Y, Funamoto M, Darville MI, Eizirik DL, et al. Activation of signal transducer and activator of transcription 3 protects cardiomyocytes from hypoxia/reoxygenation-induced oxidative stress through the upregulation of manganese superoxide dismutase. Circulation. 2001;104(9):979–81.
19. Halkein J, Tabruyn SP, Ricke-Hoch M, Haghikia A, Nguyen NQN, Scherr M, et al. MicroRNA-146a is a therapeutic target and biomarker for peripartum cardiomyopathy. J Clin Invest. 2013;123(5):2143–54.
20. Aryan L, Medzikovic L, Umar S, Eghbali M. Pregnancy-associated cardiac dysfunction and the regulatory role of microRNAs. Biol Sex Differ. 2020;11(1):1–17.

21. Shahul S, Medvedofsky D, Wenger JB, Nizamuddin J, Brown SM, Bajracharya S, et al. Circulating anti-angiogenic factors and myocardial dysfunction in hypertensive disorders of pregnancy. Hypertension. 2016;67(6):1273–80.
22. Patten IS, Rana S, Shahul S, Rowe GC, Jang C, Liu L, et al. Cardiac angiogenic imbalance leads to peripartum cardiomyopathy. Nature. 2012;485(7398):333–8.
23. Elkayam U, Goland S, Pieper PG, Silverside CK. High-risk cardiac disease in pregnancy: part I. J Am Coll Cardiol. 2016;68(4):396–410.
24. Regitz-Zagrosek V, Roos-Hesselink JW, Bauersachs J, Blomström-Lundqvist C, Cífková R, De Bonis M, et al. 2018 ESC guidelines for the management of cardiovascular diseases during pregnancy. Eur Heart J. 2018;39:3165–241.
25. Bozkurt B, Colvin M, Cook J, Cooper LT, Deswal A, Fonarow GC, et al. Current diagnostic and treatment strategies for specific dilated cardiomyopathies: a scientific statement from the American Heart Association. Circulation. 2016;134:579–646.
26. McDonagh TA, Metra M, Adamo M, Gardner RS, Baumbach A, Böhm M, et al. 2021 ESC guidelines for the diagnosis and treatment of acute and chronic heart failure. Eur J Heart Fail. 2022;24(1):4–131. https://doi.org/10.1002/ejhf.2333.
27. Heidenreich PA, Bozkurt B, Aguilar D, Allen LA, Byun JJ, Colvin MM, et al. 2022 AHA/ACC/HFSA guideline for the management of heart failure. Circulation. 2022;145(18):e876–94. https://doi.org/10.1161/CIR.0000000000001062.
28. Sliwa K, Blauwet L, Tibazarwa K, Libhaber E, Smedema JP, Becker A, et al. Evaluation of bromocriptine in the treatment of acute severe peripartum cardiomyopathy: a proof-of-concept pilot study. Circulation. 2010;121:1465–73.
29. Yaméogo NV, Kagambèga LJ, Seghda A, Owona A, Kaboré O, Kaboré E, et al. Bromocriptine in management of peripartum cardiomyopathy: a randomized study on 96 women in Burkina Faso. J Cardiol Clin Res. 2017;5:1098.
30. Hilfiker-Kleiner D, Haghikia A, Berliner D, Vogel-Claussen J, Schwab J, Franke A, et al. Bromocriptine for the treatment of peripartum cardiomyopathy: a multicentre randomized study. Eur Heart J. 2017;38:2671–9.
31. Tremblay-Gravel M, Marquis-Gravel G, Avram R, Desplantie O, Ducharme A, Bibas L, et al. The effect of bromocriptine on left ventricular functional recovery in peripartum cardiomyopathy: insights from the BRO-HF retrospective cohort study. ESC Heart Fail. 2019;6:27–36.
32. Davis MB, Arany Z, McNamara DM, Goland S, Elkayam U. Peripartum cardiomyopathy: JACC state-of-the-art review. J Am Coll Cardiol. 2020;75(2):207–21. https://doi.org/10.1016/j.jacc.2019.11.014.
33. McNamara DM, Elkayam U, Alharethi R, Damp J, Hsich E, Ewald G, et al. Clinical outcomes for peripartum cardiomyopathy in North America: results of the IPAC Study (Investigations of Pregnancy-Associated Cardiomyopathy). J Am Coll Cardiol. 2015;66:905–14.
34. Briasoulis A, Mocanu M, Marinescu K, Qaqi O, Palla M, Telila T, et al. Longitudinal systolic strain profiles and outcomes in peripartum cardiomyopathy. Echocardiography. 2016;33:1354–60.
35. Harper MA, Meyer RE, Berg CJ. Peripartum cardiomyopathy: population-based birth prevalence and 7-year mortality. Obstet Gynecol. 2012;120:1013–9.
36. Felker GM, Jaeger CJ, Klodas E, Thiemann DR, Hare JM, Hruban RH, et al. Myocarditis and long-term survival in peripartum cardiomyopathy. Am Heart J. 2000;140:785–91.
37. Pillarisetti J, Kondur A, Alani A, Reddy M, Reddy M, Vacek J, et al. Peripartum cardiomyopathy: predictors of recovery and current state of implantable cardioverter-defibrillator use. J Am Coll Cardiol. 2014;63:2831–9.
38. Mahowald MK, Basu N, Subramaniam L, Scott R, Davis MB. Long-term outcomes in peripartum cardiomyopathy. Open Cardiovasc Med J. 2019;13:13–23.
39. Cooper LT, Mather PJ, Alexis JD, Pauly DF, Torre-Amione G, Wittstein IS, et al. Myocardial recovery in peripartum cardiomyopathy: prospective comparison with recent onset cardiomyopathy in men and nonperipartum women. J Card Fail. 2012;18:28–33.
40. Amos AM, Jaber WA, Russell SD. Improved outcomes in peripartum cardiomyopathy with contemporary. Am Heart J. 2006;152:509–13.
41. Elkayam U, Tummala PP, Rao K, Akhter MW, Karaalp IS, Wani OR, et al. Maternal and fetal outcomes of subsequent pregnancies in women with peripartum cardiomyopathy. JACC Heart Fail. 2013;23(1):1–7.
42. Hilfiker-Kleiner D, Haghikia A, Masuko D, Nonhoff J, Held D, Libhaber E, et al. Outcome of subsequent pregnancies in patients with a history of peripartum cardiomyopathy. Eur J Heart Fail. 2017;19(12):1723–8.
43. Pachariyanon P, Bogabathina H, Jaisingh K, Modi M, Modi K. Long-term outcomes of women with peripartum cardiomyopathy having subsequent pregnancies. J Am Coll Cardiol. 2023;82(1):16–26. https://doi.org/10.1016/j.jacc.2023.04.043.

Cardiac Rehabilitation in Women

Lis Neubeck, Robyn Gallagher, and Tone M. Norekvål

Abstract

Cardiac rehabilitation (CR) programmes include a range of medical and lifestyle interventions, such as exercise training, dietary advice, stress management, medication adherence, and education on heart-healthy living. The programmes are typically supervised by a multidisciplinary team of healthcare professionals and are designed to address risk factors such as high blood pressure, high cholesterol, diabetes, smoking and depression. Participation in CR decreases morbidity and mortality and has therefore a class 1A recommendation in international guidelines. Despite this strong recommendation, participation in CR is low and women are poorly represented. There are barriers at an individual level (co-morbidities, pelvic floor changes following pregnancy and menopause, depression, family responsibilities) and at a system level (distance to CR centres, educational attainment, belonging to an ethnic minority group, and lack of physician referral). Increasing referral, enrolment and participation should be a high priority. Automatic or systematic referral has been shown to increase the number of participants in CR, and adherence to CR may be higher if remote or home-based interventions are included. Carer involvement can play a crucial role in the success of CR.

Keywords

Cardiac rehabilitation · Exercise training · Dietary advice · Stress management · Medication adherence

L. Neubeck
School of Health and Social Care, Edinburgh Napier University, Edinburgh, Scotland, UK
e-mail: L.Neubeck@napier.ac.uk

R. Gallagher
Faculty of Medicine and Health, The University of Sydney, Charles Perkins Centre, Camperdown, NSW, Australia
e-mail: robyn.gallagher@sydney.edu.au

T. M. Norekvål (✉)
Department of Heart Disease, Haukeland University Hospital, Bergen, Norway
e-mail: tone.merete.norekval@helse-bergen.no

A. H.E.M. Maas, E. Gerdts (eds.), *Manual of Cardiovascular Disease in Women*,
https://doi.org/10.1007/978-3-031-65952-2_27

Test your learning and check your understanding of this book's contents: use the "Springer Nature Flashcards" app to access questions using ▶ https://sn.pub/51ny7m
To use the app, please follow the instructions in chapter 1.

1 Introduction

Cardiac rehabilitation (CR) is a comprehensive service that aims to improve the health and well-being of people suffering from heart disease, often taking place after an acute event and when treated with interventional procedures or cardiac surgery. The programme includes a range of medical and lifestyle interventions, such as exercise training, dietary advice, stress management, medication adherence, and education on heart-healthy living, and is underpinned by theories of behaviour change. CR programmes are typically supervised by a multidisciplinary team of healthcare professionals, including cardiologists, nurses, physiotherapists, exercise specialists, dietitians, and psychologists (Fig. 1). The programme is designed to help patients recover from heart disease and improve their cardiovascular health by addressing risk factors such as high blood pressure, high cholesterol, and diabetes. CR also aims to reduce the risk of complications, such as heart failure or stroke. Participation in CR improves physical fitness, reduces symptoms of chest pain and shortness of breath, and helps the adoption of healthy lifestyle behaviours. Cohort studies show a lower risk of major adverse events with CR participation [1] and a lower risk of death [2]. Furthermore there appears to be a dose response, with no upper ceiling for benefit of CR [1]. Multiple systematic reviews demonstrate that participation in CR decreases morbidity and mortality, and therefore CR has a class 1A recommendation in international guidelines for people who have experienced a cardiac event [3].

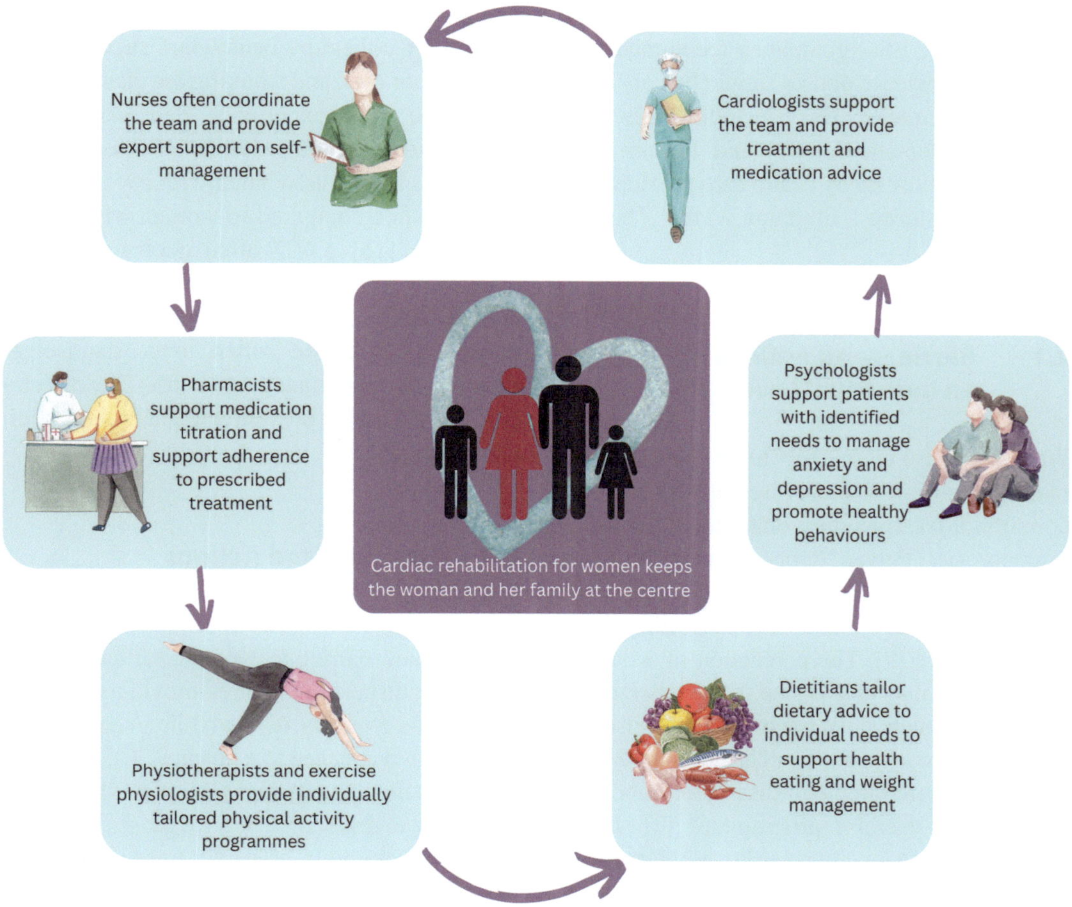

Fig. 1 Guideline based cardiac rehabilitation is interdisciplinary and multimodal

2 Cardiac Rehabilitation Referral, Enrolment and Participation

Despite the Class IA recommendation, global participation in CR is low. When we split participation by sex, we find that women are particularly poorly represented. Women are less likely to be referred to CR, less likely to be enrolled in CR, and less likely to complete a programme once enrolled. Indeed, only 39.6% of women are referred to CR, compared to 49.4% of men (odds ratio 0.68, 95% confidence interval 0.62–0.75) [4]. Similarly, women have significantly lower enrolment (odds ratio, 0.64; 95% confidence interval, 0.57–0.72) [5]. In a systematic review of global CR trials, less than 15% of women globally were found to be offered CR [6]. Lack of physician referral is highlighted as one key reason that women do not attend CR, perhaps due to a low recognition of the value of CR, or due to assumptions about women's ability to participate. This is despite strong evidence that women who do attend CR have improved outcomes at least equivalent to men [7].

Increasing referral, enrolment and participation is therefore a high priority. Automatic or systematic referral has been shown to increase the number of participants in CR [4], which might overcome perceptions that people are 'not suitable' for CR. CR enrolment is also higher if patients are seen face-to-face by a trained nurse or allied healthcare provider. However, adherence to CR may be higher if remote or home-based interventions are included [8]. Consequently, ESC guidelines recommend that methods to increase uptake should be considered (level of evidence IIa), including electronic prompts, automatic referral and liaison visits, structured follow-up by health care providers and early programme initiation after hospital discharge.

2.1 Barriers and Actions at an Individual Level

Women are also more likely to be older at the age of enrolment to CR and consequently have more co-morbidities, including diabetes, arthritis, and osteoporosis. Pelvic floor changes following pregnancy and menopause and associated urinary incontinence may make exercise difficult or uncomfortable [9]. The perception of women is that exercise may exacerbate these existing conditions, although it is likely that exercise will actually improve their overall health [10]. Women also report more fatigue or discomfort when participating in exercise programmes [7]. Indeed women live longer after cardiovascular disease (CVD) diagnosis than men, and consequently spend approximately twice as many years with a decreased quality of life as measured by loss of productivity, functional limitations, and emotional distress. Women are also more likely to experience intimate partner violence, which precludes them from participating in CR. Intimate partner violence leads to increased rates of hypertension, obesity, and hyperlipidaemia [11, 12]. Furthermore, insecure partner attachment has been shown to predict more extensive use of overprotective support strategies, which in turn predicted lower patient self-efficacy for exercise and less-frequent CR programme attendance [13].

Depression and anxiety are underdiagnosed and undertreated in women with CVD. Up to 30% of all patients with CVD will experience mild depression following a CVD event, while 11% will experience moderate to severe depression. Women experiencing depression and anxiety are less like to be motivated to participate in CR or independent physical activity activities. Other unhealthy behaviours such as overeating, poor diet, and smoking are also common in people who experience depression [14]. Women are the main providers of informal care and this is highly associated with psychological distress when compared to women who are not caregivers [15]. CVD often occurs at a time when women may be responsible for caring for ageing partners, or grandchildren. Women are known to prioritise others over themselves when it comes to managing health. These sociocultural roles may prevent women from participating in CR.

2.2 Barriers and Actions on a System Level

Another key barrier to women participating in CR is the distance to centres providing this service. CR is typically delivered in a centre-based facility often attached to a hospital. This means it can be challenging to find transport, women are less likely to drive, own or have access to a vehicle and accessibility of public transport may be more problematic for women. In a large registry of participants in the United States, geographic access predicted both enrolment and completion of CR [16].

In Western countries, educational attainment opportunities for women began to change for people born in the 1960s onwards. Prior to this, cultural norms, as well as laws, prevented women from participating in many educational programmes [17]. This means that the current participants in CR are much less likely to have had the same educational opportunities as men. In countries where women are precluded from education, such as Afghanistan, this problem persists to this day. There are also stark differences in educational attainment in low and middle-income countries [18]. This is important because educational attainment is a significant predictor of the number of CR sessions completed and is also associated with less improvement in cardiorespiratory fitness even when adjusted for other variables [19].

Belonging to an ethnic minority group is another predictor of lower uptake of CR. A recent scoping review identified that barriers exist in three key domains: referral, enrolment, adherence and completion. As before, a lack of physician referral remains a key obstacle to engagement. In addition, the language spoken is a barrier across all three domains. Knowledge and beliefs, as well as lack of family support, preclude adherence and completion, and the practical and logistical barriers to participation in CR are amplified in ethnic minority groups [20].

2.3 Exercise Training: A Specific Barrier

There is a persistent belief amongst women participating in CR that the programmes are a type of "men's club" [21]. Indeed, the majority of participants in CR are men aged in their mid-60s who are White and generally well-educated. But there are other notable challenges to participation in CR for women. One of these is gender-based exercise preferences. In a large leisure centre dataset, female participants were more likely to choose fitness classes, such as yoga and Zumba, compared to men, who were more likely to choose to go to the gym [22]. Despite this, the majority of CR services make use of a circuit-based programme typical of the gym environment. In a systematic review that examined CR provision for women, only 18% of programmes offered an alternative to the traditional gym-based format (including Tai Chi, dance, aerobics, yoga, Qigong, and water aerobics) [23]. In this review, only 40% of programmes provide any form of women-focused CR, with the majority of programmes not providing any tailored advice or information for women during the CR programme. Another review highlights the appealing nature of dance as a form of exercise for women. Importantly, dance improves physical activity levels, cardiorespiratory function, functional capacity, and balance [24]. Adherence rates in programmes that included Zumba and folk dancing were reported to be greater than 80%.

Resistance and flexibility training are particularly important for women in CR to help maintain muscle strength and joint mobility. As women age, they tend to experience a loss of muscle mass and bone density, which can lead to an increased risk of falls and fractures. Resistance training can help to slow down this loss and even increase muscle mass, which can help to maintain mobility and independence.

Flexibility training is also crucial for women as it helps to maintain joint range of motion, reducing the risk of injury and improving overall mobility. Regular stretching exercises can also help to improve posture and reduce muscle stiffness, making everyday tasks easier and more comfortable. Even small amounts of resistance and flexibility training can have a big impact on overall health and wellbeing and can help to prevent many of the age-related declines in muscle strength and flexibility.

CR programmes have been developed that are women-tailored, women-focused and women-only, and are usually designed to have alternative forms of exercise and/or additional psychosocial content. Women-tailored programmes result in better health-related quality of life than mixed-sex programmes, although women should not be presumed to prefer these programmes above convenient times and delivery methods of mixed sex programmes [23].

3 Clinical Practice

3.1 Addressing Risk Factors

Although men and women have many of the same risk factors, the effect on women is greater, from the same risks, such as diabetes and hypertension. Diet and weight are frequently listed as targets for treatment in CR (Fig. 2). Despite this, very few CR programmes (8%) include a behavioural weight loss component. This is particularly important for women. Both sexes experience mid-life weight gain, and although menopause per se is not thought to be the chief cause of weight-gain, it often coincides with weight gain. In particular, women experience an increase in

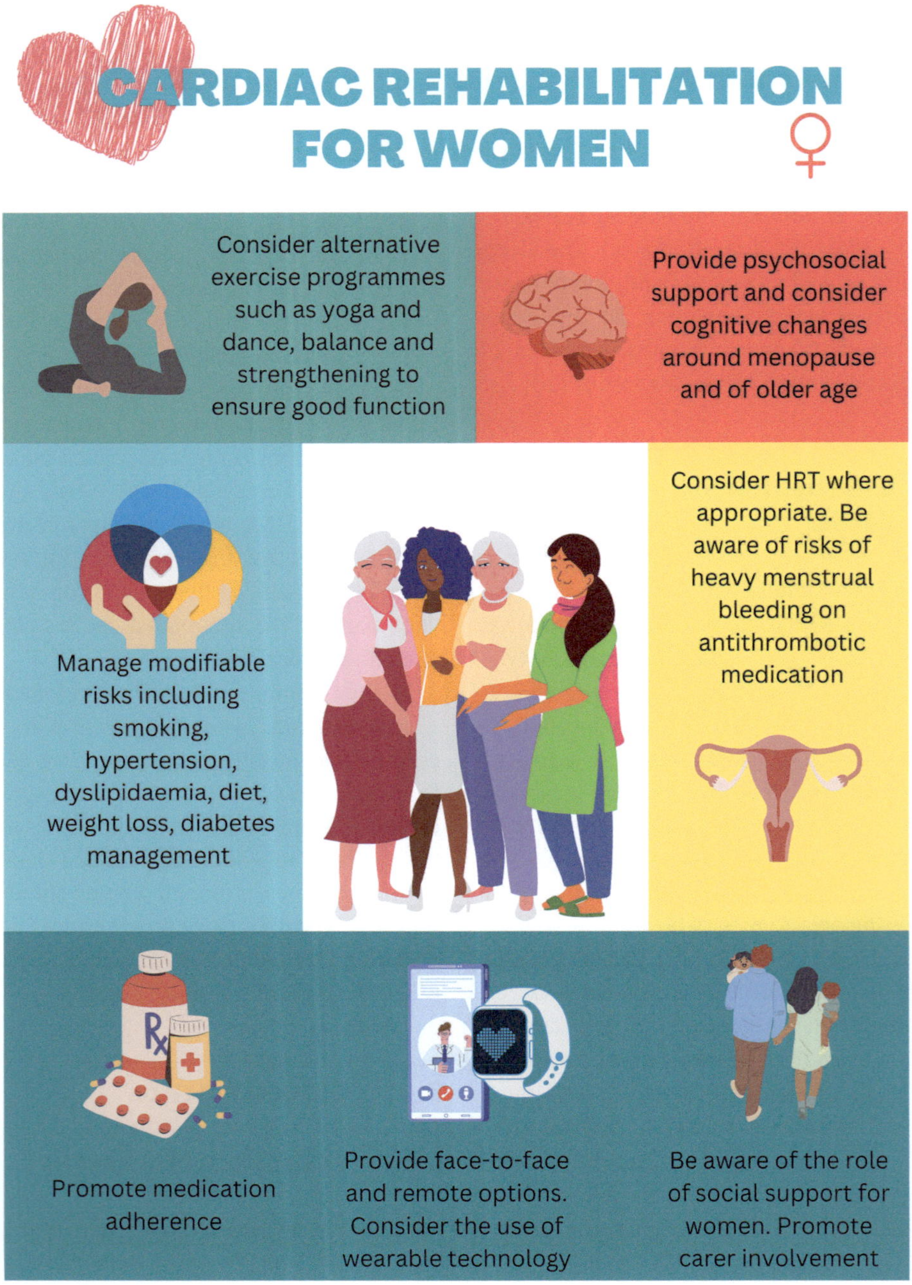

Fig. 2 Actions to overcome barriers and promote heart health in cardiac rehabilitation

central obesity, which in turn increases lipid levels, hypertension, and glucose levels [25]. Weight gain also increases the risk of cancer, arthritis, mood disorders, and sexual dysfunction. Menopause increases the risk of mood disorders and sleep disturbance, as well as brain fog. The cognitive challenges of menopause are a reported cause of distress in women. Up to 25% of women will experience severe symptoms of menopause, while 75% will experience some symptoms. Around 11% of menopausal women miss work due to menopause symptoms every year, with others reporting reduced working hours, employment loss, or early retirement. These reduce the likelihood of participating in a healthy lifestyle recommended through CR. Consequently, particular focus on menopause symptoms, including mid-life weight gain is highly recommended as a component of CR.

Conversely, for women who are still menstruating, antiplatelet and anticoagulant drugs increase the risk of heavy menstrual bleeding, defined as blood loss of greater than 80 ml per menstrual cycle. CR professionals need to understand treatment options for women who are experiencing excess bleeding, and to be able to discuss treatment.

Tobacco consumption remains the leading preventable cause of morbidity and mortality globally. While men are more likely to smoke, women suffer greater adverse effects as a result of smoking. Cigarette smoking in women enhances the risk of atherosclerosis by lowering high-density lipoprotein cholesterol levels, triglycerides, and increasing insulin resistance. Smoking cessation is complex, as there are multiple factors that contribute to the likelihood of smoking behaviours, and it is a potent addiction. Women tend to say that the main reasons for smoking are psychological such as stress and emotion. Women may benefit from targeted smoking cessation programmes that address specific challenges such as stress, social pressures, and weight management. Contrary to men, women seem to prefer non-coercive interventions such as group base support and positivity [26].

3.2 Medication Adherence

Medication adherence remains a key challenge for both men and women in CR. The World Health Organisation defines medication adherence as taking the medications as prescribed more than 80% of the time. However, adherence to medication is generally poor. One Canadian study found that only 36% of older adults with CVD were still taking their cholesterol lowering treatment at 2 years following the cardiac event. Medication non-adherence is associated with lower education attainment, and as discussed previously in this chapter, this disproportionately affects women. Adherence to medications requires both cognitive ability (orientation to time and place) and prospective memory, and a positive belief about the medication. With cardiovascular medications, adherence decreases with the increasing number of medications prescribed. The use of polypills (combined fixed does of a variety of cardioprotective drugs) is strongly associated with increased medication adherence, and consequently reduction in cardiovascular risk factors, and morbidity and mortality [27]. Despite this, translation into clinical practice is slow, and most patients will still be faced with polypharmacy challenges. Another potential solution may be the use of medication reminder apps, which appear promising to promote adherence and may be one way to address the cognitive load with medication adherence [28]. CR also has a key role to place in addressing the beliefs about medication, which may be barriers to adherence. Some people believe that medication is overprescribed and that doctors are too quick to prescribe medication as a first line of treatment. They may be sceptical of medication and prefer to try 'natural remedies' or lifestyle changes before resorting to medication. Concern about negative side effects is frequently reported. This has been particularly notable for statins and concerns over muscle pain. Patients may even believe that medication is addictive and can lead to dependence or abuse [28]. As well as CR staff providing support, family and carer support in medication adherence is critical.

3.3 Carer Involvement

Carer involvement can play a crucial role beyond medication adherence in the success of CR. Carers can provide emotional support to patients during CR, helping them to manage stress and anxiety. Carers can encourage patients to attend rehabilitation sessions and make lifestyle changes. There is a high degree of lifestyle concordance amongst spouses, and as well as motivating their partners, they can also benefit from lifestyle changes. Furthermore, unless partners are fully engaged in CR, and the lifestyle changes that are desirable, they can make it much harder for the woman in CR to maintain changes. For example, if the woman's partner continues to smoke at home, this will significantly reduce her chance of successfully quitting smoking. For women, having a partner involved may also make transportation to a CR site more feasible. CR professionals also need to be aware of the profound changes to a couple's relationship brought about by the cardiac event. Overprotectiveness may be part of these changes. There may also be a change to sex drive. It is noted that men are much more likely than women to resume sexual activity in the first month after a myocardial infarction. Women express a lack of sexual desire, difficulty lubricating, and a feeling of being unable to breathe during sexual intercourse. Despite this, CR tends to focus on men's sexual health and largely ignore the needs of women. Women need to receive information from CR providers about sex, including information about safety, and CR should specifically address these needs. This suggests a need for CR providers to have training in how to discuss sex and sexuality and healthcare providers frequently express embarrassment, or concerns that they are invading the patient's privacy when raising intimate topics of discussion.

3.4 Stress Management

There is a clear link between stress, depression and worse outcomes following a cardiac event and these problems are worse in women. Stress management and resilience training shows promise in protecting women from these effects [29]. However, psychological interventions have only been demonstrated to be effective when included in a comprehensive CR programme [30, 31], indicating a holistic approach is needed. For instance, the positive effect of regular exercise, as included in CR, on psychological distress is well-established. A group-based approach to stress management including relaxation training, methods for self-monitoring and cognitive reframing for stress experienced from family and work, and self-care (SWITCHD) demonstrated three-fold reduction in deaths and better quality of life. However, these programmes require specialised staff to deliver, in the absence of such staff, screening for stress, anxiety and depression is recommended followed by referral to specific providers. Regardless, positive self-care approaches including mindfulness, relaxation techniques should be recommended [32].

Women have difficulties accessing CR in person due to family responsibilities and transport issues, so a flexible schedule using alternative methods of delivery should be discussed based on women's specific needs. After accounting for age and employment amongst other factors, women eligible for CR use mobile apps as often as men and express similar preferences, although women were more interested in an emotional wellbeing focus. Telehealth and mHealth delivery of CR have demonstrated equivalent outcomes to in-person delivery in systematic reviews [33], although the benefits for women are rarely differentiated. Many studies on the use of apps and telehealth CR in women demonstrate acceptability and feasibility in single studies but are not adequately designed to assess effectiveness. Wearable activity trackers are important tools for all types of CR but have additional benefits for telehealth delivered CR through objective monitoring and prompting motivation [34]. Activity trackers have proven accuracy in measuring different types of physical activity and are useful in both women and men [35], but women may experience additional benefits fitting their incidental activity into carer duties and other responsibilities shown to hamper exercise in women [36]. Sophisticated activity trackers are available that also measure sedentary time, sleep and heart rate response to exercise, aspects that are important to overall health.

4 Conclusions

Adherence to guideline recommendations for CR in women is low. Increasing referral, enrolment, and participation of women in CR should be a high priority. Automatic or systematic referral can be considered, along with specific information targeting women. Some barriers can be mitigated by introducing remote or home-based interventions as an option, including wearable activity trackers. However, particular attention should be paid to the complexity brought on by co-morbidities and challenges after childbirth and menopause. Gender-based exercise preferences make CR more attractive to women and increase adherence rates (Fig. 2). CR needs to be tailored and comprehensive addressing all risk factors, including dietary advice, stress management, medication adherence, and education on heart-healthy living at large. Carer involvement can play a crucial role in the success of CR.

Key Issues

- CR includes a range of medical and lifestyle interventions, and has a class 1A recommendation in international guidelines.
- Participation in CR is low, and in particular in women. Women are less likely to be referred to CR, less likely to be enrolled, and less likely to complete a CR programme once enrolled.
- There is strong evidence that women who do attend CR have improved outcomes that are at least equivalent to men.
- Women have specific barriers to CR participation on both an individual and system level.

Questions and Answers

1. A 75-year old woman is referred to cardiac rehabilitation following an ST-elevation Myocardial Infarction (STEMI). During her exercise assessment she comments that despite knowing the benefits of exercise, she has found it more difficult to walk over the last few years. What conditions may affect her participation in the CR exercise program?
   (A) Musculoskeletal conditions that are painful and/or affect balance
   (B) Pelvic floor dysfunction including urine leakage
   (C) Depression and depressive symptoms
   (D) All of the above

   Correct answer: D

   Women present to cardiac rehabilitation at an older age than men and their older age factor contributes to the increased incidence of comorbid conditions. Comorbidities common to women at 75 years of age include musculoskeletal conditions that make exercise more uncomfortable or difficult to do and/or enjoy, pelvic floor conditions arising post-menopause or from pregnancy and depression and depressive symptoms that create sometimes overwhelming symptoms of fatigue. Women should be screened for all of these conditions at entry to cardiac rehabilitation and there should be a discussion regarding any associated difficulties they experience exercising in the cardiac rehabilitation setting and at home. Exercise can be prescribed that is graduated, accommodates these conditions, and enables women to enjoy exercise more.
2. A 42-year old woman is referred to cardiac rehabilitation following primary coronary angioplasty for acute coronary syndrome to help recovery and address her multiple cardiovascular risk factors. She visits the cardiac rehabilitation program and notes that most of the participants are men and she wonders if there are real benefits for her when she has little time free from family and work duties. What exercise benefits are there for women in attending comprehensive cardiac rehabilitation?
   (A) Women have improved quality of life but few gains in exercise capacity
   (B) Men exercise harder in cardiac rehabilitation so have more exercise benefits
   (C) Women improve their quality of life and exercise capacity
   (D) Men and women have exactly the same improvements in quality of life

   Correct answer: C

   Both women and men have significant and clinically important improvements in exercise capacity from cardiac rehabilitation regardless of men's greater capacity at commencement. Women and men may undertake exercise differently during cardiac rehabilitation sessions but there is no evidence to suggest that the overall effort differs. Both women and men have significant and clinically important improvements in overall and multiple domains quality of life from cardiac rehabilitation, but the domains may differ a little. Flexible program attendance should be discussed with women to promote attendance.

3. Two women starting cardiac rehabilitation discuss the activity trackers that they see some of the other participants wearing. One woman states confidently that these trackers are good because the device can alert her when her heart is not working properly, which raises concerns about always being alerted for the other woman. What are the benefits for women of using activity trackers during recovery?
   (A) Monitor and track incidental physical activity outside of the program
   (B) Accurate assessment of heart rhythm and alerts for arrhythmias
   (C) Automated prompts to be active to meet a pre-set goal
   (D) A and B

   Correct answer: C

   Several wearable activity trackers have proven accuracy for tracking physical activity duration and categories of intensity, which can help women to monitor their exercise participation at any time. Exercise monitoring outside of supervised sessions in cardiac rehabilitation is important for establishing a sustainable exercise habit and to incorporate a variety of physical activities. Many activity trackers can be set with the assistance of cardiac rehabilitation staff, if needed, to provide prompts to meet a pre-set daily goal, which can help with motivation and planning. While there are activity trackers that include heart rate monitoring and can alert when preset heart rates are exceeded, there are few trackers that have accurately detect arrhythmias. Cardiac rehabilitation staff should provide general advice on the use of activity trackers as well as benefits and limitations.

References

1. Medina-Inojosa JR, Grace SL, Supervia M, et al. Dose of cardiac rehabilitation to reduce mortality and morbidity: a population-based study. J Am Heart Assoc. 2021;10(20):e021356.
2. Eijsvogels TM, Maessen MF, Bakker EA, et al. Association of cardiac rehabilitation with all-cause mortality among patients with cardiovascular disease in the Netherlands. JAMA Netw Open. 2020;3(7):e2011686.
3. Visseren FL, Mach F, Smulders YM, et al. 2021 ESC guidelines on cardiovascular disease prevention in clinical practice: developed by the Task Force for cardiovascular disease prevention in clinical practice with representatives of the European Society of Cardiology and 12 medical societies with the special contribution of the European Association of Preventive Cardiology (EAPC). Eur J Prev Cardiol. 2022;29(1):5–115.
4. Colella TJ, Gravely S, Marzolini S, et al. Sex bias in referral of women to outpatient cardiac rehabilitation? A meta-analysis. Eur J Prev Cardiol. 2020;22(4):423–41. https://doi.org/10.1177/2047487314520783.
5. Samayoa L, Grace SL, Gravely S, et al. Sex differences in cardiac rehabilitation enrollment: a meta-analysis. Can J Cardiol. 2014;30(7):793–800. https://doi.org/10.1016/j.cjca.2013.11.007.
6. Dibben G, Faulkner J, Oldridge N, et al. Exercise-based cardiac rehabilitation for coronary heart disease. Cochrane Database Syst Rev. 2021;11(11):CD001800. https://doi.org/10.1002/14651858.
7. Smith JR, Thomas RJ, Bonikowske AR, et al. Sex differences in cardiac rehabilitation outcomes. Circ Res. 2022;130(4):552–65.
8. Pio CSA, Chaves G, Davies P, et al. Interventions to promote patient utilization of cardiac rehabilitation: Cochrane systematic review and meta-analysis. J Clin Med. 2019;8(2):189.
9. Luk JKH, Chiu PKC, Chu LW. Gender differences in rehabilitation outcomes among older Chinese patients. Arch Gerontol Geriatr. 2011;52(1):28–32.
10. Grace SL, Gravely-Witte S, Kayaniyil S, et al. A multisite examination of sex differences in cardiac rehabilitation barriers by participation status. J Womens Health. 2009;18(2):209–16.
11. Constantino RE, Angosta AD, Reyes AT, et al. Is intimate partner violence a risk factor for cardiovascular disease in women? A review of the preponderance of the evidence. Health. 2019;11(06):841.
12. Stubbs A, Szoeke C. The effect of intimate partner violence on the physical health and health-related behaviors of women: a systematic review of the literature. Trauma Violence Abuse. 2022;23(4):1157–72.

13. O'Bertos SE, Holmberg D, Shields CA, et al. Partners' attachment styles and overprotective support as predictors of patient outcomes in cardiac rehabilitation. Rehabil Psychol. 2020;65(3):258.
14. Rao A, Zecchin R, Newton PJ, et al. The prevalence and impact of depression and anxiety in cardiac rehabilitation: a longitudinal cohort study. Eur J Prev Cardiol. 2020;27(5):478–89.
15. Lacey RE, McMunn A, Webb E. Informal caregiving patterns and trajectories of psychological distress in the UK Household Longitudinal Study. Psychol Med. 2019;49(10):1652–60.
16. Ritchey MD, Maresh S, McNeely J, et al. Tracking cardiac rehabilitation participation and completion among Medicare beneficiaries to inform the efforts of a national initiative. Circ Cardiovasc Qual Outcomes. 2020;13(1):e005902.
17. Herd P, Freese J, Sicinski K, et al. Genes, gender inequality, and educational attainment. Am Sociol Rev. 2019;84(6):1069–98.
18. Graetz N, Woyczynski L, Wilson KF, et al. Mapping disparities in education across low- and middle-income countries. Nature. 2020;577(7789):235–8. https://doi.org/10.1038/s41586-019-1872-1.
19. Gaalema DE, Savage PD, O'Neill S, et al. The association of patient educational attainment with cardiac rehabilitation adherence and health outcomes. J Cardiopulm Rehabil Prev. 2022;42(4):227–34.
20. Vanzella LM, Oh P, Pakosh M, et al. Barriers to cardiac rehabilitation in ethnic minority groups: a scoping review. J Immigr Minor Health. 2021;23:824–39.
21. Khadanga S, Gaalema DE, Savage P, et al. Underutilization of cardiac rehabilitation in women: barriers and solutions. J Cardiopulm Rehabil Prev. 2021;41(4):207.
22. Bell J, Neubeck L, Jin K, et al. Understanding leisure centre-based physical activity after physical activity referral: evidence from scheme participants and completers in Northumberland UK. Int J Environ Res Public Health. 2021;18(6):2957.
23. Mamataz T, Ghisi GL, Pakosh M, et al. Nature, availability, and utilization of women-focused cardiac rehabilitation: a systematic review. BMC Cardiovasc Disord. 2021;21(1):1–20.
24. Vidal-Almela S, Czajkowski B, Prince SA, et al. Lessons learned from community-and home-based physical activity programs: a narrative review of factors influencing women's participation in cardiac rehabilitation. Eur J Prev Cardiol. 2021;28(7):761–78.
25. Kapoor E, Collazo-Clavell ML, Faubion SS. Weight gain in women at midlife: a concise review of the pathophysiology and strategies for management. Mayo Clin Proc. 2017;92(10):1552–8. https://doi.org/10.1016/j.mayocp.2017.08.004.
26. Dieleman LA, van Peet PG, Vos HM. Gender differences within the barriers to smoking cessation and the preferences for interventions in primary care a qualitative study using focus groups in The Hague, The Netherlands. BMJ Open. 2021;11(1):e042623.
27. Rao S, Jamal Siddiqi T, Khan MS, et al. Association of polypill therapy with cardiovascular outcomes, mortality, and adherence: a systematic review and meta-analysis of randomized controlled trials. Prog Cardiovasc Dis. 2022;73:48–55. https://doi.org/10.1016/j.pcad.2022.01.005.
28. Al-Ganmi AH, Perry L, Gholizadeh L, et al. Cardiovascular medication adherence among patients with cardiac disease: a systematic review. J Adv Nurs. 2016;72(12):3001–14. https://doi.org/10.1111/jan.13062. [Published Online First: 20160728].
29. Arabadjian M, Duberstein ZT, Sperber SH, et al. Role of resilience in the psychological recovery of women with acute myocardial infarction. J Am Heart Assoc. 2023;12(8):e027092.
30. Richards SH, Anderson L, Jenkinson CE, et al. Psychological interventions for coronary heart disease: Cochrane systematic review and meta-analysis. Eur J Prev Cardiol. 2018;25(3):247–59.
31. Orth-Gomér K, Schneiderman N, Wang H-X, et al. Stress reduction prolongs life in women with coronary disease: the Stockholm Women's Intervention Trial for Coronary Heart Disease (SWITCHD). Circ Cardiovasc Qual Outcomes. 2009;2(1):25–32.
32. Amiss E, Cottrell M. Evaluation of a novel step training mobile app intervention in cardiopulmonary rehabilitation: a single-arm prospective cohort study. Games Health J. 2022;11(5):330–6.
33. Gallagher R, Parker H, Zhang L, et al. Target audience and preferences related to an Australian coronary heart disease specific mobile app: a mixed methods study. Heart Lung Circ. 2020;29(5):696–702.
34. Andraos C, Arthur HM, Oh P, et al. Women's preferences for cardiac rehabilitation program model: a randomized controlled trial. Eur J Prev Cardiol. 2015;22(12):1513–22.
35. Alharbi M, Bauman A, Alabdulaali M, et al. Comparison of different physical activity measures in a cardiac rehabilitation program: a prospective study. Sensors. 2022;22(4):1639.
36. Broers ER, Gavidia G, Wetzels M, et al. Usefulness of a lifestyle intervention in patients with cardiovascular disease. Am J Cardiol. 2020;125(3):370–5.

Part IV

Miscellaneous Topics in Cardiology for Women

Cardiotoxicity in Breast Cancer Treatment

Berlinde A. von Kemp

Abstract

Breast cancer is the most frequently diagnosed malignancy in women worldwide. Therapeutic advances have significantly improved cancer outcomes resulting in a growing cohort of breast cancer survivors. However, these improved treatments are counterbalanced by not only an increased risk of on-treatment cardiotoxicity (cancer therapy-related cardiovascular toxicity, CTR-CVT), but also by an increased risk of long-term toxicity as well as a predisposition for premature cardiovascular disease (CVD). Appropriate surveillance is recommended in all patients undergoing potentially cardiotoxic treatments, especially anthracyclines and HER2-targeted therapies. Cardio-oncological care should start at the initiation of cancer treatment by means of a comprehensive baseline cardiovascular (CV) assessment in order to estimate the risk of CTR-CVT. Further toxicity surveillance should take place in parallel to the cancer treatment, using pre-defined surveillance protocols and toxicity definitions, in order to allow for timely detection and treatment of new-onset toxicity. Upon completing breast cancer treatment, an end-of-treatment reassessment is recommended, followed by structured, albeit less intensive, long-term CV follow-up.

Keywords

Breast cancer · Oncology · Cardio-oncology · Cardiotoxicity · CTRCD

Test your learning and check your understanding of this book's contents: use the "Springer Nature Flashcards" app to access questions using ▶ https://sn.pub/51ny7m
To use the app, please follow the instructions in chapter 1.

B. A. von Kemp (✉)
Department of Cardiology, Universitair Ziekenhuis Brussel, Centrum Hart- en Vaatziekten, Brussels, Belgium
e-mail: berlinde.vonkemp@uzbrussel.be

A. H.E.M. Maas, E. Gerdts (eds.), *Manual of Cardiovascular Disease in Women*,
https://doi.org/10.1007/978-3-031-65952-2_28

1 Introduction

Worldwide, breast cancer is the most frequently diagnosed malignancy, globally responsible for 685,000 deaths in 2020 [1]. Improving cancer care including surgical as well as medical innovations but also the development of government-led screening programs, has led to a significant improvement in cancer survival, with a reduction in breast cancer mortality of 40% between the 1980s and 2020 [1]. Current data in non-metastatic breast cancer suggest a 5-year survival of ±91% and a 10-year survival of 84–85%, and the World Health Cancer (WHO) Global Breast Cancer Initiative (GBCI) aims at a further reduction of breast cancer mortality by ±2.5% per year [1].

As more patients survive their cancer, the development of long-term treatment-related side effects becomes more and more relevant and particular attention should be paid to new-onset cardiovascular (CV) disease (CVD) in breast cancer survivors as this becomes the leading cause of death in this population [2]. Since breast cancer treatment involves a variety of therapeutic strategies that may cause CV toxicity (CTR-CVT: cancer therapy-related cardiovascular toxicity) during or after treatment, the development and implementation of cardio-oncological care pathways is urgently needed [2, 3]. These care pathways should encompass the entire oncological trajectory of the breast cancer patient, from a baseline CV evaluation prior to treatment initiation, over on-treatment surveillance as well as a long-term follow-up in cancer survivors [3].

2 Theory

2.1 Epidemiology of Breast Cancer

Breast cancer is worldwide the most frequently diagnosed malignancy. According to WHO data, in 2020, 2.3 million women were diagnosed with and 685,000 women died of this disease [1]. Since the establishment of governmentally organized screening programs in several countries, nowadays, the diagnosis is made earlier, allowing for earlier treatment and better outcomes [1].

The single most important risk factor for the development of breast cancer is female gender [1, 4]. Breast cancer in men is particularly rare, making up approximately 0.5–1% of all breast cancers [1, 4]. Other risk factors include older age, obesity, alcohol abuse, smoking, family history of breast cancer and previous radiation exposure, as well as postmenopausal hormone therapy and reproductive history (age at first menstruation and age at first pregnancy) [1, 4]. Importantly, a negative family history for breast cancer does not imply a reduced risk [1, 4].

2.2 Treatment Options in Breast Cancer

Current treatment options after breast cancer diagnosis are plentiful, and mainly depend on the extent of the tumor (using tumor staging according to the TNM classification) as well as on the immune-histochemical characteristics of the tumor: surface expression of Human Epidermal growth factor receptor 2 (HER2), oestrogen receptor status (ER) and progesterone receptor status (PR) define susceptibility or resistance of the tumor for certain treatments (e.g. trastuzumab and other HER2-targeted treatments in breast cancers with HER2-overexpression on the tumor cell surface) [5].

In the majority of cases, a combined treatment approach is preferred, which may consist of surgery, radiotherapy, and different kinds of systemic therapy. This latter category may include 'classical' chemotherapy (e.g. epirubicin, cyclophosphamide, paclitaxel, occasionally methotrexate and 5-fluorouracil), targeted therapy (e.g. HER2-targeted molecules as trastuzumab and pertuzumab), hormonotherapy (selective oestrogen-receptor modulators as tamoxifen, estrogen-receptor antagonists as fulvestrant and aromatase-inhibitors as letrozole, anastrozole and exemestane) [5]. In more advanced disease and/or selected cases, other treatment categories may be used (e.g. PARP-inhibitors, CDK4/6-inhibitors, and immune checkpoint inhibitors) as well [6].

Considering the surgical treatment options, a tissue-sparing technique is generally performed whenever possible and may be followed by reconstruction or implantation of a tissue expander (to allow for later reconstruction) [6]. Furthermore, sentinel lymph node dissection and/or (targeted) axillary lymph node resection may be required [6].

Radiotherapy is commonly prescribed in many breast cancer patients and has undergone significant technological improvement over the past decades, aiming at reducing radiation exposure to the surrounding non-target tissues [7]. This involves not only technical aspects such as the chosen energy source, target volume mapping, reducing total radiation dose as well as fraction doses and CT- or even MRI-guided shielding techniques, but also other aspects that allow dose reduction to the surrounding tissues [3, 7]. Particularly in breast cancer, the radiation dose delivered to the heart and the pericardium is attempted to be kept to an absolute minimum [3, 7]. In order to achieve this goal, other techniques are applied as well, such as deep inspirational breath hold (DIBH): performing breath hold at end-inspiration, the heart is positioned in a slightly more vertical position in the thoracic cavity, resulting in lower volumes exposed to ionizing radiation [3, 7]. This may be further accomplished by administering radiotherapy in a left lateral semi recumbent position.

Most non-metastatic breast cancer treatments will consist of a neo-adjuvant phase (systemic treatment prior to surgery in order to obtain tumor volume reduction), followed by surgery and consecutive adjuvant treatment ('consolidation treatment') after surgery in order to avoid disease recurrence [6]. The widespread use of combined treatment modalities has proven to be highly efficient but comes with the caveat of exposure to different potentially cardiotoxic molecules and the subsequent risk of developing CTR-CVT [3, 6].

2.3 What Is CTR-CVT?

Most breast cancer patients undergo a multimodal treatment, where different treatments are administered concomitantly and/or consecutively [3]. Each specific treatment confers a risk of side effects, particularly the development of CTR-CVT [3].

Cancer therapy-related cardiovascular toxicity is a general denominator for the wide range of CV manifestations that may result from all different kinds of cancer treatments [3]. According to the 2022 European Society of Cardiology (ESC) Guidelines on Cardio-Oncology, this includes heart failure (cancer treatment-related cardiac dysfunction, CTRCD), pericardial diseases, myocarditis, arrhythmias, coronary artery disease, valvular heart disease and arterial hypertension (AHT), as well as acute thrombotic disease (both arterial and venous) under the denominator of 'cancer-associated thrombosis' (CAT) [3].

Importantly, CTR-CVT encompasses a spectrum of disease manifestations that may present throughout the continuum of cancer care, therefore requiring longitudinal follow-up from diagnosis to long-term survivorship care [3]. During this extensive timeframe, the individual patient's risk of developing CTR-CVT may fluctuate significantly, so timely re-evaluation and intervention are mandatory [3]. This includes not only risk stratification, identification and treatment of cardiovascular risk factors (CVRFs) at treatment initiation but also the implementation of a patient-tailored surveillance plan throughout active cancer treatment in order to allow early identification and appropriate treatment of eventual new CV complications [3].

As a more general term, the word 'cardiotoxicity' is frequently used: usually this term refers to CTRCD but more and more commonly, it is also used to cover the different CV manifestations that may develop under active cancer treatment [3].

2.4 Commonly encountered CTR-CVT in Breast Cancer Treatment

In the following section, we will discuss the most frequently used treatments in breast cancer, and the cardiotoxic manifestations that may occur on treatment (Table 1). Different treatments may imply different CV toxicities, as well as important differences in time to onset of toxicity [3]. Of paramount importance is the notion that the development of new CTR-CVT does not necessarily require cancer treatment interruption but should rather prompt multidisciplinary team discussion with the treating oncologist and/or other specialists prior to treatment interruption or adaptation [3]. As a general rule of thumb, earlier diagnosis of CTR-CVT is associated with a higher likelihood of reversibility, thus highlighting the importance of a pre-defined surveillance strategy as well as early confirmation and treatment of new-onset CTR-CVT [3].

Table 1 Frequently used treatments in breast cancer patients and potential CTR-CVT

Frequently used treatments in breast cancer patients and potential CTR-CVT	
Chemotherapy	
Anthracyclines (epirubicin, doxorubicin)	CTRCD (HF/LVSD), arrhythmias (AF, ↑QTc), pericardial disease
Cyclophosphamide	HF, AF, coronary vasospasm, myocarditis, pericardial disease
Taxanes (paclitaxel, docetaxel)	Coronary vasospasm, bradycardia, ventricular arrhythmias
Fluoropyrimidines (5-fluorouracil, capecitabine)	Coronary vasospasm, AF, myocarditis, pericarditis
Targeted therapy	
HER2-targeted therapy (trastuzumab, pertuzumab)	CTRCD (HF/LVSD)
Other targeted therapies (PARP-inhibitors, CDK4/6-inhibitors)	CTRCD (HF/LVSD), AHT, arrhythmias (AF, ↑QTc)
Immune checkpoint inhibitors	
PD1-inhibitors (pembrolizumab)	Myocarditis, pericarditis, ACS, arrhythmias, TTCMP
Hormonotherapy	
Selective estrogen receptor modulators (SERMs, tamoxifen)	VTE (DVT/PE)
Aromatase inhibitors (letrozole, anastrozole, exemestane)	HF, atherosclerotic CAD, AHT, hypercholesterolemia
Radiotherapy	
Acute toxicity	Pericarditis
Late toxicity	CAD, VHD, conduction disease, constrictive pericarditis, HFpEF

ACS acute coronary syndrome, *AF* atrial fibrillation, *AHT* arterial hypertension, *CAD* coronary artery disease, *CDK4/6* cyclin-dependent kinase, *CTR-CVT* cancer therapy-related cardiovascular toxicity, *CTRCD* cancer therapy-related cardiac dysfunction, *DVT* deep vein thrombosis, *HER2* human epidermal growth factor receptor type 2, *HF* heart failure, *HFpEF* heart failure with preserved ejection fraction, *LVSD* left ventricular systolic dysfunction, *PARP* poly-ADP ribose polymerase, *PE* pulmonary embolism, *TTCMP* Tako Tsubo cardiomyopathy, *VHD* valvular heart disease, *VTE* venous thrombo-embolism

2.4.1 Chemotherapy

Anthracyclines

For most breast cancers, anthracycline-based chemotherapy forms the backbone of systemic therapy: usually, epirubicin is administered concomitantly with cyclophosphamide in either a standard or a dose-dense regimen [6]. Best known for their cardiotoxic potential, anthracycline-induced CTRCD is cumulative, dose-dependent and irreversible [3, 8]. Specifically for epirubicin, a cumulative dose of >312.5 mg/m^2 (equivalent to >250 mg/m^2 of doxorubicin) is considered a cut-off dose above which the risk of CTRCD significantly increases, and therefore requires closer surveillance [3]. Historically, anthracycline cardiotoxicity is known as 'type I cardiotoxicity'.

From a pathophysiological point of view, anthracyclines induce cardiomyocyte apoptosis and necrosis by several mechanisms, most of which involve oxidative stress, membrane lipid peroxidation and interference with DNA transcription and protein synthesis, as well as interference with calcium handling in the sarcoplasmic reticulum [3, 8]. Cardiomyocyte damage initially develops subclinically, with cellular damage resulting in troponin release and other biochemical alterations, followed only later by functional abnormalities as detected by deformation imaging (abnormal global longitudinal strain—GLS—values) and still later by regression of the left ventricular ejection fraction (LVEF) with subsequent development of heart failure (HF) symptoms [3, 8].

Less frequently, anthracyclines may induce arrhythmias (atrial fibrillation, conduction abnormalities, QT prolongation) as well as pericardial effusions and pericarditis [3, 9] (Table 1).

Cyclophosphamide

Despite being one of the oldest alkylating agents, cyclophosphamide is still the mainstay of breast cancer chemotherapy in coadministration with epirubicin: as such, the CV toxicity profile is dominated by the anthracycline-induced toxicity risk. Nevertheless, cyclophosphamide in itself may also result in CV complications such as (hemorrhagic) myocarditis, acute HF, atrial fibrillation (AF), coronary vasospasm and pericarditis or pericardial effusions [3, 9] (Table 1).

Taxanes (Paclitaxel and Docetaxel)

Usually administered in the neo-adjuvant setting, paclitaxel is the more commonly used taxane in breast cancer. Cardiovascular complications are less common than in the other cytostatic therapies, but may include coronary vasospasm, bradycardia and conduction disease as well as ventricular arrhythmias [3, 9] (Table 1).

Fluoropyrimidines (5-Fluorouracil and Capecitabine)

Antimetabolites are included in the older FEC chemotherapy regimen (5-fluorouracil, epirubicin, cyclophosphamide) and in the CMF regimen (cyclophosphamide, methotrexate, 5-fluorouracil), but are not by default included in standard treatment regimens [5, 9]. However, in patients in whom anthracyclines are avoided or contra-indicated (usually because of underlying CVD or old age), CMF is the first choice of non-anthracycline-based chemotherapy in breast cancer. Coronary vasospasm is the most feared but also the most common CV side-effect, generally manifesting during treatment administration as acute chest pain, mimicking acute myocardial infarction [3, 9]. Other, albeit less common cardiotoxic events include myocarditis, pericarditis and AF [3, 9] (Table 1).

2.4.2 Targeted Therapy

HER2-Targeted Therapy (Trastuzumab and Pertuzumab + Drug Conjugates Emtansine and Deruxtecan)

The development of trastuzumab and other HER2-targeted therapies has revolutionized breast cancer treatment and prognosis in patients with documented overexpression of human epidermal growth factor receptor type 2 (HER2) on the surface of breast cancer cells [3, 5, 10, 11]. Though highly efficient, this treatment is known to induce CTRCD [3, 10, 11].

Contrary to anthracycline-induced cardiotoxicity, anti-HER2-induced CTRCD is dose-independent and reversible ('type II cardiotoxicity') owing to the induction of cardiomyocyte dysfunction through a (still incompletely elucidated) interplay of multiple pathophysiological mechanisms rather than apoptosis and necrosis [10, 11]. However, ongoing undiagnosed cardiotoxicity may still result in progression towards irreversible cardiomyocyte damage, highlighting the importance of regular surveillance, particularly in patients at increased cardiotoxicity risk [3, 10, 11].

Patients developing CTRCD on HER2-targeted treatment, mostly do so during treatment or within the first year after treatment [10, 11]. Late toxicity as well as other non-heart failure CTR-CVT in anti-HER2-based therapies are rare [9–11].

In terms of cardiotoxic potential, trastuzumab is usually considered the most cardiotoxic molecule in the anti-HER2 category [10, 11]. According to literature, cardiotoxicity on pertuzumab is far less common, and therefore the addition of pertuzumab to trastuzumab-based treatments, does not significantly increase the risk of developing CTRCD [10, 11]. Drug conjugates such as trastuzumab emtansine (trastuzumab + antimicrotubule agent) or trastuzumab deruxtecan (trastuzumab + topoisomerase inhibitor) do not seem to carry an increased CTRCD risk, though literature data are relatively sparse [10–12]. Nevertheless, since all these treatments include a trastuzumab treatment backbone, baseline evaluation and regular surveillance are strongly recommended [3].

Other Targeted Therapies

In more advanced breast cancer, other targeted therapies may be used, such as mTOR inhibitors (e.g. everolimus), CDK4/6 inhibitors (e.g. the tyrosine kinase inhibitors ribociclib, abemaciclib), and PARP-inhibitors (e.g. olaparib, niraparib, both tyrosine kinase inhibitors) [12]. As a drug class, all tyrosine kinase inhibitors inherently imply a risk of CTR-CVT under the form of CTRCD, but they also carry a risk of developing AHT and QTc-prolongation, thus increasing the risk of arrhythmias (especially AF) [3, 9] (Table 1). However, these therapies are generally only used in selected patients, who have often already undergone several other treatment lines and who should therefore be considered to be at a relatively higher CTR-CVT risk [3].

2.4.3 Immune Checkpoint Inhibitor Therapy

Of increasing relevance in the treatment of a multitude of cancers, immune checkpoint inhibitors (ICIs) are also gaining importance in breast cancer patients, in particular in the neo-adjuvant and adjuvant setting in triple-negative breast cancer. These monoclonal antibodies exert their anticancer effect by 'unleashing' the immune system (mainly T-lymphocytes) against cancer cells ('host-versus-tumor' effect) through inhibition of the immune brakes that usually mitigate excessive immune responses [3, 13].

However, immune-related adverse events (irAEs) also occur frequently in non-cancerous tissues, and may lead to a range of potentially life-threatening CV complications such as myocarditis, pericarditis, acute coronary syndromes, arrhythmias, as well as Takotsubo syndrome and non-inflammatory left ventricular dysfunction (NILVD) [3, 13]. Although rare (according to literature occurring in 0.1–1% of patients, more commonly in patients undergoing dual ICI therapy), ICI-related myocarditis implies a very high fatality rate (up to 50%), thus requiring prompt recognition and treatment [3, 13]. Furthermore, data also suggest a higher risk of acute cerebrovascular disease and hypercholesterolemia, highlighting the importance of strict CVRF management [3, 13, 14].

Treatment of CV irAEs generally requires (temporary) treatment interruption and systemic corticosteroid administration [3, 13]. Particularly in suspected ICI-related myocarditis, early steroid administration is warranted, as well as early escalation to second-line immune suppressive treatment in case of a lack of treatment response [3, 13].

2.4.4 Hormonotherapy

Upon diagnosis, breast cancer hormone receptor status (ER and PR expression on cancer cell surface) is evaluated in order to identify patients eligible for endocrine therapy (generally referred to as hormonotherapy) [5]. Up to 65–70% of all early and metastatic breast cancer patients are hormone-receptor positive [1, 4]. Depending on menopausal status, relapse risk and pre-existing CVRFs, hormonotherapy may consist of selective oestrogen receptor modulators (SERM, e.g. tamoxifen) or aromatase-inhibitors (AI, e.g. letrozole, anastrozole or exemestane), each with a particular CTR-CVT risk profile [3, 5, 6]. The use of SERM significantly increases the risk of venous thromboembolic events (VTE: deep vein thrombosis and pulmonary embolism) and should therefore be avoided in patients with a baseline increased thrombotic risk [3, 15]. Aromatase inhibitors are associated with an increased risk of HF, coronary artery disease and CV events as compared to tamoxifen, and may aggravate or induce metabolic syndrome, dyslipidemia, and AHT [3, 16]. Nevertheless, the absolute benefit of preventing breast cancer recurrence outweighs the risk of CTR-CVT: rather than denying high-risk patients a potentially life-saving cancer treatment, initiation of homonotherapy should prompt a stringent revision and treatment optimization of pre-existing CVRFs and/or pre-existing CVD [3].

2.4.5 Radiotherapy

More than 50% of all breast cancer patients undergo radiotherapy (RT) as an adjuvant treatment after surgery [3–5, 17]. Exposure of CV structures to ionizing radiation increases the risk of developing subsequent CVD through different pathophysiological mechanisms, some of which are still incompletely understood. Importantly, the risk of developing RT-related CVD (RTRCD) has subsided over time with major technological advances in current RT practice, but it has not disappeared [3, 17]. Calculating the radiation dose administered to CV structures (mean heart dose, MHD) allows for CTRCD risk categorization, but this is an imperfect metric: of paramount importance is the notion that there is no 'safe heart dose' [3, 17]. Acute RT-induced pericarditis used to be common but has become relatively rare, occurring during or shortly after RT administration [3, 9, 17, 18]. Predisposing to an increased risk of developing RT-induced constrictive pericarditis at long term, timely diagnosis and appropriate treatment are crucial [3, 9, 17, 18]. Other RT-induced CV complications may develop at the level of every CV structure including the pericardium (constrictive pericarditis), myocardium (HF, particularly HF with preserved ejection fraction—HFpEF), coronary arteries (ischemic cardiomyopathy), valvular apparatus (aortic valve stenosis and mitral valve regurgitation) and conduction system (both Brady- and tachyarrhythmias) [3, 9, 17]. Unique in RTRCD is the extremely long latency period between RT exposure and the development of RTRCD, which may manifest only after 5–10 years [3, 9, 17, 18]. This highlights the importance of long-term follow-up of cancer patients after termination of cancer treatment, even when oncological follow-up has ended [3].

Surgery

Generally, the surgical approaches in breast cancer do not confer a specific risk of CTR-CVT, taking into account the fact that in general, the most tissue-sparing surgical option is preferred [5]. According to the 2022 ESC Guidelines on CV assessment and management of patients undergoing noncardiac surgery, breast surgery as well as reconstructive surgery are considered low-risk surgical interventions with an estimated 30-day risk of CV death, myocardial infarction, and stroke of <1% [19]. This forms a striking contrast with the majority of other oncological surgical interventions, which are considered at least intermediate (1–5%) or high-risk (>5%) surgery [19].

2.5 Organization of on-Treatment Cardio-Oncological Care in Breast Cancer Patients

Considering the risk of CTR-CVT during and after breast cancer treatment, cardio-oncological surveillance should be organized in parallel with cancer treatment administration [3, 20] (Table 2).

In order to optimize a patient-tailored approach, individual CTR-CVT risk should be calculated upon treatment initiation ('baseline evaluation') and the surveillance strategy should be implemented according to this risk stratification [3, 20]. For this purpose, the ESC guidelines on Cardio-Oncology propose different baseline risk stratification proformas, depending on the

Table 2 Current definitions of CTRCD

CTRCD definitions	
Symptomatic CTRCD (HF)	
Very severe	HF requiring inotropic support, mechanical circulatory support, consideration of transplantation
Severe	HF hospitalization
Moderate	Outpatient intensification of diuretic and HF therapy
Mild	Mild HF symptoms not requiring therapy intensification
Asymptomatic CTRCD (LVSD)	
Severe	New LVEF reduction to <40%
	New LVEF reduction by ≥10 percentage points to LVEF 40–49%
Moderate	OR
	New LVEF reduction by <10 percentage points to LVEF 40–49% AND either new GLS regression by >15% from baseline OR new rise in cardiac biomarkers (troponin T, natriuretic peptides)
Mild	LVEF ≥50% AND new GLS regression by >15% from baseline AND/OR new rise in cardiac biomarkers (troponin T, natriuretic peptides)

Considering the importance of anthracyclines and HER2-targeted therapy in breast cancer, with CTRCD as most important manifestation of CTR-CVT, clear definitions have been published. Adequate classification of toxicity will allow for appropriate management. *CTRCD* cancer therapy-related cardiac dysfunction, *GLS* global longitudinal strain, *HF* heart failure, *LVEF* left ventricular ejection fraction, *LVSD* left ventricular systolic dysfunction planned treatment (with different proformas for anthracyclines and for HER2-targeted therapies) [3, 20]. These proformas are available for several frequently used cancer treatments, and allow for risk stratification into low, intermediate, high or very high risk of developing cardiotoxicity, corresponding respectively to <2%, 2–9%, 10–19% and >20% risk [3, 20]. Factors taken into account include previous CVD (e.g. pre-existing HF, ischemic heart disease or arrhythmias), cardiac imaging characteristics (LVEF), cardiac biomarkers (troponin T and natriuretic peptides), age, CVRFs, lifestyle risk factors, current cancer treatment and previous cancer treatment exposure [3, 20].

Based on this risk stratification, the ESC Guidelines propose detailed on-treatment surveillance strategies for the different treatment modalities, where a more intensive follow-up will be proposed in (very) high risk patients compared to low-risk patients, highlighting the importance of a thorough CV evaluation prior to treatment initiation [3, 20].

On-treatment surveillance strategies vary depending on the planned treatment, the baseline risk stratification and the expected CV toxic manifestations for this treatment, and may consist of clinical surveillance, combined with electrocardiographic, echocardiographic and biomarker follow-up [3, 20].

2.6 Organization of Long-Term Cardio-Oncological Follow-Up in Breast Cancer Patients

Ongoing improvements in breast cancer treatment invariably result in a growing cohort of breast cancer survivors, who still have a long-life expectancy after cancer treatment [2, 3]. After finalizing systemic breast cancer therapy, oncological follow-up will be less frequent, even if a long-term hormonotherapy is still ongoing [3]. When no more potentially cardiotoxic treatments are being administered, the CTR-CVT risk will be lower, but it does not disappear completely [3]. Particularly throughout the first year after treatment a late cardiotoxicity risk persists (e.g. in trastuzumab-treated patients), highlighting the relevance of a comprehensive end-of-treatment evaluation and follow-up [3]. Beyond the first year, long-term surveillance should be planned in order to allow not only early detection of new-onset CVD, but also timely detection of (very) late toxicity [3].

As in on-treatment surveillance of asymptomatic cancer survivors, the frequency of follow-up visits is tailored to the individual patient's risk of long-term CTR-CVT, taking into account the administered MHD as well as the total cumulative dose of doxorubicin (or equivalent anthracycline dose) [3].

Irrespective of long-term risk stratification, all cancer survivors should undergo annual CV risk assessment and CVRF optimization as well as cardiology (or cardio-oncology) referral upon the development of new CV symptoms [3]. Every 5 years, re-stratification of toxicity risk should be performed [3]. For low-risk breast cancer survivors, other investigations are not required [3]. For moderate-risk survivors, current guidelines recommend transthoracic echocardiography (TTE) every 5 years, and for high- and very high-risk patients this is even recommended at 1, 3 and 5 years after treatment completion, and every 5 years thereafter [3].

Crucial in long-term follow-up is also patient education, drawing attention to a balanced diet, regular physical activity as well as maximal primary prevention measures [3].

For cancer survivors who developed symptomatic CTR-CVT, a targeted pathology-specific follow-up should be foreseen [3] (Table 2).

3 Clinical Practice

3.1 Baseline CV Evaluation Before Breast Cancer Treatment Initiation

As previously mentioned, a comprehensive baseline CV evaluation prior to initiation of cancer treatment, is crucial in order to establish a patient-tailored cardiotoxicity surveillance strategy [3, 20]. This baseline evaluation should encompass not only pre-existing CVD and CVRF but also the patients age, sex, lifestyle risk factors and family history, as well as previous exposure to cardiotoxic treatments [3, 20]. Depending on the planned treatment strategy (in breast cancer mainly anthracyclines or HER2-targeted treatment), specific risk stratification proformas allow for an easy estimation of cardiotoxicity risk (low, intermediate, high or very high risk), taking into account all previously mentioned elements [3, 20].

Besides the aforementioned risk stratification proformas, the ESC guidelines provide general recommendations on which CV investigations should be performed in which treatment and in which patient [3]. Before anthracycline treatment, TTE (transthoracic echocardiography) is recommended in all patients (recommendation class I), and CV biomarkers (cardiac troponin and natriuretic peptides) in very high risk patients [3]. In low- and moderate-risk patients, the evidence to support baseline biomarker assessment is less well established, but evaluation should be considered (recommendation class IIa) [3]. The same recommendations apply for HER2-targeted therapies, with even less evidence for biomarker testing—nevertheless, a baseline evaluation may be considered (recommendation class IIb) [3].

Importantly, this baseline assessment should not have the intention of denying patients a potentially life-saving treatment, but rather of identifying the patients at the highest toxicity risk in order to optimize CV treatment, consider cardioprotective treatment (CPT) initiation in parallel with the cancer treatment, and plan on-treatment surveillance [3, 20]. In most cases, pre-existing CVD automatically identifies the patient as high-risk, but in patients without CVD, an accumulation of CVRFs may also result in stratification into a high-risk category [3, 20].

3.2 Cardio-Oncological Follow-Up Throughout Treatment

On-treatment CTR-CVT surveillance is recommended in all patients undergoing potentially cardiotoxic treatments, especially for anthracyclines and HER2-targeted therapy [3]. A patient-tailored follow-up is recommended, and should be organized after baseline evaluation, where patients at higher risk of developing CTR-CVT, require a more intensive follow-up (both in terms of frequency of visits and type of surveillance) [3]. Detailed surveillance protocols are available for anthracyclines and HER2-targeted treatments as well as for several other frequently used therapies [3]. The purpose of this surveillance is to allow for timely detection of cardiotoxicity, particularly CTRCD in breast cancer patients, considering the higher reversibility of myocardial damage when identified and treated immediately [3, 21]. In breast cancer, surveillance strategies are best studied for the most cardiotoxic treatments, but this does not imply that other, non-HER2-targeted and non-anthracycline-based therapies cannot result in CV adverse events: particularly patients with pre-existing CVD should be considered as high-risk patients for the development of CTR-CVT, even when undergoing less notoriously toxic treatments [3, 21].

3.3 Long-Term Follow-Up After Treatment

Upon termination of cancer treatment (in breast cancer patients, this is considered the moment of the last trastuzumab or anthracycline administration), oncological follow-up visits are significantly less frequent as compared to the on-treatment follow-up, particularly in patients undergoing long-term hormonotherapy as single remaining adjuvant treatment [3]. While CTR-CVT risk is the highest throughout active treatment, it will not return to zero at the end of treatment [3]. Not only do most treatments carry to some extent a risk of late cardiotoxicity, but research has also demonstrated that breast cancer survivors exhibit up to a 32% increased risk of developing CVD as compared to non-cancer patients, highlighting the relevance of long-term surveillance in this patient cohort, as well as the importance of a comprehensive end-of-treatment CV evaluation [3, 22, 23].

This end-of-treatment evaluation will help in planning long-term follow-up and may be considered the 'new baseline evaluation' after treatment completion. High-risk patients can be identified based on clinical characteristics (high or very high baseline risk), development of on-treatment CTR-CVT (both symptomatic and asymptomatic) and new abnormalities (biomarker and/or TTE) throughout surveillance [3]. Specific breast cancer treatment-related risk factors that identify high-risk patients are cumulative doxorubicin (or equivalent) dose of ≥250 mg/m^2, RT with MHD >15 Gy, combination of anthracyclines with RT (doxorubicin ≥100 mg/m^2 + RT with MHD 5–15 Gy) [3]. Furthermore, end-of-treatment assessment of troponin levels in anthracycline-treated patients may further help identify patients at increased risk of future CTR-CVT, in whom cardioprotective therapy may prove valuable alongside standard follow-up measures [3].

Considering CTR-CVT risk, 'long-term follow-up' can be divided into two different time strata: the first year after cancer treatment completion, and the long-term follow-up after this first year. Patients who developed CTR-CVT during cancer treatment require the most intensive follow-up, by means of TTE and biomarker assessment at 3, 6 and 12 months after treatment termination [3]. For asymptomatic high-risk patients, CV follow-up including TTE and biomarker assessment is recommended at 3 and 12 months after treatment completion. In other, low-risk patients, TTE and biomarker surveillance at 12 months may suffice [3]. Beyond the first year after treatment completion, yearly clinical evaluation is recommended, with repeat imaging (TTE) every 5 years in asymptomatic cancer survivors [3]. The onset of new CV symptoms should prompt earlier reevaluation in any cancer survivor [3].

3.4 New-Onset Cardiotoxicity During Treatment

In the 2022 ESC Guidelines on Cardio-oncology, CTRCD is defined, differentiating between symptomatic and asymptomatic CTRCD, which can be mild, moderate and (very) severe (see Table 2) [3]. In breast cancer patients, most commonly encountered on-treatment CTR-CVT will be CTRCD after exposure to anthracyclines and HER2-targeted therapy [3, 24]. For both treatments, detailed flowcharts are available describing which strategy is recommended in which degree of CTRCD, distinguishing between the cardiological and the oncological approach [3]. A main point of interest is the central role of a multidisciplinary team discussion between cardiologist and oncologist before deciding to interrupt potentially lifesaving cancer treatments [3]. Furthermore, treatment interruption is only recommended in a small minority of cases (symptomatic moderate to severe CTRCD and asymptomatic severe CTRCD) [3, 24, 25]. In most cases of mild CTRCD, cancer treatment may be continued under intensified surveillance, and on cardioprotective treatment (usually consisting of beta-blocker (BB) and angiotensin converting enzyme-inhibitor (ACEi) or angiotensin receptor blocker (ARB)) [3, 24, 25]. In all other CTRCD cases, guideline-directed HF therapy is recommended [3].

3.5 New-Onset Cardiotoxicity After Treatment

Late cardiotoxicity after breast cancer treatment completion, especially CTRCD, is not uncommon, and mainly presents within the first year after termination of treatment [3]. However, in patients who underwent RT, very late CTR-CVT may manifest up to decades after RT administration [3, 17]. In these cases, CTR-CVT will present in the shape of valvular heart disease (especially mitral valve regurgitation and aortic valve stenosis), conduction disease (particularly bradyarrhythmias) and coronary artery disease [3, 17]. Particularly this very late presentation emphasizes the importance of long-term follow-up, since most patients will no longer be followed by an oncologist [3, 17].

4 Conclusions

Breast cancer is by far the most frequently diagnosed cancer in women, and both earlier detection strategies as well as efficient treatments, have significantly improved survival outcomes in these patients [1–4]. However, these benefits are counterbalanced by an increased risk of developing CTR-CVT during or after treatment, as well as an increased risk of premature CVD after exposure to a multitude of potentially cardiotoxic molecules such as anthracyclines, HER2-targeted therapy and radiotherapy [2, 3, 7, 9–11, 17, 22].

Therefore, breast cancer patients require not only a comprehensive CV evaluation prior to cancer treatment initiation, but also a specific CV follow-up throughout and after their cancer trajectory [3]. This follow-up should be tailored to the individual patient's cardiotoxicity risk, taking into account CVRFs, lifestyle risk factors, pre-existing CVD, previous cancer treatment exposure as well as cardiac biomarkers and echocardiography findings [3, 20]. Furthermore, this strategy may also help in identifying high-risk patients who may benefit from cardioprotective treatments [3, 20].

A structured toxicity surveillance using the recently updated definitions of CTR-CVT, allows for timely detection, confirmation and treatment of new-onset cardiotoxicity, resulting in higher probability of successful cancer treatment completion but also of (at least partial) recovery of left ventricular function [3, 20]. Optimization of the treatment of pre-existing CVD and a meticulous treatment of all CVRFs may help in mitigating the risk of long-term CTR-CVT and premature CVD in cancer survivors [3].

In conclusion, breast cancer patients make up a specific population requiring dedicated cardio-oncological care throughout the entirety of their cancer treatment as well as beyond treatment fulfillment, with a focus on pre-treatment risk stratification, early diagnosis and treatment of CTR-CVT and appropriate management of pre-existing CVD and CVRFs [3].

Key Issues

- **Pre-existing CVD and (very) high cardiotoxicity risk**
  - Identify the high-risk patients using baseline risk stratification proformas and plan on-treatment surveillance.
  - Pre-existing CVD and the presence of multiple CVRFs automatically results in stratification as (very) high risk patient: guideline-directed treatment of pre-existing CVD and optimal CVRF control is recommended
  - Consider initiation of cardioprotective treatments (e.g. BB and ACEi/ARBs) in high-risk patients, but a high-risk stratification should not by default exclude a patient from undergoing potentially lifesaving cancer treatments—unless the left ventricular function is altogether too poor (LVEF <40%) [3, 24, 25].
- **New-onset cardiotoxicity on-treatment**
  - Upon a suspicion of new-onset CTR-CVT (mainly CTRCD), early confirmation is crucial before any decisions are made concerning cancer treatment (dis-)continuation [3, 24].
  - CTRCD grading depends on GLS values, LVEF values and biomarker levels, and the recommended approach depends on the type of cancer treatment as well as on the severity of CTRCD at diagnosis [3, 24, 25].
  - Mild cardiotoxicity warrants initiation of cardioprotective therapy but no interruption of cancer treatment [3, 24, 25].
  - In severe cardiotoxicity, treatment interruption (albeit temporary or definitively) should be discussed in a multidisciplinary team, considering other available treatment options, and guideline-directed HF treatment should be initiated [3, 24, 25]. Consider permissive cardiotoxicity in order

to allow for completion of cancer treatment to optimize cancer prognosis, under the condition of a more intensive CV surveillance [3, 24, 25].

- **Late cardiotoxicity**
  - Late cardiotoxicity (new-onset CTR-CVT after termination of cancer treatment) is most common during the first year after treatment: plan end-of-treatment assessment and intensive surveillance throughout the first year in high-risk patients [3, 22].
  - During long-term follow-up, optimize CVRF management and beware of new CV symptoms and of premature CVD [3, 22].
- **New symptoms of CVD in breast cancer patients**
  - New symptoms suspect of CVD in patients undergoing active cancer therapy and in cancer survivors, should prompt further diagnostic workup [3].
  - Symptoms suggestive of HF in patients receiving anthracyclines or HER2-targeted therapy are alarming and require a short-term reevaluation [3, 24].

Questions and Answers

1. Are all breast cancer patients at increased risk for the development of CVD?
   (A) No, only HER2-positive patients undergoing trastuzumab treatment.
   (B) No, only patients undergoing anthracycline-based therapy or HER2-targeted therapy.
   (C) Yes, except when there is no systemic treatment involved.
   (D) Yes, even when the treatment does not involve systemic therapies or radiotherapy.
   Correct answer: D
   Cancer and CVD share common risk factors, so in general, cancer patients are indeed at increased risk for developing CVD. This highlights the importance of guideline-based management of CVRFs in this population. Particularly breast cancer patients treated with anthracyclines, HER2-targeted therapy, aromatase inhibitors as well as radiotherapy are at increased risk.
2. Which breast cancer patient needs 3-monthly echocardiography evaluation?
   (A) A 28-years old patient undergoing adjuvant treatment with trastuzumab/pertuzumab for HER2-positive breast cancer, who has no other comorbidities.
   (B) A 66-years old patient undergoing neoadjuvant treatment with epirubicin-cyclophosphamide, with medical history consisting of arterial hypertension, type II diabetes, hypercholesterolemia, obesity (BMI 32 kg/m^2) and active smoking (± 50 py). Baseline LVEF 53%, troponin T undetectable, NT pro-BNP 78 ng/L.
   (C) A + B.
   (D) Neither A nor B.
   Correct answer: A
   Depending on the prescribed treatment and the cardiotoxicity risk stratification at baseline evaluation, surveillance intervals may be defined for each patient. However, for most patients treated with anthracyclines or anti-HER2-based treatment, a 3-monthly TTE is indeed recommended during active treatment. For other systemic and endocrine treatments, recommendations for imaging reevaluation are less stringent. For this question, patient A is indeed at low risk for cardiotoxicity but requires 3-monthly evaluation nonetheless, while patient B is at high-risk, requiring evaluation after every 2 cycles of anthracyclines (± every 6 weeks).
3. Who is at high cardiotoxicity risk?
   (A) A 59-year-old breast cancer patient who underwent CABG 2 years ago, with current LVEF of 56%.
   (B) A 34-year-old breast cancer patient who was treated for Hodgkin's lymphoma at the age of 17 (including doxorubicin, bleomycin, vincristine, dacarbazine and involved field radiotherapy).
   (C) A + B.
   (D) None of them, patient A is at very high risk and patient B is only at intermediate risk.
   Correct answer: C

For most frequently used cancer treatments, risk stratification proformas are readily available and allow easy baseline evaluation. Any pre-existing CVD will automatically categorize the patient as high-risk, requiring a close cardio-oncological surveillance and strict optimization of the pre-existing CVD.

4. Which preventive measures can be taken in order to reduce the risk of cardiotoxicity?
   (A) Add acetyl-salicylic acid to the treatment.
   (B) Start ACE-inhibition and beta-blockers in all patients undergoing anthracycline- or HER2-targeted therapy.
   (C) Optimize all cardiovascular risk factors upon treatment initiation.
   (D) All of the above.

   Correct answer: C

   Current data concerning cardioprotective strategies are still somewhat limited to date. In high-risk patients, beta blockers and angiotensin converting enzyme inhibitors or angiotensin receptor blockers may be considered as cardioprotective treatments, besides general measures as regular physical activity (whether or not in a training program) and a balanced diet. Furthermore, the use of dexrazoxane may prove valuable as well as the use of liposomal or PEGylated anthracyclines.

5. In whom do we have to stop cancer treatment?
   (A) Never stop cancer treatment. It saves lives.
   (B) Any breast cancer patient on anthracycline-based treatment in whom LVEF drops below 40%, regardless of baseline value. Discuss alternatives in multidisciplinary team.
   (C) Any breast cancer patient on HER2-targeted treatment in whom LVEF drops below 40% regardless of baseline value. Discuss alternatives in multidisciplinary team.
   (D) B + C.

   Correct answer: D

   Cancer treatment interruption or discontinuation has important prognostic implications for the patient in terms of survival outcomes. Therefore, interruption of potentially life-saving cancer treatments is a last-resort solution and should always be preceded by a multidisciplinary team discussion concerning the risks of treatment continuation versus temporary or definite treatment interruption. Alternative treatment strategies should be considered, such as switching to a different line of cancer treatment, or permissive cardiotoxicity under close cardio-oncology surveillance. In general, the only situations requiring discussion concerning treatment interruption are in cases of severe or moderate (a-)symptomatic CTRCD on anthracyclines, and in cases of either severe asymptomatic or moderate to (very) severe symptomatic CTRCD on HER2-targeted therapies.

6. Do breast cancer patients need a life-long follow-up after treatment completion?
   (A) Yes, but the frequency and the type of follow-up may differ from patient to patient.
   (B) Yes, annual ECG, TTE and biomarkers are the minimum.
   (C) No, patients at low cardiotoxicity risk don't need any kind of follow-up.
   (D) No, only the patients that developed cardiotoxicity need long-term follow-up.

   Correct answer: A

   Considering the increased risk of premature CVD in cancer patients and the exposure to one or more potentially cardiotoxic treatments, annual CV reevaluation is recommended after completion of cancer treatment, with particular attention to optimal management of CVRFs and new symptoms. Imaging reevaluation may be reduced in frequency to a 5-yearly TTE in most patients.

   Breast cancer patients receiving aromatase inhibitor-based hormonotherapy require particular attention, considering the fact that these very long-term treatments (5–10 years) inevitably imply a very long-term exposure as well as multiple cardiometabolic alterations.

References

1. Breast cancer [Internet]. United States of America (USA): World Health Organization; 2023 [updated 2023; cited 25 Sep 2023]. https://www.who.int/news-room/fact-sheets/detail/breast-cancer.
2. Patnaik JL, Byers T, DiGuiseppi C, Dabelea D, Denberg T. Cardiovascular disease competes with breast cancer as the leading cause of death for older females diagnosed with breast cancer: a retrospective cohort study. Breast Cancer Res. 2011;13:R64.
3. Lyon AR, Lopez-Fernandez T, Couch LS, Asteggiano R, Aznar M, et al. 2022 ESC guidelines on cardio-oncology developed in collaboration with the European Hematology Association (EHA), the European Society for Therapeutic Radiology and Oncology (ESTRO) and the International Cardio-Oncology Society (IC-OS). Eur Heart J. 2022;43(41):4229–361.
4. Cijfers over borstkanker [Internet]. Belgium (BE): Pink Ribbon; 2023 [Updated 2023, cited 25 Sep 2023]. https://pink-ribbon.be/over-borstkanker/cijfers-over-borstkanker-1#:~:text=Vandaag%20sterven%207%20vrouwen%20in,over%201%20op%207%20gesproken.
5. Overview of the treatment of newly diagnosed invasive, non-metastatic breast cancer [Internet]. United Stated of America (USA): UpToDate; 2023 [updated 2023; cited 25 Sep 2023]. https://www.uptodate.com/contents/overview-of-the-treatment-of-newly-diagnosed-invasive-non-metastatic-breast-cancer?search=breast%20cancer%20treatment&source=search_result&selectedTitle=1~150&usage_type=default&display_rank=1.
6. Overview of the approach to metastatic breast cancer [Internet]. United Stated of America (USA): UpToDate; 2023 [updated 2023; 25 Sep 2023]. https://www.uptodate.com/contents/overview-of-the-approach-to-metastatic-breast-cancer?search=metastatic%20breast%20cancer%20treatment&source=search_result&selectedTitle=2~150&usage_type=default&display_rank=2.
7. Meattini I, Poortmans PM, Aznar MC, Becherini C, Bonzano E, Cardinale D, et al. Association of breast cancer irradiation with cardiac toxic effects. A narrative review. JAMA Oncol. 2021;7(6):924–32.
8. Sawyer DB. Anthracyclines and heart failure. N Engl J Med. 2013;368:1154–6.
9. Gevaert SA, Halvorsen S, Sinnaeve P, Sambola A, Gulati G, et al. Evaluation and management of cancer patients presenting with acute cardiovascular disease: a consensus document of the Acute CardioVascular Care (ACVC) association and the ESC council of cardio-oncology—part 1: acute coronary syndromes and acute pericardial diseases. Eur Heart J Acute Cardiovasc Care. 2021;10:947–59.
10. Yu AF, Moskowitz CS, Lee Chuy K, Yang J, Dang CT, et al. Cardiotoxicity surveillance and risk of heart failure during HER2 targeted therapy. J Am Coll Cardiol CardioOncol. 2020;2(2):166–75.
11. Barish R, Gates E, Barac A. Trastuzumab-induced cardiomyopathy. Cardiol Clin. 2019;37:407–18.
12. Jacobs AT, Castaneda-Cruz DM, Rose MM, Connelly L. Targeted therapy for breast cancer: an overview of drug classes and outcomes. Biochem Pharmacol. 2022;204:115209.
13. Mahmood SS, Fradley MG, Cohen JV, Nohria A, Reyolds KL, et al. Myocarditis in patients treated with immune checkpoint inhibitors. J Am Coll Cardiol. 2018;71:1755–64.
14. Dolladille C, Akroun J, Morice PM, Dompmartin A, Ezine E, et al. Cardiovascular immunotoxicities associated with immune checkpoint inhibitors: a safety meta analysis. Eur Heart J. 2021;42:4964–77.
15. Xu X, Chlebowski RT, Shi J, Barac A, Haque R. Aromatase inhibitor and tamoxifen use and the risk of venous thromboembolism in breast cancer survivors. Breast Cancer Res Treat. 2018;174(3):785–94.
16. Khosrow-Khavar F, Filion KB, Bouganim N, Suissa S, Azoulay L. Aromatase inhibitors and the risk of cardiovascular outcomes in women with breast cancer. A population-based cohort study. Circulation. 2020;141:549–59.
17. Mitchell JD, Cehic DA, Morgia M, Bergom C, Toohey J, et al. Cardiovascular manifestations from therapeutic radiation. A multidisciplinary expert consensus statement from the International Cardio-Oncology Society. J Am Coll Cardiol CardioOncol. 2021;3(3):360–80.
18. Szpakowski N, Desai MY. Radiation-associated pericardial disease. Curr Cardiol Rep. 2019;21:97–107.
19. Halvorsen S, Mehilli J, Cassese S, Hall TS, Abdelhamid M, et al. 2022 ESC guidelines on cardiovascular assessment and management of patients undergoing non-cardiac surgery. Eur Heart J. 2022;43(39):3826–924.
20. Lyon AR, Dent S, Stanway S, Earl H, Brezden-Masley C, et al. Baseline cardiovascular risk assessment in cancer patients scheduled to receive cardiotoxic cancer therapies: a position statement and new risk assessment tools from the Cardio-Oncology Study Group of the Heart Failure Association of the European Society of Cardiology in collaboration with the International Cardio-Oncology Society. Eur J Heart Fail. 2020;22:1945–60.
21. Demissei BG, Adusumalli S, Hubbard RA, Denduluri S, Narayan V, et al. Cardiology involvement in patients with breast cancer treated with trastuzumab. J Am Coll Cardiol CardioOncol. 2020;2(2):179–89.
22. Koric A, Chang CP, Mark B, Rowe K, Snyder J, et al. Cardiovascular disease risk in long-term breast cancer survivors: a population-based cohort study. Cancer. 2022;128:2862–35.
23. Puckett LL, Saba SG, Henry S, Rosen S, Rooney E, et al. Cardiotoxicity screening of long-term breast cancer survivors—the CAROLE (Cardiac-

Related Oncologic Late Effects) Study. Cancer Med. 2021;10(15):5051–61.
24. Blaes A, Manisty C, Barac A. How to follow, manage and treat cardiac dysfunction in patients with Her2+ breast cancer. J Am Coll Cardiol CardioOncol. 2020;2(4):661–5.
25. Leong DP, Cosman T, Alhussein MM, Kumar Tyagi N, Karampatos S, et al. Safety of continuing trastuzumab despite mild cardiotoxicity. J Am Coll Cardiol CardioOncol. 2019;1(1):1–10.

Cardiovascular Genetics in Women

Yilong Lin and Nabila Bouatia-Naji

Abstract

Cardiovascular diseases are the leading cause of global morbidity and mortality in men and women. Women may exhibit a heightened susceptibility to some cardiovascular diseases due to their distinctive physiological characteristics and during critical life milestones. Some cardiovascular diseases specific to pregnancy and others showing women-predominance present specific genetic features. Cardiovascular risk factors such as obesity, blood pressure, and hormonal changes are also under genetic control that is increasingly investigated for specific risk in women, not only during pregnancy. The majority of cardiovascular diseases present a complex genetic underpinning involving rare and common genetic variants that contribute to the risk through cumulative and potentially interacting effects with non-genetic risk factors. Understanding the genetic architecture of CVDs and cardiometabolic traits in women is crucial to expect the implementation of sex and gender equality in precision medicine. This review aims to provide an overview of the current knowledge about the genetics cardiovascular diseases in women, with the objective of enhancing awareness and understanding of their pathophysiology.

Keywords

Genetic risk · Heredity · Genetic susceptibility · GWAS · Exome sequencing · Polygenic risk score

Test your learning and check your understanding of this book's contents: use the "Springer Nature Flashcards" app to access questions using ▶ https://sn.pub/51ny7m
To use the app, please follow the instructions in chapter 1.

Y. Lin · N. Bouatia-Naji (✉)
Université Paris Cité, PARCC, INSERM, Paris, France
e-mail: yilong.lin@inserm.fr; nabila.bouatia-naji@inserm.fr

A. H.E.M. Maas, E. Gerdts (eds.), *Manual of Cardiovascular Disease in Women*,
https://doi.org/10.1007/978-3-031-65952-2_29

1 Introduction

Cardiovascular diseases (CVDs) present differently in man and women mostly due to multiple physiological differences mainly influenced by sex hormones fluctuations in women, especially during pregnancy and transition to menopause. More generally, sex differences in CVDs can manifest as sex-specific disease manifestations in terms of incidence, prevalence, etiology, symptomology, treatment response, morbidity, and mortality [1]. The pathogenesis of CVDs has a substantial heritable component that involves complex interactions between environmental and genetic factors. Heritable cardiovascular conditions cover multiple if not all clinical entities, i.e. cardiomyopathies, hypertension, aortopathies, coronary artery disease, valvular heart disease, congenital heart disease, dyslipidemia and arrhythmias [2]. Main risk factors for CVDs are also highly heritable traits and their genetic risk factors are likely to potentially influence women's predisposition to some forms for CVDs, especially in the context of gene by behavior interactions.

In the past 20 years, huge progress was made in our understanding of the genetics of CVDs and cardiometabolic traits. Initially, genetic investigations relied on studies conducted in families to investigate the role of candidate genes and pathways involved in women's specific risk for CVDs. Genome-wide association study (GWAS), exome and genome sequencing became affordable thanks to the advent of low cost and high throughput technology that enables access a large and dense maps of rare and common genetic variation [3]. Some of these studies investigated the role of genetic variations specifically in women CVDs. We note that most CVDs are under a polygenic, multifactorial and complex genetic model where individual genetic risk variants have small individual effect sizes, with reported odds ratios under 1.50 for risk allele carriers. The currently available knowledge about CVDs genetics is only partially covered by the available GWAS for instance, and most of the data lack sex-stratified analyses. Nonetheless, there is increasing interest in the field of cardiovascular genetics to understand the possible specific genetic context of CVDs in women.

There is a clear need to provide a systematic understanding of the CVDs specifically in women through genetic investigation. Genetically determined mechanisms may at least partially explain the differential risk in women, and will set the stage for efficient and validated precision medicine that also consider the sex and hormonal specific to women.

In this chapter, we provide a brief descriptive of the methodology employed and study designs applied in cardiovascular genetics (Table 1) prior

Table 1 Summary of the main genetic methodology reported in this chapter

Methodology	Brief description	Applied technique	Advantage
Family-based study	Explores inheritable factors of traits or diseases within families by collecting genetic data from multiple family members to identify genetic variants segregating with the trait of interest. Provides insights into familial mechanisms contributing to cardiovascular diseases	Genetic data collection, exome or genome sequencing, and analysis within families	Provides insights into familial mechanisms contributing to cardiovascular diseases, potential to identify rare variants with large effects
Population-based study	Examines the frequency and distribution of genetic variants in a diverse population to identify common genetic factors associated with a trait or disease. Collects genetic data from unrelated individuals to understand genetic factors in the general population	Genetic data collection, genotyping using arrays or sequencing and analysis in diverse populations	Provides insights into the frequency and distribution of genetic variants, potential to identify common variants with small effects
Genome-Wide Association Study (GWAS)	Observational genetic studies (cohort or case control settings) aiming to discern potential associations between genetic variants and specific traits or diseases. Focuses on establishing links between single-nucleotide polymorphisms (SNPs) and human diseases	Analysis of a large number of genetic variants or polygenic risk scores (PRS) across the genome using genotyping or sequencing in case-control or cohort study settings	Enables the investigation of numerous traits and diseases, provides insights into the genetic architecture of complex polygenic diseases

to summarize the current knowledge related to the genetic causes of chronic and common CVDs in women. We first report genetic studies related to diseases related to pregnancy, followed by studies where specific genetic investigation was conducted in women about cardiometabolic risk traits, including obesity and blood pressure, and major chronic and acute CVDs. Finally, we describe genetic results related to CVDs with higher prevalence in women.

2 Methodology

Over the last few decades, multiple epidemiology studies have proved that genetic factors contribute to complex diseases such as cancer and cardiovascular diseases. In order to investigate the role of genetic factors in these diseases, the use of appropriate research strategies is imperative. Family-based studies focus on genetic information within families to explore the inheritable factors of traits or diseases. These studies often involve collecting data from multiple family members, such as siblings, parents, and grandparents. The goal is to seek whether a particular genetic variant segregates with the trait of interest within families. The primary predisposing factor in the development of cardiovascular disease is a family history of the condition. Familial mechanisms contributing to cardiovascular diseases can be diverse and specific to each family [3]. However, findings from family-based studies may not be easily generalized to the broader population since they focus on specific families with a history of the trait or disease under investigation. Environmental factors may be difficult to identify since family members live in similar environments. In addition, recruiting well-characterized family cohorts can be logistically challenging and time-consuming, especially family members may reside dispersed across the country or even in foreign locations [4].

In the early stages of genetic research on CVDs, study cohorts primarily consisted of families with a predisposition to familial inherited CVDs [5–7]. While those family-based GWAS have provided valuable insights, it is acknowledged that these studies often account for only a small proportion of the total genetic variance associated with most diseases, which require larger sample sizes to identify additional genetic variants contributing to the complex natures of these diseases [8].

Population-based studies involve examining the genetic information of individuals within a larger and more diverse population. These studies aim to understand the frequency and distribution of genetic variants in a broader context. Researchers collect genetic data from unrelated individuals, often from different geographic regions and ethnic backgrounds, to identify common genetic factors associated with a trait or disease in the general population.

Nevertheless, population-based studies may struggle to identify rare genetic variants associated with a trait or disease due to the low frequency of these variants in the general population.

Recent advances in research field of CVDs have provided cardiovascular epidemiology with powerful methods for studying the genetic architecture of complex polygenic diseases. Since 2005, genome-wide association studies (GWAS) have been used to investigate numerous traits and diseases. GWAS are observational studies of a comprehensive array of genetic variants throughout an assortment of individuals, aiming to discern any potential associations between any variant and a specific trait. Typically, GWAS concentrate on establishing links between single-nucleotide polymorphisms (SNPs), which represent the most common fraction of human genetic variability and the easiest to be genotyped, and traits like human diseases and clinically relevant phenotypes.

The advancement of sequencing technologies and the development of analytical tools have expanded the scope of GWAS, enabling the study of larger populations. Thus, allowing research cohorts to shift towards population-based studies while concurrently driving investigations into rare CVDs, which often exhibit a more complex genetic architecture [9, 10]. Deep whole-genome sequencing is widely recognized as the definitive method for comprehensive genetic variation assessment. Despite its status as the gold standard, its application encounters impracticality in large-scale studies due to the substantial costs [11]. In population-based GWAS, researchers typically rely on genotyping arrays, a class of high-throughput platforms designed to assess hundreds of thousands to millions of SNPs throughout the genome [12]. In contrast, whole-genome sequencing and exome sequencing, more commonly employed in family-based studies, play pivotal roles in the construction of genetic models. However, it is important to recognize their limited versatility because the identified genetic factors may be unique to certain familial contexts [4].

Large-scale biobank datasets have emerged as a critical component in the analysis of CVDs through GWAS. These datasets typically encompass detailed phenotypic information, including questionnaires, health records, laboratory measurements, and imaging data, collected from diverse voluntary participants [13]. Moreover, they incorporate genetic characterization through SNP array genotyping and, in many cases, whole-exome or whole-genome sequencing. The establishment of biobanks facilitates centralized storage and shared utilization of research cohorts, significantly enhancing the efficiency of disease research. The large scale of clinical and genetic data allows the investigation of the role of polygenic risk scores (PRS), which are generated by summing the risk alleles of established variants at risk of a given disease or trait variability as estimated from GWAS. Meanwhile, biobank data is subject to several limitations. Biobanks often rely on volunteers or individuals who choose to participate, leading to a potential bias in the population represented. The data may lack comprehensive phenotypic information, including lifestyle factors, environmental exposures, cardiac imaging and detailed clinical data. Incomplete phenotypic information can limit the ability to explore gene-environment interactions. Hopefully, more and more information will soon be available thanks to deep learning.

3 Main Body

3.1 Pregnancy and CVD Risk

Pregnancy-associated cardiovascular complications are the leading cause of maternal and fetal morbidity and mortality. Hypertensive disorders of pregnancy (HDP) are a major health issue for women and their enfants, which include preeclampsia (PE), eclampsia, pregnancy chronic hypertension, gestational hypertension, and preeclampsia superimposed on chronic hypertension [14]. Other important and common pregnancy complications that increase CVD risk are gestational diabetes, peripartum cardiomyopathy, connective tissue disorders, and venous thromboembolism.

3.1.1 Preeclampsia/Eclampsia and CVD Risk

PE is characterized by onset of hypertension after 20 weeks gestation, affecting 4–5% of pregnancies worldwide [15]. Several family studies have provided evidence for a maternal gene model in the context of PE. Numerous early case reports and systematic family studies support the idea that maternal genetic influence plays a significant role in the development of PE. However, the impact of maternal genetic factors on the predisposition to PE remain unanswered [16]. A systematic review of controlled studies showed that a family history of PE increases the risk of PE, indicating the genetic predisposition of PE [17]. The first GWAS of offspring from preeclamptic pregnancies, included 4380 cases and 310,238 controls and reported a genome-wide significant association of PE with a genetic variant located on chromosome 13 near the FLT1 gene, which encodes Fms-like tyrosine kinase 1 [18]. The soluble isoform of this protein is associated with the onset of PE.

In a meta-analysis performed in an Australian and New Zealand familial cohort, the authors identified 4 independent SNPs: LCT (rs2322659), LRP1B (rs35821928), RND3 (rs115015150) and GCA (rs17783344) on chromosome 2q22 [19].

These SNPs emphasized the polygenic feature of PE and provide potential shared genetic mechanisms that linked to both PE and other CVDs risk factors. In a case-control cohort of Finnish preeclamptic women, genetic predisposition to elevated BP is significantly associated with an increased risk of PE, recurrent PE, and PE with severe features. Moreover, PRS for higher BP in women suggested a higher BP value during pregnancy [20]. This implies that women have genetically predisposed to hypertension might face an increased risk of experiencing PE [19]. Further related study in an independent Australian population-based cohort found that the GCA SNP exhibited a significant association with a reduced risk of adolescents being born from a pregnancy complicated by PE ($P = 0.003$) and having a mother with prior PE ($P = 0.033$) [21]. However, these findings only partially support the shared genetic mechanisms of PE and CVDs.

The latest multi-ancestry meta-analysis of PE/eclampsia and gestational hypertension identified 18 loci, with 12 of them are new (i.e., WNT3A, NPR3 and PGR). These loci have also found to be associated with various pathways such as natriuretic peptide signaling, angiogenesis, trophoblast development and immune dysregulation. Additionally, the authors described PE/eclampsia and gestational hypertension are independent of clinical risk factors with genome-wide PRS prediction [22]. These collective findings underscore the genetic complexity of PE/eclampsia and gestational hypertension and allow the polygenic prediction of the HDPs.

3.1.2 Gestational Hypertension and CVD Risk

Gestational hypertension used to be considered as a subtype of preeclampsia. However, gestational hypertension is likely to be chronic hypertension masked by the normal reduction of blood pressure in early pregnancy. Roberts pointed out that gestational hypertension is probably best considered as non-syndromic increased blood pressure during pregnancy [23]. Several case-control studies have identified genes that significantly associated with gestational hypertension. Notably, AGT rs3789678 demonstrated a significant association with gestational hypertension in Chinese population [24]. Polymorphisms within TGFβR2 have been implicated as potential contributor in the pathologic process of gestational hypertension [25]. Grandi and colleagues summarized from nine studies that women with gestational hypertension have a 67% higher risk of subsequent CVD [26]. A genome-wide screen of Icelandic families, including 343 affected women, revealed a significant locus on 2p13, meeting the criteria for the first reported genome-wide significant locus for gestational hypertension [27]. However, while this analysis provided valuable insights, there is still a relative lack of GWAS of gestational hypertension.

3.1.3 Gestational Diabetes and CVD Risk

Diabetes during pregnancy is considered an important complication with severe health outcomes for both pregnant women and newborns. The causes of this common pregnancy complication are complex. Multiple genetic investigation have demonstrated the strong correlation between gestational diabetes and type 2 diabetes (T2D) reporting the same genetic risk loci overall (e.g. *MTNR1B*, *TCF7L2*, among others) [28, 29]. Considering the well-established link between T2D and CVD, a recent systematic review revealed that gestational diabetes is independently associated with a twofold increased risk of cardiovascular events postpartum (RR 1.98 [95% CI 1.57, 2.50]), and this risk persists irrespective of the development of T2D. This increased risk is evident within the first decade post-pregnancy, underscoring the importance of early monitoring and risk modification for women with gestational diabetes [30].

3.1.4 Peripartum Cardiomyopathy and CVD Risk

Peripartum cardiomyopathy (PPCM) is a life-threatening disease that occurs in women late in pregnancy, during delivery or in the postpartum months, causing substantial maternal and neonatal morbidity [31]. Recent new knowledge on PPCM has widely improved our understanding of its genetic predisposition.

Multiple studies have described genetic overlaps between PPCM and dilated cardiomyopathy (DCM) [32–34], a form of cardiac muscle disease that is characterized by ventricular dilation. An early genetic analysis of PPCM patients in 90 DCM families revealed a mutation (c.149A>G, p.Gln50Arg) in the gene encoding cardiac troponin C (TNNC1) segregating with disease in a DCM family with a member with PPCM, suggesting that family history and genetic factors play a role in the pathogenesis of PPCM [35]. Twenty-six rare truncating variants have been identified among 172 women with PPCM, two-third of which were clustered in the gene TTN, which encodes the sarcomere protein titin, a major mutated gene in DCM [34]. Furthermore, the authors observed a significant association between the TTN truncating variants and a lower ejection fraction at 1-year follow-up, within a clinical cohort including 83 women with PPCM [34]. Karolina et al. conducted a genetic testing on a female patient with severe course of PPCM and identified a novel TTN truncating mutation (NM_001267550: p. Leu 23499fs/c.70497_40498insT). Remarkably, this variant was also detected in the patient's mother. Given the fact that no other traditional risk factors were found in the patient, it was suggested that the identified TTN variant played a significant role in elucidating the genetic cause of PPCM [36].

Recent studies have identified mutations in BAG3, an important molecular chaperone, in patients with PPCM. The formation of BAG3 and heat shock proteins (Hsps) complex might be critically protective of the heart [37]. Horne et al. performed a GWAS analysis involving a cohort of 31 women with PPCM and 49 locally-matched controls and revealed a potential association between SNP rs258415, located on chromosome 12p11.22 near the PTHLH gene (encoding parathyroid hormone-related protein), and PPCM [38]. However, further investigation is warranted to elucidate the biological significance of this association. Overall, genetic investigation supports PPCM to genetically overlap with DCM, prompting exploration into their potential interplay, which may offer insights for elucidating the biological mechanism of specifically related to PPCM onset.

3.1.5 Pregnancy and Connective Tissue Disorders

Pregnancy represents a physiological condition imposing cardiac stress [39], marked by various alterations, including hormonally mediated changes, elevated heart rate, and vasodilation of maternal blood vessels. Women with connective tissue disorders, such as Marfan syndrome (MFS), Ehlers–Danlos syndrome, or other aortic abnormalities, have a higher risk to develop pregnancy-related complications [40]. Genetic defaults in structural proteins such as fibrillin, collagens and elements of the TGF beta signaling are likely to exacerbate vascular dysfunctions during pregnancy. A study conducted on a Canadian cohort revealed a significant association between MFS and increased likelihood of preterm birth and small-for-gestational-age infants [41]. While MFS remains acknowledged as a predominant contributor to pregnancy-related acute dissections [42], comprehensive genetic investigations on the disorder remain limited in pregnancy context.

3.1.6 Pregnancy and Venous Thromboembolism

Pregnancy is also considered as a thrombogenic state, and venous thromboembolism (VTE) is a serious pregnancy complication that can lead to severe maternal morbidity and mortality [43]. Previous family studies have shown that VTE has a strong genetic predisposition and is influenced by environmental factors [44]. Two prevalent polymorphic variants Factor V Leiden (FVL), Prothrombin G20210A (PT G20210A) have been shown to be associated with increased genetic risk of VTE in the pregnant population [45]. In women without prior thrombosis, the risk of pregnancy-associated thrombosis is relatively low, approximately 1 in 400, particularly when the prothrombin gene harbors a heterozygous Factor V Leiden (FVL) or heterozygous G20210A mutation, underscoring the polygenic nature of this condition [46]. In addition, research on genetic effects of heterozygous and homozygous carriers in relation to FVL and G20210A did not justify stratification of heterozygous as "lower risk" over homozygous mutants [45]. Many of our present knowledge of the genetic risk factor for VTE in pregnant or postpartum women is described from family studies, potentially resulting in an overestimation of the risk for women without preselection for these complications. As large-scale population-based studies rapidly expand, the insights from such studies are poised to enrich and advance our comprehension of the diseases, including in pregnant women.

3.2 Cardiometabolic Diseases

Under the currently increasing epidemic of obesity and diabetes, CVD complications account for the majority of mortality in affected patients. Women with diabetes tend to present worse clinical presentation and experience higher risk of CVD morbidity and mortality compared with men [47]. On the other hand, increased blood pressure and its associated complications, mainly stroke, are more prevalent in women compared to men. Here we report recent studies where women-specific genetic studies were conducted to understand the risk for cardiometabolic diseases, namely T2D, hypertension and stroke.

3.2.1 Diabetes-Related CVDs in Women

The investigation of diabetes sex-specific genetics in an emerging field of research. For instance, the coronary risk in diabetes (CoRDia) trial, which compared the effectiveness of usual diabetes care with a self-management intervention, with and without personalized risk information (including genetics) was underpowered to investigate sex-stratified effects on coronary risk in the 210 participants [48, 49]. One of the early reported sex-specific association with CVD risk in diabetes was reported for one common variant in the superoxide dismutase 2 gene (*SOD2*), involved in mitochondrial antioxidant enzyme activity. In this study, the risk for coronary heart disease in diabetics patients was reported to be only significant in women, although this findings will need further replication in larger samples [50]. More recently, several coronary artery disease risk genes were found to be modified by T2D in the development of subclinical atherosclerosis. *ATP1B1, ARVCF,* and *LIPG* associated with coronary artery calcification and *ABCG8 and EIF2B2* associated with carotid intima-media thickness and carotid plaque [51]. However, sex-specific risk was not covered in this study. A network analysis involving over 15,000 women across three diverse ethnicities used GWAS to reveal eight common pathways and gene networks, including cardiomyopathy, calcium signaling, and cell adhesion, across all ethnicities in CVD risk in diabetes [52]. Interestingly, ethnicity-specific pathways were described, with cell cycle to be specific for Hispanic and Caucasian Americans, while tight junction in CVD and combined CVD and T2D in Hispanic Americans [52]. These studies emphasized the importance of understanding specific genetic risk of CVD in diabetes, although we are still missing well-powered sex-specific studies to address the numerous clinical and behavioral specificities of cardiovascular outcomes among diabetic women.

3.2.2 Blood Pressure and Related Cardiovascular Complications

Blood Pressure Genetics

Being a major CVD risk factor, the genetics of blood pressure (BP) traits and hypertension was extensively studies in the past, but little investigation is available where women-specific genetic risk was assessed. The most recent large-scale GWAS meta-analysis that investigate the genetics of BP over 1000 risk loci, supporting its highly polygenic feature, with most genes involved in biological mechanisms influencing atherosclerosis, inflammation and vascular remodeling [53]. Kurniansyah et al. [54] evaluated polygenic risk scores (PRSs) for blood pressure in diverse populations, comparing different construction methods and sex-stratified prediction power. In the All of Us cohort, PRSs demonstrate superior predictive ability in females, emphasizing their efficacy in blood pressure prediction for women [54]. An additional study examined a Korean population comprising 13,926 participants in a sex-balanced distribution (men = 6402, women = 7524) to investigate sex-specific genetic susceptibility to hypertension. Independent GWASs and heterogeneity analyses identified significant loci, including rs11066015 of ACAD10 and rs2074356 of HECTD4, elucidating sex-specific effects on hypertension [55]. Shetty and colleagues [56] investigated the genetic contributions to hypertension in a diverse US population, revealing sex-specific differences. In a cohort of 212,669 individuals, females exhibited higher odds of hypertension per standard deviation increase in SBP polygenic risk scores compared to males. Stratifying by genetic risk, high-risk females had elevated odds of hypertension, while low-risk females had lower odds compared to their male counterparts. These findings underscore the sex-specific impact of genetic factors on hypertension susceptibility, shedding light on potential avenues for targeted interventions in women.

Stroke Genetics

The largest and most recent GWAS meta-analysis (67,162 cases and 454,450 controls) reported 32 stroke-associated risk loci, with the majority of these loci sharing genetic variations related to blood pressure, cardiac traits, and venous thromboembolism [57]. The enrichment of these loci varies across different subtypes of ischemic stroke, although, shared genetic variations were also evident across different stroke subtypes, such as *SH2B3* (encoding cytokine signaling-related protein) and ABO encoding blood group-related protein [57].

Most existing genetic studies on stroke lack explicit sex and gender investigation. Traylor et al. examined genetic influences on stroke across age and sex cohorts, utilizing data from four GWAS datasets [58]. The results indicated a noteworthy genetic correlation with age at stroke onset, indicating a potential heightened genetic influence in women [58]. Also, the study suggested the presence of distinct genetic factors impacting stroke susceptibility, especially in women [58]. Zhang et al. conducted a small-scale case-control study (591 cases and 553 controls) in the Chinese population that showed that CASZ1 genetic variants (rs4845941 and rs778228) were significantly associated with an increased risk of stroke, and the existence or interaction with sex with higher prevalence of the risk allele in women with stroke [59]. The CASZ1 gene plays a role in the development of the central nervous system, and has previously been considered to influence the risk of stroke [60]. More studies leveraging larger-scale GWASs are needed to unveil additional female-specific genetic associations with stroke.

3.3 Predominant Diseases in Women

Several CVDs manifest with a high sex-bias toward women that is not fully understood. Here we will cite recent progress in the genetics of most common female-predominant vascular diseases, namely fibromuscular dysplasia, spontaneous coronary artery disease, myocardial infarction with non-obstructive coronary arteries and Takotsubo syndrome.

3.3.1 Fibromuscular Dysplasia

Fibromuscular dysplasia (FMD) has been considered a rare neglected vascular disease related to hypertension and its most common complication, stroke. FMD genetics has gained momentum in the very recent years thanks to a shift in its genetic model and through the investigation of rare and common genetic variants. In a study investigating the role of common variants in ~1000 FMD cases, *PHACTR1*, a pleiotropic genetic risk locus reported previously in other common CVDs, including coronary artery disease and migraine, was first reported as associated with increased risk for FMD [61]. Richer et al. have identified a very rare variant within the COL5A1 gene, also involved in classical Ehlers Danlos syndrome, from four independent patients with FMD, but also involving arterial aneurysms, dissections and tortuosity [62]. Sequencing of unrelated FMD patients revealed enrichment for a rare variant in the prostaglandin receptor gene (*PTGIR*) suggesting a role of this important pathway for vasodilation and constriction, with relevance to stenosis and aneurysm in FMD [63]. A recent comprehensive GWAS involving 1556 FMD cases and 7100 controls identified several genetic risk loci for FMD, including the previously reported PHACTR1, and for the first time *LRP1, ATP2B1, SLC24A3* and *LIMA1*. The genes prioritized in these risk loci are involved in vascular contraction mechanisms and extracellular matrix regulation suggesting these mechanisms as important for arterial integrity [64]. At present, genetic research on FMD remains limited, with identified variations insufficient to fully elucidate the whole genetic spectrum of this complex condition. Further studies are anticipated to provide additional data and support in unraveling more genetic mechanisms, especially to explain the important female bias.

3.3.2 Spontaneous Coronary Artery Dissection

Spontaneous coronary artery dissection (SCAD) presents in the context of rare connective tissue disorders but also in pregnancy, with pregnancy SCAD representing ~5% of SCAD cases [9]. Whole-exome sequencing (WES) into familial or sporadic patients with SCAD have revealed the association of several genes. For instance, with the TLN1 gene, which encodes a protein responsible for bridging the cellular cytoskeleton and the extracellular matrix [65], and TSR1 gene encoding TSR1 ribosome maturation factor as a potential candidate gene for SCAD in this specific ethnic background [66].

SCAD has been reported to associate clinically with other CVDs presenting female-bias like hypertension, migraine, and FMD. Thus, the first genetic locus involving common genetic variants to be reported to associate with SCAD was *PHACTR1*, investigated after the establishment of its role in FMD [67]. GWAS has hugely contributed to understand the genetic risk for SCAD. The most comprehensive GWAS meta-analysis was recently published involving 1917 cases and 9292 controls where we reported 16 risk loci associated with SCAD [68]. Genes located near GWAS risk loci were mostly involved in extracellular matrix biology, with one locus involving the tissue-mediated coagulation factor gene *F3* that showed evidence for association with SCAD genetic risk only [68]. This study included an intriguing an opposite genetic correlation between SCAD and coronary artery disease (CAD), indicating shared biological processes between SCAD and CAD, albeit with distinct underlying mechanisms that deserves deeper investigation [68].

3.3.3 Myocardial Infarction with Non-obstructive Coronary Arteries

Myocardial infarction with non-obstructive coronary arteries (MINOCA) results from various causes, including coronary microvascular dysfunction (CMD). More than 50% of patients with INOCA and MINOCA have CMD [69], the majority of whom are women [70]. MINOCA can be observed in certain hematologic disorders associated with specific genetic mutations, such as chronic myeloproliferative Philadelphia-negative neoplasms (cMPNs) [69]. The Janus kinase 2 V617F mutation is present in over 70% of cMPN patients, and this variant may potentially lead to endothelial dysfunction and coronary artery spasms [71]. The higher prevalence of microcirculatory dysfunction has the potential to increase the risk of experiencing acute coronary syndrome (ACS), MI, stroke, and recurrent cardiovascular surgeries in patients [72]. Currently, three associated genetic variations have been identified in men: 5′-nucleotidase ecto (NT5E) (encoding lymphocyte differentiation-related protein), myosin heavy chain 15 (MYH15) (encoding myosin heavy-chain polypeptide), and VEGF-A (encoding endothelial function-related protein) [69]. Notably, MYH15 has been implicated in an increased risk of CMD. However, the relationship between SNPs and the risk of microcirculatory diseases in women remains unclear. Overall, little is known about women's specific risk for microvascular disease in general, and MINOCAs in particular.

3.3.4 Takotsubo Syndrome

The first family cases of Takotsubo syndrome TTS were reported in two sisters in 2004, supporting the potential genetic predisposition of TTS [73]. Nevertheless, the underlying mechanisms are vastly unknown. A systematic review summarized the genetic variants of ADRB1, GRK5 and BAG3 genes, or variants of APOE, MFGE8, ALB, APOB, SAA1, A2M, and C3 genes, associated with cardiomyopathies, to associate with the risk of TTS [74]. These variants are likely to interact with environmental factor, emotional and physical stress, which are thought to be important triggering factors of TTS. In previous clinical research, patients with TTS were considered to have a higher risk of cardiac complications, and subsequent high mortality [75]. Eitel et al. performed the first GWAS analysis of TTS in 2017, with an Illy-powered study population consisting of 96 TTS patients and 475 healthy controls, reporting 18 suggestively associated loci [76]. The authors pointed out several of these risk SNPs to be at risk for blood pressure and thyroid stimulating hormone. Despite a growing number of studies focusing on TTS and its emphasis on genetic predisposition, most of the existing genetic researches are still in the preliminary phases, supporting the need for further exploration encompassing specific genetic variants and functional pathways to this intriguing condition with high relevance to women's cardiovascular risk.

4 Conclusions

To summarize, the field of cardiovascular genetics in women has made some strides in understanding the genetic underpinnings of cardiovascular diseases and risk factors specific to women (Table 2). The evidence presented in this review underscores the importance of considering sex-specific genetic factors in the development, progression, and treatment of cardiovascular diseases. It is evident that genetic determinants play a crucial role in shaping the differential risk profiles observed in women, and a deeper understanding of these genetic mechanisms holds great promise for the advancement of precision medicine tailored to women's cardiovascular health.

Moving forward, it is imperative to continue exploring the genetic landscape of cardiovascular diseases in women through comprehensive research methodologies such as GWAS, including in more diverse ethnic backgrounds. Additionally, the integration of large-scale biobank datasets and advanced sequencing technologies will be instrumental in unraveling the complex genetic architecture of cardiovascular diseases in women. The development of analytical methods capable to cope with genetic by environment interactions will facilitate the integration of circulating female hormonal levels, and other important environmental factors that are needed to integrate to fully address women's specific cardiovascular genetic risk.

In essence, the insights gained from cardiovascular genetics research in women have the potential to revolutionize the way we approach risk assessment, diagnosis, and treatment of cardiovascular diseases. By embracing a sex-specific and genetically informed approach, we can pave the way for a more equitable and effective cardiovascular healthcare landscape for women. The ongoing necessity for research and clinical translation is emphasized, aiming to fully harness the potential of precision medicine in addressing the unique cardiovascular health needs of women.

Table 2 Major genetic research articles dedicated to cardiovascular diseases in women

Section.	Methodology	Number	Main findings	References
Preeclampsia/ eclampsia and CVD risk	GWAS	Preeclampsia: 20,064 cases and 703,117 controls Gestational hypertension: 11,027 cases and 412,788 controls	18 independent loci were identified associated with PE/eclampsia and/or gestational hypertension, 12 of which are new (*MECOM, FGF5, SH2B3, FLT1, FTO, ZNF831, MTHFR–CLCN6, WNT3A, NPR3, PGR and RGL3*)	[22]
Preeclampsia/ eclampsia and CVD risk	GWAS	4380 cases and 310,238 controls	The first genome-wide significant susceptibility locus (rs4769613; $P = 5.4 \times 10^{-11}$) was identified. This locus is near the FLT1 gene encoding Fms-like tyrosine kinase 1	[18]
Gestational diabetes and CVD risk	GWAS	1399 cases and 2025 controls	Two loci (rs7754840, rs10830962) known to be associated with type 2 diabetes had a genome-wide significant association with GDM	[28]
Peripartum cardiomyopathy and CVD risk	GWAS	31 cases and 49 controls	Revealed a potential association between SNP rs258415 and PPCM	[38]
Diabetes-related CVDs in women	GWAS	15,346 individuals	Eight common pathways and gene networks, including cardiomyopathy, calcium signalling, and cell adhesion, across all ethnicities are identified. Ethnicity-specific pathways are also identified. Key driver genes, such as COL1A1, COL3A1, and ELN, are validated in mouse models	[52]
Blood pressure genetics	GWAS	Over one million people	Identified 535 new loci associated with blood pressure traits	[53]
Blood pressure genetics	GWAS	13,926 participants	Identified significant loci, including rs11066015 of *ACAD10* and rs2074356 of *HECTD4*, elucidating sex-specific effects on hypertension	[55]
Stroke genetics	GWAS	110,182 cases and 1,503,898 controls	Reported 32 stroke-associated risk loci, with the majority of these loci sharing genetic variations related to blood pressure, cardiac traits, and venous thromboembolism	[57]
Fibromuscular dysplasia	GWAS	1556 cases and 7100 controls	Identified four significantly genetic risk loci (*PHACTR1*, *LRP1*, *ATP2B1*, and *LIMA1*) with FMD and those genetic variants linked to these loci were found to be associated with vascular constriction mechanisms	[64]
Spontaneous coronary artery dissection	GWAS	1917 cases and 9292 controls	Identified 16 risk loci associated with SCAD, with one of the locus involving *F3* encoding tissue factor suggesting a specific association with SCAD risk	[68]
Takotsubo syndrome	GWAS	96 cases (5 men, 91 women) and 475 controls (268 men, 207 women)	Identified 18 loci included top SNPs. Two out of 18 SNPs are associated with some traits such as blood pressure and thyroid stimulating hormone	[76]

(continued)

Table 2 (continued)

Section.	Methodology	Number	Main findings	References
Preeclampsia/ eclampsia and CVD risk	Candidate genes	1246 mothers and 1404 of their now adolescent offspring	Nominal associations (P < 0.05) with cardiovascular risk factors were detected for all four SNPs (rs2322659 (*LCT*), rs35821928 (*LRP1B*), rs115015150 (RND3) and rs17783344 (GCA))	[21]
Diabetes-related CVDs in women	Candidate genes	776 cases	The TT genotype of rs4880 SOD2 variant is associated with increased CHD risk	[50]
Stroke genetics	Candidate genes	591 cases and 553 controls	CASZ1 genetic variants (rs4845941 and rs778228) were significantly associated with an increased risk of stroke. rs778228 of CASZ1 were found to have higher prevalence in women with stroke	[59]
Peripartum cardiomyopathy and CVD risk	Candidate genes	172 cases	Twenty-six rare truncating variants have been identified, two-third of which were clustered in the gene TTN	[34]
Preeclampsia/ eclampsia and CVD risk	Exome sequencing	48 cases	Four independent SNP associations satisfied our gene-centric multiple testing correction criteria: (rs2322659 (LCT), rs35821928 (LRP1B), rs115015150 (RND3) and rs17783344 (GCA))	[19]
Peripartum cardiomyopathy and CVD risk	Exome sequencing	90 DCM families	Revealed a mutation (c.149A>G, p. Gln50Arg) in the gene encoding cardiac troponin C (*TNNC1*) segregating with disease in a DCM family with a member with PPCM	[35]
Gestational hypertension and CVD risk	Linkage in families	343 cases	Reported the first significant locus on 2p13 for gestational hypertension	[27]

Questions and Answers

1. What are the advantages of family-based studies
   (A) They allow to distinguish between genetic and environmental factors
   (B) Large and multi-generation families are frequently seen for late-onset CVDs
   (C) Family studies are very powerful to identify rare genetic variants with large effects through co-segregation between the genetic variant and disease status.
   (D) Findings from family-studies can be generalized to the general population

   Correct answer: C

   In the genome sequencing era, family studies have gained interest from geneticists in the cardiovascular field to investigate the role of rare and highly penetrant mutations through the study of their segregation with diverse type of disease. However, given the huge investment needed to collect large and multi-generational families, with the cost of including many non-affected and few affected members from the same family, and the limited number of informative carriers (affected individuals) for late onset diseases such as CVDs, this design is only applied in early onset forms of CVDs, mainly pediatric cardiomyopathies for instance.
2. What are the main pathways represented by the genes to be near the 18 GWAS signals of pre-eclampsia/eclampsia and gestational hypertension?
   (A) Natriuretic peptide signaling, angiogenesis, trophoblast development, and immune dysregulation
   (B) Angiotensin, TGF beta signaling, and autoimmune system

(C) Glucose homeostasis, vascular smooth muscle cells proliferation, and erythropoiesis
(D) Angiogenesis, TGF beta signaling, autoimmune system and erythropoiesis

Correct answer: A

Among the genes cited we report WNT3A, NPR3 and PGR. The authors performed a pathway analysis that highlighted the pathways cited in this answer.

3. What is the first genetic locus reported to associate with SCAD involving common genetic variants?
(A) TSR1 identified by exome sequencing
(B) PHACTR1, identified by GWAS
(C) LRP1, first reported to associate with fibromuscular dysplasia and then investigated in SCAD
(D) PHACTR1, first reported to associate with fibromuscular dysplasia and then investigated in SCAD

Correct answer: D

PHACTR1 was identified in fibromuscular dysplasia using a GWAS but was investigated in SCAD as a candidate locus. The following GWAS conducted in SCAD all confirmed that common genetic variants in this locus do associate with the risk of SCAD.

References

1. Shufelt CL, Pacheco C, Tweet MS, Miller VM. Sex-specific physiology and cardiovascular disease. In: Kerkhof PLM, Miller VM, editors. Sex-specific analysis of cardiovascular function. Cham: Springer; 2018. p. 433–54. (Advances in Experimental Medicine and Biology; vol. 1065). http://link.springer.com/10.1007/978-3-319-77932-4_27.
2. Laing N, Kraus SM, Shaboodien G, Ntusi NAB. An overview of the genetic basis of cardiovascular disease. S Afr Med J. 2019;109(6):364.
3. Mansour-Chemaly M, Haddy N, Siest G, Visvikis S. Family studies: their role in the evaluation of genetic cardiovascular risk factors. Clin Chem Lab Med. 2002;40(11):1085–96.
4. Hopper JL, Bishop DT, Easton DF. Population-based family studies in genetic epidemiology. Lancet. 2005;366(9494):1397–406.
5. Myers RH, Kiely DK, Cupples LA, Kannel WB. Parental history is an independent risk factor for coronary artery disease: the Framingham Study. Am Heart J. 1990;120(4):963–9.
6. Christophersen IE, Ravn LS, Budtz-Joergensen E, Skytthe A, Haunsoe S, Svendsen JH, et al. Familial aggregation of atrial fibrillation: a study in Danish twins. Circ Arrhythm Electrophysiol. 2009;2(4):378–83.
7. Marenberg ME, Risch N, Berkman LF, Floderus B, de Faire U. Genetic susceptibility to death from coronary heart disease in a study of twins. N Engl J Med. 1994;310(15):1041–6.
8. Benyamin B, Visscher PM, McRae AF. Family-based genome-wide association studies. Pharmacogenomics. 2009;10(2):181–90.
9. Hayes SN, Tweet MS, Adlam D, Kim ESH, Gulati R, Price JE, et al. Spontaneous coronary artery dissection. J Am Coll Cardiol. 2020;76(8):961–84.
10. Sen-Chowdhry S, Jacoby D, Moon JC, McKenna WJ. Update on hypertrophic cardiomyopathy and a guide to the guidelines. Nat Rev Cardiol. 2016;13(11):651–75.
11. Quick C, Anugu P, Musani S, Weiss ST, Burchard EG, White MJ, et al. Sequencing and imputation in GWAS: cost-effective strategies to increase power and genomic coverage across diverse populations. Genet Epidemiol. 2020;44(6):537–49.
12. Samuels DC, Below JE, Ness S, Yu H, Leng S, Guo Y. Alternative applications of genotyping array data using multivariant methods. Trends Genet. 2020;36(11):857–67.
13. Walsh R, Jurgens SJ, Erdmann J, Bezzina CR. Genome-wide association studies of cardiovascular disease. Physiol Rev. 2023;103(3):2039–55.
14. Hypertension in pregnancy. Report of the American College of Obstetricians and Gynecologists' task force on hypertension in pregnancy. Obstet Gynecol. 2013;122(5):1122–31.
15. Phipps EA, Thadhani R, Benzing T, Karumanchi SA. Pre-eclampsia: pathogenesis, novel diagnostics and therapies. Nat Rev Nephrol. 2019;15(5):275–89.
16. Lachmeijer AMA, Dekker GA, Pals G, Aarnoudse JG, Ten Kate LP, Arngrímsson R. Searching for preeclampsia genes: the current position. Eur J Obstet Gynecol Reprod Biol. 2002;105(2):94–113.
17. Duckitt K, Harrington D. Risk factors for preeclampsia at antenatal booking: systematic review of controlled studies. BMJ. 2005;330(7491):565.
18. The FINNPEC Consortium, The GOPEC Consortium, McGinnis R, Steinthorsdottir V, Williams NO, Thorleifsson G, et al. Variants in the fetal genome near FLT1 are associated with risk of preeclampsia. Nat Genet. 2017;49(8):1255–60.
19. Johnson MP, Brennecke SP, East CE, Dyer TD, Roten LT, Proffitt JM, et al. Genetic dissection of the preeclampsia susceptibility locus on chromosome 2q22 reveals shared novel risk factors for cardiovascular disease. Mol Hum Reprod. 2013;19(7):423–37.
20. Kivioja A, Toivonen E, Tyrmi J, Ruotsalainen S, Ripatti S, Huhtala H, et al. Increased risk of preeclampsia in women with a genetic predisposition to

elevated blood pressure. Hypertension. 2022;79(9): 2008–15.
21. Løset M, Johnson MP, Melton PE, Ang W, Huang RC, Mori TA, et al. Preeclampsia and cardiovascular disease share genetic risk factors on chromosome 2q22. Pregnancy Hypertens Int J Womens Cardiovasc Health. 2014;4(2):178–85.
22. Honigberg MC, Truong B, Khan RR, Xiao B, Bhatta L, Vy HMT, et al. Polygenic prediction of preeclampsia and gestational hypertension. Nat Med. 2023;29(6):1540–9.
23. Roberts JM, Rich-Edwards JW, McElrath TF, Garmire L, Myatt L, For the Global Pregnancy Collaboration. Subtypes of preeclampsia: recognition and determining clinical usefulness. Hypertension. 2021;77(5):1430–41.
24. Li X, Tan H, Zhou S, Hu S, Zhang T, Li Y, et al. Renin–angiotensin–aldosterone system gene polymorphisms in gestational hypertension and preeclampsia: a case–control gene-association study. Sci Rep. 2016;6(1):38030.
25. Li X, Tan H, Chen M, Zhou S. Transforming growth factor beta 1 related gene polymorphisms in gestational hypertension and preeclampsia: a case-control candidate gene association study. Pregnancy Hypertens. 2018;12:155–60.
26. Grandi SM, Filion KB, Yoon S, Ayele HT, Doyle CM, Hutcheon JA, et al. Cardiovascular disease-related morbidity and mortality in women with a history of pregnancy complications: systematic review and meta-analysis. Circulation. 2019;139(8):1069–79.
27. Arngrimsson R, Siguroarottir S, Frigge ML, Bjarnaottir RI, Jonsson T, Stefansson H, et al. A genome-wide scan reveals a maternal susceptibility locus for pre-eclampsia on chromosome 2p13. Hum Mol Genet. 1999;8(9):1799–805.
28. Kwak SH, Kim SH, Cho YM, Go MJ, Cho YS, Choi SH, et al. A genome-wide association study of gestational diabetes mellitus in Korean women. Diabetes. 2012;61(2):531–41.
29. Lauenborg J, Grarup N, Damm P, Borch-Johnsen K, Jørgensen T, Pedersen O, et al. Common type 2 diabetes risk gene variants associate with gestational diabetes. J Clin Endocrinol Metab. 2009;94(1):145–50.
30. Kramer CK, Campbell S, Retnakaran R. Gestational diabetes and the risk of cardiovascular disease in women: a systematic review and meta-analysis. Diabetologia. 2019;62(6):905–14.
31. Sliwa K, Bauersachs J, Arany Z, Spracklen TF, Hilfiker-Kleiner D. Peripartum cardiomyopathy: from genetics to management. Eur Heart J. 2021;42(32):3094–102.
32. Goli R, Li J, Brandimarto J, Levine LD, Riis V, McAfee Q, et al. Genetic and phenotypic landscape of peripartum cardiomyopathy. Circulation. 2021;143(19):1852–62.
33. Morales A, Painter T, Li R, Siegfried JD, Li D, Norton N, et al. Rare variant mutations in pregnancy-associated or peripartum cardiomyopathy. Circulation. 2010;121(20):2176–82.
34. Ware JS, Li J, Mazaika E, Yasso CM, DeSouza T, Cappola TP, et al. Shared genetic predisposition in peripartum and dilated cardiomyopathies. N Engl J Med. 2016;374(3):233–41.
35. Van Spaendonck-Zwarts KY, Van Tintelen JP, Van Veldhuisen DJ, Van Der Werf R, Jongbloed JDH, Paulus WJ, et al. Peripartum cardiomyopathy as a part of familial dilated cardiomyopathy. Circulation. 2010;121(20):2169–75.
36. Kryczka KE, Dzielińska Z, Franaszczyk M, Wojtkowska I, Henzel J, Śpiewak M, et al. Severe course of peripartum cardiomyopathy and subsequent recovery in a patient with a novel TTN gene-truncating mutation. Am J Case Rep. 2018;19:820–4.
37. Spracklen TF, Chakafana G, Schwartz PJ, Kotta MC, Shaboodien G, Ntusi NAB, et al. Genetics of peripartum cardiomyopathy: current knowledge, future directions and clinical implications. Genes. 2021;12(1):103.
38. Horne BD, Rasmusson KD, Alharethi R, Budge D, Brunisholz KD, Metz T, et al. Genome-wide significance and replication of the chromosome 12p11.22 locus near the *PTHLH* gene for peripartum cardiomyopathy. Circ Cardiovasc Genet. 2011;4(4):359–66.
39. Chung E, Leinwand LA. Pregnancy as a cardiac stress model. Cardiovasc Res. 2014;101(4):561–70.
40. Van Hagen IM, Roos-Hesselink JW. Aorta pathology and pregnancy. Best Pract Res Clin Obstet Gynaecol. 2014;28(4):537–50.
41. Ramage K, Grabowska K, Silversides C, Quan H, Metcalfe A. Maternal, pregnancy, and neonatal outcomes for women with Marfan syndrome. Birth Defects Res. 2020;112(20):1802–8.
42. Goland S, Elkayam U. Pregnancy and Marfan syndrome. Ann Cardiothorac Surg. 2017;6(6):642–53.
43. Varrias D, Spanos M, Kokkinidis DG, Zoumpourlis P, Kalaitzopoulos DR. Venous thromboembolism in pregnancy: challenges and solutions. Vasc Health Risk Manag. 2023;19:469–84.
44. Heit JA, Phelps MA, Ward SA, Slusser JP, Petterson TM, De Andrade M. Familial segregation of venous thromboembolism. J Thromb Haemost. 2004;2(5):731–6.
45. Ziakas PD, Poulou LS, Pavlou M, Zintzaras E. Thrombophilia and venous thromboembolism in pregnancy: a meta-analysis of genetic risk. Eur J Obstet Gynecol Reprod Biol. 2015;191:106–11.
46. Zotz RB, Gerhardt A, Scharf RE. Inherited thrombophilia and gestational venous thromboembolism. Best Pract Res Clin Haematol. 2003;16(2):243–59.
47. Broni EK, Ndumele CE, Echouffo-Tcheugui JB, Kalyani RR, Bennett WL, Michos ED. The diabetes-cardiovascular connection in women: understanding the known risks. Outcomes, and implications for care. Curr Diab Rep. 2022;22(1):11–25.
48. Beaney KE, Ward CE, Bappa DAS, McGale N, Davies AK, Hirani SP, et al. A 19-SNP coronary heart disease gene score profile in subjects with type 2 diabetes: the coronary heart disease risk in type 2 dia-

betes (CoRDia study) study baseline characteristics. Cardiovasc Diabetol. 2016;15(1):141.
49. Davies AK, McGale N, Humphries SE, Hirani SP, Beaney KE, Bappa DAS, et al. Effectiveness of a self-management intervention with personalised genetic and lifestyle-related risk information on coronary heart disease and diabetes-related risk in type 2 diabetes (CoRDia): study protocol for a randomised controlled trial. Trials. 2015;16(1):547.
50. Jones DA, Prior SL, Tang TS, Bain SC, Hurel SJ, Humphries SE, et al. Association between the rs4880 superoxide dismutase 2 (C>T) gene variant and coronary heart disease in diabetes mellitus. Diabetes Res Clin Pract. 2010;90(2):196–201.
51. Hasbani NR, Westerman KE, Kwak SH, Chen H, Li X, Di Corpo D, et al. Type 2 diabetes modifies the association of CAD genomic risk variants with subclinical atherosclerosis. Circ Genomic Precis Med. 2023;16(6):e004176. https://www.ahajournals.org/doi/10.1161/CIRCGEN.123.004176.
52. Chan KHK, Huang YT, Meng Q, Wu C, Reiner A, Sobel EM, et al. Shared molecular pathways and gene networks for cardiovascular disease and type 2 diabetes mellitus in women across diverse ethnicities. Circ Cardiovasc Genet. 2014;7(6):911–9.
53. The Million Veteran Program, Evangelou E, Warren HR, Mosen-Ansorena D, Mifsud B, Pazoki R, et al. Genetic analysis of over 1 million people identifies 535 new loci associated with blood pressure traits. Nat Genet. 2018;50(10):1412–25.
54. Kurniansyah N, Goodman MO, Khan AT, Wang J, Feofanova E, Bis JC, et al. Evaluating the use of blood pressure polygenic risk scores across race/ethnic background groups. Nat Commun. 2023;14(1):3202.
55. Cho SB, Jang J. A genome-wide association study of a Korean population identifies genetic susceptibility to hypertension based on sex-specific differences. Genes. 2021;12(11):1804.
56. Shetty NS, Pampana A, Patel N, Yerabolu K, Patel G, Irvin MR, Natarajan P, Lin HJ, Guo X, Rich SS, Rotter JI, Li P, Arora G, Arora P. Sex differences in the association of multiethnic genome-wide blood pressure polygenic risk score with population-level systolic blood pressure trajectories. Circ Genom Precis Med. 2024;17(2):e004515.
57. Mishra A, Malik R, Hachiya T, Jürgenson T, Namba S, Posner DC. Stroke genetics informs drug discovery and risk prediction across ancestries. Nature. 2022;611(7934):115–23.
58. Traylor M, Rutten-Jacobs LCA, Holliday EG, Malik R, Sudlow C, Rothwell PM, et al. Differences in common genetic predisposition to ischemic stroke by age and sex. Stroke. 2015;46(11):3042–7.
59. Zhang F, Fu C, Deng Y, Zhang M, Peng H, Li W, et al. Association of CASZ1 genetic variants with stroke risk in the Chinese population. J Stroke Cerebrovasc Dis. 2023;32(8):107169.
60. Mo XB, Zhang H, Wang AL, Xu T, Zhang YH. Integrative analysis identifies the association between *CASZ1* methylation and ischemic stroke. Neurol Genet. 2020;6(5):e509.
61. Kiando SR, Tucker NR, Castro-Vega LJ, Katz A, D'Escamard V, Tréard C, et al. PHACTR1 is a genetic susceptibility locus for fibromuscular dysplasia supporting its complex genetic pattern of inheritance. PLoS Genet. 2016;12(10):e1006367.
62. Richer J, Hill HL, Wang Y, Yang ML, Hunker KL, Lane J, et al. A novel recurrent *COL5A1* genetic variant is associated with a dysplasia-associated arterial disease exhibiting dissections and fibromuscular dysplasia. Arterioscler Thromb Vasc Biol. 2020;40(11):2686–99.
63. Georges A, Albuisson J, Berrandou T, Dupré D, Lorthioir A, D'Escamard V, et al. Rare loss-of-function mutations of *PTGIR* are enriched in fibromuscular dysplasia. Cardiovasc Res. 2021;117(4):1154–65.
64. Georges A, Yang ML, Berrandou TE, Bakker MK, Dikilitas O, Kiando SR, et al. Genetic investigation of fibromuscular dysplasia identifies risk loci and shared genetics with common cardiovascular diseases. Nat Commun. 2021;12(1):6031.
65. Turley TN, Theis JL, Sundsbak RS, Evans JM, O'Byrne MM, Gulati R, et al. Rare missense variants in *TLN1* are associated with familial and sporadic spontaneous coronary artery dissection. Circ Genomic Precis Med. 2019;12(4):e002437.
66. Sun Y, Chen Y, Li Y, Li Z, Li C, Yu T, et al. Association of TSR1 variants and spontaneous coronary artery dissection. J Am Coll Cardiol. 2019;74(2):167–76.
67. Adlam D, Olson TM, Combaret N, Kovacic JC, Iismaa SE, Al-Hussaini A, et al. Association of the PHACTR1/EDN1 genetic locus with spontaneous coronary artery dissection. J Am Coll Cardiol. 2019;73(1):58–66.
68. Adlam D, Berrandou TE, Georges A, Nelson CP, Giannoulatou E, Henry J, et al. Genome-wide association meta-analysis of spontaneous coronary artery dissection identifies risk variants and genes related to artery integrity and tissue-mediated coagulation. Nat Genet. 2023;55(6):964–72.
69. Severino P, D'Amato A, Prosperi S, Myftari V, Colombo L, Tomarelli E, et al. Myocardial infarction with non-obstructive coronary arteries (MINOCA): focus on coronary microvascular dysfunction and genetic susceptibility. J Clin Med. 2023;12(10):3586.
70. Ford TJ, Ong P, Sechtem U, Beltrame J, Camici PG, Crea F, et al. Assessment of vascular dysfunction in patients without obstructive coronary artery disease. JACC Cardiovasc Interv. 2020;13(16):1847–64.
71. Pósfai É, Marton I, Borbényi Z, Nemes A. Myocardial infarction as a thrombotic complication of essential thrombocythemia and polycythemia vera. Anatol J Cardiol. 2016;16(6):397–402.
72. Pacheco Claudio C, Quesada O, Pepine CJ, Merz CNB. Why names matter for women: MINOCA/INOCA (myocardial infarction/ischemia and no

obstructive coronary artery disease). Clin Cardiol. 2018;41(2):185–93.
73. Masarone D, Maddaloni V, Rubino M, Fratta F, Cirillo A, Spinelli Barrile L, et al. Pathogenesis of takotsubo syndrome. Cardiogenetics. 2017;6(1):5973.
74. Ferradini V, Vacca D, Belmonte B, Mango R, Scola L, Novelli G, et al. Genetic and epigenetic factors of takotsubo syndrome: a systematic review. Int J Mol Sci. 2021;22(18):9875.
75. Murakami T, Yoshikawa T, Maekawa Y, Ueda T, Isogai T, Konishi Y, et al. Characterization of predictors of in-hospital cardiac complications of takotsubo cardiomyopathy: multi-center registry from Tokyo CCU Network. J Cardiol. 2014;63(4):269–73.
76. Eitel I, Moeller C, Munz M, Stiermaier T, Meitinger T, Thiele H, et al. Genome-wide association study in takotsubo syndrome—preliminary results and future directions. Int J Cardiol. 2017;236:335–9.

Aortic Pathology and Peripheral Arterial Disease in Women

M. Teraa and C. E. V. B. Hazenberg

Abstract

Cardiovascular diseases (CVD) represent a major health care burden and are the leading cause of mortality in Western Society. Of the CVD lower limb peripheral arterial disease (PAD) is understudied despite its high global prevalence (>230 million people), which is expected to increase substantially in the next decades, and its excessively high risk of major adverse cardiovascular (MACE) and limb events (MALE). Another vascular disease that has major impact on survival, despite a global declining prevalence, are abdominal aortic aneurysms (AAA). Both PAD and AAA have sex-specific characteristics.

In general women are less likely to receive secondary preventive medical management according to guidelines. Although prevalence of PAD in women is at least similar to that in men, women present more often with atypical symptoms. Moreover, women are less likely to undergo revascularization for PAD, and often at a later stage and older age. Furthermore, they tend to undergo less open revascularizations than men. Despite these differences reported sex-specific prognosis of PAD is divergent.

The prevalence of AAA is lower in women than in men, however women with AAA do much worse than men. AAA in women tend to grow faster and women are more often not suitable for regular endovascular aneurysm repair (EVAR). Furthermore, women have higher complication and mortality rates after both elective and emergent repair (both open and endovascular).

Undoubtedly, sex plays an important role in the prevalence, management and outcome of both PAD and AAA. Female specific data is often lacking and women are underrepresented in clinical studies. Future studies should aim to increase the engagement of women in clinical trials and at least report sex-specific data to improve knowledge on and outcome of CVD in women.

Keywords

Aortic pathology · Aneurysm · Peripheral arterial disease · Women · Sex-specific

M. Teraa (✉) · C. E. V. B. Hazenberg
Department of Vascular Surgery, University Medical Center Utrecht, Utrecht, The Netherlands
e-mail: m.teraa@umcutrecht.nl; c.e.v.b.hazenberg@umcutrecht.nl

A. H.E.M. Maas, E. Gerdts (eds.), *Manual of Cardiovascular Disease in Women*,
https://doi.org/10.1007/978-3-031-65952-2_30

Test your learning and check your understanding of this book's contents: use the "Springer Nature Flashcards" app to access questions using ▶ https://sn.pub/51ny7m
To use the app, please follow the instructions in chapter 1.

1 Introduction

Cardiovascular diseases (CVD) represent a major global health care burden and are the leading cause of death in Western Society [1]. Moreover, atherosclerotic vascular disease is the major cause of myocardial infarction, stroke, and limb amputation. There are three major manifestations of atherosclerosis: coronary (CAD), cerebrovascular (CeVD), and peripheral arterial disease (PAD). As compared to CAD and CeVD, PAD is under-studied, despite the fact that it affects over 230 million people worldwide [2] and is associated with the highest morbidity and mortality rates. Compared to CAD, PAD patients face 1.5–2.0 times higher risk of major adverse cardiovascular (MACE) or limb events (MALE) [3]. PAD is a growing health issue with a global prevalence increasing >20% over the past decade with even steeper increases expected for the next decade [2]. Although the prevalence is higher in high-income countries, the bulk of the disease burden resides in low- and middle-income countries [2].

Despite the fact that CAD, CeVD, and PAD are often considered the main clinical presentations of CVD, aortic pathology is another important vascular disease with considerable global impact. The aorta can be affected by a wide range of pathologies, however the most common are the abdominal aortic aneurysm (AAA) and the acute aortic syndrome (AAS). In general AAS consist of acute aortic dissection (AAD), intramural hematoma (IMH), and penetrating aortic ulcer (PAU) [4]. In contrast to PAD the prevalence of AAAs are declining the past decades and current prevalence in men >65 years of age varies roughly between 1% and 5% based on data of several screening programs [5]. This decline in prevalence goes hand in hand with a reduction in the number of acute (ruptured) AAAs [5]. However, despite these facts the disease has an important impact on cardiovascular prognosis with the highest risk of recurrent cardiovascular events (defined as myocardial infarction, ischemic stroke, or cardiovascular death) compared to CAD, CeVD and PAD [6].

Sex-specific differences have been widely described in a wide range of diseases and have also been considered a factor in CVD. However, its role has been underrated and only recently received increasing attention as an important factor in epidemiology, modifier of risk and treatment effect (both medical as well as invasive interventions), prognostic factor and also determinant of treatment decisions [7]. And sex does not only influence prevalence of well-known risk factors, such as age, smoking, hypertension, and diabetes mellitus, but adds an extra layer by modifying the impact of these risk factors in development and progression of CVD [7]. Despite the sex-related influences in CVD, women are understudied and data often extrapolated from studies in predominantly male. To improve treatment and ultimate prognosis of CVD in women it is of utmost importance to appreciate these differences in basic science and augment female participation in translational and clinical studies [8].

The aim of this book chapter is to discuss the role of sex on epidemiology, treatment decisions, and outcome of interventions for and general prognosis of aortic pathology and PAD. For the purpose of this chapter we will focus on the biological phenomenon of sex rather than the psychosocial construct of gender, unless otherwise specified [9]. Furthermore, PAD is used to refer to lower-extremity PAD unless stated differently and the chapter does not focus on congenital or soft tissue disease-related aortic pathology.

2 Secondary Prevention and Medical Management

Medical therapy should be initiated in all patients that suffer from CVD in order to reduce its adverse effects and hence improve prognosis of the presenting disease, but also to reduce risk of recurring cardiovascular events. Cornerstone of secondary prevention are smoking cessation, optimal glucose regulation, antithrombotic, lipid-lowering, and anti-hypertensive drugs. However, current guidelines are mainly based on data derived from men, as women are generally and still underrepresented in studies and clinical trials [10, 11]. Moreover, sex-specific results are often not reported, which further hampers knowledge of treatment effects in women per se.

The fact that women are underrepresented in studies on secondary prevention of CVD leads to lack of knowledge on sex-specific effects. This is important since effects of risk factors and of therapeutic interventions are not necessarily identical in women and men. For instance smoking and hypertension are associated with a higher risk of developing PAD in women than in men [12–14]. On the other hand presence of diabetes seems to elevate the risk of limb amputation more excessively in men than in women [15], but risk of CVD-related mortality is higher in women with diabetes [16, 17]. Furthermore, differential effects of antihypertensive [18] and antithrombotic drugs [19] have been reported in men and women. All these factors underline that sex-specific data are essential to optimal medical management of CVD in women.

Although the risk of CVD and recurrent events in women is at least as high as in men [20], women are less likely to meet guideline-directed therapy. Several studies and reviews have shown that secondary prevention in men was more often in line with guidelines than in women. The suboptimal management in women was displayed along the whole spectrum of secondary prevention, i.e. antihypertensive drugs, statins, antithrombotic drugs [19, 20]. Moreover, this difference persisted even after revascularization in PAD [21, 22] and even in those patients with premature atherosclerotic CVD [23]. These data underline the need for increased awareness of CVD in women and sex-specific effects in CVD management in order to optimize CVD treatment and hence outcomes in women.

3 Aortic Pathology in Women

The sex-specific differences in aortic pathology and related etiology, preoperative standard of care and rupture risk, and perioperative outcome after (acute) repair is not fully understood and the center of interest the last two decades [24].

3.1 Epidemiology

Abdominal aortic aneurysm (AAA) is 4–6 times less common in women than in men (prevalence men 7.6% vs women 1.3%) [25, 26]. However, its nature seems to be more aggressive in terms of progression; growth rate is twice as fast in women [27–29]. Furthermore, women are at a higher age at diagnosis and therapy, and consequently have a greater number of comorbidities [30]. The role of hormonal, genetic, and anatomical differences in women and men are still largely unresolved.

In general, AAA prevalence and incidence rates declined worldwide [5, 31, 32] and consequently a decrease of ruptured AAA (rAAA) has been reported in the last two decades, partially due to a decline in smoking, optimization of cardiovascular risk management and population screening programs [33–35].

3.2 Treatment

Large national vascular registries and databases showed that preoperative standard of care for AAA, in terms of waiting times, receipt of perioperative medication and secondary cardiac prevention was inferior in women in the US compared with men [36], and that women in the UK were less likely to undergo an intervention for AAA [36]. AAA repair should be considered in women with an aortic diameter of 5.0 cm according to international guidelines (European Society for Vascular Surgery (ESVS) 5.0 cm [5]; Society for Vascular Surgery (SVS) 5.0–5.4 cm) [37]. This sex-specific threshold in women is smaller compared with men (5.5 cm) and is probably the result of (baseline) disparities in aortic anatomy, the aortic diameter measurements being circa 2–6 mm smaller in women compared to men [38, 39].

Compared with elective open AAA repair (OAR), endovascular repair (EVAR) is less invasive and results in a lower peri-operative mortality risk and better outcome during the first 6 months [40]. Regarding morphological suitability for endovascular repair (EVAR), a smaller proportion of women are eligible for EVAR (estimation 34% according the manufacturers' instruction for use (IFU)) compared with men [41]. Hostile aneurysm necks (short and angulated) and more narrow access iliac arteries are more often present in women, which may be an explanation why a higher portion of women are not offered intervention [41]. To overcome these issues, newer generation or sex-dedicated endografts have been developed the last decade. Technical advances in endograft design have led to lower profile introduction systems, increased conformability and wider IFUs. The relation of sex and unfavorable aneurysm morphology present in women are not well studied and further endograft development and future studies are an important element in optimized AAA intervention in women.

3.3 Outcomes and Prognosis

Peri-operative mortality is much higher in women, and mid- and long-term survival rate is lower, after both OAR and EVAR, and both in the emergency as well as the elective setting. A recent systematic review and meta-analysis showed that women had a higher incidence of transfusion, pulmonary and bowel complications after elective EVAR and AOR [42], which presumably contribute to higher 30 days mortality rate compared with men. In particular post-EVAR women encounter more cardiac, arterial injury and thrombo-embolic complications resulting in bowel, renal and limb ischemia. Also long term data seem to show that women fare worse after elective EVAR with respect to overall (5-year) survival [43]. The same unfavorable trend has been observed for women after complex endovascular aortic repair (fenestrated-branched EVAR for pararenal aortic aneurysm). In one recent multicenter study as well as two monocenter studies, female sex was associated with worse outcomes in terms of technical success (e.g. target vessel patency) [44–46]. Furthermore, both single center studies reported that female sex was an independent predictor of peri-operative complications and in-hospital mortality (OR 2.836, 95% CI: 1.510–5.328 [46] and OR 10.135, 95% CI 2.264–45.369 [45]), in contrast to the multicenter study which reports similar 30-day mortality rates. Further studies should be conducted to demonstrate sex differences in outcomes after OAR and EVAR of abdominal aneurysms for further optimization of treatment outcomes in women.

3.4 Acute Aortic Syndrome

Another entity, acute aortic syndromes (AAS) including acute aortic dissection (AAD, Stanford type A and B), intramural hematoma (IMH), and penetrating aortic ulcer (PAU), is associated with high mortality risk and require immediate diagnosis and treatment [4]. AAD is the most prevalent form of AAS. As in thoracic aortic aneurysms, the minority of AAD patients are women (approximately 30–40%) [47–50]. Women present at an older age than men, and experience a delay in presentation and diagnosis, possibly because the onset of symptoms in AAD in women is less acute and seem to be less ominous at presentation [51]. Sex-specific data in AAD and AAS in general and its management are scarce. A better understanding of the sex differences is warranted in the near future for guidance towards a more tailor made and optimal management of AAS.

4 Peripheral Arterial Disease in Women

4.1 Epidemiology

Traditionally PAD has been considered a disease of the male, but prevalence of PAD in women seems at least equal to that in men [2, 52]. True prevalence of PAD is likely to be higher than the reported rates as PAD is often asymptomatic or patients present with atypical symptoms, which is more often present in women [53]. This could lead to a more pronounced underestimation of the PAD burden in women. PAD is related to the worst outcomes of the atherosclerotic CVD, with highest risk of MACE and MALE [3] and recurrent cardiovascular events [6]. Moreover, prevalence of PAD seems to increase more rapid in women than in men [54, 55] and they might experience more negative PAD-related effects, such as PAD-related mortality and disability [56]. Despite these figures women are undertreated not only medically, but also with respect to revascularization for PAD.

4.2 Revascularization Strategies

In line with data on secondary prevention contemporary sex-specific revascularization patterns and outcomes are still poorly understood and understudied. Women are not only underrepresented in drug trials, but also in studies that focus on revascularization for PAD [20]. Despite more focus on sex-specific differences the underrepresentation of women in interventional studies has not changed over time, for instance the percentage of women included in the recently published BASIL-2 and BEST-CLI trials that studied endovascular compared to open revascularization in CLTI varied between 17% and 28% [57, 58].

In general there are data that suggest a differential approach to revascularization in women compared to men. Data suggest that women are less likely to undergo revascularization, often at an older age and at a more advanced stage of the disease [59, 60]. A large registry-study from the United States based on over one million hospitalizations for vascular surgery showed that—corrected for severity of disease—women are up to 30% less likely to be revascularized than men [61]. A large VASCUNET analysis showed that this pattern is consistent over countries, although large regional differences exist [59].

Not only the likelihood to undergo and the stage at which revascularization is performed for PAD is influenced by sex. Also the method used for revascularization, either open or endovascular, is influenced by sex. Most studies have shown that women, when revascularized, tend to undergo more often endovascular than open surgical revascularization compared to their male counterparts [59, 61–63]. The exact reasons for this disparity are not clear, but they might be influenced by anatomical factors, disease stage at which they present, and perceived risk of open surgery. Future studies should help elucidate these differences.

4.3 Outcomes and Prognosis

Some of the data on sex differences are quite consistent, but some are more contradictive, which is true for outcomes of PAD. Outcomes of patients that undergo revascularization for PAD have not been reported unequivocally worse in women [64–66] or in men [60, 67, 68]. For instance a recent French registry-study in almost 250,000 patients that underwent revascularization for PAD showed that 1 year risk of mortality was higher in women (7.7% vs 5.9%, $p < 0.001$) and that of amputation was lower (3.7% vs 3.9%, $p = 0.005$) in univariate analyses. However, after adjustment for potential confounding factors risk of both amputation and mortality was lower for women (adjusted OR 1.20; 95%CI 1.15–1.26 and OR 1.13; 95%CI 1.09–1.17) [60]. On the other hand a recently published meta-analysis that studied outcomes after endovascular intervention for CLTI suggested worse outcomes with respect to limb loss and MALE in women [66]. Moreover, there are also data that suggests that sex-differences post-revascularization might depend on the stage of the disease (intermittent claudication vs CLTI) [69]. Overall, this suggests that sex influences treatment and outcome of PAD, but also underlines the immense knowledge gap.

The influence of sex on outcomes of PAD after revascularization is obviously not that simple. Results depend on the type of intervention and outcome considered, but also the study cited [70]. The discrepant results are likely due to factors, such as selection of the patient population, regional differences, co-morbidities, baseline characteristics, concurrent medical treatment, and analytical methods. While the exact reasons are not entirely clear, they do underline the importance for studies to focus on female patients and to also report sex-specific outcomes to further increase insight in the sex differences with respect to outcomes in PAD and to elucidate the underlying mechanisms.

5 Conclusions

Women with PAD and AAA are not simple copies of their male counterparts, but represent a separate entity and would require a dedicated approach. Women are underrepresented in clinical studies and data from studies including predominantly men are extrapolated to women. Because of the important differences future studies should focus on increased engagement of women in clinical studies and at least report female specific data in order to increase knowledge on CVD in women and ultimately improve their clinical management and treatment outcomes.

Key Issues

- CVD has an important global health impact on women.
- Women are underrepresented in clinical studies on PAD and AAA.
- Women are less likely to meet guideline-directed secondary prevention than men.
- AAA prevalence is lower in women, but their outcomes are worse for both open and endovascular repairs.
- Prevalence of PAD is at least similar in women and men.
- Women with PAD more often present with atypical leg symptoms.
- Women with PAD are less likely to undergo revascularization, and at an older age and later stage.
- Future studies in CVD should focus more on sex-specific data and increased engagement of women in clinical studies.

Questions and Answers

1. Do smoking and hypertension have a more pronounced effect on the development of PAD in men?

   Correct answer: Smoking and hypertension are associated with a higher risk of developing PAD in women than in men [12–14].
2. Although secondary prevention in women is less often in line with treatment guidelines, this differences compared to men disappear after revascularization. True or false?

   Correct answer: The suboptimal management in women was displayed along the whole spectrum of secondary prevention, i.e. antihypertensive drugs, statins, antithrombotic drugs [19, 20]. Moreover, this difference persisted even after revascularization in PAD [21, 22] and even in those patients with premature atherosclerotic CVD [23].
3. If women with PAD are compared to men they undergo more often open or endovascular revascularization?

   Correct answer: Most studies have shown that women, when revascularized, tend to undergo more often endovascular than open surgical revascularization compared to their male counterparts [59, 61–63].
4. Which is true for the relation of women and AAA:
   (A) Prevalence of AAA is higher in women
   (B) Women are less likely to meet EVAR's instruction for use (IFU)
   (C) Women do better after open repair than men
   (D) Peri-operative mortality after EVAR is higher in women, but long-term outcomes are better
   (E) Both B and D are true

   Correct answer: B

Regarding morphological suitability for endovascular repair (EVAR), a smaller proportion of women are eligible for EVAR (estimation 34% according the manufacturers' instruction for use (IFU)) compared with men [41].

References

1. Virani SS, Alonso A, Aparicio HJ, Benjamin EJ, Bittencourt MS, Callaway CW, et al. Heart disease and stroke statistics-2021 update: a report from the American Heart Association. Circulation. 2021;143(8):e254–743. http://www.ncbi.nlm.nih.gov/pubmed/33501848.
2. Song P, Rudan D, Zhu Y, Fowkes FJI, Rahimi K, Fowkes FGR, et al. Global, regional, and national prevalence and risk factors for peripheral artery disease in 2015: an updated systematic review and analysis. Lancet Glob Health. 2019;7(8):e1020–30. http://www.ncbi.nlm.nih.gov/pubmed/31303293.
3. Eikelboom JW, Connolly SJ, Bosch J, Dagenais GR, Hart RG, Shestakovska O, et al. Rivaroxaban with or without aspirin in stable cardiovascular disease. N Engl J Med. 2017;377(14):1319–30. https://pubmed.ncbi.nlm.nih.gov/28844192/.
4. Writing Committee Members, Isselbacher EM, Preventza O, Hamilton Black Iii J, Augoustides JG, Beck AW, et al. 2022 ACC/AHA guideline for the diagnosis and management of aortic disease: a report of the American Heart Association/American College of Cardiology Joint Committee on clinical practice guidelines. J Am Coll Cardiol. 2022;80(24):e223–393.
5. Wanhainen A, Verzini F, Van Herzeele I, Allaire E, Bown M, Cohnert T, et al. Editor's choice—European Society for Vascular Surgery (ESVS) 2019 clinical practice guidelines on the management of abdominal aorto-iliac artery aneurysms. Eur J Vasc Endovasc Surg. 2019;57(1):8–93. http://www.ncbi.nlm.nih.gov/pubmed/30528142.
6. Burger PM, Pradhan AD, Dorresteijn JAN, Koudstaal S, Teraa M, de Borst GJ, et al. C-reactive protein and risk of cardiovascular events and mortality in patients with various cardiovascular disease locations. Am J Cardiol. 2023;197:13–23. http://www.ncbi.nlm.nih.gov/pubmed/37218417.
7. Wenger NK, Lloyd-Jones DM, Elkind MSV, Fonarow GC, Warner JJ, Alger HM, et al. Call to action for cardiovascular disease in women: epidemiology, awareness, access, and delivery of equitable health care: a presidential advisory from the American Heart Association. Circulation. 2022;145(23):e1059–71. http://www.ncbi.nlm.nih.gov/pubmed/35531777.
8. Boulware LE, Corbie G, Aguilar-Gaxiola S, Wilkins CH, Ruiz R, Vitale A, et al. Combating structural inequities—diversity, equity, and inclusion in clinical and translational research. N Engl J Med. 2022;386(3):201–3. http://www.ncbi.nlm.nih.gov/pubmed/35029847.
9. Rossi AM, Pilote L. Let's talk about sex and gender! Circ Cardiovasc Qual Outcomes. 2016;9(2 Suppl 1):S100–1. http://www.ncbi.nlm.nih.gov/pubmed/26908854.
10. Hirsch AT, Allison MA, Gomes AS, Corriere MA, Duval S, Ershow AG, et al. A call to action: women and peripheral artery disease: a scientific statement from the American Heart Association. Circulation. 2012;125(11):1449–72. http://www.ncbi.nlm.nih.gov/pubmed/22343782.
11. Mayor JM, Preventza O, McGinigle K, Mills JL, Montero-Baker M, Gilani R, et al. Persistent underrepresentation of female patients in United States trials of common vascular diseases from 2008 to 2020. J Vasc Surg. 2022;75(1):30–6. http://www.ncbi.nlm.nih.gov/pubmed/34438003.
12. Gerhard M, Baum P, Raby KE. Peripheral arterial-vascular disease in women: prevalence, prognosis, and treatment. Cardiology. 1995;86(4):349–55. http://www.ncbi.nlm.nih.gov/pubmed/7553710.
13. Hiramoto JS, Katz R, Weisman S, Conte M. Gender-specific risk factors for peripheral artery disease in a voluntary screening population. J Am Heart Assoc. 2014;3(2):e000651. http://www.ncbi.nlm.nih.gov/pubmed/24627420.
14. Kannel WB, McGee DL. Update on some epidemiologic features of intermittent claudication: the Framingham Study. J Am Geriatr Soc. 1985;33(1):13–8. http://www.ncbi.nlm.nih.gov/pubmed/3965550.
15. Fan L, Wu XJ. Sex difference for the risk of amputation in diabetic patients: a systematic review and meta-analysis. PLoS One. 2021;16(3):e0243797. http://www.ncbi.nlm.nih.gov/pubmed/33705430.
16. Huxley RR, Peters SAE, Mishra GD, Woodward M. Risk of all-cause mortality and vascular events in women versus men with type 1 diabetes: a systematic review and meta-analysis. Lancet Diabetes Endocrinol. 2015;3(3):198–206. http://www.ncbi.nlm.nih.gov/pubmed/25660575.
17. Gregg EW, Gu Q, Cheng YJ, Narayan KMV, Cowie CC. Mortality trends in men and women with diabetes, 1971 to 2000. Ann Intern Med. 2007;147(3):149–55. http://www.ncbi.nlm.nih.gov/pubmed/17576993.
18. Kalibala J, Pechère-Bertschi A, Desmeules J. Gender differences in cardiovascular pharmacotherapy-the example of hypertension: a mini review. Front Pharmacol. 2020;11:564. http://www.ncbi.nlm.nih.gov/pubmed/32435193.
19. Gasecka A, Zimodro JM, Appelman Y. Sex differences in antiplatelet therapy: state-of-the art. Platelets. 2023;34(1):2176173. http://www.ncbi.nlm.nih.gov/pubmed/36809993.
20. Pabon M, Cheng S, Altin SE, Sethi SS, Nelson MD, Moreau KL, et al. Sex differences in peripheral artery disease. Circ Res. 2022;130(4):496–511. http://www.ncbi.nlm.nih.gov/pubmed/35175843.

21. Altin SE, Castro-Dominguez YS, Kennedy KF, Orion KC, Lanksy AJ, Abbott JD, et al. Predictors of underutilization of medical therapy in patients undergoing endovascular revascularization for peripheral artery disease. JACC Cardiovasc Interv. 2020;13(24):2911–8. http://www.ncbi.nlm.nih.gov/pubmed/33357529.
22. Singh N, Ding L, Magee GA, Shavelle DM, Kashyap VS, Garg PK. Discharge prescription patterns for antiplatelet therapy following lower extremity peripheral vascular intervention. Circ Cardiovasc Interv. 2020;13(8):e008791. http://www.ncbi.nlm.nih.gov/pubmed/32791948.
23. Lee MT, Mahtta D, Ramsey DJ, Liu J, Misra A, Nasir K, et al. Sex-related disparities in cardiovascular health care among patients with premature atherosclerotic cardiovascular disease. JAMA Cardiol. 2021;6(7):782–90. http://www.ncbi.nlm.nih.gov/pubmed/33881448.
24. Hoel AW, Kayssi A, Brahmanandam S, Belkin M, Conte MS, Nguyen LL. Under-representation of women and ethnic minorities in vascular surgery randomized controlled trials. J Vasc Surg. 2009;50(2):349–54.
25. Starr JE, Halpern V. Abdominal aortic aneurysms in women. J Vasc Surg. 2013;57(4 Suppl):3S–10S.
26. Pleumeekers HJ, Hoes AW, van der Does E, van Urk H, Hofman A, de Jong PT, et al. Aneurysms of the abdominal aorta in older adults. The Rotterdam Study. Am J Epidemiol. 1995;142(12):1291–9.
27. Lo RC, Schermerhorn ML. Abdominal aortic aneurysms in women. J Vasc Surg. 2016;63(3):839–44.
28. Cheung K, Boodhwani M, Chan KL, Beauchesne L, Dick A, Coutinho T. Thoracic aortic aneurysm growth: role of sex and aneurysm etiology. J Am Heart Assoc. 2017;6(2):e003792.
29. Mofidi R, Goldie VJ, Kelman J, Dawson ARW, Murie JA, Chalmers RTA. Influence of sex on expansion rate of abdominal aortic aneurysms. Br J Surg. 2007;94(3):310–4.
30. Stoberock K, Kölbel T, Atlihan G, Debus ES, Tsilimparis N, Larena-Avellaneda A, et al. Gender differences in abdominal aortic aneurysm therapy—a systematic review. Vasa. 2018;47(4):267–71.
31. Sampson UKA, Norman PE, Fowkes FGR, Aboyans V, Song Y, Harrell FE, et al. Estimation of global and regional incidence and prevalence of abdominal aortic aneurysms 1990 to 2010. Glob Heart. 2014;9(1):159–70.
32. Sidloff D, Stather P, Dattani N, Bown M, Thompson J, Sayers R, et al. Aneurysm global epidemiology study: public health measures can further reduce abdominal aortic aneurysm mortality. Circulation. 2014;129(7):747–53.
33. Dreyer SB, Burns P. Ruptured abdominal aortic aneurysms: decreasing incidence may reduce the impact of a Scottish screening programme. Scott Med J. 2015;60(1):23–8.
34. Laine MT, Laukontaus SJ, Kantonen I, Venermo M. Population-based study of ruptured abdominal aortic aneurysm. Br J Surg. 2016;103(12):1634–9.
35. Schermerhorn ML, Bensley RP, Giles KA, Hurks R, et al. Changes in abdominal aortic aneurysm rupture and short-term mortality, 1995-2008: a retrospective observational study. Ann Surg. 2012;256(4):651–8.
36. Pouncey AL, Sweeting MJ, Bicknell C, Powell JT. Sex-specific differences in the standard of care for infrarenal abdominal aortic aneurysm repair, and risk of major adverse cardiovascular events and death. Br J Surg. 2023;110(4):481–8.
37. Chaikof EL, Dalman RL, Eskandari MK, Jackson BM, Lee WA, Mansour MA, et al. The Society for Vascular Surgery practice guidelines on the care of patients with an abdominal aortic aneurysm. J Vasc Surg. 2018;67(1):2–77.e2.
38. Wanhainen A, Themudo R, Ahlström H, Lind L, Johansson L. Thoracic and abdominal aortic dimension in 70-year-old men and women--a population-based whole-body magnetic resonance imaging (MRI) study. J Vasc Surg. 2008;47(3):504–12.
39. Rogers IS, Massaro JM, Truong QA, Mahabadi AA, Kriegel MF, Fox CS, et al. Distribution, determinants, and normal reference values of thoracic and abdominal aortic diameters by computed tomography (from the Framingham Heart Study). Am J Cardiol. 2013;111(10):1510–6.
40. Antoniou GA, Antoniou SA, Torella F. Editor's choice—Endovascular vs. open repair for abdominal aortic aneurysm: systematic review and meta-analysis of updated peri-operative and long term data of randomised controlled trials. Eur J Vasc Endovasc Surg. 2020;59(3):385–97.
41. Ulug P, Sweeting MJ, von Allmen RS, Thompson SG, Powell JT, SWAN Collaborators. Morphological suitability for endovascular repair, non-intervention rates, and operative mortality in women and men assessed for intact abdominal aortic aneurysm repair: systematic reviews with meta-analysis. Lancet. 2017;389(10088):2482–91.
42. Pouncey AL, David M, Morris RI, Ulug P, Martin G, Bicknell C, et al. Editor's choice—Systematic review and meta-analysis of sex specific differences in adverse events after open and endovascular intact abdominal aortic aneurysm repair: consistently worse outcomes for women. Eur J Vasc Endovasc Surg. 2021;62(3):367–78.
43. Corsi T, Ciaramella MA, Palte NK, Carlson JP, Rahimi SA, Beckerman WE. Female sex is associated with reintervention and mortality following elective endovascular abdominal aortic aneurysm repair. J Vasc Surg. 2022;76(6):1494–1501.e1.
44. Edman NI, Schanzer A, Crawford A, Oderich GS, Farber MA, Schneider DB, et al. Sex-related outcomes after fenestrated-branched endovascular aneurysm repair for thoracoabdominal aortic aneurysms in the U.S. Fenestrated and Branched Aortic Research Consortium. J Vasc Surg. 2021;74(3):861–70.
45. Behrendt CA, Panuccio G, Kuchenbecker J, Rohlffs F, Heidemann F, Debus ES, et al. How does female sex affect complex endovascular aortic repair? A

single centre cohort study. Eur J Vasc Endovasc Surg. 2021;62(6):849–56.
46. Gontarz B, Majeed R, Staff I, DeMartino R, Jain A, Aitcheson E, et al. Female sex is associated with worse outcomes following complex fenestrated or branched endovascular aortic repair. Ann Vasc Surg. 2022;87:113–23.
47. Cote CL, De Waard D, Kivell M, Fagan A, Horne G, Hassan A, et al. Sex differences in trends in incidence of thoracic aortic aneurysm repair and aortic dissection: 2005-2015. CJC Open. 2022;4(12):1081–9.
48. DeMartino RR, Sen I, Huang Y, Bower TC, Oderich GS, Pochettino A, et al. Population-based assessment of the incidence of aortic dissection, intramural hematoma, and penetrating ulcer, and its associated mortality from 1995 to 2015. Circ Cardiovasc Qual Outcomes. 2018;11(8):e004689.
49. Nienaber CA, Fattori R, Mehta RH, Richartz BM, Evangelista A, Petzsch M, et al. Gender-related differences in acute aortic dissection. Circulation. 2004;109(24):3014–21.
50. Norton EL, Kim KM, Fukuhara S, Wu X, Patel HJ, Deeb GM, et al. Differences among sexes in presentation and outcomes in acute type A aortic dissection repair. J Thorac Cardiovasc Surg. 2023;165(3):972–81.
51. Bhatt N, Chung JCY. Gender differences in acute aortic syndromes. Curr Opin Cardiol. 2023;38(2):75–81.
52. Higgins JP, Higgins JA. Epidemiology of peripheral arterial disease in women. J Epidemiol. 2003;13(1):1–14. http://www.ncbi.nlm.nih.gov/pubmed/12587608.
53. Porras CP, Teraa M, Bots ML, de Boer AR, Peters SAE, van Doorn S, et al. The frequency of primary healthcare contacts preceding the diagnosis of lower-extremity arterial disease: do women consult general practice differently? J Clin Med. 2022;11(13):3666. http://www.ncbi.nlm.nih.gov/pubmed/35806951.
54. Sigvant B, Wiberg-Hedman K, Bergqvist D, Rolandsson O, Andersson B, Persson E, et al. A population-based study of peripheral arterial disease prevalence with special focus on critical limb ischemia and sex differences. J Vasc Surg. 2007;45(6):1185–91. http://www.ncbi.nlm.nih.gov/pubmed/17543683.
55. Walker JP, Hiramoto JS. Diagnosis and management of peripheral artery disease in women. Int J Womens Health. 2012;4:625–34. http://www.ncbi.nlm.nih.gov/pubmed/23277744.
56. Sampson UKA, Fowkes FGR, McDermott MM, Criqui MH, Aboyans V, Norman PE, et al. Global and regional burden of death and disability from peripheral artery disease: 21 world regions, 1990 to 2010. Glob Heart. 2014;9(1):145–158.e21. http://www.ncbi.nlm.nih.gov/pubmed/25432124.
57. Bradbury AW, Moakes CA, Popplewell M, Meecham L, Bate GR, Kelly L, et al. A vein bypass first versus a best endovascular treatment first revascularisation strategy for patients with chronic limb threatening ischaemia who required an infra-popliteal, with or without an additional more proximal infra-inguinal revascularisation procedure to restore limb perfusion (BASIL-2): an open-label, randomised, multicentre, phase 3 trial. Lancet. 2023;401(10390):1798–809. http://www.ncbi.nlm.nih.gov/pubmed/37116524.
58. Farber A, Menard MT, Conte MS, Kaufman JA, Powell RJ, Choudhry NK, et al. Surgery or endovascular therapy for chronic limb-threatening ischemia. N Engl J Med. 2022;387(25):2305–16. http://www.ncbi.nlm.nih.gov/pubmed/36342173.
59. Behrendt CA, Sigvant B, Kuchenbecker J, Grima MJ, Schermerhorn M, Thomson IA, et al. Editor's choice—International variations and sex disparities in the treatment of peripheral arterial occlusive disease: a report from VASCUNET and the International Consortium of Vascular Registries. Eur J Vasc Endovasc Surg. 2020;60(6):873–80. http://www.ncbi.nlm.nih.gov/pubmed/33004283.
60. Raffort J, Lareyre F, Pradier C, Fabre R, Behrendt CA, Bailly L. Editor's choice—Impact of sex on the outcomes of patients undergoing repair for lower extremity peripheral arterial disease in France. Eur J Vasc Endovasc Surg. 2023;65(6):905–6. http://www.ncbi.nlm.nih.gov/pubmed/36858253.
61. McGinigle KL, Browder SE, Strassle PD, Shalhub S, Harris LM, Minc SD. Sex-related disparities in intervention rates and type of intervention in patients with aortic and peripheral arterial diseases in the National Inpatient Sample Database. J Vasc Surg. 2021;73(6):2081–2089.e7. http://www.ncbi.nlm.nih.gov/pubmed/33301865.
62. Lo RC, Bensley RP, Dahlberg SE, Matyal R, Hamdan AD, Wyers M, et al. Presentation, treatment, and outcome differences between men and women undergoing revascularization or amputation for lower extremity peripheral arterial disease. J Vasc Surg. 2014;59(2):409–18.e3. http://www.ncbi.nlm.nih.gov/pubmed/24080134.
63. Freisinger E, Malyar NM, Reinecke H, Unrath M. Low rate of revascularization procedures and poor prognosis particularly in male patients with peripheral artery disease—a propensity score matched analysis. Int J Cardiol. 2018;255:188–94. http://www.ncbi.nlm.nih.gov/pubmed/29329771.
64. Brothers TE, Zhang J, Mauldin PD, Tonnessen BH, Robison JG, Vallabhaneni R, et al. Predicting outcomes for infrapopliteal limb-threatening ischemia using the Society for Vascular Surgery Vascular Quality Initiative. J Vasc Surg. 2016;63(1):114–24.e5. http://www.ncbi.nlm.nih.gov/pubmed/26432282.
65. Lee MHY, Li PY, Li B, Shakespeare A, Samarasinghe Y, Feridooni T, et al. A systematic review and meta-analysis of sex- and gender-based differences in presentation severity and outcomes in adults undergoing major vascular surgery. J Vasc Surg. 2022;76(2):581–94.e25. http://www.ncbi.nlm.nih.gov/pubmed/35257798.
66. Farag N, Pham BL, Aldilli L, Bourque ML, Zigui M, Nauche B, et al. A systematic review and meta-analysis on sex-based disparities in patients with chronic limb threatening ischemia undergoing revas-

cularization. Ann Vasc Surg. 2023;95:317–29. http://www.ncbi.nlm.nih.gov/pubmed/37075836.
67. Gallagher KA, Meltzer AJ, Ravin RA, Graham A, Connolly P, Escobar G, et al. Gender differences in outcomes of endovascular treatment of infrainguinal peripheral artery disease. Vasc Endovascular Surg. 2011;45(8):703–11. http://www.ncbi.nlm.nih.gov/pubmed/21914680.
68. Heidemann F, Kuchenbecker J, Peters F, Kotov A, Marschall U, L'Hoest H, et al. A health insurance claims analysis on the effect of female sex on long-term outcomes after peripheral endovascular interventions for symptomatic peripheral arterial occlusive disease. J Vasc Surg. 2021;74(3):780–7.e7. http://www.ncbi.nlm.nih.gov/pubmed/33647437.
69. Ramkumar N, Suckow BD, Behrendt CA, Mackenzie TA, Sedrakyan A, Brown JR, et al. Association between sex and long-term outcomes of endovascular treatment for peripheral artery disease. Catheter Cardiovasc Interv. 2023;101(5):877–87. http://www.ncbi.nlm.nih.gov/pubmed/36924009.
70. Kim S, Pendleton AA, McGinigle KL. Women's vascular health: peripheral artery disease in female patients. Semin Vasc Surg. 2022;35(2):155–61. http://www.ncbi.nlm.nih.gov/pubmed/35672105.

Cardiovascular Therapy in Women with Hypertension or Heart Failure

Juan Tamargo and Eva Delpón

Abstract

There are sex/gender-related differences (SGRDs) in epidemiology, risk factors, pathophysiology, treatment, and outcomes of cardiovascular diseases as well as in body composition, sex hormonal regulation and drug pharmacokinetics (absorption, distribution, metabolism, and excretion). Thus, it shouldn't be a surprise that women and men may respond differently to guideline-recommended drugs for the treatment of hypertension or heart failure (HTN/HF). However, the clinical relevance of SGRDs in the efficacy, safety and dosing of some guideline-recommended drugs remains uncertain because women were traditionally underrepresented and a sex/gender-specific analysis of clinical results was not regularly performed in many randomized clinical trials. Therefore, many trials were underpowered to examine SGRDs in drug efficacy and safety even if they do exist. As a result, clinical practice guidelines recommend the same drugs and doses for the treatment of women and men with HTN/HF. Despite this recommendation, there is evidence of SGRDs in the clinical efficacy, safety (women develop more frequent and serious adverse reactions) and doses of some drugs used in these patients. A better understanding of the potential SGRDs, the pathophysiological mechanisms involved, and its clinical relevance is critical to optimize the treatment of HTN/HF and improve clinical outcomes in women. This chapter briefly summarizes SGRDs in the pharmacokinetics, efficacy, safety, and optimal doses of guideline-recommended drugs for the treatment of HTN/HF.

Keywords

Sex/gender-related differences · Hypertension
Heart failure · Clinical trials · Adverse drug reactions

J. Tamargo (✉) · E. Delpón
Department of Pharmacology and Toxicology, School of Medicine, Universidad Complutense, Instituto de Investigación Sanitaria Gregorio Marañón, CIBERCV, Madrid, Spain
e-mail: jtamargo@med.ucm.es; edelpon@ucm.es

A. H.E.M. Maas, E. Gerdts (eds.), *Manual of Cardiovascular Disease in Women*,
https://doi.org/10.1007/978-3-031-65952-2_31

Test your learning and check your understanding of this book's contents: use the "Springer Nature Flashcards" app to access questions using ▶ https://sn.pub/51ny7m
To use the app, please follow the instructions in chapter 1.

1 Introduction

Cardiovascular diseases (CVDs) are the leading cause of death and disability wordwide [1–3]. In women, arterial hypertension (HTN) represents the leading modifiable risk factor for all-cause death and early development of cardiovascular disease [4–6], and heart failure (HF) causes ~35% of deaths for cardiovascular causes [7, 8]. Unfortunately, quite often women and heathcare providers underestimate this increased CV risk due to a misperception that women are protected against CVDs which contributes to undertreatment of cardiovascular risk factors and CVDs in women [9, 10].

There are important sex/gender-related differences (SGRDs) in the epidemiology, risk factors, pathophysiology, diagnosis, treatment, and outcomes of CVDs [11–13]. A recent sex-pooled analysis of BP trajectories in a sex-stratified fashion found that, in contrast with the notion that CVDs in women lag behind men by 10–20 years, they present a steeper increase in blood pressure (BP) that started in the third decade of life and continued throughout the life course [14, 15]. Other studies confirmed the SGRDs in BP trajectories from early life, so that the steeper rise in BP throughout their life course may set the stage for later-life CVDs that tend to present differently in women and men [16–20]. Thus, it is not yet known whether hypertension should be differently managed in women and men, including BP thresholds to initiate treatment, treatment goals and choice and dosages of antihypertensive drugs to reduce the risk of organ damage associated with high BP in women [17–20]. There are also SGRDs in HF phenotypes. Indeed, although the overall lifetime risk of HF is fairly comparable between men and women, the risk of developing HF with reduced EF (HFrEF) is higher in men than women, while the lifetime risk of developing HF with preserved ejection fraction (HFpEF) is similar in men and women [7, 8, 21, 22]. Accordingly, HFpEF is the most common phenotype in women increasing with age and hypertension represents the most common comorbidity [21, 23, 24].

Because of all these differences, SGRDs in the pharmacokinetics (absorption, distribution, biotransformation, and elimination), pharmacodynamics (relationship between drug concentration at the site of action and the resulting pharmacologic or toxicologic response) and optimal dosing of some guideline-recommended drugs (GRDs) for the treatment of HTN/HTN do not come as a surprise [25–27].

The aims of this chapter are to review the main SGRDs in the pharmacokinetics, efficacy, and safety of GRDs for the treatment of HTN/HF and draw recommendations to optimize the pharmacological therapy and minimize the incidence of adverse drug reactions (ADRs) in women. Throughout the text, the terms "sex" (which refers to the different biological and physiological characteristics of females, males, and intersex persons, such as chromosomes, genes, hormones and reproductive organs) and "gender" (which comprises social, environmental, cultural, and behavioral factors and choices that influence a person's self-identity and health) were used as synonyms [28].

2 Theory

2.1 Differences in Drug Pharmacokinetics and Pharmacodynamic

SGRDs in the drug efficacy and safety can be related to differences body composition and physiology (changes in sex hormone levels during menstrual cycle/pregnancy/menopause) and/or in the pharmacokinetics and pharmacodynamics (Table 1), and clinical outcomes (Table 2) of some GRDs for the treatment of HTN and/or HF [25–27, 44, 86–90].

Table 1 Sex/gender-related differences in pharmacokinetics and pharmacodynamics of guideline-recommended drugs for the treatment of hypertion and heart failure

Drug class	Pharmacokinetics	Pharmacodynamics
Angiotensin-converting enzyme inhibitors	• Captopril is better absorbed in W when administered on an empty stomach	• No mortality benefit in W with asymptomatic LV systolic dysfunction [29] • W with HFrEF may have the lowest risk of death or HFH at half the guideline-recommended doses compared with M [30]
Angiotensin receptor blockers	• SGRDs in the PK of candesartan, eprosartan, irbesartan and valsartan disappear after normalizing the dose for body weight [31, 32] • C_{max} for losartan and telmisartan are twice as high in W than in M; the renal Cl of irbesartan decreases in elderly W. However, dose modifications in W are not recommended [31]	• No SGRDs in antihypertensive response [27, 31] • W with HFrEF on ARBs had significantly better survival than those on ACEIs; no differences in survival in men prescribed ARBs compared to ACEIs [33] • W with HFrEF may have the lowest risk of death or HFH at half the guideline-recommended doses compared with M [30] • W has greater sensitivity to RAS blockade [27] and may require lower dosages of ARBs than M
Beta-blockers: • Metoprolol, propranolol	• Higher exposure (50–80%) of metoprolol and propranolol in W due to a lower Vd and slower Cl [34, 35] • OCs increase metoprolol exposure [36] • A 50 mg dose in adult W provides a similar exposure to metoprolol than 100 mg dose in adult M [37]	• In hypertensives, they produced a greater decrease in BP and a smaller increase in heart rate during exercise in W than in M [34, 35, 38] • The optimal effect of propranolol and metoprolol may be achieved with lower doses in W than in M [35, 37] • W with HFrEF may have the lowest risk of death or HFH at half the guideline-recommended doses compared with M [30]
CYP2D6-dependent β-blockers	• Higher exposure of these β-blockers (carvedilol, metoprolol, nebivolol, propranolol) in W due to a lower Vd and reduced metabolism [39]	• The interaction between these β-blockers and bradycardic drugs (digoxin, diltiazem, verapamil) is significantly higher in W. No SGRDs with CYP2D6-independent β-blockers (sotalol, bisoprolol, atenolol) [39]
Calcium channel blockers	• Faster oral clearance and lower exposure of nifedipine and verapamil in W, probably due to the higher activity of CYP3A4 and/or lower activity of P-gp [40, 41] • Amlodipine and verapamil clearance decreases in W with aging [41, 42]	• Older W experience more effective BP reduction than do younger W treated with verapamil or amlodipine [41, 42] • Verapamil decreases BP with greater heart rate increases in W [40] • Amlodipine produces more pronounced BP reduction in elderly W [42]
Digoxin	• Higher SDC in W due to reduced Vd and lower Cl [43] • Digoxin Cl increases during pregnancy [44]	• Higher mortality in W with HFrEF [45]. They require lower SDC (0.5–0.9 ng/mL) [7, 8]

(continued)

Table 1 (continued)

Drug class	Pharmacokinetics	Pharmacodynamics
Diuretics: Thiazides and loop diuretics	• No SGRDs in the PK of hydrochlorothiazide [27] • W present higher exposure (40–50%) of torasemide (and probably of other loop diuretics) due to reduced Cl than in M [46]	• Higher diuretic, natriuretic, and kaliuretic effects of furosemide in female rats as compared with males probably due to a lower expression of OAT1 in the tubular basolateral membrane [46, 47] and of the Na^+-K^+-$2Cl^-$ cotransporter in the loop of Henle and a lower drug Cl [48] • The expression of thiazide-sensitive Na^+-Cl^- cotransporter in the distal convoluted tubule is two-fold higher in female than in male rats [49] • Bendroflumethiazide increases renal excretion of Na^+ and Cl^- more in female than in male rats, but decreases the excretion of Ca^{2+} by 50% only in female rats [49, 50]
Iron	• Greater drug absorption [51]	
Isosorbide dinitrate/ hydralazine		• Survival was better in W in the I/H arm than in the placebo arm; the difference was of lesser magnitude in M [52]
Ivabradine	• No SGRDs in pharmacokinetics [26]	• No SGRDs in pharmacodynamics [53]
Mineralocorticoid receptor antagonists	• No SGRDs in the PK of spironolactone or eplerenone [26, 27]	• In a model of MI, eplerenone reduces cardiac remodeling and phenotypic alterations of gene expression in female but not in male rats [54] • Serum aldosterone is positively associated with a LV geometric pattern suggestive of concentric remodeling in W but not in M [55]
Sacubitril-valsartan	• No SGRDs in the PK [27]	• Significantly reduces the risk of HFH in W but mot in M with HFpEF [56] • W with HFpEF may have a greater natriuretic peptide deficiency and a reduced cGMP-PKG signalling than M. Neprilysin inhibition may increase the levels of atrial natriuretic peptides and cGMP-PKG signalling more in W than in M [56, 57]

ACEIs angiotensin-converting enzyme inhibitors, *ARBs* angiotensin AT1 receptor blockers, *BP* blood pressure, *cGMP* cyclic guanosine monophosphate, *Cl* clearance, C_{max} peak plasma concentrations, *CYP* cytochrome P450 isoforms, *HF* heart failure, *HFH*, heart failure hospitalization, *HFpEF* heart failure with preserved ejection fraction, *HFrEF* heart failure with reduced ejection fraction, *I/H* isosorbide dinitrate/hydralazine, *LV* left ventricular, *M* men, *MI* myocardial infarction, *OAT1* organic anion transporter 1, *OC* oral contraceptives, *P* pregnancy, *P-gp* P-glycoprotein, *PK* pharmacokinetics, *PKG* protein kinase G, *RAS* renin-angiotensin system, *SDC* serum digoxin concentrations, *SGRDs* sex/gender-related differences, *TD* thiazide diuretics, *Vd*: volume of distribution, *W* women

Table 2 Sex/gender-related differences in the main clinical endpoints of clinical trials and meta-analysis of drugs recommended for the treatments of hypertension and heart failure

Study, references and treatment	Sample (n) (Women, %)	End point	Men (HR/RR, 95% CI)	Women (HR/RR, 95% CI)	P (M vs W)
Trials in hypertensive patients					
ALLHAT [58–60] Chlortalidone, amlodipine and lisinopril	33,357 (46.8%) Hypertension and at least another CVD risk factor	Stroke outcome	No SGRDs	Stroke rate significantly higher in W on lisinopril compared to chlorthalidone (HR 1.21) and amlodipine (HR 1.45)	

(continued)

Table 2 (continued)

Study, references and treatment	Sample (n) (Women, %)	End point	Men (HR/RR, 95% CI)	Women (HR/RR, 95% CI)	P (M vs W)
ACCOMPLISH [61] Benazepril + amlodipine vs benazepril + HCTZ	11,506 (39.5)	Composite of CV death, nonfatal MI, nonfatal stroke, hospitalization for angina, resuscitation after sudden cardiac arrest, and coronary revascularization	HR 0.80 (0.69–0.91; $P < 0.001$)	HR 0.83 (0.68–1.01; NS)	
ACCT [42] Amlodipine	380/704 Mild-moderate HTN	Patients reaching goal BP response	83%	91.4%	$P \leq 0.001$
Fan et al. [62] Atenolol, HCTZ, captopril, or sustained-released nifedipine	3535 (65%) Aged 40–75 years	SGRDs in BP response to antihypertensive drugs		W had better DBP response to HCTZ than M Atenolol decreases mean SBP more in W than M	$P < 0.05$ $P < 0.05$
HOT [63]	18,790 (47%) Aged 50–80 years	Relationship between target office DBP (≤80 or ≤85 mmHg) and MI	Achieving target DBP ≤80 mmHg did not reduce MI (0.81; 0.49–1.31; NS)	Achieving target DBP ≤80 mmHg reduced MI (0.58; 0.41–0.81; $P = 0.034$)	
INCLUSIVE [64] Irbesartan/HCTZ	736 (52%) Uncontrolled BP on monotherapy	Mean change in SBP from baseline		W had a mean of 3.0 ± 0.9 mmHg greater reduction than M	0.002
INDANA database [65] β-blockers and thiazide diuretics	40,777 (48.9)	Subgroup meta-analysis of individual patient data according to sex	Treatment effect was statistically significant for all events (total and specific mortality, all coronary events, all strokes, and major CV events)	Treatment effect was statistically significant for stroke (fatal strokes and all strokes) and for major CV events	
LIFE (post-hoc analysis) [66, 67] Losartan + HCTZ vs atenolol + HCTZ	9.193 (54) Adults with HTN and ECG signs of LVH	Losartan vs atenolol:			
		• CV death, MI, or stroke	0.91 (0.78–1.06; NS)	0.82 (0.68–0.98; $P = 0.03$)	
		• Stroke	0.80 (0.63–1.01; NS)	0.71 (0.55–0.90; $P = 0.005$)	
		• Total mortality	1.02 (0.85–1.23; NS)	0.77 (0.63–0.95; $P = 0.014$).	
		Angina hospitalization in the losartan group	0.93 (0.70–1.23)	1.70 (1.16–2.51)	0.012

(continued)

Table 2 (continued)

Study, references and treatment	Sample (n) (Women, %)	End point	Men (HR/RR, 95% CI)	Women (HR/RR, 95% CI)	P (M vs W)
OSCAR study Group [68] Olmesartan vs CCBs (amlodipine or azelnidipine) + olmesartan	1164 (56%) High-risk elderly Japanese patients	Composite of CV events and non-CV death	SBP and CV events (HR = 1.86) were higher in the ARB group (P = 0.03)	No differences in SBP between groups or in primary outcome events (HR = 0.97; P = 0.92)	Pint = 0.17
ANBP2 [69] ACEI vs diuretic treatment	6083 (51%) elderly patients	All-CV events or total death	0.83 (0.71–0.97; P = 0.02)	1.00 (0.83–1.21; NS)	NA
		1st CV event or total death	0.83 (0.71–0.97; P = 0.02)	1.00 (0.83–1.20; NS)	
		All CV events	0.83 (0.71–0.97; P = 0.02)	1.00 (0.83–1.21; NS)	
SPRINT [70] SBP target <130 mmHg (intensive) vs <140 mmHg (standard)	9361 (35.6) Adults ≥50 years with HTN and increased CV risk	Composite of MI, acute CHD, stroke, HF or death from CV causes	0.72 (0.59–0.88; P = 0.001)	0.84 (0.61–1.11; P = 0.20)	P_{inter} 0.45 [71] P = 0.001 [72]
VALUE [73] Valsartan vs amlodipine-based regimens	15,314 (42.4) HTN and high-risk of cardiac events	Composite of cardiac mortality and morbidity Secondary endpoint: HFH	Amlodipine does not reduce the primary endpoint in M M, but not W, have a lower incidence of HF with valsartan (P < 0.0001)	Amlodipine is more effective than valsartan to reduce SBP and reduces the primary endpoint in W than in M. P = 0.016)	
Turnbull et al. [74] Analysis of 31 RCTs	190,617 (45%)	Stroke prevention	All drug classes were equally effective in stroke prevention	CCBs were more effective than ACEIs (HR 1.27, 1.05–1.55; P = 0.05)	
Trials in patients with heart failure					
A-HeFT [52] Isosorbide dinitrate/ hydralazine	1050 (40) Black patients with HFrEF	Mortality	0.79 (0.46–1.35; P = 0.38)	0.33 (0.16–0.71; P = 0.003)	P_{int} = 0.470
		Event free survival	0.67 (0.49–0.92; P = 0.013)	0.58 (0.39–0.86; P = 0.007)	
		CV mortality (vs PCB)	18 vs 28 (P = 0.36)	8 vs 17 (P = 0.023)	
ATLAS [75] High (32.5–35 mg/day) vs low (2.5–5 mg/day) doses of lisinopril	3164 (20.5) HFrEF	All-cause mortality or hospitalization with the higher dose of lisinopril	0.89 (0.79–1.00; P = 0.05)	1.05 (0.82–1.35; NS)	

(continued)

Table 2 (continued)

Study, references and treatment	Sample (n) (Women, %)	End point	Men (HR/RR, 95% CI)	Women (HR/RR, 95% CI)	P (M vs W)
CHARM Program [76]	7599 (31.5) HF with a broad spectrum of LVEF	All-cause mortality		0.77 (0.69–0.86) vs M	<0.001
		CV death or HFH		0.83 (0.76–0.91) vs M	<0.001
		CV death		0.78 (0.69–0.88) vs M	<0.001
		Deaths due to HF		0.72 (0.58–0.89) vs M	0.002
		HF hospitalizations		0.87 (0.78–0.97) vs M	0.012
CHART-2 study [77]	4683 (32) All-cause mortality	β-blockers in HFrEF	0.87 (0.63–1.1; P = 0.40)	0.45 (0.23–0.88; P = 0.021)	0.04
		RAASIs in HFpEF	0.70 (0.56–0.86; P = 0.001)	0.96 (0.72–1.28; P = 0.79)	0.053
CIBIS-II [78] Bisoprolol	2467 (24) HFrEF	All-cause mortality		0.64 (0.47–0.86) vs M	0.003
		CV mortality		0.64 (0.45–0.91) vs M	0.013
		Pump failure death		0.30 (0.13–0.70) vs M	0.005
CONSENSUS-1 [79]	253 (29) HFrEF	Reduction in 6-month mortality	51% (P < 0.001)	6% (NS)	
DIG [80] Digoxin	6800 (22.4%) HFrEF	All-cause mortality	0.93 (0.85–1.02)	1.23 (1.02–1.47)	0.014
Subanalysis of the DIG trial [81]	757 women All-cause death	SDC 0.5–0.9 ng/mL SDC 1.2–2.0 ng/mL	.80 (0.70–0.92; P = 0.002) 1.18 (0.99–1.139; P = 0.060)	0.84 (0.62–1.13; P = 0.24) 1.33 (1.00–1.76; P = 0.49)	
I-PRESERVE [82] Irbesartan, HFpEF	4128 (60)	All-cause death		0.70 (0.59–0.83) vs M	<0.001
		Hospitalizations or death		0.80 (0.72–0.89) vs M	<0.001
		CV hospitalization or death		0.81 (0.72–0.92) vs M	0.001
		Non-CV hospitalization or death		0.78 (0.69–0.90) vs M	<0.001
		All-cause hospitalizations		0.80 (0.76–0.84) vs M	P < 0.0001
PARAGON-HF [56] Sacubitril/valsartan vs valsartan	4822 (51) HFpEF	HFH and CV death	1.03 (0.85–1.25)	0.73 (0.59–0.90)	0.017
		Primary composite outcome + urgent HF visits	0.99 (0.81–1.20)	0.74 (0.61–0.91)	0.044
		Total HFH	1.07 (0.84–1.34)	0.67 (0.54–0.84)	0.004

(continued)

Table 2 (continued)

Study, references and treatment	Sample (n) (Women, %)	End point	Men (HR/RR, 95% CI)	Women (HR/RR, 95% CI)	P (M vs W)
TOPCAT Americas [83] Spironolactone	1767 (49.9%) HFpEF	All-cause mortality	1.06 (0.81–1.39; P = 0.68)	0.66 (0.48–0.90; P = 0.01)	P_{inter} 0.02
		Multivariate HR for mortality	0.80 (NS)	0.57 (0.39–0.83; P = 0.003)	
TRACE [84] Trandolapril	6676 (28%) HFrEF	All-cause death	0.74 (0.62–0.89)	0.90 (0.69–1.18)	0.02
Meta-analysis/pooled analysis in patients with HF					
ACEIs vs ARBs [33] Administrative database from Quebec	16,698 (51.6) HFrEF	Survival: ARBs vs ACEIs	1.10 (0.95–1.30; P = 0.21)	0.69 (0.59–0.80; P < 0.0001	<0.0001
		With hypertension	0.86 (0.64–1.15; NS)	0.65 (0.52–0.8); P < 0.0001	NS
		Without hypertension	1.20 (1.01–1.43; P < 0.03)	0.72 (0.59–0.90; P < 0.002	<0.03
ACEIs [85] 32 RCTs	7105 (14.5%) HFrEF	Total mortality	0.76 (0.65–0.88; P < 0.05)	0.79 (0.59–1.06; NS)	NA
		Total mortality or HFH	0.63 (0.55–0.73; P < 0.05)	0.78 (0.59–1.04; NS)	NA
ACEIs and β-blockers [29] 12 RCTs	4497 (24%) Symptomatic HFrEF	Mortality from HF	0.80 (0.68–0.93)	0.90 (0.78–1.05) RRR 1.15 (0.88–1.51)	0.07
	8015 (16%) Asymptomatic HFrEF	Mortality from HF	0.83 (0.71–0.96)	0.96 (0.75–1.22) RRR 1.25 (0.94–1.65)	NA

ACEIs angiotensin-converting enzyme inhibitors, *ARBs* angiotensin AT1 receptor antagonists, *BP* blood pressure, *CCBs* calcium channel blockers, *CI* confidence interval, *CV* cardiovascular, *CVD* cardiovascular disease, *DBP* diastolic blood pressure, *HCTZ* hydrochlorothiazide, *HF* heart failure, *HFH* heart failure hospitalization, *HFrEH* heart failure with reduced ejection fraction, *HFpEF* heart failure with preserved ejection fraction, *HR* hazard ratio, *HTN* hypertension, *LVEF* left ventricular ejection fraction, *LVH* left ventricular hypertrophy, *M* men, *MI* myocardial infarction, *NA* not available, *NS* not significant, P_{inter} P for interaction, *RCTs* randomized clinical trials, *RAASIs* renin-angiotensin-aldosterone system inhibitors, *RR* relative risk, *RRR* relative risk reduction, *SBP* systolic blood pressure, *SDC* serum digoxin concentration, *W* women

ACCT The Amlodipine Cardiovascular Community Trial, *ACCOMPLISH* Avoiding Cardiovascular Events Through Combination Therapy in Patients Living With Systolic Hypertension, *A-HeFT* African American Heart Failure Trial, *ALLHAT* Antihypertensive and Lipid-Lowering Treatment to Prevent Heart Attack Trial, *ANBP2* Second Australian National Blood Pressure Study, *ATLAS* Assessment of Treatment with Lisinopril and Survival, *CHARM* Candesartan in Heart Failure Assessment of Reduction in Mortality and morbidity, *CHART-2* Chronic Heart Failure Analysis and Registry in the Tohoku District-2, *CIBIS II* Cardiac Insufficiency BIsoprolol Study II, *CONSENSUS* Cooperative North Scandinavian Enalapril Survival Study, *DIG* Digitalis Investigation Group, *HOT* The Hypertension Optimal treatment trial, *INCLUSIVE* Irbesartan/Hydrochlorothiazide Blood Pressure Reductions in Diverse Patient Populations, *INDANA* INdividual Data ANalysis of Antihypertensive intervention trials, *I-PRESERVE* Irbesartan in Heart Failure with Preserved Ejection Fraction Study, *LIFE* Losartan Intervention For Endpoint reduction in hypertension, *OSCAR* OlmeSartan and Calcium Antagonists Randomized study, *PARAGON-HF* Prospective Comparison of ARNI with ARB Global Outcomes in HF With Preserved Ejection Fraction, *SPRINT* Systolic Blood Pressure Intervention Trial, *TOPCAT* Treatment of Preserved Cardiac Function Heart Failure With an Aldosterone Antagonist Trial, *TRACE* Trandolapril Cardiac Evaluation, *VALUE* Valsartan Antihypertensive Long-term Use Evaluation

2.1.1 Differences in Pharmacokinetics

There are SGRDs in the pharmacokinetic properties of GRDs for the treatment of HTN/HF. Drug distribution depends on body composition, organ blood flow and tissue and plasma protein binding. Women have higher proportion of body fat but lower body weight/size, plasma volume, cardiac output, organ blood flow and volume of distribution (Vd). This explains the higher Vd and prolonged duration of action of lipophilic drugs in women and why drugs requiring loading-dosages (i.e., digoxin) can reach higher peak plasma levels and produce a higher incidence of ADRs in women [25, 44]. Hepatic clearance is a function of cardiac output and blood flow which are lower in women, and the activity of drug metabolizing enzymes and transporters which play a major role in pharmacokinetic variability. The activity of cytochromes P450 (CYP) 3A4 and 2D6 responsible for the metabolism of many cardiovascular drugs increases, while the activity of the transporter P-glycoprotein decreases in women [44, 88, 89]. Drugs substrates for both CYP3A4 and P-glycoprotein typically had higher clearance in women due to the lower P-glycoprotein activity [91]. Women also presents lower estimated glomerular filtration rate (eGFR) and tubular secretion/reabsorption, so that drugs excreted mainly unchanged in urine (digoxin) present a slower clearance and longer half-life [44, 87, 89]. Interestingly, most SGRDs in pharmacokinetics disappear when doses are adjusted for body weight or eGFR, but this is not common practice as CPGs recommend administering the same doses to men and women with HTN/HF.

2.1.2 Differences in Pharmacodynamics

There are SGRDs in the efficacy of some GRDs used for the treatment of HTN/HF, but their clinical relevance is considered moderate or remains uncertain because: in many randomized clinical trials (RCTs) women were underrepresented; randomization was not stratified by sex/gender; and a pre-specified sex/gender evaluation of drug efficacy and safety was not performed. Indeed, women represent only 36% of the population recruited in RCTs supporting the approval of cardiovascular drugs from 2005 to 2018 and were underrepresented (24–29%) in HF trials [92–94]. In the ESC-HF-LT registry only 28.8% of patients were women [95]. Additionally, among 156 cardiovascular trials (30.6% women), only one-third reported sex-specific results [93]. In another analysis of 2046 studies evaluating in 1,348,172 adults the effect of the major antihypertensive drug groups until May 2020, the mean percentage of women was 38.1%, but only 75 (3.7%) presented sex-stratified outcome data [96]. As a result, in many trials women represent a subgroup not representative of the patient population to treat (sample selection bias) which prevents generalization of trial results [94] and were underpowered to examine SGRDs in drug efficacy and safety of cardiovascular drugs even if they do exist [93, 94, 97]. Under these conditions, data obtained mainly from middle-aged men were extrapolated to the whole population and information on SGRDs derived mainly from retrospective studies, subgroup and *post-hoc* analyses subjected to numerous potential sources of error [98], or meta-analyses enrolling women with different baseline characteristics [92, 94, 99]. Therefore, the limited information on SGRDs in drug pharmacodynamics is the result of RCTs not designed to detect such differences rather than a true absence of difference. Consequently, major CPGs based on the results of RCTs do not present sex/gender-specific recommendations and concluded that there is currently no evidence of SGRDs in the efficacy and doses of the drugs used for the treatment of HTN [5, 6] (except for pregnancy) or HF [7, 8] (except for digoxin) even in the absence of robust evidence to support this claim. A recent study quantified the sex/gender-based medicine content in the two mayor hypertension guidelines. Pregnancy represented 2.4–3% of the total words, but there was minimal coverage of any other life periods [100]. Additionally, SGRDs are not mentioned on prescribing labels [26, 27].

2.2 SGRDs in Patients with Hypertension and Heart Failure with Preserved Ejection Fraction

2.2.1 Beta-Blockers

Compared with other first-line antihypertensives β-blockers are equivalent in preventing major CV events but provide less effective prevention of stroke. They are recommended in hypertensive women with ischemic heart disease, HFrEF or atrial fibrillation, and represent an alternative to angiotensin-converting enzyme inhibitors (ACEIs) or angiotensin receptor blockers (ARBs), in hypertensive women planning pregnancy or with child-bearing potential [5, 6, 8].

Metoprolol and propranolol exposure is up to 80–100% higher in women compared to men due to higher oral bioavailability, lower Vd and slower clearance via CYP2D6, resulting in a more pronounced decrease in systolic blood pressure (SBP) and heart rate during exercise [34, 35, 38]. Higher metoprolol exposure persisted after normalisation for bodyweight and increased by oral contraceptives and CYP2D6 inhibitors [34, 36]. In pharmacokinetic simulations, metoprolol doses resulting a similar exposure in healthy young males administered 50 mg tablet were 15 mg for elderly women and 25 mg for elderly men [37]. Based on these results, a 50% dose reduction for metoprolol was recommended in women.

Some trials showed that β-blockers improved survival in men, but not in women, with hypertension [101] or coronary artery disease [102], while contradictory results were reported in patients with HFrEF. MERIT-HF and COPERNICUS trials did not find a beneficial effect on mortality in women probably because women were underrepresented in these trials, present lower event rates and were older and sicker than men. Conversely, in the US Carvedilol Heart Failure Study and CIBIS II trials a significant reduction in all-cause mortality was observed in women compared with men [25, 26, 78, 103, 104]. When pooling mortality from these trials, β-blockers significantly reduced all-cause mortality in both women and men [105]. Other meta-analysis confirmed that β-blockers significantly reduced all-cause mortality/hospitalizations in man and women with HFrEF [106, 107], asymptomatic or symptomatic LV systolic dysfunction [29] or post-myocardial infarction (MI) [108, 109].

2.2.2 Calcium Channel Blockers (CCBs)

CCBs undergo extensive first-pass metabolism in the liver, and are substrates of CYP3A4 [40, 110]. Women present faster clearance and lower exposure to verapamil [40, 41] and nifedipine [110] than men, probably due to the lower body weight, higher activity of CYP3A4 and/or lower activity of P-glycoprotein [111]. In hypertensive women, verapamil reduces BP with greater heart rate increases than in men [40, 41] and because aging decreases drug clearance, older women experience more effective BP reduction than younger women or elderly men [25, 41].

A large open study found that, even after dose adjustment for body weight, the antihypertensive response to amlodipine was significantly greater in women than in men and in women ≥65 years [42], and some RCTs showed a greater antihypertensive effect of CCBs in women than in men (Table 2). Additionally, in a sex-specific analysis of the HOT trial, where patients received felodipine as basal therapy in combination with other antihypertensives, the incidence of MI decreased in women with the lower diastolic BP (≤80–85 mmHg), but this benefit was not found in men [63]. Additionally, in a meta-analysis of 31 RCTs, among women, CCBs were more effective than ACEIs in stroke prevention [39]. However, major RCTs with CCBs in hypertensive patients did not find SGRDs in clinical outcomes [27].

CCBs are not recommended in patients with HFrEF, but amlodipine and felodipine can be added to standard therapy in patients with uncontrolled angina or hypertension. However, no sex-specific analysis of their efficacy or safety was performed [7, 8].

2.2.3 Renin-Angiotensin-Aldosterone System Inhibitors

Sex hormones modulate the activity of the renin-angiotensin-aldosterone system (RAAS). Estrogens inhibit, while androgens increase the RAAS, so that the premenopausal cardioprotective effects of estrogens might result, in part, from inhibition of the RAAS, an effect that is lost after menopause [112, 113]. However, how sex hormonal changes modulate effectiveness and safety of RAAS inhibitors [ACEIs, ARBs, mineralocorticoid receptor antagonists (MRAs), sacubitril-valsartan] remains uncertain.

There are no major SGRDs in the pharmacokinetics of RAASIs and similar doses are recommended in both men and women [25–27, 31, 44].

2.2.4 Angiotensin-Converting Enzyme Inhibitors

Several RCTs reported SGRDs in the antihypertensive effects of ACEIs (Table 2). In the Second Australian National Blood Pressure Study initiation of antihypertensive treatment with ACEIs led to better outcomes than treatment with diuretic agents only in men, despite similar reductions of BP in both sexes [69]. In a systematic review of 21 trials that used ACEIs or ARBs for the treatment of hypertension, only 9 trials reported sex-specific outcome data (74,105 patients, 39% women). Although the majority of trials did not have adequate power to evaluate SGRDs, in 7 of the 9 trials there was a trend suggesting that ACEIs and ARBs may be more effective in men [114]. However, since the magnitude of these differences in most trials was small further studies are needed to confirm or not these results.

Early RCTs (CONSENSUS-1, SAVE, SOLVD) enalapril and captopril reduced mortality and HF hospitalizations (HFH) much less in women than in men with HFrEF, but because women were underrepresented (<20%), they were underpowered to examine SGRDs on clinical outcomes [44, 104, 115]. Later trials (AIRE and HOPE trials) reported no SGRDs in the secondary prevention of cardiovascular events in high-risk patients [24, 44, 116]. An overview of 32 RCTs found comparable benefits of ACEIs on total mortality in men and women with HFrEF, but on the combined endpoint of death or HFH, the reduction was significant in men (37%), but not in women (22%) [85]. Interestingly, in another meta-analysis, women and men with symptomatic HFrEF benefit from ACEIs, while women with asymptomatic LV dysfunction did not achieve a mortality benefit when treated with ACEIs [29]. Thus, it remains uncertain whether ACEIs produce the same benefit in men and women with HFrEF.

2.2.5 Angiotensin AT1 Receptor Blockers

No SGRDs were reported with ARBs on clinical outcomes in trials recruiting patients with hypertension (LIFE, VALUE), HFrEF (CHARM, ELITE I and II, RESOLVD, Val-HeFT, VALUE) and post-MI (OPTIMAAL, VALIANT) [24, 26, 27]. However, in a retrospective population-based study, women with HFrEF on ARBs had better survival than those on ACEIs whether they are hypertensive or not, but no differences in survival were observed in men prescribed ARBs or ACEIs [33]. Among hypertensive men, those treated with ACEIs show longer survival than do those treated with ARBs. Importantly, in an analysis of the CHARM program, compared to men, women have lower risk of cardiovascular death or HFH that were not explained by LVEF or origin of HF [76] (Table 2). These surprising findings which were never replicated and merit further investigation.

2.2.6 Mineralocorticoid Receptor Antagonists

African Americans (AA) develop HTN earlier and present lower rates of BP control than other ethnicities [117]. In a small trial, AA women taking spironolactone had lower BP levels and the proportion with uncontrolled HTN was significantly less than in women not prescribed spironolactone. However, these benefits were not observed in AA men or white females [118]. No SRDs were described with spironolactone in patients with severe ischemic and non-ischemic HFrEF [119] or with eplerenone in patients with acute MI complicated by LV dysfunction and HF [120] or HFrEF and mild symptoms [121]. In patients with LV dysfunction post-MI, eplerenone showed a trend towards a reduction in all-cause mortality in women at 30 days, but not at 16 months after randomization [122]. However, once again, because of the low inclusion of women (<30%), these studies were underpowered to detect SGRDs. A recent meta-analysis of 3 RCTs (RALES, EMPHASIS-HF, TOPCAT-Americans) recruiting patients with different HF phenotypes concluded that there were no SGRDs in the benefits of MRAs on cardiovascular death or HFH [123], but this mix-up of underpowered trials can not be accepted as evidence of the absence of SGRDs [26].

2.2.7 Sacubitril-Valsartan

No SGRDs on CV death or HFH hospitalisations were described with sacubitril-valsartan in patients with HFrEF [124].

2.2.8 Nitrates

In a *post-hoc* analysis of the A-HeFT trial, women (but not men) treated with hydralazine and isosorbide dinitrate appeared to have a survival benefit, but there was no significant treatment interaction by sex/gender [52].

2.2.9 Ivabradine

No SGRDs in PK, efficacy or safety were observed in patients with chronic stable angina [53] or symptomatic chronic HFrEF and heart rate ≥ 70 bpm [125].

2.2.10 Digoxin

Pivotal trials (DIG, PROVED, RADIANCE) with digoxin did not perform a sex/gender-specific analysis in patients with HFrEF [26]. However, a *post-hoc* analysis of the DIG trial found that digoxin increased all-cause mortality in women, but not in men [45]. This increase was related to: (1) higher serum digoxin concentrations (SDCs between 1.5 and 2.0 ng/mL) due to the lower Vd and slower renal Cl in women compared to men [43, 44, 126]. Indeed, a beneficial effect of digoxin on morbidity without an increased mortality was reported in women at low SDCs (0.5–0.9 ng/mL), whereas SDCs ≥1.2 mg/mL were harmful [81]. (2) A reduced expression of Na^+,K^+-ATPase in women, leading to SGRDs in cellular Na^+ and Ca^{2+} handling which might predispose to fatal arrhythmias [26].

However, the *post-hoc* analysis of the DIG trial was underpowered to determine SGRDs in drug safety, SDCs were measured in less than a third of the participants, and digoxin was prescribed more frequently in elderly women at higher mortality risk (prescription biases) [43]. Additionally, other studies [127–129] and a recent Cochrane Review reported a neutral effect of digoxin on mortality and a significant reduction in HFH in patients with HFrEF who are sinus rhythm [130]. Two ongoing trials examine the effects of digoxin in patients with advanced HFrEF (DIGIT-HF, EudraCT 2013–005326-38) and whether low SDCs (0.5–0.9 ng/mL) are beneficial in HF with reduced or mid-range (<50%) ejection fraction (DECISION-NCT03783429) [131].

2.2.11 Loop and Thiazide Diuretics

Thiazide diuretics (TD) are more frequently prescribed in hypertensive women [132–134] and thiazide and loop diuretics in women with HF as compared to men (see below) [26]. Torasemide exposure is 40–50% higher in women than in men due a reduced drug clearance, and SGRDs in the diuretic effects of thiazides and furosemide (and probably other loop diuretics) were described in experimental models (Table 1) [46, 135, 136]. Although SGRDs on diuretic efficacy have not been evaluated in HF patients, some SGRDs were observed in hypertensive patients (Table 2). In a sex-specific meta-analysis of the INDANA database, TD treatment significantly improved stroke and major cardiovascular events in women, while in men improved all categories of events (total and specific mortality, all coronary events, all strokes, and major cardiovascular events) [65]. In Chinese patients, women obtained better BP control with hydrochlorothiazide and atenolol and experience more ADRs with nifedipine and captopril than men [62]. Additionally, SBP reduction in response to indapamide was significantly greater in women than in men and increased by 3 mm Hg every 10 years of age gradient in women [137].

ADRs, including electrolyte disturbances leading to hospitalization are more frequent in women [46, 135], but no sex-specific dose adjustments for diuretics are recommended in CPG or Rx labels.

2.2.12 Sodium-Glucose Cotransporter 2 Inhibitors (SGLT2Is)

Although some meta-analysis reported that SGLT2Is reduced major cardiac outcomes in men but not in women [138, 139] or suggested a progressive decremental benefit when the percentage of women in the SGLT2I arm was >50% [140], no SGRDs were reported in patients with or without type 2 diabetes in the EMPA-REG OUTCOME, CANVAS Program, DECLARE TIMI-58 and CREDENCE trials in patients with HFrEF [141–143]. Nevertheless, women only represented ~35% of the population in RCTs and women with diabetes or at cardiorenal risk are less likely to receive SGLT2Is than men [144, 145]. Thus, further effort is needed to increase the prescription of SGLT2Is in women.

3 Clinical Practice

3.1 SGRDs in Patients with Heart Failure with Preserved Ejection Fraction

HFpEF occurs more commonly in women and comprises over 80% of incident HF cases among elderly women [2, 21, 24]. Pivotal trials with β-blockers in patients with HFpEF were underpowered to assess SGRDs [94, 146]. However, no RGRDs were reported in a pre-specified subanalysis of the SENIORS trial where the effect of nebivolol was similar in patients with HFrEF and HFpEF [147], or in a large Swedish cohort study where the use of β-blockers in patients with HFpEF was associated with lower all-cause mortality, but not with combined all-cause mortality or HFH [148]. Conversely, a small prospective observational study suggested that beta-blocker therapy may be associated with a higher risk of HF rehospitalization in women with HFpEF [149]. However, because a larger proportion of women discharged on β-blockers were not on sinus rhythm at the time of admission, the failure of treatment to control the arrhythmia may be the cause of readmissions not the β-blockade.

No SGRDs in clinical outcomes were reported with digoxin [150, 151], with candesartan in the CHARM Program [76] or in the only 2 RCTs with ACEIs or ARBs that performed a sex-prespecified analysis of the results (I-PRESERVE, CHARM-Preserved) [94]. In a sex-specific Japanese trial, β-blockers improved mortality in women but not men with HFrEF, while RAASIs (particularly ACEIs) were not associated with improved mortality in women with LVEF ≥50% but were in men [77]. Despite CPGs strongly recommend the use of diuretics [7, 8], the existence of SGRD has not been studied in patients with HFpEF.

In the TOPCAT trial, spironolactone did not reduce the primary cardiovascular outcome in patients with HFpEF [152]. However, in a *post hoc*, non-pre-specified, analysis of this trial enrolling only patients from the Americas, spironolactone significantly reduced all-cause mortality in women but not in men (Table 2), although no SGRDs were found on non-cardiovascular mortality and cardiovascular/non-CV hospitalizations [83]. Whether this beneficial effect can be related to the greater impact of MRAs on cardiac remodeling in women as described in preclinical studies is uncertain [54]. Thus, further prospective RCTs are needed to confirm that spironolactone improves outcomes in women with HFpEF.

In a sex-prespecified subgroup analysis of the PARAGON-HF trial enrolling patients with HFpEF (51.8% women), sacubitril/valsartan significantly reduced the composite of total HFH and cardiovascular death only in women; this benefit was attributable to a reduction in HFH (Table 2) [56]. Furthermore, in a recent analysis of the CHARM Programme, TOPCAT, PARADIGM-HF and PARAGON-HF trials the treatment benefit seemed to extend to a higher LVEF (40–49% or even to the lower part of the LVEF range currently categorized as HFpEF) only in women, but there were no SGRDs in drug efficacy in patients with HFrEF [153].

No SGRDs were reported with empagliflozin [154] or dapagliflozin [155] in patients with HFpEF, i.e. there were no SGRDs in the effects of SGLT2Is across the range of ejection fraction.

Thus, although some evidence suggests the existence of SGRDs in the response to MRAs and sacubitril-valsartan in patients with HFpEF, further RCTs are needed to confirm this possibility and to determine possible SGRDs in the response to GRDs across the spectrum of LVEF.

3.2 SGRDs in Drug Safety

Women have a higher risk of developing ADRs to most cardiovascular drugs and sometimes they are more severe and different than in men [44, 156–158]. Similarly, during postmarketing surveillance ADRs are more commonly reported in women [159]. ADRs reduce therapeutic adherence and increase morbidity, mortality and healthcare costs in women compared to men [160–162]. SGRDs in ADRs produced by GRDs for the treatment of HTN/HF are summarized in Table 3. Only MRAs produce a higher prevalence of ADRs in men [135, 163].

Table 3 Sex/gender-related differences in adverse drug reactions

Drug class	Adverse drug reactions
Angiotensin-converting enzyme inhibitors[a]	• Cough, dysgeusia, skin rash, increase in serum creatinine and gastrointestinal upset are more frequent in W [163–167] • Majority of W discontinue ACEI therapy due to cough, men because of hypotension [166] • The incidence of angioedema is higher in W with HFrEF, particularly in the first 30 days of therapy [168, 169]
Angiotensin receptor blockers[a]	• No SDRDs in hyperkalemia, or hypotension in patients with HFrEF [26] • Angioedema is more frequent in M than in W [164] • W are less persistent to ACEIs than to ARBs; M are more persistent to ACEIs than to ARBs [33]
Beta-blockers	• ADRs caused by CYP2D6-dependent β-blockers (carvedilol, metoprolol, nebivolol, propranolol) are significantly higher in W. No SGRDs were described with CYP2D6-independent β-blockers (sotalol, bisoprolol, atenolol) [39] • BP lowering and heart rate reduction produced by metoprolol and propranolol are higher in W [38]
Calcium channel blockers	• Flushing, headache and ankle edema are more common in W, particularly in elderly W [42, 62, 170, 171]
Digoxin	• Cardiac disorders are more frequent in W [167]. Higher mortality in W with HFrEF [45]. SDC ≤0.9 ng/mL are recommended in W [7, 8]
Diuretics: • Thiazides and loop diuretics	• W experience more electrolyte disturbances and higher rates of hospitalizations due to hypo-osmolarity, hypokalaemia and hyponatraemia than M [46, 135, 136, 156, 170]. However, no dose adjustments are recommended in W • Higher risk of QT-related arrhythmias in W in the presence of hypokalemia or when combined with QT-prolonging drugs [51, 136] • W are less likely to experience hyperuricemia and gout in response to thiazide diuretics than M [27, 172]
Hydralazine (± dinitrate isosorbide)	• Women with HFrEF reported more ADRs (headache or dizziness); no SGRDs in hypotension [52, 163] • Systemic lupus erythematosus more common in W [173]
Ivabradine	• Sex-stratified data are not available in patients with HFrEF [163]. In the VigiBase there were more nonserious ADRs in W [26]
Mineralocorticoid receptor antagonists[a]	• Higher drug discontinuation because of ADRs (hyperkalemia, deterioration of renal function, gynecomastia) in M than in W with HFrEF [119, 135, 163, 174]. Only 1 out of 18 articles reported sex-specific ADRs data with MRAs in patients with HF [163] • Eplerenone produces greater increases in serum potassium and serum creatinine in W [83]
Sacubitril-valsartan[a]	• Bradykinin production after neprilysin inhibition is higher in W than in M and W are more likely to develop angioedema when treated with sacubitril-valsartan [169]. ADRs were not analysed by sex in pivotal RCTs [26, 27]
SGLT2 inhibitors	• Urosepsis and genital mycotic infections are more frequent in W, especially premenopausal W [175, 176]. Acute renal failure is less common in W [141]

ACEIs angiotensin-converting enzyme inhibitors, *ADRs* adverse drug reactions, *ARBs* angiotensin AT1 receptor blockers, *CYP* cytochrome P450 isoforms, *HF* heart failure, *HFrEF* heart failure with reduced ejection fraction, *LV* left ventricular, *M* men, *MRAs* mineralocorticoid receptor antagonists, *RCTs* randomized clinical trials, *SDC* serum digoxin concentrations, *SGLT2Is* sodium-glucose-like transport-2 inhibitors, *SGRDs* sex/gender-related differences. *W* women

[a] Contraindicated in pregnancy due to the risk of fetal abnormalities

The reasons for the higher incidence of ADRs include:

- SGRDs in pharmacokinetics. Because women present lower body weight/size and eGFR, the administration of the same doses in women and men frequently result in higher drug exposure, potentially leading to a higher risk of ADRs than in men [25, 44, 157, 177, 178].
- SGRDs in pharmacodynamics, including changes in drug-target expression, drug-receptor affinity and/or in signal transduction pathways, immunological and hormonal factors [37, 51, 178].
- Women present more comorbidities and consume more medications than men, including over-the-counter medications, herbal remedies, and vitamins and polypharmacy which increases the risk of ADRs and drug-drug interactions [51, 178].
- SGRDs on reporting, as women are more likely to seek healthcare and report more ADRs than men [157].

But despite the evidence of SGRDs in drug safety, most RCTs also do not present their results in a sex/gender-disaggregated manner. In a review of 155 RCTs performed with CPG-recommended HF drugs, only 11 (7%) reported ADRs stratified by sex and women experience more ADRs than men [163]. Unfortunately, SGRDs in ADRs are rarely mentioned in CPGs and Rx labels. The development of sex/gender-specific pharmacological guidelines represents an effective strategy to minimize the higher incidence of ADRs in women.

3.3 Which Are the Right Doses in Women?

CPGs for the treatment of HNT/HF make no distinction in the doses prescribed in women and man, but we described that there are SGRDs in the exposure of some drugs (metoprolol, propranolol, verapamil or torasemide) [34, 37, 41, 46] and in the response to low vs. high doses of digoxin, lisinopril or losartan (Table 2). These findings raised the possibility that lower doses of these drugs should be used in women. Indeed, a *post-hoc* analysis of the BIOSTAT-CHF trial found that in men with HFrEF the lowest hazards of all-cause death or HFH occurred at 100% of CPG-recommended doses of ACEIs, ARBs or β blockers, while women showed ~30% lower risk at only 40–60% of CPG-recommended doses of these drugs, and no additional benefit was gained when doses were up-titrated in women [30]. These findings which were validated in the ASIAN-HF cohort suggest that women may need up to 50% lower doses of these drugs than those recommended in CPGs. Therefore, despite some of these drugs were marketed decades ago, their optimal dosing in women remains undefined. Meanwhile, they will continue to receive overdoses that may result in higher incidence of ADRs [26]. Notably, neither pharmaceutical industries nor scientific societies seem interested in clinical trials to define the optimal doses of cheap generic drugs in women.

3.4 SGRDs in the Prescription of Guideline-Recommended Drugs

Women take more medications (prescribed or not), present lower drug adherence in their use of use of chronic GRDs (possibly due to the higher incidence of ADRs or prevalence of comorbidities) and are less likely to receive GRDs for the treatment of HTN/HF than men at similar risk [26, 27, 178]. Real-world data confirm that treatment of HTN/HF differs between men and women. Hypertensive women receive less antihypertensive drugs, are more frequently prescribed diuretics and ARBs, but less frequently ACEIs, β-blockers and CCBs than men despite comparable BP levels, and BP control (<140/90 mmHg) is more difficult to achieve in elderly women than in men [27, 170, 179, 180]. Hypertensive women with coronary heart disease receive more ARBs and MRAs but less ACEIs than men [181], and hypertensive women with chronic kidney disease receive more ARBs probably because they are better tolerated, but less

ACEIs, β-blockers and CCBs [182]. Although the lower use of ACEIs in young women may be related to their potential teratogenic effects, this bias persists at all ages probably because of the higher incidence of ADRs. Women with HF are more likely receive diuretics probably because they present more congestion, digoxin (despite its use may be associated with higher mortality risk) and ARBs, but are less frequently treated with ACEIs, MRAs, or β-blockers than men even after adjusting for all known variables [23, 24, 26, 183, 184]. Thus, women with HF are less likely to receive GRDs which may contribute to persistent symptoms).

The lower adherence to GRDs represents a significant obstacle to improve patient outcomes, while SGRDs in the intensity of and the likelihood of receiving GRDs confirms the need for a more personalized drug selection to improve clinical outcomes in women [160, 161, 178, 185].

4 Conclusions

There are SGRDs in the efficacy, dosage, and, particularly, in the safety profile of some GRDs for the treatment of HTN or HF. However, because in many RCTs women were underrepresented and sex-specific analyses of clinical data were not performed, the clinical impact of these differences is considered moderate or uncertain and their translation into clinical practice is slow. Indeed, major CPGs recommend (with a few exceptions) to treat women with HTN/HF like men. Consequently, treatment choices may be less optimal for women, leading to more frequent ADRs and suboptimal outcomes (Fig. 1).

Prospective RCTs should be specifically designed to analyze the potential SGRDs in dosing, efficacy, and safety of GRDs, understand the mechanisms involved and determine its clinical

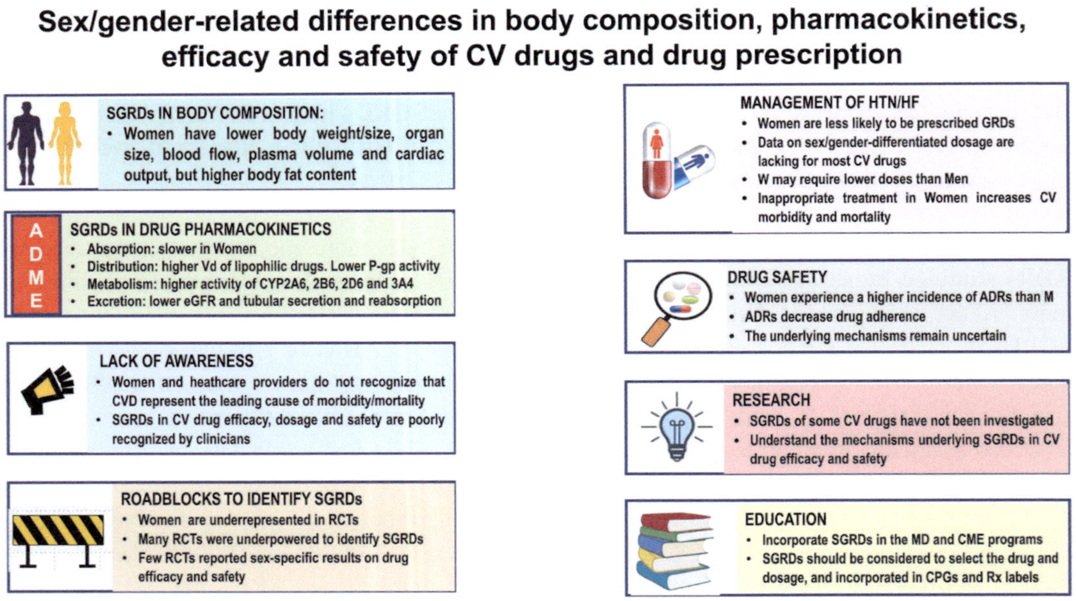

Fig. 1 Sex/gender-related differences in body composition, pharmacokinetics, efficacy and safety of CV drugs and CV drug prescription. *ADRs* adverse drug reactions, *CV* cardiovascular, *CME* continuing medical education, *CVDs* cardiovascular diseases, *eGFR* estimated glomerular filtration rate, *GRDs* guideline recommended drugs, *HF* heart failure, *HTN* hypertension, *MD* medical doctor, *RCTs* randomized clinical trials, *P-gp* P-glycoprotein, *SGRDs* sex/gender-related differences

relevance. SGRDs in cardiovascular drug efficacy and safety should be part of medical education and included on drug labels, and sex-specific guidelines to treat CVDs should be developed to optimize the treatment of women and minimize the higher incidence of ADRs. A better understanding of SGRDs of the efficacy and safety of GRDs is the first step for the design of a more personalized treatment of CVDs in women and men.

Key Issues

- There are SGRDs in the efficacy safety and optimal doses of some drugs recommended in clinical guidelines for the treatment of HTN or HF
- Treatment of HTN/HF differs between men and women. Women are less likely to receive guideline-recommended drugs than men at similar risk
- Spironolactone and sacubitril may be more effective in women than in men with HFpEF
- Optimal doses of some guideline-recommended drugs remain uncertain in women. Digoxin, metoprolol, propranolol, verapamil or torasemide exposure is higher in women and may require lower doses to reduce the risk of ADRs. In women with HFrEF the lowest hazards of all-cause death or HFH occurred at 40–60% of guideline-recommended doses of ACEIs, ARBs or β blockers; in men at 100% of the recommended dose.
- Women experience more ADRs than men, but most trials do not report ADRs stratified by sex/gender. SGRDs in drug safety should be mentioned in guidelines and Rx labels.
- SGRDs in drug efficacy and safety should be part of medical education and included on drug labels
- A better understanding of SGRDs in the efficacy and safety of GRDs is the first step to design a more personalized pharmacological treatment and improve clinical outcomes in women

Questions and Answers

1. Indicate which of the following drugs have demonstrated to reduce hospitalizations in women, but not in men, with heart failure with preserved ejection fraction
   (A) Metoprolol
   (B) Eplerenone
   (C) Enalapril
   (D) Sacubitril-valsartan
   (E) Candesartan
   Correct answer: D
2. Which of the following statements is **incorrect**
   (A) Metoprolol exposure increases in women as compared with men
   (B) Loop diuretics produce more electrolyte abnormalities in women than in men
   (C) In hypertensive patients, calcium channel blockers reduce the incidence of stroke more in men than in women
   (D) Doses of digoxin that achieve a plasma concentration of the drug in the range of 0.5–0.9 ng/mL are recommended
   (E) Espironolatone produce more adverse reactions in men than in women
   Correct answer: C
3. Indicate which of the following statements is **incorrect**
   (A) The BIOSTAT-CHF study suggests that women with HFrEF might need higher doses of ACE inhibitors or angiotensin receptor blockers and β blockers than men
   (B) Torasemide exposure is significantly higher in women as compared with men
   (C) In many randomized clinical trials (RCTs) enrolling patients with heart failure women were underrepresented
   (D) Many RCTs are underpowered to identify sex/gender-related differences in the efficacy of cardiovascular drugs
   (E) Hypertensive women are more frequently prescribed diuretics and angiotensin receptor blockers, but less frequently angiotensin converting enzyme inhibitors, β-blockers and calcium channel blockers
   Correct answer: A

4. Indicate which of the following statements is **incorrect**
   (A) Women presents a lower glomerular filtration rate (GFR) and tubular secretion/reabsorption than men
   (B) Women present lower activity of CYP (cytochrome P450) 3A4 and 2D6
   (C) Women present lower activity of glycoprotein P
   (D) Women present a higher proportion of body fat
   (E) Many sex/gender-related differences in drug pharmacokinetics disappear when doses are adjusted to body weight or GFR

   Correct answer: B
5. Among these statements, which is true?
   (A) No mortality benefits of angiotensin-converting enzyme inhibitors were reported in women with asymptomatic LV systolic dysfunction
   (B) In hypertensive patients, metoprolol produces a greater decrease in blood pressure and a smaller increase in heart rate during exercise in men than in women
   (C) Young women present higher blood pressure reduction in response to verapamil than old women
   (D) Women with heart failure are more likely to receive angiotensin converting enzyme inhibitors, mineralocorticoid receptor antagonists or β-blockers than men
   (E) Women receive more SGLT2 inhibitors than men with heart failure with reduced ejection fraction

   Correct answer: A

Acknowledgments This manuscript was funded by grants from the Ministerio de Ciencia e Innovación (PID2020-118694RB-I00) and Comunidad de Madrid (P2022/BMD-722).

Declaration of Competing Interest The authors declare that there are no conflicts of interest.

References

1. Timmis A, Vardas P, Townsend N, Torbica A, Katus H, De Smedt D, et al. European Society of Cardiology: cardiovascular disease statistics 2021. Eur Heart J. 2022;43(8):716–99.
2. Tsao CW, Aday AW, Almarzooq ZI, Alonso A, Beaton AZ, Bittencourt MS, et al. Heart disease and stroke statistics-2022 update: a report from the American Heart Association. Circulation. 2022;145(8):e153–639.
3. Lindstrom M, DeCleene N, Dorsey H, Fuster V, Johnson CO, LeGrand KE, et al. Global burden of cardiovascular diseases and risks collaboration, 1990-2021. J Am Coll Cardiol. 2022;80(25):2372–425.
4. Yusuf S, Joseph P, Rangarajan S, Islam S, Mente A, Hystad P, et al. Modifiable risk factors, cardiovascular disease, and mortality in 155 722 individuals from 21 high-income, middle-income, and low-income countries (PURE): a prospective cohort study. Lancet. 2020;395(10226):795–808.
5. Whelton PK, Carey RM, Aronow WS, Casey DE, Collins KJ, Dennison Himmelfarb C, et al. 2017 ACC/AHA/AAPA/ABC/ACPM/AGS/APhA/ASH/ASPC/NMA/PCNA guideline for the prevention, detection, evaluation, and management of high blood pressure in adults: a report of the American College of Cardiology/American Heart Association task force on clinical practice guidelines. J Am Coll Cardiol. 2018;71(19):e127–248.
6. Williams B, Mancia G, Spiering W, Agabiti Rosei E, Azizi M, Burnier M, et al. 2018 ESC/ESH guidelines for the management of arterial hypertension. Eur Heart J. 2018;39(33):3021–104.
7. Heidenreich PA, Bozkurt B, Aguilar D, Allen LA, Byun JJ, Colvin MM, et al. 2022 AHA/ACC/HFSA guideline for the management of heart failure: a report of the American College of Cardiology/American Heart Association Joint Committee on clinical practice guidelines. J Am Coll Cardiol. 2022;79(17):e263–421.
8. McDonagh TA, Metra M, Adamo M, Gardner RS, Baumbach A, Böhm M, et al. 2021 ESC guidelines for the diagnosis and treatment of acute and chronic heart failure. Eur Heart J. 2021;42(36):3599–726.
9. Bairey Merz CN, Andersen H, Sprague E, Burns A, Keida M, Walsh MN, et al. Knowledge, attitudes, and beliefs regarding cardiovascular disease in women: the Women's Heart Alliance. J Am Coll Cardiol. 2017;70(2):123–32.
10. Maas AH, van der Schouw YT, Regitz-Zagrosek V, Swahn E, Appelman YE, Pasterkamp G, et al. Red alert for women's heart: the urgent need for more research and knowledge on cardiovascular disease in women: proceedings of the workshop held in Brussels on gender differences in cardiovascular disease, 29 September 2011. Eur Heart J. 2011;32(11):1362–8.

11. Connelly PJ, Azizi Z, Alipour P, Delles C, Pilote L, Raparelli V. The importance of gender to understand sex differences in cardiovascular disease. Can J Cardiol. 2021;37(5):699–710.
12. EUGenMed Cardiovascular Clinical Study Group, Regitz-Zagrosek V, Oertelt-Prigione S, Prescott E, Franconi F, Gerdts E, et al. Gender in cardiovascular diseases: impact on clinical manifestations, management, and outcomes. Eur Heart J. 2016;37(1):24–34.
13. Townsend N, Kazakiewicz D, Lucy Wright F, Timmis A, Huculeci R, Torbica A, et al. Epidemiology of cardiovascular disease in Europe. Nat Rev Cardiol. 2022;19(2):133–43.
14. Ji H, Niiranen TJ, Rader F, Henglin M, Kim A, Ebinger JE, et al. Sex differences in blood pressure associations with cardiovascular outcomes. Circulation. 2021;143(7):761–3.
15. Ji H, Kim A, Ebinger JE, Niiranen TJ, Claggett BL, Bairey Merz CN, et al. Sex differences in blood pressure trajectories over the life course. JAMA Cardiol. 2020;5(3):19–26.
16. Kringeland E, Tell GS, Midtbø H, Haugsgjerd TR, Igland J, Gerdts E. Factors associated with increase in blood pressure and incident hypertension in early midlife: the Hordaland Health Study. Blood Press. 2020;29(5):267–75.
17. Shen W, Zhang T, Li S, Zhang H, Xi B, Shen H, et al. Race and sex differences of long-term blood pressure profiles from childhood and adult hypertension: the Bogalusa Heart Study. Hypertension. 2017;70(1):66–74.
18. O'Keeffe LM, Simpkin AJ, Tilling K, Anderson EL, Hughes AD, Lawlor DA, et al. Sex-specific trajectories of measures of cardiovascular health during childhood and adolescence: a prospective cohort study. Atherosclerosis. 2018;278:190–6.
19. Wenger NK, Arnold A, Bairey Merz CN, Cooper-DeHoff RM, Ferdinand KC, Fleg JL, et al. Hypertension across a woman's life cycle. J Am Coll Cardiol. 2018;71(16):1797–813.
20. Gerdts E, Sudano I, Brouwers S, Borghi C, Bruno RM, Ceconi C, et al. Sex differences in arterial hypertension. Eur Heart J. 2022;43(46):4777–88.
21. Pepine CJ, Merz CNB, El Hajj S, Ferdinand KC, Hamilton MA, Lindley KJ, et al. Heart failure with preserved ejection fraction: similarities and differences between women and men. Int J Cardiol. 2020;304:101–8.
22. Pandey A, Omar W, Ayers C, LaMonte M, Klein L, Allen NB, et al. Sex and race differences in lifetime risk of heart failure with preserved ejection fraction and heart failure with reduced ejection fraction. Circulation. 2018;137(17):1814–23.
23. Dewan P, Rørth R, Jhund PS, Shen L, Raparelli V, Petrie MC, et al. Differential impact of heart failure with reduced ejection fraction on men and women. J Am Coll Cardiol. 2019;73(1):29–40.
24. Regitz-Zagrosek V. Sex and gender differences in heart failure. Int J Heart Fail. 2020;2(3):157–81.
25. Jochmann N, Stangl K, Garbe E, Baumann G, Stangl V. Female-specific aspects in the pharmacotherapy of chronic cardiovascular diseases. Eur Heart J. 2005;26(16):1585–95.
26. Tamargo J, Caballero R, Delpón E. Sex-related differences in the pharmacological treatment of heart failure. Pharmacol Ther. 2022;229:107891.
27. Tamargo J, Caballero R, Mosquera ED. Sex and gender differences in the treatment of arterial hypertension. Expert Rev Clin Pharmacol. 2023;16(4):329–47.
28. Clayton JA, Gaugh MD. Sex as a biological variable in cardiovascular diseases: JACC focus seminar 1/7. J Am Coll Cardiol. 2022;79(14):1388–97.
29. Shekelle PG, Rich MW, Morton SC, Atkinson CSW, Tu W, Maglione M, et al. Efficacy of angiotensin-converting enzyme inhibitors and beta-blockers in the management of left ventricular systolic dysfunction according to race, gender, and diabetic status: a meta-analysis of major clinical trials. J Am Coll Cardiol. 2003;41(9):1529–38.
30. Santema BT, Ouwerkerk W, Tromp J, Sama IE, Ravera A, Regitz-Zagrosek V, et al. Identifying optimal doses of heart failure medications in men compared with women: a prospective, observational, cohort study. Lancet. 2019;394(10205):1254–63.
31. Israili ZH. Clinical pharmacokinetics of angiotensin II (AT1) receptor blockers in hypertension. J Hum Hypertens. 2000;14(Suppl 1):S73–86.
32. Cabaleiro T, Román M, Ochoa D, Talegón M, Prieto-Pérez R, Wojnicz A, et al. Evaluation of the relationship between sex, polymorphisms in CYP2C8 and CYP2C9, and pharmacokinetics of angiotensin receptor blockers. Drug Metab Dispos. 2013;41(1):224–9.
33. Hudson M, Rahme E, Behlouli H, Sheppard R, Pilote L. Sex differences in the effectiveness of angiotensin receptor blockers and angiotensin converting enzyme inhibitors in patients with congestive heart failure—a population study. Eur J Heart Fail. 2007;9(6–7):602–9.
34. Luzier AB, Killian A, Wilton JH, Wilson MF, Forrest A, Kazierad DJ. Gender-related effects on metoprolol pharmacokinetics and pharmacodynamics in healthy volunteers. Clin Pharmacol Ther. 1999;66(6):594–601.
35. Walle T, Walle UK, Cowart TD, Conradi EC. Pathway-selective sex differences in the metabolic clearance of propranolol in human subjects. Clin Pharmacol Ther. 1989;46(3):257–63.
36. Kendall MJ, Quarterman CP, Jack DB, Beeley L. Metoprolol pharmacokinetics and the oral contraceptive pill. Br J Clin Pharmacol. 1982;14(1):120–2.
37. Eugene AR. Gender based dosing of metoprolol in the elderly using population pharmacokinetic modeling and simulations. Int J Clin Pharmacol Toxicol. 2016;5(3):209–15.
38. Hendriksen LC, Omes-Smit G, Koch BCP, Ikram MA, Stricker BH, Visser LE. Sex-based difference in the effect of metoprolol on heart rate and brady-

cardia in a population-based setting. J Pers Med. 2022;12(6):870.
39. Thürmann PA, Haack S, Werner U, Szymanski J, Haase G, Drewelow B, et al. Tolerability of beta-blockers metabolized via cytochrome P450 2D6 is sex-dependent. Clin Pharmacol Ther. 2006;80(5):551–3.
40. Krecic-Shepard ME, Barnas CR, Slimko J, Jones MP, Schwartz JB. Gender-specific effects on verapamil pharmacokinetics and pharmacodynamics in humans. J Clin Pharmacol. 2000;40(3):219–30.
41. Schwartz JB, Capili H, Wainer IW. Verapamil stereoisomers during racemic verapamil administration: effects of aging and comparisons to administration of individual stereoisomers. Clin Pharmacol Ther. 1994;56(4):368–76.
42. Kloner RA, Sowers JR, DiBona GF, Gaffney M, Wein M. Sex- and age-related antihypertensive effects of amlodipine. The Amlodipine Cardiovascular Community Trial Study Group. Am J Cardiol. 1996;77(9):713–22.
43. Rathore SS, Curtis JP, Wang Y, Bristow MR, Krumholz HM. Association of serum digoxin concentration and outcomes in patients with heart failure. JAMA. 2003;289(7):871–8.
44. Tamargo J, Rosano G, Walther T, Duarte J, Niessner A, Kaski JC, et al. Gender differences in the effects of cardiovascular drugs. Eur Heart J Cardiovasc Pharmacother. 2017;3(3):163–82.
45. Rathore SS, Wang Y, Krumholz HM. Sex-based differences in the effect of digoxin for the treatment of heart failure. N Engl J Med. 2002;347(18):1403–11.
46. Werner U, Werner D, Heinbüchner S, Graf B, Ince H, Kische S, et al. Gender is an important determinant of the disposition of the loop diuretic torasemide. J Clin Pharmacol. 2010;50(2):160–8.
47. Vormfelde SV, Schirmer M, Hagos Y, Toliat MR, Engelhardt S, Meineke I, et al. Torsemide renal clearance and genetic variation in luminal and basolateral organic anion transporters. Br J Clin Pharmacol. 2006;62(3):323–35.
48. Brandoni A, Villar SR, Torres AM. Gender-related differences in the pharmacodynamics of furosemide in rats. Pharmacology. 2004;70(2):107–12.
49. Chen Z, Vaughn DA, Fanestil DD. Influence of gender on renal thiazide diuretic receptor density and response. J Am Soc Nephrol. 1994;5(4):1112–9.
50. Verlander JW, Tran TM, Zhang L, Kaplan MR, Hebert SC. Estradiol enhances thiazide-sensitive NaCl cotransporter density in the apical plasma membrane of the distal convoluted tubule in ovariectomized rats. J Clin Invest. 1998;101(8):1661–9.
51. Tamargo J, Agarwall NR, Tamargo M. Sex differences in cardiac diseases. Cambridge: Elsevier; 2021. p. 597–641.
52. Taylor AL, Lindenfeld J, Ziesche S, Walsh MN, Mitchell JE, Adams K, et al. Outcomes by gender in the African-American Heart Failure Trial. J Am Coll Cardiol. 2006;48(11):2263–7.
53. Tendera M, Borer JS, Tardif JC. Efficacy of I(f) inhibition with ivabradine in different subpopulations with stable angina pectoris. Cardiology. 2009;114(2):116–25.
54. Kanashiro-Takeuchi RM, Heidecker B, Lamirault G, Dharamsi JW, Hare JM. Sex-specific impact of aldosterone receptor antagonism on ventricular remodeling and gene expression after myocardial infarction. Clin Transl Sci. 2009;2(2):134–42.
55. Vasan RS, Massaro JM, Wilson PWF, Seshadri S, Wolf PA, Levy D, et al. Antecedent blood pressure and risk of cardiovascular disease: the Framingham Heart Study. Circulation. 2002;105(1):48–53.
56. McMurray JJV, Jackson AM, Lam CSP, Redfield MM, Anand IS, Ge J, et al. Effects of sacubitril-valsartan versus valsartan in women compared with men with heart failure and preserved ejection fraction: insights from PARAGON-HF. Circulation. 2020;141(5):338–51.
57. Novella S, Pérez-Cremades D, Mompeón A, Hermenegildo C. Mechanisms underlying the influence of oestrogen on cardiovascular physiology in women. J Physiol. 2019;597(19):4873–86.
58. Oparil S, Davis BR, Cushman WC, Ford CE, Furberg CD, Habib GB, et al. Mortality and morbidity during and after Antihypertensive and Lipid-Lowering Treatment to Prevent Heart Attack Trial: results by sex. Hypertension. 2013;61(5):977–86.
59. Yamal JM, Oparil S, Davis BR, Alderman MH, Calhoun DA, Cushman WC, et al. Stroke outcomes among participants randomized to chlorthalidone, amlodipine or lisinopril in ALLHAT. J Am Soc Hypertens. 2014;8(11):808–19.
60. ALLHAT Officers and Coordinators for the ALLHAT Collaborative Research Group. The Antihypertensive and Lipid-Lowering Treatment to Prevent Heart Attack Trial. Major outcomes in high-risk hypertensive patients randomized to angiotensin-converting enzyme inhibitor or calcium channel blocker vs diuretic: the Antihypertensive and Lipid-Lowering Treatment to Prevent Heart Attack Trial (ALLHAT). JAMA. 2002;288(23):2981–97.
61. Jamerson K, Weber MA, Bakris GL, Dahlöf B, Pitt B, Shi V, et al. Benazepril plus amlodipine or hydrochlorothiazide for hypertension in high-risk patients. N Engl J Med. 2008;359(23):2417–28.
62. Fan X, Han Y, Sun K, Wang Y, Xin Y, Bai Y, et al. Sex differences in blood pressure response to antihypertensive therapy in Chinese patients with hypertension. Ann Pharmacother. 2008;42(12):1772–81.
63. Kjeldsen SE, Warnold I, Hansson L, HOT Study Group. Hypertension Optimal Treatment Study Group. Influence of gender on prevention of myocardial infarction by antihypertensives and acetylsalicylic acid: the HOT study. J Gend Specif Med. 2000;3(8):35–8.
64. Saunders E, Cable G, Neutel J. Predictors of blood pressure response to angiotensin receptor blocker/diuretic combination therapy: a secondary analy-

sis of the irbesartan/hydrochlorothiazide blood pressure reductions in diverse patient populations (INCLUSIVE) study. J Clin Hypertens (Greenwich). 2008;10(1):27–33.

65. Gueyffier F, Boutitie F, Boissel JP, Pocock S, Coope J, Cutler J, et al. Effect of antihypertensive drug treatment on cardiovascular outcomes in women and men. A meta-analysis of individual patient data from randomized, controlled trials. The INDANA Investigators. Ann Intern Med. 1997;126(10):761–7.
66. Os I, Franco V, Kjeldsen SE, Manhem K, Devereux RB, Gerdts E, et al. Effects of losartan in women with hypertension and left ventricular hypertrophy: results from the Losartan Intervention for Endpoint Reduction in Hypertension Study. Hypertension. 2008;51(4):1103–8.
67. Okin PM, Gerdts E, Kjeldsen SE, Julius S, Edelman JM, Dahlöf B, et al. Gender differences in regression of electrocardiographic left ventricular hypertrophy during antihypertensive therapy. Hypertension. 2008;52(1):100–6.
68. Matsui K, Kim-Mitsuyama S, Ogawa H, Jinnouchi T, Jinnouchi H, Arakawa K, et al. Sex differences in response to angiotensin II receptor blocker-based therapy in elderly, high-risk, hypertensive Japanese patients: a subanalysis of the OSCAR study. Hypertens Res. 2014;37(6):526–32.
69. Wing LMH, Reid CM, Ryan P, Beilin LJ, Brown MA, Jennings GLR, et al. A comparison of outcomes with angiotensin-converting—enzyme inhibitors and diuretics for hypertension in the elderly. N Engl J Med. 2003;348(7):583–92.
70. SPRINT Research Group, Wright JT, Williamson JD, Whelton PK, Snyder JK, Sink KM, et al. A randomized trial of intensive versus standard blood-pressure control. N Engl J Med. 2015;373(22):2103–16.
71. Foy CG, Lovato LC, Vitolins MZ, Bates JT, Campbell R, Cushman WC, et al. Gender, blood pressure, and cardiovascular and renal outcomes in adults with hypertension from the Systolic Blood Pressure Intervention Trial. J Hypertens. 2018;36(4):904–15.
72. Ochoa-Jimenez R, Viquez-Beita K, Daluwatte C, Zusterzeel R. Sex differences of patients with systemic hypertension (from the analysis of the Systolic Blood Pressure Intervention Trial [SPRINT]). Am J Cardiol. 2018;122(6):985–93.
73. Zanchetti A, Julius S, Kjeldsen S, McInnes GT, Hua T, Weber M, et al. Outcomes in subgroups of hypertensive patients treated with regimens based on valsartan and amlodipine: an analysis of findings from the VALUE trial. J Hypertens. 2006;24(11):2163–8.
74. Turnbull F, Woodward M, Neal B, Barzi F, Ninomiya T, Chalmers J, et al. Do men and women respond differently to blood pressure-lowering treatment? Results of prospectively designed overviews of randomized trials. Eur Heart J. 2008;29(21):2669–80.
75. Packer M, Poole-Wilson PA, Armstrong PW, Cleland JG, Horowitz JD, Massie BM, et al. Comparative effects of low and high doses of the angiotensin-converting enzyme inhibitor, lisinopril, on morbidity and mortality in chronic heart failure. ATLAS Study Group. Circulation. 1999;100(23):2312–8.
76. O'Meara E, Clayton T, McEntegart MB, McMurray JJV, Piña IL, Granger CB, et al. Sex differences in clinical characteristics and prognosis in a broad spectrum of patients with heart failure: results of the Candesartan in Heart failure: Assessment of Reduction in Mortality and morbidity (CHARM) program. Circulation. 2007;115(24):3111–20.
77. Sakata Y, Miyata S, Nochioka K, Miura M. Sex differences in patients with chronic heart failure with reference to left ventricular ejection fraction: a report from the CHART-2 study. Gender Genome. 2018;2:27–42.
78. Simon T, Mary-Krause M, Funck-Brentano C, Jaillon P. Sex differences in the prognosis of congestive heart failure: results from the Cardiac Insufficiency Bisoprolol Study (CIBIS II). Circulation. 2001;103(3):375–80.
79. CONSENSUS Trial Study Group. Effects of enalapril on mortality in severe congestive heart failure. Results of the Cooperative North Scandinavian Enalapril Survival Study (CONSENSUS). N Engl J Med. 1987;316(23):1429–35.
80. Digitalis Investigation Group. The effect of digoxin on mortality and morbidity in patients with heart failure. N Engl J Med. 1997;336(8):525–33.
81. Adams KF, Patterson JH, Gattis WA, O'Connor CM, Lee CR, Schwartz TA, et al. Relationship of serum digoxin concentration to mortality and morbidity in women in the digitalis investigation group trial: a retrospective analysis. J Am Coll Cardiol. 2005;46(3):497–504.
82. Lam CSP, Carson PE, Anand IS, Rector TS, Kuskowski M, Komajda M, et al. Sex differences in clinical characteristics and outcomes in elderly patients with heart failure and preserved ejection fraction: the Irbesartan in Heart Failure with Preserved Ejection Fraction (I-PRESERVE) trial. Circ Heart Fail. 2012;5(5):571–8.
83. Merrill M, Sweitzer NK, Lindenfeld J, Kao DP. Sex differences in outcomes and responses to spironolactone in heart failure with preserved ejection fraction: a secondary analysis of TOPCAT trial. JACC Heart Fail. 2019;7(3):228–38.
84. Køber L, Torp-Pedersen C, Carlsen JE, Bagger H, Eliasen P, Lyngborg K, et al. A clinical trial of the angiotensin-converting-enzyme inhibitor trandolapril in patients with left ventricular dysfunction after myocardial infarction. Trandolapril Cardiac Evaluation (TRACE) Study Group. N Engl J Med. 1995;333(25):1670–6.
85. Garg R, Yusuf S. Overview of randomized trials of angiotensin-converting enzyme inhibitors on mortality and morbidity in patients with heart failure. Collaborative Group on ACE Inhibitor Trials. JAMA. 1995;273(18):1450–6.
86. Gandhi M, Aweeka F, Greenblatt RM, Blaschke TF. Sex differences in pharmacokinetics and pharmacodynamics. Annu Rev Pharmacol Toxicol. 2004;44:499–523.

87. Franconi F, Campesi I. Pharmacogenomics, pharmacokinetics, and pharmacodynamics: interaction with biological differences between men and women. Br J Pharmacol. 2014;171(3):580–94.
88. Soldin OP, Chung SH, Mattison DR. Sex differences in drug disposition. J Biomed Biotechnol. 2011;2011:187103.
89. Nicolas JM, Espie P, Molimard M. Gender and interindividual variability in pharmacokinetics. Drug Metab Rev. 2009;41(3):408–21.
90. Mangoni AA, Jarmuzewska EA. The influence of heart failure on the pharmacokinetics of cardiovascular and non-cardiovascular drugs: a critical appraisal of the evidence. Br J Clin Pharmacol. 2019;85(1):20–36.
91. Cummins CL, Wu CY, Benet LZ. Sex-related differences in the clearance of cytochrome P450 3A4 substrates may be caused by P-glycoprotein. Clin Pharmacol Ther. 2002;72(5):474–89.
92. Scott PE, Unger EF, Jenkins MR, Southworth MR, McDowell TY, Geller RJ, et al. Participation of women in clinical trials supporting FDA approval of cardiovascular drugs. J Am Coll Cardiol. 2018;71(18):1960–9.
93. Melloni C, Berger JS, Wang TY, Gunes F, Stebbins A, Pieper KS, et al. Representation of women in randomized clinical trials of cardiovascular disease prevention. Circ Cardiovasc Qual Outcomes. 2010;3(2):135–42.
94. Levinsson A, Dubé MP, Tardif JC, de Denus S. Sex, drugs, and heart failure: a sex-sensitive review of the evidence base behind current heart failure clinical guidelines. ESC Heart Fail. 2018;5(5):745–54.
95. Crespo-Leiro MG, Anker SD, Maggioni AP, Coats AJ, Filippatos G, Ruschitzka F, et al. European Society of Cardiology Heart Failure Long-Term Registry (ESC-HF-LT): 1-year follow-up outcomes and differences across regions. Eur J Heart Fail. 2016;18(6):613–25.
96. Mohseni-Alsalhi Z, Vesseur MAM, Wilmes N, Laven SAJS, Meijs DAM, van Luik EM, et al. The representation of females in studies on antihypertensive medication over the years: a scoping review. Biomedicines. 2023;11(5):1435.
97. Wang W, Ma Y, Huang Y, Chen H. Generalizability analysis for clinical trials: a simulation study. Stat Med. 2017;36(10):1523–31.
98. Yusuf S, Wittes J, Probstfield J, Tyroler HA. Analysis and interpretation of treatment effects in subgroups of patients in randomized clinical trials. JAMA. 1991;266(1):93–8.
99. Nguyen QD, Peters E, Wassef A, Desmarais P, Rémillard-Labrosse D, Tremblay-Gravel M. Evolution of age and female representation in the most-cited randomized controlled trials of cardiology of the last 20 years. Circ Cardiovasc Qual Outcomes. 2018;11(6):e004713.
100. Griffin BL, Bolch CA, Bourjeily G, Madsen TE, Hasnain M, McGregor AJ, et al. Hypertension: are current guidelines inclusive of sex and gender? J Womens Health (Larchmt). 2022;31(10):1391–6.
101. Fletcher A, Beevers DG, Bulpitt C, Butler A, Coles EC, Hunt D, et al. Beta adrenoceptor blockade is associated with increased survival in male but not female hypertensive patients: a report from the DHSS Hypertension Care Computing Project (DHCCP). J Hum Hypertens. 1988;2(4):219–27.
102. A randomized trial of propranolol in patients with acute myocardial infarction. I. Mortality results. JAMA. 1982;247(12):1707–14.
103. Effect of metoprolol CR/XL in chronic heart failure: Metoprolol CR/XL Randomised Intervention Trial in Congestive Heart Failure (MERIT-HF). Lancet. 1999;353(9169):2001–7.
104. Seeland U, Regitz-Zagrosek V. Sex and gender differences in cardiovascular drug therapy. Handb Exp Pharmacol. 2012;214:211–36.
105. Ghali JK, Piña IL, Gottlieb SS, Deedwania PC, Wikstrand JC, MERIT-HF Study Group. Metoprolol CR/XL in female patients with heart failure: analysis of the experience in Metoprolol Extended-Release Randomized Intervention Trial in Heart Failure (MERIT-HF). Circulation. 2002;105(13):1585–91.
106. López-Sendón J, Swedberg K, McMurray J, Tamargo J, Maggioni AP, Dargie H, et al. Expert consensus document on beta-adrenergic receptor blockers. Eur Heart J. 2004;25(15):1341–62.
107. Kotecha D, Manzano L, Krum H, Rosano G, Holmes J, Altman DG, et al. Effect of age and sex on efficacy and tolerability of β blockers in patients with heart failure with reduced ejection fraction: individual patient data meta-analysis. BMJ. 2016;353:i1855.
108. Olsson G, Wikstrand J, Warnold I, Manger Cats V, McBoyle D, Herlitz J, et al. Metoprolol-induced reduction in postinfarction mortality: pooled results from five double-blind randomized trials. Eur Heart J. 1992;13(1):28–32.
109. Gottlieb SS, McCarter RJ, Vogel RA. Effect of beta-blockade on mortality among high-risk and low-risk patients after myocardial infarction. N Engl J Med. 1998;339(8):489–97.
110. Krecic-Shepard ME, Park K, Barnas C, Slimko J, Kerwin DR, Schwartz JB. Race and sex influence clearance of nifedipine: results of a population study. Clin Pharmacol Ther. 2000;68(2):130–42.
111. Kang D, Verotta D, Krecic-Shepard ME, Modi NB, Gupta SK, Schwartz JB. Population analyses of sustained-release verapamil in patients: effects of sex, race, and smoking. Clin Pharmacol Ther. 2003;73(1):31–40.
112. Fischer M, Baessler A, Schunkert H. Renin angiotensin system and gender differences in the cardiovascular system. Cardiovasc Res. 2002;53(3):672–7.
113. Komukai K, Mochizuki S, Yoshimura M. Gender and the renin-angiotensin-aldosterone system. Fundam Clin Pharmacol. 2010;24(6):687–98.
114. Rabi DM, Khan N, Vallee M, Hladunewich MA, Tobe SW, Pilote L. Reporting on sex-based analysis in clinical trials of angiotensin-converting enzyme inhibitor and angiotensin receptor blocker efficacy. Can J Cardiol. 2008;24(6):491–6.

115. Bourassa MG, Gurné O, Bangdiwala SI, Ghali JK, Young JB, Rousseau M, et al. Natural history and patterns of current practice in heart failure. The Studies of Left Ventricular Dysfunction (SOLVD) Investigators. J Am Coll Cardiol. 1993;22(4 Suppl A):14A–9A.
116. Lonn E, Roccaforte R, Yi Q, Dagenais G, Sleight P, Bosch J, et al. Effect of long-term therapy with ramipril in high-risk women. J Am Coll Cardiol. 2002;40(4):693–702.
117. Virani SS, Alonso A, Aparicio HJ, Benjamin EJ, Bittencourt MS, Callaway CW, et al. Heart disease and stroke statistics-2021 update: a report from the American Heart Association. Circulation. 2021;143(8):e254–743.
118. Clemmer JS, Faulkner JL, Mullen AJ, Butler KR, Hester RL. Sex-specific responses to mineralocorticoid receptor antagonism in hypertensive African American males and females. Biol Sex Differ. 2019;10(1):24.
119. Pitt B, Zannad F, Remme WJ, Cody R, Castaigne A, Perez A, et al. The effect of spironolactone on morbidity and mortality in patients with severe heart failure. Randomized Aldactone Evaluation Study Investigators. N Engl J Med. 1999;341(10):709–17.
120. Pitt B, Remme W, Zannad F, Neaton J, Martinez F, Roniker B, et al. Eplerenone, a selective aldosterone blocker, in patients with left ventricular dysfunction after myocardial infarction. N Engl J Med. 2003;348(14):1309–21.
121. Zannad F, McMurray JJV, Krum H, van Veldhuisen DJ, Swedberg K, Shi H, et al. Eplerenone in patients with systolic heart failure and mild symptoms. N Engl J Med. 2011;364(1):11–21.
122. Pitt B, White H, Nicolau J, Martinez F, Gheorghiade M, Aschermann M, et al. Eplerenone reduces mortality 30 days after randomization following acute myocardial infarction in patients with left ventricular systolic dysfunction and heart failure. J Am Coll Cardiol. 2005;46(3):425–31.
123. Rossello X, Ferreira JP, Pocock SJ, McMurray JJV, Solomon SD, Lam CSP, et al. Sex differences in mineralocorticoid receptor antagonist trials: a pooled analysis of three large clinical trials. Eur J Heart Fail. 2020;22(5):834–44.
124. McMurray JJV, Packer M, Desai AS, Gong J, Lefkowitz MP, Rizkala AR, et al. Angiotensin-neprilysin inhibition versus enalapril in heart failure. N Engl J Med. 2014;371(11):993–1004.
125. Swedberg K, Komajda M, Böhm M, Borer JS, Ford I, Dubost-Brama A, et al. Ivabradine and outcomes in chronic heart failure (SHIFT): a randomised placebo-controlled study. Lancet. 2010;376(9744):875–85.
126. White J, Tannenbaum C, Klinge I, Schiebinger L, Clayton J. The integration of sex and gender considerations into biomedical research: lessons from international funding agencies. J Clin Endocrinol Metab. 2021;106(10):3034–48.
127. Ahmed A, Rich MW, Love TE, Lloyd-Jones DM, Aban IB, Colucci WS, et al. Digoxin and reduction in mortality and hospitalization in heart failure: a comprehensive post hoc analysis of the DIG trial. Eur Heart J. 2006;27(2):178–86.
128. Freeman JV, Yang J, Sung SH, Hlatky MA, Go AS. Effectiveness and safety of digoxin among contemporary adults with incident systolic heart failure. Circ Cardiovasc Qual Outcomes. 2013;6(5):525–33.
129. Flory JH, Ky B, Haynes K, Brunelli M, et al. Observational cohort study of the safety of digoxin use in women with heart failure. BMJ Open. 2012;2(2):e000888.
130. Hood WB, Dans AL, Guyatt GH, Jaeschke R, McMurray JJV. Digitalis for treatment of heart failure in patients in sinus rhythm. Cochrane Database Syst Rev. 2014;2014(4):CD002901.
131. Boorsma EM, Rienstra M, van Veldhuisen DJ, van der Meer P. Residual confounding in observational studies: new data from the old DIG trial. Eur Heart J. 2019;40(40):3342–4.
132. Musini VM, Nazer M, Bassett K, Wright JM. Blood pressure-lowering efficacy of monotherapy with thiazide diuretics for primary hypertension. Cochrane Database Syst Rev. 2014;2014(5):CD003824.
133. Olde Engberink RHG, Frenkel WJ, van den Bogaard B, Brewster LM, Vogt L, van den Born BJH. Effects of thiazide-type and thiazide-like diuretics on cardiovascular events and mortality: systematic review and meta-analysis. Hypertension. 2015;65(5):1033–40.
134. Suchard MA, Schuemie MJ, Krumholz HM, You SC, Chen R, Pratt N, et al. Comprehensive comparative effectiveness and safety of first-line antihypertensive drug classes: a systematic, multinational, large-scale analysis. Lancet. 2019;394(10211):1816–26.
135. Rydberg DM, Mejyr S, Loikas D, Schenck-Gustafsson K, von Euler M, Malmström RE. Sex differences in spontaneous reports on adverse drug events for common antihypertensive drugs. Eur J Clin Pharmacol. 2018;74(9):1165–73.
136. Sharabi Y, Illan R, Kamari Y, Cohen H, Nadler M, Messerli FH, et al. Diuretic induced hyponatraemia in elderly hypertensive women. J Hum Hypertens. 2002;16(9):631–5.
137. Gueyffier F, Subtil F, Bejan-Angoulvant T, Zerbib Y, Baguet JP, Boivin JM, et al. Can we identify response markers to antihypertensive drugs? First results from the IDEAL trial. J Hum Hypertens. 2015;29(1):22–7.
138. Singh AK, Singh R. Gender difference in cardiovascular outcomes with SGLT-2 inhibitors and GLP-1 receptor agonist in type 2 diabetes: a systematic review and meta-analysis of cardio-vascular outcome trials. Diabetes Metab Syndr. 2020;14(3):181–7.
139. Mishriky BM, Okunrintemi V, Jain S, Sewell KA, Powell JR, Cummings DM. Do GLP-1RAs and SGLT-2is reduce cardiovascular events in women with type 2 diabetes? A systematic review and meta-analysis. Diabetes Metab. 2021;47(1):101160.
140. Mahmoud AN, Elgendy IY, Saad M, Elgendy AY, Barakat AF, Mentias A, et al. Does gender influence the cardiovascular benefits observed with

sodium glucose co-transporter-2 (SGLT-2) inhibitors? A meta-regression analysis. Cardiol Ther. 2017;6(1):129–32.
141. Raparelli V, Elharram M, Moura CS, Abrahamowicz M, Bernatsky S, Behlouli H, et al. Sex differences in cardiovascular effectiveness of newer glucose-lowering drugs added to metformin in type 2 diabetes mellitus. J Am Heart Assoc. 2020;9(1):e012940.
142. Rådholm K, Zhou Z, Clemens K, Neal B, Woodward M. Effects of sodium-glucose co-transporter-2 inhibitors in type 2 diabetes in women versus men. Diabetes Obes Metab. 2020;22(2):263–6.
143. Pruett JE, Lirette ST, Romero DG, Yanes Cardozo LL. Sodium-glucose cotransporter-2 inhibition benefits in cardiorenal risk in men and women. J Endocr Soc. 2022;7(2):bvac191.
144. Eberly LA, Yang L, Eneanya ND, Essien U, Julien H, Nathan AS, et al. Association of race/ethnicity, gender, and socioeconomic status with sodium-glucose cotransporter 2 inhibitor use among patients with diabetes in the US. JAMA Netw Open. 2021;4(4):e216139.
145. Khedagi A, Hoke C, Kelsey M, Coviello A, Jones WS, Jackson LR, et al. Call to action: understanding the differences in the use of SGLT-2 inhibitors and GLP-1 receptor agonists. Am J Prev Cardiol. 2023;13:100477.
146. Patel K, Fonarow GC, Ekundayo OJ, Aban IB, Kilgore ML, Love TE, et al. Beta-blockers in older patients with heart failure and preserved ejection fraction: class, dosage, and outcomes. Int J Cardiol. 2014;173(3):393–401.
147. van Veldhuisen DJ, Cohen-Solal A, Böhm M, Anker SD, Babalis D, Roughton M, et al. Beta-blockade with nebivolol in elderly heart failure patients with impaired and preserved left ventricular ejection fraction: data from SENIORS (Study of Effects of Nebivolol Intervention on Outcomes and Rehospitalization in Seniors With Heart Failure). J Am Coll Cardiol. 2009;53(23):2150–8.
148. Lund LH, Benson L, Dahlström U, Edner M, Friberg L. Association between use of β-blockers and outcomes in patients with heart failure and preserved ejection fraction. JAMA. 2014;312(19):2008–18.
149. Farasat SM, Bolger DT, Shetty V, Menachery EP, Gerstenblith G, Kasper EK, et al. Effect of Beta-blocker therapy on rehospitalization rates in women versus men with heart failure and preserved ejection fraction. Am J Cardiol. 2010;105(2):229–34.
150. Ahmed A, Rich MW, Fleg JL, Zile MR, Young JB, Kitzman DW, et al. Effects of digoxin on morbidity and mortality in diastolic heart failure: the ancillary digitalis investigation group trial. Circulation. 2006;114(5):397–403.
151. Deswal A, Bozkurt B. Comparison of morbidity in women versus men with heart failure and preserved ejection fraction. Am J Cardiol. 2006;97(8):1228–31.
152. Pitt B, Pfeffer MA, Assmann SF, Boineau R, Anand IS, Claggett B, et al. Spironolactone for heart failure with preserved ejection fraction. N Engl J Med. 2014;370(15):1383–92.
153. Dewan P, Jackson A, Lam CSP, Pfeffer MA, Zannad F, Pitt B, et al. Interactions between left ventricular ejection fraction, sex and effect of neurohumoral modulators in heart failure. Eur J Heart Fail. 2020;22(5):898–901.
154. Butler J, Filippatos G, Siddiqi TJ, Ferreira JP, Brueckmann M, Bocchi E, et al. Effects of empagliflozin in women and men with heart failure and preserved ejection fraction. Circulation. 2022;146(14):1046–55.
155. Wang X, Vaduganathan M, Claggett BL, Hegde SM, Pabon M, Kulac IJ, et al. Sex differences in characteristics, outcomes, and treatment response with dapagliflozin across the range of ejection fraction in patients with heart failure: insights from DAPA-HF and DELIVER. Circulation. 2023;147(8):624–34.
156. Rodenburg EM, Stricker BHC, Visser LE. Sex-related differences in hospital admissions attributed to adverse drug reactions in the Netherlands. Br J Clin Pharmacol. 2011;71(1):95–104.
157. Watson S, Caster O, Rochon PA, den Ruijter H. Reported adverse drug reactions in women and men: aggregated evidence from globally collected individual case reports during half a century. EClinicalMedicine. 2019;17:100188.
158. Yu Y, Chen J, Li D, Wang L, Wang W, Liu H. Systematic analysis of adverse event reports for sex differences in adverse drug events. Sci Rep. 2016;6:24955.
159. Parekh A, Fadiran EO, Uhl K, Throckmorton DC. Adverse effects in women: implications for drug development and regulatory policies. Expert Rev Clin Pharmacol. 2011;4(4):453–66.
160. Rasmussen AA, Wiggers H, Jensen M, Berg SK, Rasmussen TB, Borregaard B, et al. Patient-reported outcomes and medication adherence in patients with heart failure. Eur Heart J Cardiovasc Pharmacother. 2021;7(4):287–95.
161. Burnier M, Egan BM. Adherence in hypertension. Circ Res. 2019;124(7):1124–40.
162. Biffi A, Rea F, Iannaccone T, Filippelli A, Mancia G, Corrao G. Sex differences in the adherence of antihypertensive drugs: a systematic review with meta-analyses. BMJ Open. 2020;10(7):e036418.
163. Bots SH, Groepenhoff F, Eikendal ALM, Tannenbaum C, Rochon PA, Regitz-Zagrosek V, et al. Adverse drug reactions to guideline-recommended heart failure drugs in women: a systematic review of the literature. JACC Heart Fail. 2019;7(3):258–66.
164. Alharbi FF, Kholod AAV, Souverein PC, Meyboom RH, de Groot MCH, de Boer A, et al. The impact of age and sex on the reporting of cough and angioedema with renin-angiotensin system inhibitors: a case/noncase study in VigiBase. Fundam Clin Pharmacol. 2017;31(6):676–84.
165. Vukadinović D, Vukadinović AN, Lavall D, Laufs U, Wagenpfeil S, Böhm M. Rate of cough during treat-

ment with angiotensin-converting enzyme inhibitors: a meta-analysis of randomized placebo-controlled trials. Clin Pharmacol Ther. 2019;105(3):652–60.
166. Shah MR, Granger CB, Bart BA, McMurray JJ, Petrie MC, Michelson EL, et al. Sex-related differences in the use and adverse effects of angiotensin-converting enzyme inhibitors in heart failure: the study of patients intolerant of converting enzyme inhibitors registry. Am J Med. 2000;109(6):489–92.
167. Bots SH, Schreuder MM, Roeters van Lennep JE, Watson S, van Puijenbroek E, Onland-Moret NC, et al. Sex differences in reported adverse drug reactions to angiotensin-converting enzyme inhibitors. JAMA Netw Open. 2022;5(4):e228224.
168. Do TP, Seetasith A, Belleli R, Schlienger RG, Corda S, Burudpakdee C, et al. A database cohort study to assess the risk of angioedema among patients with heart failure initiating angiotensin-converting enzyme inhibitors in the USA. Am J Cardiovasc Drugs. 2018;18(3):205–11.
169. Kostis WJ, Shetty M, Chowdhury YS, Kostis JB. ACE inhibitor-induced angioedema: a review. Curr Hypertens Rep. 2018;20(7):55.
170. Cadeddu C, Franconi F, Cassisa L, Campesi I, Pepe A, Cugusi L, et al. Arterial hypertension in the female world: pathophysiology and therapy. J Cardiovasc Med (Hagerstown). 2016;17(4):229–36.
171. Messerli FH. Vasodilatory edema: a common side effect of antihypertensive therapy. Am J Hypertens. 2001;14(9 Pt 1):978–9.
172. Igho Pemu P, Ofili E. Hypertension in women: part I. J Clin Hypertens (Greenwich). 2008;10(5):406–10.
173. Vedove CD, Del Giglio M, Schena D, Girolomoni G. Drug-induced lupus erythematosus. Arch Dermatol Res. 2009;301(1):99–105.
174. DeFilippis EM, Desai AS. Treatment of hyperkalemia in heart failure. Curr Heart Fail Rep. 2017;14(4):266–74.
175. Zinman B, Inzucchi SE, Wanner C, Hehnke U, George JT, Johansen OE, et al. Empagliflozin in women with type 2 diabetes and cardiovascular disease—an analysis of EMPA-REG OUTCOME®. Diabetologia. 2018;61(7):1522–7.
176. McGill JB, Subramanian S. Safety of sodium-glucose co-transporter 2 inhibitors. Am J Cardiol. 2019;124(Suppl 1):S45–52.
177. Ueno K, Sato H. Sex-related differences in pharmacokinetics and pharmacodynamics of anti-hypertensive drugs. Hypertens Res. 2012;35(3):245–50.
178. Manteuffel M, Williams S, Chen W, Verbrugge RR, Pittman DG, Steinkellner A. Influence of patient sex and gender on medication use, adherence, and prescribing alignment with guidelines. J Womens Health (Larchmt). 2014;23(2):112–9.
179. Muntner P, Miles MA, Jaeger BC, Hannon Iii L, Hardy ST, Ostchega Y, et al. Blood pressure control among US adults, 2009 to 2012 through 2017 to 2020. Hypertension. 2022;79(9):1971–80.
180. Osude N, Durazo-Arvizu R, Markossian T, Liu K, Michos ED, Rakotz M, et al. Age and sex disparities in hypertension control: the multi-ethnic study of atherosclerosis (MESA). Am J Prev Cardiol. 2021;8:100230.
181. Ljungman C, Kahan T, Schiöler L, Hjerpe P, Hasselström J, Wettermark B, et al. Gender differences in antihypertensive drug treatment: results from the Swedish Primary Care Cardiovascular Database (SPCCD). J Am Soc Hypertens. 2014;8(12):882–90.
182. Muiesan ML, Ambrosioni E, Costa FV, Leonetti G, Pessina AC, Salvetti M, et al. Sex differences in hypertension-related renal and cardiovascular diseases in Italy: the I-DEMAND study. J Hypertens. 2012;30(12):2378–86.
183. Lainščak M, Milinković I, Polovina M, Crespo-Leiro MG, Lund LH, Anker SD, et al. Sex- and age-related differences in the management and outcomes of chronic heart failure: an analysis of patients from the ESC HFA EORP Heart Failure Long-Term Registry. Eur J Heart Fail. 2020;22(1):92–102.
184. Crousillat DR, Ibrahim NE. Sex differences in the management of advanced heart failure. Curr Treat Options Cardiovasc Med. 2018;20(11):88.
185. Ferdinand KC, Senatore FF, Clayton-Jeter H, Cryer DR, Lewin JC, Nasser SA, et al. Improving medication adherence in cardiometabolic disease: practical and regulatory implications. J Am Coll Cardiol. 2017;69(4):437–51.

Sex Differences in Pharmacokinetics, Pharmacodynamics, and Adverse Drug Reactions of Cardiovascular Drugs

A. Evelo, E. Leegwater, and L. E. Visser

Abstract

Although the number of trials enrolling women has increased, women are still consistently underrepresented. This is especially notable in cardiovascular drug trials, where only 20–30% of participants are women. In addition, sex-specific analyses on the efficacy and safety of drugs are not always performed, or not performed correctly. A consequence of this sex inequality is that most drugs are prescribed to women and men at the same dose, and the information on efficacy and safety at the time of market access is rather limited in women. In the meantime, cardiovascular drugs appear to account for the most pronounced differences in adverse drug reactions between men and women. There are several well-established pharmacokinetic sex differences. Female and male bodies distribute, metabolize and excrete drugs differently, leading to sex differences in drug disposition. Sex-determined variations in pharmacodynamics have traditionally been more difficult to quantify, but several studies have explored these differences for cardiovascular drugs. This chapter examines the biological basis of differences in pharmacokinetics and pharmacodynamics between the sexes for cardiovascular drugs and summarizes studies that have addressed these differences.

Keywords

Sex differences · Pharmacokinetics · Pharmacodynamics · Adverse drug reactions · Cardiovascular drugs

A. Evelo
Department of Hospital Pharmacy, Haga Teaching Hospital, The Hague, The Netherlands

Department of Hospital Pharmacy, Erasmus Medical Center, Rotterdam, The Netherlands
e-mail: a.evelo@hagaziekenhuis.nl

E. Leegwater
Department of Hospital Pharmacy, Rijnstate Hospital, Arnhem, The Netherlands

Department of Infectious Diseases, Leiden University Medical Centre, Leiden, The Netherlands
e-mail: eleegwater@rijnstate.nl

L. E. Visser (✉)
Department of Hospital Pharmacy, Haga Teaching Hospital, The Hague, The Netherlands

Department of Hospital Pharmacy, Erasmus Medical Center, Rotterdam, The Netherlands
e-mail: l.e.visser@hagaziekenhuis.nl

A. H.E.M. Maas, E. Gerdts (eds.), *Manual of Cardiovascular Disease in Women*,
https://doi.org/10.1007/978-3-031-65952-2_32

Test your learning and check your understanding of this book's contents: use the "Springer Nature Flashcards" app to access questions using ▶ https://sn.pub/51ny7m
To use the app, please follow the instructions in chapter 1.

1 Introduction

In the past, drug testing on women, particularly on women of childbearing age, was not recommended by the US Food and Drug Administration (FDA), and, thus, women tended to be underrepresented in clinical trials [1]. As a consequence, sex differences in efficacy and safety had a higher risk of not being identified. Moreover, in the late 1990s, the FDA withdrew 10 drugs from the U.S. market of which 8 showed greater health risks in women [2]. Since 1993, the Guideline for the Study and Evaluation of Gender Differences in the Clinical Evaluation of Drugs by the FDA states that women should be included in all phases of clinical trials [3]. Although the participation of women in clinical trials has improved, a study from 2022 showed that women are still underrepresented in early-phase and cardiovascular drug trials [4]. Reasons to decline trial participation for women are for example transportation problems and a perceived higher risk of harm from trial participation than men [5]. In addition to the underrepresentation, sex-specific analyses on the efficacy and safety of drugs are not always performed, or not performed correctly [6]. It is known that there are differences between female and male distribution, metabolism and excretion of drugs [7]. In addition, women report and experience more adverse drug reactions than men [8, 9]. Therefore, this chapter will give insight into the effect of sex differences on pharmacokinetics, pharmacodynamics, and adverse drug reactions of cardiovascular drugs.

2 Sex Differences in Pharmacokinetics

Several sex-based physiological differences contribute to differences in pharmacokinetics, Fig. 1. Pharmacokinetics is the study of the relationship between drug dosage and the concentration of drug over time in blood or plasma, or preferably, in cells and tissues, which may be more representative of the site of action. Sex-based differences in the four major factors that contribute to interindividual pharmacokinetic variability—absorption, distribution, metabolism and elimination—are explored in greater depth below.

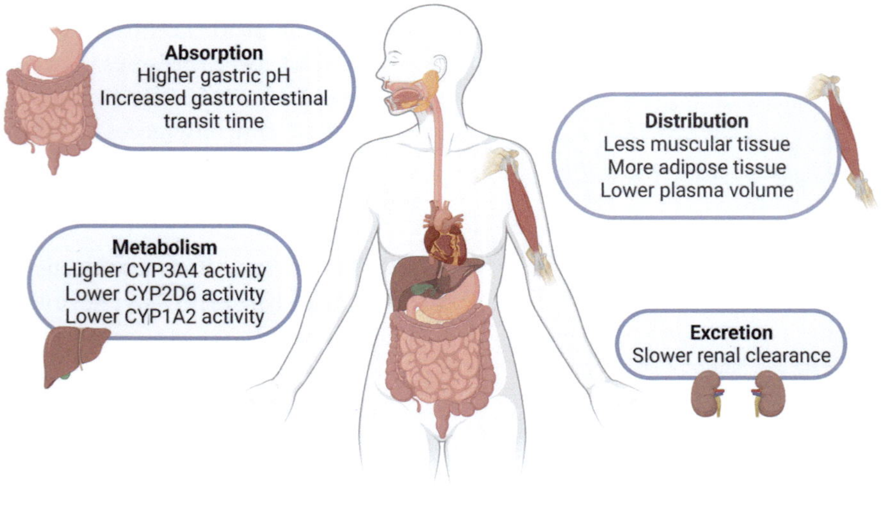

Fig. 1 Drug processing in women influenced by physiological sex differences (created with Biorender.com)

2.1 Drug Absorption

Drug absorption describes the process of administration of a drug into the systemic circulation. The influence of sex on the absorption of drugs is determined by the route of administration. This paragraph focuses predominantly on oral drug absorption, as this is the most common method of administration of cardiovascular drugs. Oral drug absorption is dependent on drug characteristics and can be influenced by several processes including gastric acid secretion, gastric emptying time, gastrointestinal transit rate, gastrointestinal blood flow, and first-pass effect [10]. Gastric acid secretion is lower in women than men, resulting in a higher gastric pH (pH 2.59 versus pH 1.92) [10]. Gastric pH influences the portion of the drug that is charged versus uncharged. Drugs that are uncharged will be better able to diffuse through a lipid cellular membrane and enter the bloodstream. Thus, gastric pH can influence the solubility and bioavailability of oral drugs. In addition, women have an increased gastrointestinal transit time, which leads to a prolonged absorption window and increased absorption [11–13]. These differences increase even further after a meal and suggest women should wait longer after eating than men before taking drugs that should be administered on an empty stomach [14]. For only a few drugs the influence of sex on absorption is studied. For example, enteric-coated acetylsalicylic acid shows delayed absorption in women, especially after food intake [14]. Luzier et al. found increased absorption of metoprolol in women [15]. This could be caused by the increased gastrointestinal transit time which leads to metoprolol residing in the gastrointestinal tract for a longer time, thus being available for absorption for a longer period of time. Even though pharmacokinetic studies described these sex-specific differences in drug absorption, they did not lead to sex-specific dose adjustments in cardiovascular drugs.

2.2 Drug Distribution

Once absorbed and in circulation, drugs are distributed over the body. The distribution of a drug is affected by drug characteristics like protein binding, lipophilicity, and affinity for certain tissues and drug transporters. Sex differences in drug distribution might be expected because of the differences in physical composition. Women have a lower body weight, relatively less muscular and more adipose tissue, smaller organ sizes, lower plasma volume and lower blood flow rate compared to men [16, 17]. For example, due to the lower body weight, women treated with isosorbide-5-mononitrate had significantly higher serum plasma concentrations compared to men [18]. Because of the differences in body composition, hydrophilic drugs have a lower volume of distribution in women producing higher peak plasma levels, while lipophilic drugs have a higher volume of distribution in women, often leading to a longer duration of action [16, 17].

Although the clinical significance of the sex-specific distribution differences has yet to be determined, it suggests rather than fixed-doses, dosing should be titrated to the required clinical effect, aimed at blood target levels or be based on body weight. Loading doses should be adjusted for drugs with a small therapeutic range to prevent adverse events in women. For antiarrhythmics (such as intravenous amiodarone, lidocaine, procainamide) and heparin, weight-based dose adjustment is routinely recommended [17, 19, 20]. However, sex-specific distribution differences can remain even after adjustment for body weight. For example, women have a smaller volume of distribution for metoprolol even after correction for body weight possibly due to sex-related differences in muscle mass and body composition [15].

In addition, drug-protein binding may also be influenced by sex. Albumin and alpha(1)-acid glycoprotein are the main binding proteins for drugs in plasma. Some reports show lower alpha(1)-acid glycoprotein levels in women, while albumin levels are not affected by sex [21–24]. However, the clinical impact of the lower alpha(1)-acid glycoprotein remains unclear.

2.3 Drug Metabolism

Drug metabolism describes the process of chemical alteration of a drug to make it more suitable for elimination. The liver is the main site for drug metabolism. Hepatic clearance of drugs is a function of liver blood flow and hepatic enzyme activity. Although cardiac output and hepatic blood flow are lower in women than men, sex differences in hepatic enzymes seem to play the major role in determining pharmacokinetic variability by sex. Hepatic drug metabolism is divided into two, usually sequential, enzymatic reactions: phase I reactions include oxidation, reduction, and hydrolysis and are mediated through the cytochrome (CYP) P450 system, phase II reactions include glucuronidation, sulfation, acetylation, or methylation to form polar conjugates for renal excretion. Important sex differences in some of the key cytochrome P450 enzymes have been demonstrated. CYP3A4-enzymes have a higher metabolic activity for numerous CYP3A4 substrates in women. For example, intravenously administered nifedipine and verapamil clearance is higher in women than in men [25–27]. The increased clearance could be due to higher CYP3A4 activity but also due to lower activity of the transmembrane efflux transporter P-glycoprotein (P-gp), which would result in increased intrahepatic substrate for CYP3A4 [25–28]. However, Krecic-Shepard et al. reported lower clearance after oral administration of verapamil in women [25, 28]. An explanation for this contrasting result between oral and intravenous administration could be sex differences in intestinal CYP3A4 and P-gp activity [28, 29]. CYP2D6 activity seems to be higher in men [30]. In accordance, healthy women, who were CYP2D6 extensive metabolisers (EM) showed a higher exposure and slower metoprolol clearance rate than EM men [15]. For CYP2C9 and CYP2C19, there seems to be no difference in enzyme activity between men and women. CYP1A2 activity, which influences the metabolism of a few antipsychotics among others, is lower in women than men.

2.4 Drug Elimination

The predominant route of elimination for cardiovascular drugs is renal clearance. Renal clearance of drugs that are not actively secreted or reabsorbed is dependent on glomerular filtration rate (GFR), which is directly proportional to body weight and consequently higher on average in men than women [23, 31, 32]. Hence, sex differences in rates of renal excretion are for most drugs likely attributable to weight differences [22]. This is the case for digoxin, which has a 14% slower clearance in women [33]. The lower clearance and reduced volume of distribution of digoxin in women contribute to higher serum levels. However, dose adjustment based on weight and renal function is sufficient and sex-differential dose adjustment seems unnecessary [34]. Drugs that are actively secreted by the kidney may also show differences in excretion. Torsemide, a loop diuretic which is actively secreted by the proximal tubules, showed a reduced elimination in women, leading to a 30–40% higher Cmax and AUC compared to men [35]. These pharmacokinetic differences remained even after adjustment for age, BMI and estimated GFR and could be due to the impact of sex hormones on the expression of renal organic anion transporters. Although these sex differences in torsemide pharmacokinetics are likely to contribute to a higher rate of ADRs in women, which has, for example, been observed in a German Pharmacovigilance Project with 66% of hospitalizations due to torsemide ADRs occurring in women, these differences have not led to sex-based dose recommendations.

2.5 Hormonal Influences

Hormonal influences play a key role in several aspects of pharmacological response. In women, oral absorption, distribution, metabolism and elimination can be influenced by the menstrual cycle phase, pregnancy, lactation, and fluctuations in concentrations of sexual steroids. Furthermore, the use of oral contraceptives or hormonal replacement therapy can influence these processes.

During pregnancy, physiology changes in a time-dependent manner, and these changes alter pharmacokinetics. Absorption is affected because of an increase in gastric and intestinal emptying time and a reduction in gastric acid secretion which leads to an increased gastric pH [36]. This increased emptying time is possible due to increased plasma progesterone levels [36, 37]. At the same time, nausea and vomiting may cause lower bioavailability. Drug distribution is also altered as a result of total body water expansion. As the plasma volume expands, a physiological dilutional hypoalbuminaemia is created, leading to a decreased binding capacity for albumin and, thus, an increased unbound drug fraction [36]. For example, the unbound fraction of diazepam, phenytoin and valproic acid were in vitro elevated during pregnancy [38]. Liver enzymes involved in drug metabolism are increased in expression and activity, resulting in enhanced drug metabolism. For example, pregnancy induces CYP2D6, resulting in increased metabolism of metoprolol, and thus plasma levels of metoprolol are reduced in women who are pregnant compared with women who are not pregnant [39]. Furthermore, the glomerular filtration rate is increased by 50% starting in the second semester and until 3 months postpartum. Therefore, during pregnancy, the clearance of drugs that are excreted unchanged in the urine, such as heparin, is increased [39].

3 Sex Differences in Pharmacodynamics

Pharmacodynamic disparities in drug response based on sex have not been studied as extensively as pharmacokinetic differences, partially because pharmacologic effects can be difficult to quantify. Sex-related effects on pharmacodynamics are distinguished from differences in pharmacokinetics by demonstrating that the same plasma concentration of a drug in both sexes does not yield the same pharmacologic outcome. Examples of studies that have examined pharmacodynamics differences with widely used cardiovascular drugs between men and women are summarized below.

3.1 Acetylsalicylic Acid

Acetylsalicylic acid (ASA) is an antiplatelet drug, given to prevent major cardiovascular events. Sex-specific meta-analyses showed that ASA for primary prevention significantly reduces the risk of myocardial infarction (MI) in men, however, ASA did not significantly change the risk of stroke in men [40, 41]. In contrast, ASA was ineffective as primary prevention of MI in women but showed significant protection against ischaemic stroke [40, 41]. In addition, subgroup analysis of the Women's Health study showed that only women of 65 years and older benefit from primary prevention with ASA, as it significantly reduced the risk of major cardiovascular events, ischaemic stroke and MI in this subgroup [42]. Although differences in efficacy are seen, ASA increased the risk of major bleeding to the same degree (approximately 70%) in both men and women when compared to placebo [40].

Secondary prevention with ASA reduces serious cardiovascular events (non-fatal MI, non-fatal stroke, or vascular death), irrespective of sex [43]. This was confirmed in a meta-analysis that compared long-term ASA treatment on serious vascular events (MI, stroke, or vascular death) and major bleeding [44]. In both primary and secondary prevention trials, the proportional reductions in the composite of these serious vascular events seemed similar for men and women [44].

Several potential reasons exist for the sex differences in the prevention of a first MI or stroke, including the previously discussed pharmacokinetic differences leading to higher plasma salicylate levels [45]. The higher clearance of ASA in men is probably due to greater activity of the glycine conjugation pathway. Oral contraceptives can stimulate these degradation pathways, as the differences in biotransformation disappear in women taking oral contraceptives [46]. In addition, sex hormones are thought to play a role. Estradiol stimulates the production of prostacyclin, thereby shifting the haemostatic balance toward inhibition of platelet aggregation [47]. Estrogen increases nitric oxide synthesis and release from vascular endothelium, resulting in potent antiplatelet effects [48]. Contrary, platelets from men are more responsive and tend to generate more thromboxane A2, possibly mediated by testosterone [49, 50]. As a result, platelets from premenopausal women are suggested to be less prothrombotic than platelets from men. The differences in outcomes between the sexes might also be affected by attenuation of ASA inhibition of epinephrine- and ADP-induced platelet aggregation after 4 weeks of ASA in women [51]. Alternatively, sex-related differences in platelet and vascular functions and disease pathogenesis between men and women could play a role. For example, women with stable ischaemic heart disease exhibit higher platelet aggregation to mental stress, while men are more likely to respond by increasing blood pressure [52]. The difference in cardioprotection may also be explained by a difference in event rates of stroke and MI between both sexes. Women have a greater proportion of strokes compared to MIs, whereas in men it is the opposite. Thus, studies are possibly not powered to find a statistically significant protective effect on the risk of MI among women and the risk of stroke in men [40].

No sex differences in the efficacy and safety outcomes were seen in women and men with ASA for secondary prevention, therefore differential treatment with ASA is not justified after a coronary heart event or stroke. Although the risk of stroke and MI differs between men and women, this is possibly due to a difference in event rates. In addition, ASA's role in primary prevention is uncertain and not recommended on a routine basis in adults older than 70 years, or at increased risk of bleeding [53]. Therefore, with the current knowledge, sex differential treatment is not advised with ASA for secondary prevention.

3.2 P2Y12 Receptor Antagonists

Another group of antiplatelet drugs are the P2Y12 receptor antagonists, they block the adenosine diphosphate (ADP) receptor, stimulate platelet activation and hinder clot formation. Clopidogrel, prasugrel, and ticagrelor are the three approved P2Y12 receptor antagonists for dual antiplatelet therapy (DAPT) in patients with acute coronary syndrome. In a meta-analysis of patients treated with (DAPT) for the prevention of cardiovascular events, women treated with clopidogrel had a reduced risk of MI whereas men had a significant risk reduction of MI, stroke, and all-cause mortality [54]. Despite these observations, there was no evidence of statistically significant heterogeneity when the effect of clopidogrel was compared between women and men, indicating that much of the difference between men and women could be explained by the play of chance. Other meta-analyses demonstrated that the efficacy and safety of potent P2Y12 inhibitors, namely, prasugrel, ticagrelor, and cangrelor, in DAPT, are comparable in women and men with stable and unstable coronary artery disease [55, 56]. In addition, these meta-analyses showed that the use of these potent antiplatelet therapies reduced the risk of both major adverse cardiac events (MACE) and all-cause mortality while the increased risk of major bleeding was similar between men and women.

As described for ASA, the reasons for potential sex differences in the effect of clopidogrel could be influenced by sex hormones on the haemostatic balance, sex-related differences in platelet and vascular functions, and disease pathogenesis.

3.3 Digoxin

Digoxin is a cardiac glycoside and is used to treat arrhythmias and heart failure. In a post hoc analysis of the DIG study, digoxin in heart failure patients increased the all-cause mortality risk among women but not among men [57]. Furthermore, a study in the Netherlands showed that women had a higher risk of hospitalization for digoxin intoxication [58]. Higher serum digoxin concentrations in women were associated with higher mortality and hospitalisation rates [59]. Women had slightly higher serum digoxin levels than men after 1 month of use, despite lower doses of digoxin per body mass index unit [53]. At low digoxin serum concentrations [0.5–0.9 ng/mL], there was no evidence that digoxin increased mortality in women [60]. Therefore, digoxin serum concentrations are recommended to be between 0.5 and 0.9 ng/mL to reduce mortality in heart failure patients regardless of sex [61].

The increased mortality risk is partly due to the previously stated differences in pharmacokinetics. As mentioned, the pharmacokinetic differences disappear when the digoxin dose is corrected for renal function and actual or ideal body weight. Because digoxin is distributed to lean body mass, the use of the BMI could overadjust body weight [34]. An alternative hypothesis involves the suggestion that women have lower P-glycoprotein expression [62], resulting in higher bioavailability of digoxin [58]. Additionally, the different effects of digoxin may be due to differences in cellular sodium and calcium handling. Women demonstrated lower Na^+ concentrations and fewer Na^+ pumps in erythrocytes and skeletal muscle than men [63–65]. Extrapolation of these data to cardiomyocytes implies that women have fewer active Na^+ pumps localized in the plasma membrane, which would predispose women to fatal arrhythmias [63].

3.4 Calcium Channel Blokkers

Calcium channel blockers (CCB) are antihypertensive agents. Dihydropyridine CCBs (e.g. nifedipine) are more vascular selective while non-dihydropyridines (e.g. diltiazem and verapamil) are more myocardial selective and tend to reduce heart rate [66]. In a systematic meta-analysis, women with hypertension treated with calcium channel blockers showed a greater blood pressure reduction than men [67]. Heart rate and left ventricular ejection fraction decreased in women while remaining unaltered in men. In addition, age influences blood pressure reduction too, as verapamil clearance decreases with age, older women show a greater antihypertensive response [68].

In an 18-week open study by Kloner et al., amlodipine reduced blood pressure more and produced a higher incidence of oedema in women than in men [69]. These effects remained even after adjustment for differences in baseline blood pressure, age, weight, and dose.

The differences in outcome could be due to the aforementioned pharmacokinetic differences in drug distribution and metabolism leading to higher exposure [25, 28], or it could be due to differences in vascular reactivity [69]. Namely, the adrenergic reactivity of macrovessels is modulated by estrogen, which results in weaker alpha-adrenergic vasoconstriction in women than in men [70]. Contrary, men have a greater sensitivity to norepinephrine compared to women, leading to more vasoconstriction in men. The release of another vasoconstrictor (endothelin-1) is also influenced by sex hormones, whereby testosterone increased endothelin-1 release and estrogen and progesterone decreased it [71].

In conclusion, women show a greater blood pressure reduction during treatment with CCBs than men. However, women do have a higher baseline blood pressure and to our knowledge, no studies described the difference between men and women reaching a target blood pressure. Therefore, sex-specific advice about dosing strategies cannot be given. However, when normalizing blood pressure, people should be aware of the influence of sex on the effects and adverse reactions of calcium channel blockers.

3.5 Renin-Angiotensin-Aldosterone System Inhibitors

Angiotensin-converting enzyme (ACE) inhibitors and angiotensin-receptor blockers (ARBs) both act by inhibiting the renin-angiotensin-aldosterone system (RAAS) and are used to treat HF and hypertension. In a meta-analysis, comparable benefits are described of ACE-inhibitors on total mortality and the combined endpoint of mortality or HF hospitalization for HF in men and women with HF [72]. Another meta-analysis showed comparable effects of ACE inhibitors on prognosis and hospitalization rate for both sexes after MI complicated by left-ventricular dysfunction [73]. In addition, Santema et al. found that women with HF treated with ACE-inhibitors have a 40% lower risk of mortality or hospitalisation than men, at 50% of the recommended dose [74]. In contrast, the lowest risk in men occurred at 100% of the recommended dose. However, women treated with ACE-inhibitors are more likely to develop and report the typically ACE-induced cough [75] and angioedema [76, 77]. For ARBs, large trials showed reduced mortality or HF hospitalization with a similar rate in both women and men with HFrEF [78–80].

Although ACE-inhibitors and ARBs have comparable benefits in both men and women, the renin-angiotensin system is regulated by sex hormones [81–83]. Estrogen increases angiotensinogen levels but decreases renin levels, angiotensin-converting enzyme activity, AT1 receptor density and aldosterone production causing vasodilatation Twee zinnen van maken. Contrary, testosterone increases renin levels and ACE-activity leading to vasoconstriction. Accordingly, pre-menopausal women demonstrate lower ACE activity than post-menopausal women [84]. Estrogen might also play a role in the sex difference in the incidence of ACE-induced cough, as estrogen induces the expression of bradykinin type 2 receptor [85]. However, it remains the question whether the higher rate of cough and angioedema in women is, in addition, influenced by a sex difference in reporting ADRs.

In conclusion, ACE-inhibitors and ARBs show comparable effects in men and women with HF although women treated with ACE inhibitors reach a lower risk of death or hospitalization for HF at 50% of the recommended dose. However, current guidelines still do not advise sex-specific target doses. A prospective sex-stratified dose-finding including clinical endpoints is needed, but it is unlikely that such a trial will be done.

3.6 Beta-Blockers

Beta-blockers are hypertensive agents, which reduce cardiac output and slow the heart rate. As discussed earlier in the paragraph about pharmacokinetics, women have higher drug exposure to metoprolol than men. These higher serum concentrations in women lead to a greater reduction in heart rate and blood pressure [15]. Despite the higher plasma levels in women, metoprolol reduces angina pectoris in men and women to the same extent [86]. Several individual trials found that beta-blockers improved survival in men but not in women with heart failure. However, two meta-analyses confirmed very similar and statistically significant survival benefits in heart failure in both women and men [87, 88]. The lack of evidence in some individual beta-blocker trials is probably due to the underrepresentation of women in these studies. Another meta-analysis showed that the reduction of metoprolol on cardiovascular death after MI was comparable in women and men [89]. The optimal effect of beta-blockers may be achieved with lower doses in women than in men as women showed the lowest risk of the composite outcome death or hospitalization at around 60% of the recommended doses, with no further decrease in risk at higher dose levels [74]. In contrast, the lowest risks for men occurred at 100% of the recommended dose.

Due to the higher drug exposure and greater efficacy of beta blockers in women, more adverse reactions among women are theoretically expected. However, a systematic review found that women and men reported similar numbers of adverse drug reactions and a similar percentage of men and women failed to reach the recommended target dose because of ADRs [90]. On the other hand, a recent study showed that women did have an increased risk of bradycardia, possibly due to higher metoprolol plasma concentrations [91].

The sex-specific differences in the pharmacodynamics of beta-blockers might be expected because of the suppressive effect of estrogens and progesterone on the cardiac expression of Beta-1 receptors [92]. This effect increases even further when women use oral contraceptives, which increase metoprolol blood levels [93]. In addition, it's speculated that higher testosterone levels in men increase enzyme expression of CYP2D6, thereby causing a greater clearance in men [15].

It is demonstrated that beta-blockers are just as effective in women or show an even greater reduction of heart rate and blood pressure, and therefore no sex-specific treatment guidelines exist. However, women have a higher drug exposure and thus true optimal dosing of beta-blockers in women, with respect to the sex-dependent risk for ADRs, should be further investigated.

3.7 PCSK9 Inhibitors

PCSK9 inhibitors are a relatively new class of drugs that lower low-density lipoprotein (LDL) and reduce the atherosclerotic risk. Guideline recommendations and consensus statements now endorse the use of PCSK9 inhibitors as appropriate second- or third-line agents or as an alternative therapy in case of complete statin intolerance, for patients with established atherosclerotic CVD or familial hypercholesterolemia with persistent hypercholesterolemia. In real-world evidence studies, women treated with PCSK9 inhibitors show less LDL-c reduction and reach LDL-C target levels less often [94–99]. Adverse drug reactions and discontinuation rates appeared to be similar in both sexes [94].

PCSK9 levels are higher in women than men and fluctuate during the menstrual cycle and with menopause status [100, 101]. Therefore, it is presumed that PCSK9 levels are influenced by estrogen, possibly through G-protein coupled estrogen receptor activation on hepatocytes [102]. Due to the decrease of estrogen in normal ageing women but especially in postmenopausal women, women have higher PCSK9 concentrations resulting in higher LDL-c levels [101].

Although the effect of PCSK9 inhibitors is dependent on sex-based pharmacodynamics and results in lower LDL-c reduction in women, it is still unknown whether the difference in LDL-C change between men and women translates into a difference in long-term cardiovascular risk. As women reach the treatment target less often, it could be argued to start with the full dose of PCSK9 inhibitors in women.

4 Adverse Drug Reactions

The incidence of ADRs is greater in women than in men and more often requires hospitalization [8, 103]. Cardiovascular drugs appear to account for the most pronounced differences in adverse drug reactions between men and women [103]. These differences may result from sex-related differences in pharmacokinetics, pharmacodynamics or from increased medication use. Women often use more drugs than men, including herbal remedies and non-prescription medication, which results in an increased risk of ADRs from herb-drug or drug-drug interactions. The risk of an ADR varies between the sexes in the type of reaction and the causative drug. Specific drug-ADR combinations are more frequently reported by men while other combinations are more frequently reported by women [104]. This paragraph focuses on cardiovascular drugs for which specific sex differences of adverse drug reactions are described while differences in effectiveness are not known.

4.1 Antiarrhythmics

Sex-specific differences in myocardial repolarization were noted more than 100 years ago since Bazett described in the 1920s that women demonstrated longer QT intervals on an ECG than men [105]. Female sex has been identified as an independent risk factor for drug-induced QT prolongation and Torsade de pointes (TdP) [106, 107]. The observed difference in risk for drug-induced long QT syndrome is partly explained by sex hormones [108]. Androgens protect against drug effects on repolarization, whereas estrogens seem to be proarrhythmic.

Seventy percent of the patients who developed TdP on a class I or III antiarrhythmic (quinidine, procainamide, disopyramide, amiodarone, sotalol, bepridil or prenylamine) appeared to be women [107]. A meta-analysis of 22 clinical trials involving

3235 patients treated with a racemic mixture of sotalol or racemic sotalol showed that women had threefold greater odds of developing TdP than men even after adjustment for risk factors (congestive heart failure, history of sustained ventricular tachycardia or fibrillation, sotalol dose >320 mg, and serum creatinine >1.4 mg/dL in women and >1.6 mg/dL in men) [106]. In addition, healthy women experienced higher peak plasma concentrations after a single 160 mg oral dose of sotalol, and had a significantly larger QTc prolongation than men [109]. Overall, female sex is a known risk factor for drug-induced QT prolongation and, therefore, should be included when assessing a patient's risk for QT prolongation. Therefore, female sex is one of the variables in the Tisdale Risk Score for QT prolongation [110].

4.2 Diuretics

Numerous studies have shown that women treated with diuretics experience more frequent electrolyte disturbances (e.g. hyponatremia and hypokalaemia) [111–114]. Women are also more likely to be hospitalized for hyponatremia due to diuretics [103, 115]. A possible explanation is that androgens in men may enhance proximal sodium reabsorption by facilitating the action of angiotensin II [116]. According to a study in rats, females have a higher expression of renal vasopressin regulation receptors, which may result in a greater sensitivity to arginine vasopressin [117]. In addition, female mice had a greater abundance and higher activity of the Na(+)/Cl(−) co-transporters [118]. Alternatively, polymorphism in the angiotensin I-converting enzyme gene is associated with variation in serum ACE activity and the response to hydrochlorothiazide [116].

Women have a higher risk of hospital admission attributed to hyponatremia due to diuretics. This risk should be considered and sodium levels monitored closely when prescribing diuretics to women.

4.3 Statins

Women are more likely to stop or switch their statin than men, and the main reason for this appeared new or worsening muscle symptoms. Although not statistically significant, a greater than twofold increase in risk for rhabdomyolysis among females was observed [119, 120]. The predisposition to statin-induced myalgia in women is possibly caused by higher frailty and higher exposure due to the smaller body frame of women [121]. The risk of statin-induced myopathy has been shown to be dose-dependent [121]. In addition, women report different types of ADRs than men while using statins. For example, women more often report alopecia, dry mouth, nausea and palpitations, while men more often report decreased libido, peripheral neuropathy, pancreatitis and tendon rupture [104].

5 Conclusions

We described sex differences in pharmacokinetics, pharmacodynamics and (type of) adverse drug reaction of multiple cardiovascular drugs. However, current guidelines still do not advise sex-differential treatment for any cardiovascular drug. The demonstrated differences are scarcely recognized possibly due to incomplete, not well-designed studies and inconsistent results. Prospective dose-finding sex-stratified studies are needed to possibly guide clinicians to sex-differential treatment.

Key Issues

- Physiological sex differences lead to sex differences in drug absorption, distribution, metabolism and excretion.
- As women are often underrepresented in trials and the role of sex hormones in the final response is often not taken into consideration, sex differences in pharmacodynamics are difficult to quantify.
- Sex hormones are thought to affect the pharmacodynamics of aspirin, P2Y12 inhibitors, CCBs, ACE inhibitors, ARBs, beta-blockers, and PCSK9 inhibitors.
- The incidence of ADRs is greater in women than in men and more often requires hospitalization, e.g. hyponatremia associated with the use of diuretics.

- Specific drug-ADR combinations are more frequently reported by men, while other drug-ADR combinations are more frequently reported by women, e.g. with statins.
- Prospective dose-finding sex-stratified studies are needed to guide clinicians to sex-differential treatment.

Questions and Answers

1. Indicate which of the following answers is incorrect.
   (A) Women have a higher gastric pH
   (B) Women have higher CYP3A4 activity
   (C) Women have a higher plasma volume
   (D) Women have an increased gastrointestinal time

   Correct answer: C

   The distribution of drugs in women is influenced by several physiological sex differences, namely less muscular tissue, more adipose tissue, and lower plasma volume.
2. Indicate which of the following answers is incorrect.
   (A) Women have higher PCSK9 levels
   (B) Women treated with PCSK9 inhibitors reach LDL-C target levels less often
   (C) The discontinuation rate of PCSK9 inhibitors is similar in both sexes
   (D) Women treated with PCSK9 inhibitors have side effects more often

   Correct answer: D

   Adverse drug reactions and discontinuation rates appear to be similar in both sexes treated with PCSK9 levels.
3. Indicate which of the following answers is incorrect.
   (A) Female sex is a risk factor for drug-induced QT prolongation
   (B) Men on statins more often report dry mouth as an adverse drug reaction than women
   (C) Women on diuretics have a higher of hospital admission because of hyponatremia
   (D) Men on statins more often report tendon rupture as an adverse drug reaction than women

   Correct answer: B

   Women report different types of ADRs than men while using statins. For example, women more often report dry mouth as adverse drug reaction than men.

References

1. FDA. Gender studies in product development: historical overview [updated 16 Feb 2018]. https://www.fda.gov/science-research/womens-health-research/gender-studies-product-development-historical-overview.
2. United States General Accounting Office. Drug safety: most drugs withdrawn in recent years had greater health risks for women 2001 [updated Jan 19]. https://www.gao.gov/assets/gao-01-286r.pdf.
3. FDA. Guideline for the study and evaluation of gender differences in the clinical evaluation of drugs; notice 1993 [updated Jul 22.1993/07/22:39406–16].
4. Sosinsky AZ, Rich-Edwards JW, Wiley A, Wright K, Spagnolo PA, Joffe H. Enrollment of female participants in United States drug and device phase 1–3 clinical trials between 2016 and 2019. Contemp Clin Trials. 2022;115:106718.
5. van Diemen J, Verdonk P, Chieffo A, Regar E, Mauri F, Kunadian V, et al. The importance of achieving sex- and gender-based equity in clinical trials: a call to action. Eur Heart J. 2021;42(31):2990–4.
6. Vorland CJ. Sex difference analyses under scrutiny. eLife. 2021;10:e74135.
7. Mauvais-Jarvis F, Berthold HK, Campesi I, Carrero JJ, Dakal S, Franconi F, et al. Sex- and gender-based pharmacological response to drugs. Pharmacol Rev. 2021;73(2):730–62.
8. Martin RM, Biswas PN, Freemantle SN, Pearce GL, Mann RD. Age and sex distribution of suspected adverse drug reactions to newly marketed drugs in general practice in England: analysis of 48 cohort studies. Br J Clin Pharmacol. 1998;46(5):505–11.
9. Watson S, Caster O, Rochon PA, den Ruijter H. Reported adverse drug reactions in women and men: aggregated evidence from globally collected individual case reports during half a century. EClinicalMedicine. 2019;17:100188.
10. Fletcher CV, Acosta EP, Strykowski JM. Gender differences in human pharmacokinetics and pharmacodynamics. J Adolesc Health. 1994;15(8):619–29.
11. Datz FL, Christian PE, Moore J. Gender-related differences in gastric emptying. J Nucl Med. 1987;28(7):1204–7.
12. Wang YT, Mohammed SD, Farmer AD, Wang D, Zarate N, Hobson AR, et al. Regional gastrointestinal transit and pH studied in 215 healthy volunteers using the wireless motility capsule: influence of age,

gender, study country and testing protocol. Aliment Pharmacol Ther. 2015;42(6):761–72.
13. Rao SS, Kuo B, McCallum RW, Chey WD, DiBaise JK, Hasler WL, et al. Investigation of colonic and whole-gut transit with wireless motility capsule and radiopaque markers in constipation. Clin Gastroenterol Hepatol. 2009;7(5):537–44.
14. Mojaverian P, Rocci ML Jr, Conner DP, Abrams WB, Vlasses PH. Effect of food on the absorption of enteric-coated aspirin: correlation with gastric residence time. Clin Pharmacol Ther. 1987;41(1):11–7.
15. Luzier AB, Killian A, Wilton JH, Wilson MF, Forrest A, Kazierad DJ. Gender-related effects on metoprolol pharmacokinetics and pharmacodynamics in healthy volunteers. Clin Pharmacol Ther. 1999;66(6):594–601.
16. Anderson GD. Sex and racial differences in pharmacological response: where is the evidence? Pharmacogenetics, pharmacokinetics, and pharmacodynamics. J Womens Health (Larchmt). 2005;14(1):19–29.
17. Tamargo J, Rosano G, Walther T, Duarte J, Niessner A, Kaski JC, et al. Gender differences in the effects of cardiovascular drugs. Eur Heart J Cardiovasc Pharmacother. 2017;3(3):163–82.
18. Vree TB, Dammers E, Valducci R. Sex-related differences in the pharmacokinetics of isosorbide-5-mononitrate (60 mg) after repeated oral administration of two different original prolonged release formulations. Int J Clin Pharmacol Ther. 2004;42(8):463–72.
19. Schwartz JB. The current state of knowledge on age, sex, and their interactions on clinical pharmacology. Clin Pharmacol Ther. 2007;82(1):87–96.
20. Stolarz AJ, Rusch NJ. Gender differences in cardiovascular drugs. Cardiovasc Drugs Ther. 2015;29(4):403–10.
21. Kishino S, Nomura A, Itoh S, Nakagawa T, Takekuma Y, Sugawara M, et al. Age- and gender-related differences in carbohydrate concentrations of alpha1-acid glycoprotein variants and the effects of glycoforms on their drug-binding capacities. Eur J Clin Pharmacol. 2002;58(9):621–8.
22. Schwartz JB. The influence of sex on pharmacokinetics. Clin Pharmacokinet. 2003;42(2):107–21.
23. Soldin OP, Mattison DR. Sex differences in pharmacokinetics and pharmacodynamics. Clin Pharmacokinet. 2009;48(3):143–57.
24. Woo J, Chan HS, Or KH, Arumanayagam M. Effect of age and disease on two drug binding proteins: albumin and alpha-1-acid glycoprotein. Clin Biochem. 1994;27(4):289–92.
25. Krecic-Shepard ME, Barnas CR, Slimko J, Jones MP, Schwartz JB. Gender-specific effects on verapamil pharmacokinetics and pharmacodynamics in humans. J Clin Pharmacol. 2000;40(3):219–30.
26. Dadashzadeh S, Javadian B, Sadeghian S. The effect of gender on the pharmacokinetics of verapamil and norverapamil in human. Biopharm Drug Dispos. 2006;27(7):329–34.
27. Krecic-Shepard ME, Park K, Barnas C, Slimko J, Kerwin DR, Schwartz JB. Race and sex influence clearance of nifedipine: results of a population study. Clin Pharmacol Ther. 2000;68(2):130–42.
28. Krecic-Shepard ME, Barnas CR, Slimko J, Schwartz JB. Faster clearance of sustained release verapamil in men versus women: continuing observations on sex-specific differences after oral administration of verapamil. Clin Pharmacol Ther. 2000;68(3):286–92.
29. Kalibala J, Pechère-Bertschi A, Desmeules J. Gender differences in cardiovascular pharmacotherapy—the example of hypertension: a mini review. Front Pharmacol. 2020;11:564.
30. Hägg S, Spigset O, Dahlqvist R. Influence of gender and oral contraceptives on CYP2D6 and CYP2C19 activity in healthy volunteers. Br J Clin Pharmacol. 2001;51(2):169–73.
31. Berg UB. Differences in decline in GFR with age between males and females. Reference data on clearances of inulin and PAH in potential kidney donors. Nephrol Dial Transplant. 2006;21(9):2577–82.
32. James GD, Sealey JE, Alderman M, Ljungman S, Mueller FB, Pecker MS, et al. A longitudinal study of urinary creatinine and creatinine clearance in normal subjects. Race, sex, and age differences. Am J Hypertens. 1988;1(2):124–31.
33. Yukawa E, Honda T, Ohdo S, Higuchi S, Aoyama T. Population-based investigation of relative clearance of digoxin in Japanese patients by multiple trough screen analysis: an update. J Clin Pharmacol. 1997;37(2):92–100.
34. Lee LS, Chan LN. Evaluation of a sex-based difference in the pharmacokinetics of digoxin. Pharmacotherapy. 2006;26(1):44–50.
35. Werner U, Werner D, Heinbüchner S, Graf B, Ince H, Kische S, et al. Gender is an important determinant of the disposition of the loop diuretic torasemide. J Clin Pharmacol. 2010;50(2):160–8.
36. Loebstein R, Lalkin A, Koren G. Pharmacokinetic changes during pregnancy and their clinical relevance. Clin Pharmacokinet. 1997;33(5):328–43.
37. Parry E, Shields R, Turnbull AC. Transit time in the small intestine in pregnancy. J Obstet Gynaecol Br Commonw. 1970;77(10):900–1.
38. Perucca E, Ruprah M, Richens A. Altered drug binding to serum proteins in pregnant women: therapeutic relevance. J R Soc Med. 1981;74(6):422–6.
39. Ansari J, Carvalho B, Shafer SL, Flood P. Pharmacokinetics and pharmacodynamics of drugs commonly used in pregnancy and parturition. Anesth Analg. 2016;122(3):786–804.
40. Berger JS, Roncaglioni MC, Avanzini F, Pangrazzi I, Tognoni G, Brown DL. Aspirin for the primary prevention of cardiovascular events in women and men: a sex-specific meta-analysis of randomized controlled trials. JAMA. 2006;295(3):306–13.
41. Xie M, Shan Z, Zhang Y, Chen S, Yang W, Bao W, et al. Aspirin for primary prevention of cardiovascular events: meta-analysis of randomized controlled

trials and subgroup analysis by sex and diabetes status. PLoS One. 2014;9(10):e90286.
42. Ridker PM, Cook NR, Lee IM, Gordon D, Gaziano JM, Manson JE, et al. A randomized trial of low-dose aspirin in the primary prevention of cardiovascular disease in women. N Engl J Med. 2005;352(13):1293–304.
43. Antithrombotic Trialists' Collaboration. Collaborative meta-analysis of randomised trials of antiplatelet therapy for prevention of death, myocardial infarction, and stroke in high risk patients. BMJ. 2002;324(7329):71–86.
44. Baigent C, Blackwell L, Collins R, Emberson J, Godwin J, Peto R, et al. Aspirin in the primary and secondary prevention of vascular disease: collaborative meta-analysis of individual participant data from randomised trials. Lancet. 2009;373(9678):1849–60.
45. Trnavská Z, Trnavský K. Sex differences in the pharmacokinetics of salicylates. Eur J Clin Pharmacol. 1983;25(5):679–82.
46. Miners JO, Grgurinovich N, Whitehead AG, Robson RA, Birkett DJ. Influence of gender and oral contraceptive steroids on the metabolism of salicylic acid and acetylsalicylic acid. Br J Clin Pharmacol. 1986;22(2):135–42.
47. Mikkola T, Turunen P, Avela K, Orpana A, Viinikka L, Ylikorkala O. 17 beta-estradiol stimulates prostacyclin, but not endothelin-1, production in human vascular endothelial cells. J Clin Endocrinol Metab. 1995;80(6):1832–6.
48. Caulin-Glaser T, García-Cardeña G, Sarrel P, Sessa WC, Bender JR. 17 beta-estradiol regulation of human endothelial cell basal nitric oxide release, independent of cytosolic Ca^{2+} mobilization. Circ Res. 1997;81(5):885–92.
49. Pinto S, Coppo M, Paniccia R, Prisco D, Gori AM, Attanasio M, et al. Sex related differences in platelet TxA2 generation. Prostaglandins Leukot Essent Fatty Acids. 1990;40(3):217–21.
50. Ajayi AA, Mathur R, Halushka PV. Testosterone increases human platelet thromboxane A2 receptor density and aggregation responses. Circulation. 1995;91(11):2742–7.
51. Friede KA, Infeld MM, Tan RS, Knickerbocker HJ, Myers RA, Dubois LG, et al. Influence of sex on platelet reactivity in response to aspirin. J Am Heart Assoc. 2020;9(14):e014726.
52. Samad Z, Boyle S, Ersboll M, Vora AN, Zhang Y, Becker RC, et al. Sex differences in platelet reactivity and cardiovascular and psychological response to mental stress in patients with stable ischemic heart disease: insights from the REMIT study. J Am Coll Cardiol. 2014;64(16):1669–78.
53. Visseren FLJ, Mach F, Smulders YM, Carballo D, Koskinas KC, Bäck M, et al. 2021 ESC guidelines on cardiovascular disease prevention in clinical practice. Eur Heart J. 2021;42(34):3227–337.
54. Berger JS, Bhatt DL, Cannon CP, Chen Z, Jiang L, Jones JB, et al. The relative efficacy and safety of clopidogrel in women and men a sex-specific collaborative meta-analysis. J Am Coll Cardiol. 2009;54(21):1935–45.
55. Lau ES, Braunwald E, Murphy SA, Wiviott SD, Bonaca MP, Husted S, et al. Potent P2Y(12) inhibitors in men versus women: a collaborative meta-analysis of randomized trials. J Am Coll Cardiol. 2017;69(12):1549–59.
56. Schreuder MM, Badal R, Boersma E, Kavousi M, Roos-Hesselink J, Versmissen J, et al. Efficacy and safety of high potent P2Y(12) inhibitors prasugrel and ticagrelor in patients with coronary heart disease treated with dual antiplatelet therapy: a sex-specific systematic review and meta-analysis. J Am Heart Assoc. 2020;9(4):e014457.
57. Rathore SS, Wang Y, Krumholz HM. Sex-based differences in the effect of digoxin for the treatment of heart failure. N Engl J Med. 2002;347(18):1403–11.
58. Aarnoudse AL, Dieleman JP, Stricker BH. Age- and gender-specific incidence of hospitalisation for digoxin intoxication. Drug Saf. 2007;30(5):431–6.
59. Rathore SS, Curtis JP, Wang Y, Bristow MR, Krumholz HM. Association of serum digoxin concentration and outcomes in patients with heart failure. JAMA. 2003;289(7):871–8.
60. Adams KF Jr, Patterson JH, Gattis WA, O'Connor CM, Lee CR, Schwartz TA, et al. Relationship of serum digoxin concentration to mortality and morbidity in women in the digitalis investigation group trial: a retrospective analysis. J Am Coll Cardiol. 2005;46(3):497–504.
61. Heidenreich PA, Bozkurt B, Aguilar D, Allen LA, Byun JJ, Colvin MM, et al. 2022 AHA/ACC/HFSA guideline for the management of heart failure: a report of the American College of Cardiology/American Heart Association Joint Committee on clinical practice guidelines. Circulation. 2022;145(18):e895–1032.
62. Schuetz EG, Furuya KN, Schuetz JD. Interindividual variation in expression of P-glycoprotein in normal human liver and secondary hepatic neoplasms. J Pharmacol Exp Ther. 1995;275(2):1011–8.
63. Blaustein MP, Robinson SW, Gottlieb SS, Balke CW, Hamlyn JM. Sex, digitalis, and the sodium pump. Mol Interv. 2003;3(2):68–72. 50
64. Smith JB, Wade MB, Fineberg NS, Weinberger MH. Influence of race, sex, and blood pressure on erythrocyte sodium transport in humans. Hypertension. 1988;12(3):251–8.
65. Green HJ, Duscha BD, Sullivan MJ, Keteyian SJ, Kraus WE. Normal skeletal muscle Na(+)-K(+) pump concentration in patients with chronic heart failure. Muscle Nerve. 2001;24(1):69–76.
66. Opie LH. Pharmacological differences between calcium antagonists. Eur Heart J. 1997;18(Suppl A):A71–9.
67. van Luik EM, Vaes EWP, Vesseur MAM, Wilmes N, Meijs DAM, Laven S, et al. Sex differences in the anti-hypertensive effect of calcium-channel blockers: a systematic review and meta-analysis. Biomedicines. 2023;11(6):1622.

68. Schwartz JB, Capili H, Daugherty J. Aging of women alters S-verapamil pharmacokinetics and pharmacodynamics. Clin Pharmacol Ther. 1994;55(5):509–17.
69. Kloner RA, Sowers JR, DiBona GF, Gaffney M, Wein M. Sex- and age-related antihypertensive effects of amlodipine. The Amlodipine Cardiovascular Community Trial Study Group. Am J Cardiol. 1996;77(9):713–22.
70. Al-Gburi S, Deussen A, Zatschler B, Weber S, Künzel S, El-Armouche A, et al. Sex-difference in expression and function of beta-adrenoceptors in macrovessels: role of the endothelium. Basic Res Cardiol. 2017;112(3):29.
71. Wilbert-Lampen U, Seliger C, Trapp A, Straube F, Plasse A. Female sex hormones decrease constitutive endothelin-1 release via endothelial sigma-1/cocaine receptors: an action independent of the steroid hormone receptors. Endothelium. 2005;12(4):185–91.
72. Garg R, Yusuf S. Overview of randomized trials of angiotensin-converting enzyme inhibitors on mortality and morbidity in patients with heart failure. Collaborative Group on ACE Inhibitor Trials. JAMA. 1995;273(18):1450–6.
73. Flather MD, Yusuf S, Køber L, Pfeffer M, Hall A, Murray G, et al. Long-term ACE-inhibitor therapy in patients with heart failure or left-ventricular dysfunction: a systematic overview of data from individual patients. ACE-Inhibitor Myocardial Infarction Collaborative Group. Lancet. 2000;355(9215):1575–81.
74. Santema BT, Ouwerkerk W, Tromp J, Sama IE, Ravera A, Regitz-Zagrosek V, et al. Identifying optimal doses of heart failure medications in men compared with women: a prospective, observational, cohort study. Lancet. 2019;394(10205):1254–63.
75. Yeşil S, Yeşil M, Bayata S, Postaci N. ACE inhibitors and cough. Angiology. 1994;45(9):805–8.
76. Alharbi FF, Kholod AAV, Souverein PC, Meyboom RH, de Groot MCH, de Boer A, et al. The impact of age and sex on the reporting of cough and angioedema with renin-angiotensin system inhibitors: a case/noncase study in VigiBase. Fundam Clin Pharmacol. 2017;31(6):676–84.
77. Do TP, Seetasith A, Belleli R, Schlienger RG, Corda S, Burudpakdee C, et al. A database cohort study to assess the risk of angioedema among patients with heart failure initiating angiotensin-converting enzyme inhibitors in the USA. Am J Cardiovasc Drugs. 2018;18(3):205–11.
78. Cohn JN, Tognoni G. A randomized trial of the angiotensin-receptor blocker valsartan in chronic heart failure. N Engl J Med. 2001;345(23):1667–75.
79. Velazquez EJ, Pfeffer MA, McMurray JV, Maggioni AP, Rouleau JL, Van de Werf F, et al. VALsartan In Acute myocardial iNfarcTion (VALIANT) trial: baseline characteristics in context. Eur J Heart Fail. 2003;5(4):537–44.
80. Dickstein K, Kjekshus J. Effects of losartan and captopril on mortality and morbidity in high-risk patients after acute myocardial infarction: the OPTIMAAL randomised trial. Optimal trial in myocardial infarction with angiotensin II antagonist losartan. Lancet. 2002;360(9335):752–60.
81. Komukai K, Mochizuki S, Yoshimura M. Gender and the renin-angiotensin-aldosterone system. Fundam Clin Pharmacol. 2010;24(6):687–98.
82. Sullivan JC. Sex and the renin-angiotensin system: inequality between the sexes in response to RAS stimulation and inhibition. Am J Physiol Regul Integr Comp Physiol. 2008;294(4):R1220–6.
83. Fischer M, Baessler A, Schunkert H. Renin angiotensin system and gender differences in the cardiovascular system. Cardiovasc Res. 2002;53(3):672–7.
84. Schunkert H, Danser AH, Hense HW, Derkx FH, Kürzinger S, Riegger GA. Effects of estrogen replacement therapy on the renin-angiotensin system in postmenopausal women. Circulation. 1997;95(1):39–45.
85. Walford HH, Zuraw BL. Current update on cellular and molecular mechanisms of hereditary angioedema. Ann Allergy Asthma Immunol. 2014;112(5):413–8.
86. Cocco G, Chu D. The anti-ischemic effect of metoprolol in patients with chronic angina pectoris is gender-specific. Cardiology. 2006;106(3):147–53.
87. Ghali JK, Piña IL, Gottlieb SS, Deedwania PC, Wikstrand JC. Metoprolol CR/XL in female patients with heart failure: analysis of the experience in Metoprolol Extended-Release Randomized Intervention Trial in Heart Failure (MERIT-HF). Circulation. 2002;105(13):1585–91.
88. Kotecha D, Manzano L, Krum H, Rosano G, Holmes J, Altman DG, et al. Effect of age and sex on efficacy and tolerability of β blockers in patients with heart failure with reduced ejection fraction: individual patient data meta-analysis. BMJ. 2016;353:i1855.
89. Olsson G, Wikstrand J, Warnold I, Manger Cats V, McBoyle D, Herlitz J, et al. Metoprolol-induced reduction in postinfarction mortality: pooled results from five double-blind randomized trials. Eur Heart J. 1992;13(1):28–32.
90. Bots SH, Groepenhoff F, Eikendal ALM, Tannenbaum C, Rochon PA, Regitz-Zagrosek V, et al. Adverse drug reactions to guideline-recommended heart failure drugs in women: a systematic review of the literature. JACC Heart Fail. 2019;7(3):258–66.
91. Hendriksen LC, Omes-Smit G, Koch BCP, Ikram MA, Stricker BH, Visser LE. Sex-based difference in the effect of metoprolol on heart rate and bradycardia in a population-based setting. J Pers Med. 2022;12(6):870.
92. Thawornkaiwong A, Preawnim S, Wattanapermpool J. Upregulation of beta 1-adrenergic receptors in ovariectomized rat hearts. Life Sci. 2003;72(16):1813–24.
93. Kendall MJ, Quarterman CP, Jack DB, Beeley L. Metoprolol pharmacokinetics and the oral contraceptive pill. Br J Clin Pharmacol. 1982;14(1):120–2.

94. Galema-Boers AMH, Mulder J, Steward K, van Lennep JER. Sex differences in efficacy and safety of PCSK9 monoclonal antibodies: a real-world registry. Atherosclerosis. 2023;384:117108.
95. Paquette M, Faubert S, Saint-Pierre N, Baass A, Bernard S. Sex differences in LDL-C response to PCSK9 inhibitors: a real world experience. J Clin Lipidol. 2023;17(1):142–9.
96. Vicente-Valor J, García-González X, Ibáñez-García S, Durán-García ME, de Lorenzo-Pinto A, Rodríguez-González C, et al. PCSK9 inhibitors revisited: effectiveness and safety of PCSK9 inhibitors in a real-life Spanish cohort. Biomed Pharmacother. 2022;146:112519.
97. Cordero A, Del Olmo MRF, Quiroga GAC, Romero-Menor C, Fácila L, Seijas-Amigo J, et al. Sex differences in low-density lipoprotein cholesterol reduction with PCSK9 inhibitors in real-world patients: the LIPID-REAL Registry. J Cardiovasc Pharmacol. 2022;79(4):523–9.
98. Leitner DR, Toplak H, Kedenko L, Steinmaurer T, Gräff V, Metzner T, et al. Efficacy and tolerability of alirocumab in Austrian clinical practice—results of the non-interventional PEARL-AT study. Curr Med Res Opin. 2020;36(9):1419–25.
99. Hollstein T, Vogt A, Grenkowitz T, Stojakovic T, März W, Laufs U, et al. Treatment with PCSK9 inhibitors reduces atherogenic VLDL remnants in a real-world study. Vascul Pharmacol. 2019;116:8–15.
100. Ferri N, Ruscica M, Coggi D, Bonomi A, Amato M, Frigerio B, et al. Sex-specific predictors of PCSK9 levels in a European population: the IMPROVE study. Atherosclerosis. 2020;309:39–46.
101. Ghosh M, Gälman C, Rudling M, Angelin B. Influence of physiological changes in endogenous estrogen on circulating PCSK9 and LDL cholesterol. J Lipid Res. 2015;56(2):463–9.
102. Jia F, Fei SF, Tong DB, Xue C, Li JJ. Sex difference in circulating PCSK9 and its clinical implications. Front Pharmacol. 2022;13:953845.
103. Rodenburg EM, Stricker BH, Visser LE. Sex-related differences in hospital admissions attributed to adverse drug reactions in the Netherlands. Br J Clin Pharmacol. 2011;71(1):95–104.
104. de Vries ST, Denig P, Ekhart C, Burgers JS, Kleefstra N, Mol PGM, et al. Sex differences in adverse drug reactions reported to the National Pharmacovigilance Centre in the Netherlands: an explorative observational study. Br J Clin Pharmacol. 2019;85(7):1507–15.
105. Bazett H. An analysis of the time-relations of electrocardiograms. Ann Noninvasive Electrocardiol. 1997;2:177–94.
106. Lehmann MH, Hardy S, Archibald D, Quart B, MacNeil DJ. Sex difference in risk of torsade de pointes with d,l-sotalol. Circulation. 1996;94(10):2535–41.
107. Makkar RR, Fromm BS, Steinman RT, Meissner MD, Lehmann MH. Female gender as a risk factor for torsades de pointes associated with cardiovascular drugs. JAMA. 1993;270(21):2590–7.
108. Hreiche R, Morissette P, Turgeon J. Drug-induced long QT syndrome in women: review of current evidence and remaining gaps. Gend Med. 2008;5(2):124–35.
109. Darpo B, Karnad DR, Badilini F, Florian J, Garnett CE, Kothari S, et al. Are women more susceptible than men to drug-induced QT prolongation? Concentration-QTc modelling in a phase 1 study with oral rac-sotalol. Br J Clin Pharmacol. 2014;77(3):522–31.
110. Tisdale JE, Jaynes HA, Kingery JR, Mourad NA, Trujillo TN, Overholser BR, et al. Development and validation of a risk score to predict QT interval prolongation in hospitalized patients. Circ Cardiovasc Qual Outcomes. 2013;6(4):479–87.
111. Hwang KS, Kim GH. Thiazide-induced hyponatremia. Electrolyte Blood Press. 2010;8(1):51–7.
112. Rydberg DM, Mejyr S, Loikas D, Schenck-Gustafsson K, von Euler M, Malmström RE. Sex differences in spontaneous reports on adverse drug events for common antihypertensive drugs. Eur J Clin Pharmacol. 2018;74(9):1165–73.
113. Toner JM, Ramsay LE. Thiazide-induced hypokalaemia; prevalence higher in women. Br J Clin Pharmacol. 1984;18(3):449–52.
114. Werner U, Werner D, Heinbüchner S, Graf B, Ince H, Kische S, et al. Gender is an important determinant of the disposition of the loop diuretic torasemide. J Clin Pharmacol. 2010;50:160–8.
115. Hendriksen LC, van der Linden PD, Herings RMC, Stricker BH, Visser LE. Women on diuretics have a higher risk of hospital admission because of hyponatremia than men. Pharmacoepidemiol Drug Saf. 2023;32(6):635–42.
116. Schwartz GL, Turner ST, Chapman AB, Boerwinkle E. Interacting effects of gender and genotype on blood pressure response to hydrochlorothiazide. Kidney Int. 2002;62(5):1718–23.
117. Liu J, Sharma N, Zheng W, Ji H, Tam H, Wu X, et al. Sex differences in vasopressin V_2 receptor expression and vasopressin-induced antidiuresis. Am J Physiol Renal Physiol. 2011;300(2):F433–40.
118. Tahaei E, Coleman R, Saritas T, Ellison DH, Welling PA. Distal convoluted tubule sexual dimorphism revealed by advanced 3D imaging. Am J Physiol Renal Physiol. 2020;319(5):F754–F64.
119. Mancini GBJ, Baker S, Bergeron J, Fitchett D, Frohlich J, Genest J, et al. Diagnosis, prevention, and management of statin adverse effects and intolerance: Canadian Consensus Working Group update (2016). Can J Cardiol. 2016;32(7 Suppl):S35–65.
120. Schech S, Graham D, Staffa J, Andrade SE, Grenade LL, Burgess M, et al. Risk factors for statin-associated rhabdomyolysis. Pharmacoepidemiol Drug Saf. 2007;16(3):352–8.
121. Chatzizisis YS, Koskinas KC, Misirli G, Vaklavas C, Hatzitolios A, Giannoglou GD. Risk factors and drug interactions predisposing to statin-induced myopathy: implications for risk assessment, prevention and treatment. Drug Saf. 2010;33(3):171–87.

MIX
Papier aus verantwortungsvollen Quellen
Paper from responsible sources
FSC® C105338

If you have any concerns about our products,
you can contact us on
ProductSafety@springernature.com

In case Publisher is established outside the EU,
the EU authorized representative is:
Springer Nature Customer Service Center GmbH
Europaplatz 3, 69115 Heidelberg, Germany

Printed by Libri Plureos GmbH
in Hamburg, Germany